THE ESSENTIAL GUIDE TO

Occupational Therapy Fieldwork Education

Resources for Educators and Practitioners, 2nd Edition

Edited by

Donna M. Costa, DHS, OTR/L, FAOTA

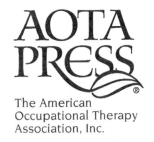

AOTA PRESS

The American
Occupational Therapy
Association, Inc.

AOTA Centennial Vision
We envision that occupational therapy is a powerful, widely recognized, science-driven, and evidence-based profession with a globally connected and diverse workforce meeting society's occupational needs.

Mission Statement
The American Occupational Therapy Association advances the quality, availability, use, and support of occupational therapy through standard-setting, advocacy, education, and research on behalf of its members and the public.

AOTA Staff
Frederick P. Somers, *Executive Director*
Christopher M. Bluhm, *Chief Operating Officer*

Chris Davis, *Director, AOTA Press*
Caroline Polk, *Digital Manager and AJOT Managing Editor*
Ashley Hofmann, *Development Editor*
Barbara Dickson, *Production Editor*
Mark Connelly, *Inventory and Cost Control Analyst*

Rebecca Rutberg, *Director, Marketing*
Amanda Goldman, *Marketing Manager*
Jennifer Folden, *Marketing Specialist*

American Occupational Therapy Association, Inc.
4720 Montgomery Lane
Bethesda, MD 20814
Phone: 301-652-AOTA (2682)
TDD: 800-377-8555
Fax: 301-652-7711
www.aota.org
To order: 1-877-404-AOTA or store.aota.org

Disclaimers
This publication is designed to provide accurate and authoritative information in regard to the subject matter covered. It is sold or distributed with the understanding that the publisher is not engaged in rendering legal, accounting, or other professional service. If legal advice or other expert assistance is required, the services of a competent professional person should be sought.

—From the Declaration of Principles jointly adopted by the American Bar Association and a Committee of Publishers and Associations

It is the objective of the American Occupational Therapy Association to be a forum for free expression and interchange of ideas. The opinions expressed by the contributors to this work are their own and not necessarily those of the American Occupational Therapy Association.

ISBN: 978-1-56900-366-4
Library of Congress Control Number: 2015946383

Cover Design by Debra Naylor, Naylor Design Inc., Washington, DC
Composition by MidAtlantic Publishing Services, Baltimore, MD
Printed by Automated Graphic Systems, Inc., White Plains, MD

CONTENTS

---

*= Included on flash drive

EXHIBITS, FIGURES, LEARNING ACTIVITIES, TABLES, APPENDIXES, AND CASE SCENARIOS

EXHIBITS

FIGURES

LEARNING ACTIVITIES

TABLES

APPENDIXES

CASE SCENARIOS

ABOUT THE EDITOR

Donna Costa, DHS, OTR/L, FAOTA, is an Associate Professor of Occupational Therapy at Touro University, Nevada. She has been an occupational therapist for more than 40 years, specializing in mental health practice, and has been teaching full-time in occupational therapy programs at several academic institutions for the past 20 years.

Donna received her Doctor of Health Sciences degree from the University of Indianapolis in 2007, a master of science degree in health care administration from the New School for Social Research in 2001, and a bachelor of arts degree in psychology and a bachelor of science degree in occupational therapy in 1973 from the University of Buffalo.

She is the editor of *The Essential Guide to Fieldwork Education* (2004), author of *Clinical Supervision in Occupational Therapy: A Guide for Fieldwork and Practice* (2007), and has written numerous articles for *OT Practice*.

Donna is the current Chair of the AOTA Special Interest Sections Council and is a fellow of the American Occupational Therapy Association. She is a frequently sought-after public speaker on topics related to fieldwork education, mindfulness, and compassion fatigue.

PREFACE

Donna Costa, DHS, OTR/L, FAOTA

This is an exciting time for the occupational therapy profession, and I am delighted to be a part of it. As the profession approaches its 100th anniversary, we are seeing unprecedented growth. Occupational therapy educational programs at the associate's degree, master's degree, and doctoral levels are expanding, and each year sees the development of new programs seeking accreditation from the Accreditation Council for Occupational Therapy Education (ACOTE®). The number of students in these programs was nearly 18,000 in 2013, according to ACOTE (2014). This growth creates a huge demand for quality fieldwork placements throughout the United States. More than ever, we need occupational therapy practitioners to commit to serving the profession by being the best fieldwork educators they can be.

Much has changed in fieldwork education since the inception of our profession in 1917. Early on, the majority of fieldwork education was completed in hospitals, particularly large psychiatric hospitals; fieldwork today takes place in a wide variety of institutional and community practice settings. However, the focus of fieldwork education remains the same—to prepare competent, entry-level practitioners by providing opportunities in which students can apply the knowledge they have learned in the classroom. We now have an abundance of educational theories and models guiding how we teach students in the classroom and a growing body of knowledge about the theoretical models that provide the foundation for fieldwork education. If we are to continue to meet the growing demand for fieldwork in the United States and internationally; we need to explore alternative models for fieldwork education, some of which are addressed in this book.

This book will help both occupational therapy fieldwork educators and academic fieldwork coordinators as they prepare to provide clinical learning fieldwork environments that maximize student learning. For practitioners new to fieldwork education, this book will provide a thorough background in relevant policies, procedures, and processes. Fieldwork remains the bridge between education and practice, where educators and clinicians collaborate to provide the education that will ensure the ongoing success of the occupational therapy profession.

Reference

Accreditation Council for Occupational Therapy Education. (2014). *ACOTE academic programs annual data report for academic year 2013/2014.* Retrieved from http://www .aota.org/-/media/Corporate/Files/EducationCareers/ Accredit/2013-2014-Annual-Data-Report.pdf

INTRODUCTION

Yvonne M. Randall, EdD, OTR/L, FAOTA

Do you remember your first day as a fieldwork educator? My recollection of my first experience as a fieldwork educator was that I placed pressure on myself to be the "expert" and "teach" the student everything I had learned during 2 years as a practitioner in just 6 weeks. In hindsight, this was a rather ambitious task! The facility fieldwork manual had already been established, so my contribution for the student related to compiling specific client information for my assigned unit. However, the fieldwork manual had no information on how to initiate or continue a supervisory relationship, and fieldwork educator mentorship was learned from observing peers while they worked with students.

I can assure you that my first day was not a success. What I did take away from that initial fieldwork educator experience was to be prepared and be flexible! My own journey as a fieldwork educator was necessary to realize that fluctuations occur with the flow of student occupational therapy progression during fieldwork just as clients fluctuate in their progression through the treatment process.

As I prepared for my first day as an academic fieldwork coordinator in a new occupational therapy educational program, I searched the American Occupational Therapy Association website for materials. *The Essential Guide to Occupational Therapy Fieldwork Education: Resources for Today's Educators and Practitioners* (Costa, 2004) became a well-worn resource on my desk. The chapters provided information that I could immediately utilize and stressed the importance of policies and

the supervisory process. It became my go-to book as I worked with fieldwork educators and students, and I routinely encouraged fieldwork educators to use the book as a template when establishing their facility fieldwork manuals.

Fieldwork educators and academic fieldwork coordinators (AFWCs) are important for the development and maintenance of the occupational therapy profession because fieldwork provides the link between education and practice (Royeen & Fazio, 2004). My experience has been that although many occupational therapy practitioners readily seek the opportunity to mentor students, some wait for others to take charge of accepting students to mentor. These practitioners have expressed that they were not prepared to take on the responsibility of mentoring a student—even though they were once students, they were not provided training on how to become an effective fieldwork supervisor.

However, mentoring students through fieldwork is one method our profession has used to determine entry-level competence. As occupational therapists, we expect our students to graduate with a level of competence that can be facilitated only through the process of fieldwork. As a result, the profession has placed a greater emphasis on fieldwork education.

The process of fieldwork enables students to take learned material from the classroom and use it in real time with clients. Fieldwork provides the necessary environment for students to work with clients on required and desired occupations to engage in life. The collaboration between the fieldwork educator and the student must be established and can be enhanced through use of the materials provided in this updated book.

About this Book

The new edition of *The Essential Guide to Occupational Therapy Fieldwork Education: Resources for Educators and Practitioners* is welcome as the profession embarks on new opportunities, such as the expansion of practice settings and a more diverse practitioner workforce. Editor Donna M. Costa, DHS, OTR/L, FAOTA, provides experience as a clinician, educator, and researcher. Her enthusiasm for fieldwork education is seen throughout the chapters. In this edition, she has included expert contributors and expanded the original text's content. The details and breadth of fieldwork information provided for readers is tremendous; however, each chapter has been synthesized to allow immediate use of the information.

Of particular interest are the expanded sections related to becoming a fieldwork educator and resources for students. Also new to this edition are chapters on setting up role-emerging fieldwork

and working with students with disabilities, and an extended chapter on the role and responsibilities of the AFWC. The appendixes on the accompanying flash drive contain valuable resources, including occupational therapy and occupational therapy assistant fieldwork manuals and a facility fieldwork manual.

Novice and experienced fieldwork educators and AFWCs will find this book essential to working with students. Students may gain a greater appreciation of the importance of fieldwork when reading this text. In addition, AFWCs of all levels can use this text as a guide when working with students and facility fieldwork educators.

References

Costa, D. M. (Ed.). (2004). *The essential guide to occupational therapy fieldwork education: Resources for today's educators and practitioners.* Bethesda, MD: AOTA Press.

Royeen, C. B., & Fazio, L. S. (2004). Introduction. In D. M. Costa (Ed.), *The essential guide to occupational therapy fieldwork education: Resources for today's educators and practitioners* (p. xiii). Bethesda, MD: AOTA Press.

Part 1.

PURPOSE OF FIELDWORK EDUCATION

OVERVIEW OF PART 1

Donna Costa, DHS, OTR/L, FAOTA

This first section of *The Essential Guide to Occupational Therapy Fieldwork Education* addresses the purpose of fieldwork education and contains several major official and other documents that affect its process. The American Occupational Therapy Association (AOTA) Commission on Education has written three of these documents: "Occupational Therapy Fieldwork Education: Value and Purpose" (Chapter 1), which defines *fieldwork education* as "the essential bridge between academic education authentic occupational therapy practice"; the "Philosophy of Occupational Therapy Education" (Chapter 2), which addresses the values inherent in the education of occupational therapy students; and "A Descriptive Review of Occupational Therapy Education" (Chapter 6), which defines the various levels of education and degrees within our profession.

The Occupational Therapy Practice Framework: Domain and Process (AOTA, 2014) is another document that shapes how fieldwork education is provided. Chapter 5, "*The Occupational Therapy Practice Framework: Domain and Process, 3rd Edition,* and Fieldwork," describes the *Framework's* intent and provides the reader with a summary. Because this document reflects the language that students learn in the classroom, it is critical for fieldwork educators to be familiar with it.

In clinical practice, numerous theories, frames of reference, and theoretical models provide a lens through which occupational therapy interventions are delivered to clients. Similarly, in academic and fieldwork education, educational and learning theories shape how students are educated. Chapter 3, "Models and Theoretical Frameworks for Fieldwork Education," provides an overview of some of the theories that are used in fieldwork education, whereas Chapter 4, "Transformative Learning: Facilitating Growth and Change Through Fieldwork," presents a detailed outline of transformative learning theory, which is particularly relevant to fieldwork education.

Current occupational therapy practice is informed by evidence, and the education of occupational therapy students includes research coursework to prepare them to be effective consumers of research. Chapter 7, "Evidence-Based Practice and How It Relates to Fieldwork," provides an overview of evidence-based practice and suggested ways that fieldwork educators can incorporate more evidence into fieldwork assignments and learning activities.

Reference

American Occupational Therapy Association. (2014). Occupational therapy practice framework: Domain and process (3rd ed.). *American Journal of Occupational Therapy, 68*(Suppl. 1), S1–S48. http://dx.doi.org/10.5014/ajot.2014.682006

Chapter 1.

OCCUPATIONAL THERAPY FIELDWORK EDUCATION: VALUE AND PURPOSE

American Occupational Therapy Association

The purpose of fieldwork education is to propel each generation of occupational therapy practitioners from the role of student to that of practitioner. Through the fieldwork experience, future practitioners achieve competence in applying the occupational therapy process and using evidence-based interventions to meet the occupational needs of a diverse client population. Fieldwork assignments may occur in a variety of practice settings, including medical, educational, and community-based programs. Moreover, fieldwork placements also present the opportunity to introduce occupational therapy services to new and emerging practice environments.

Fieldwork assignments constitute an integral part of the occupational therapy and occupational therapy assistant education curricula. Through fieldwork, students learn to apply theoretical and scientific principles learned from their academic programs to address actual client needs within the context of authentic practice environments. While on fieldwork, each student develops competency to ascertain client occupational performance needs, to identify supports or barriers affecting health and participation, and to document interventions

provided. Fieldwork also provides opportunities for the student to develop advocacy, leadership, and managerial skills in a variety of practice settings. Finally, the student develops a professional identity as an occupational therapy practitioner, aligning his or her professional judgments and decisions with the American Occupational Therapy Association (AOTA) *Standards of Practice for Occupational Therapy* (AOTA, 2005b) and the *Occupational Therapy Code of Ethics* (AOTA, 2005a).

As students proceed through their fieldwork assignments, performance expectations become progressively more challenging. *Level I fieldwork* experiences occur concurrently with academic coursework and are "designed to enrich didactic coursework through directed observation and participation in selected aspects of the occupational therapy process" (Accreditation Council for Occupational Therapy Education [ACOTE®], 2007a, 2007b, 2007c, p. 650). *Level II fieldwork* experiences occur at or near the conclusion of the didactic phase of occupational therapy curricula and are designed to develop competent, entry-level, generalist practitioners (ACOTE, 2007a, 2007b, 2007c). Level II fieldwork assignments feature in-depth experience in delivering occupational therapy services to clients, focusing on the application of purposeful and meaningful occupation and evidence-based practice through exposure to a "variety of clients across the life span and to a variety of settings" (ACOTE, 2007a, 2007b, 2007c).

The value of fieldwork transcends the obvious benefits directed toward the student. Supervising students enhances fieldwork educators' own professional development by providing exposure to current practice trends, evidence-based practice, and research. Moreover, the experience of fieldwork supervision is recognized by the National Board for Certification in Occupational Therapy (NBCOT) and many state regulatory boards as a legitimate venue for achieving continuing competency requirements for occupational therapy practitioners.

Another benefit to the fieldwork site for sponsoring a fieldwork education program is with the recruitment of qualified occupational therapy personnel. Through the responsibilities expected during Level II fieldwork, occupational therapy staff and administration are given opportunity for an in-depth view of a student's potential as a future employee. In turn, an active fieldwork program allows the student, as a potential employee, to view first-hand the agency's commitment to the professional growth of its occupational therapy personnel and to determine the "fit" of his or her professional goals with agency goals. The fieldwork program also creates a progressive, state-of-the-art image to the professional community, consumers, and other external audiences through its partnership with the academic programs.

In summary, fieldwork education is an essential bridge between academic education and authentic occupational therapy practice. Through the collaboration between academic faculty and fieldwork educators, students are given the opportunity to achieve the competencies necessary to meet the present and future occupational needs of individuals, groups, and indeed, society as a whole.

References

Accreditation Council for Occupational Therapy Education. (2007a). Accreditation standards for a doctoral-degree-level educational program for the occupational therapist. *American Journal of Occupational Therapy, 61,* 641–651. http://dx.doi .org/10.5014/ajot.61.6.641

Accreditation Council for Occupational Therapy Education. (2007b). Accreditation standards for a master's-degree-level educational program for the occupational therapist. *American Journal of Occupational Therapy, 61,* 662–671. http://dx.doi .org/10.5014/ajot.61.6.662

Accreditation Council for Occupational Therapy Education. (2007c). Accreditation standards for an educational program for the occupational therapy assistant. *American Journal of Occupational Therapy, 61,* 652–661. http://dx.doi.org/10.5014/ ajot.61.6.652

American Occupational Therapy Association. (2005a). Occupational therapy code of ethics (2005). *American Journal of Occupational Therapy, 59,* 639–642.

American Occupational Therapy Association. (2005b). Standards of practice for occupational therapy. *American Journal of Occupational Therapy, 59,* 663–665.

The Commission on Education:
René Padilla, PhD, OTR/L, FAOTA, *Chairperson*
Andrea Bilics, PhD, OTR/L
Judith C. Blum, MS, OTR/L
Paula C. Bohr, PhD, OTR/L, FAOTA
Jennifer C. Coyne, COTA/L
Jyothi Gupta, PhD, OTR/L
Linda Musselman, PhD, OTR, FAOTA
Linda Orr, MPA, OTR/L
Abbey Sipp, *ASD Liaison*
Patricia Stutz-Tanenbaum, MS, OTR
Neil Harvison, PhD, OTR/L, *AOTA Staff Liaison*

Adopted by the Representative Assembly 2009Feb-CS115

This document replaces the document *The Purpose and Value of Occupational Therapy Fieldwork Education* 2003M41.

Chapter 2.

PHILOSOPHY OF OCCUPATIONAL THERAPY EDUCATION

American Occupational Therapy Association

Preamble

Occupational therapy education prepares occupational therapy practitioners to address the occupational needs of individuals, groups, communities, and populations. The education process includes academic and fieldwork components. The philosophy of occupational therapy education parallels the philosophy of occupational therapy yet remains distinctly concerned with beliefs about knowledge, learning, and teaching.

What Are the Fundamental Beliefs of Occupational Therapy Education?

Students are viewed as occupational beings who are in dynamic transaction with the learning context and the teaching–learning process. The learning context includes the curriculum and pedagogy and conveys a perspective and belief system that includes a view of humans as occupational beings, occupation as a health determinant, and participation as a fundamental right. Education promotes clinical reasoning and the integration of professional values, theories, evidence, ethics, and skills.

This approach will prepare practitioners to collaborate with clients to achieve health, well-being, and participation in life through engagement in occupation (American Occupational Therapy Association, 2014). Occupational therapy education is the process by which practitioners acquire their professional identity.

What Are the Values Within Occupational Therapy Education?

Enacting the above beliefs to facilitate the development of a sound reasoning process that is client centered, occupation based, and theory driven while encouraging the use of best evidence and outcomes data to inform the teaching–learning experience may include supporting

- Active and diverse learning within and beyond the classroom environment;
- A collaborative process that builds on prior knowledge and experience;
- Continuous professional judgment, evaluation, and self-reflection; and
- Lifelong learning.

Reference

American Occupational Therapy Association. (2014). Occupational therapy practice framework: Domain and process (3rd ed.). *American Journal of Occupational Therapy, 68*(Suppl. 1), S1–S48. http://dx.doi.org/10.5014/ajot.2014.682006

The Commission on Education
Andrea Bilics, PhD, OTR/L, FAOTA, *Chairperson*
Tina DeAngelis, EdD, OTR/L
Jamie Geraci, MS, OTR/L
Julie McLaughlin Gray, PhD, OTR/L
Michael Iwama, PhD, OT(c)
Julie Kugel, OTD, MOT, OTR/L
Kate McWilliams
Maureen S. Nardella, MS, OTR/L
Renee Ortega, MA, COTA
Kim Qualls, MS, OTR/L

Tamra Trenary, OTD, OTR/L, BCPR
Neil Harvison, PhD, OTR/L, FAOTA, *AOTA Headquarters Liaison*

Adopted by the Representative Assembly 2014NovCO49

Note. This revision replaces the 2007 document *Philosophy of Occupational Therapy Education,* previously published and copyrighted in 2007 by the American Occupational Therapy Association in the *American Journal of Occupational Therapy, 61,* 678. http://dx.doi.org/10.5014/ajot.61.6.678

Chapter 3.

MODELS AND THEORETICAL FRAMEWORKS FOR FIELDWORK EDUCATION

Donna Costa, DHS, OTR/L, FAOTA

Just as there are many theoretical models and frames of reference to guide occupational therapy practitioners in clinical practice, so too are there numerous theoretical models to guide fieldwork educators. These models are divided into two broad categories: (1) learning theories and models and (2) supervision theories and models.

Learning theories and models provide an understanding for how students learn and can be further divided into learning theories, learning styles, and types of learning. Supervision theories and models provide a framework for how fieldwork educators engage in the supervisory process, and this category is further divided into supervision theories and supervision formats. Brief descriptions of each of these categories follow; readers are encouraged to continue independent learning in this area.

Learning Theories and Models

Learning theories and models provide a framework that explains how people learn. This helps us understand the complex process of learning and how to best structure our teaching and training. Learning theories have been broadly categorized into pedagogy and andragogy. Pedagogy originally referred to theories that explain how children learn, while andragogy is about adult learning.

Today the term *pedagogy* refers to the theories and methods that are utilized in teaching. Because the majority of occupational therapy and occupational therapy assistant students are in their early adult years, it makes the most sense for fieldwork educators to become familiar with adult learning theories and models.

Adult learning theories used in this text are those most relevant to fieldwork education. Being an effective fieldwork educator involves understanding how adults learn best. *Andragogy* is a theory that holds a set of assumptions about how adults learn and emphasizes the process of learning. Adult learning approaches are often problem-based because adult learners want to know what is in it for them. It also involves a more collaborative process between the teacher and learner compared with child learning approaches.

Malcolm Knowles (1980) made andragogy popular as a theory and model of adult learning and in it identified six principles of adult learning:

1. Adults are internally motivated and self-directed.
2. Adults bring life experiences and knowledge to learning experiences.
3. Adults are goal oriented.
4. Adults are relevancy oriented.
5. Adults are practical.
6. Adult learners like to be respected.

Andragogy and Occupational Therapy Fieldwork

The Queensland Occupational Therapy Fieldwork Collaborative (2007) applied Knowles's six adult learning principles to occupational therapy fieldwork education.

Adults Are Internally Motivated and Self-Directed

Adult learners resist learning when they feel others are imposing information, ideas, or actions on them. Your role as a fieldwork educator is to facilitate a student's movement toward being more self-directed and responsible for his or her learning and increase the student's internal motivation to learn. As a fieldwork educator, you can facilitate a student's growth by doing the following:

- Structure the fieldwork experience with graded learning, moving from more to less structure, from less to more responsibility, and from more to less direct supervision at an appropriate pace that challenges but does not overwhelm the student.
- Develop rapport with the student to increase his or her comfort level with you and with asking questions and exploring new concepts.
- Demonstrate interest in what the student is thinking and his or her opinions through use of active listening strategies.
- Facilitate the student's ability to engage in inquiry before supplying him or her with too much information.
- Provide the student with regular constructive and specific feedback, both positive and negative.

- Collaborate with the student by reviewing goals and expectations, and acknowledge when the student accomplishes goals.
- Encourage the student to use all available resources such as the library, journals, Internet sources, and department resources.
- Discover what the student is interested in learning, and assign projects or tasks for the student that reflect his or her interests and that must be completed over the course of the placement (e.g., provide an in-service on his or her topic of choice, present a case study based on one of his or her clients, design a client educational handout, lead a client group activity session).
- Use the student's preferred learning style throughout the fieldwork experience.

Adults Bring Life Experiences and Knowledge to Learning Experiences

Students come to fieldwork with a wide range of previous life experiences; as adult learners, they like to be given the opportunity to apply their life experiences and knowledge to new learning experiences. As a fieldwork educator, you can help the student use such experiences and knowledge by doing the following:

- Ask about the student's interests and past experiences (i.e., personal, work, and study related).
- Assist the student to draw on past experiences when problem solving, reflecting, and applying clinical reasoning processes.
- Engage the student in reflective learning opportunities to help him or her them integrate existing biases or habits based on life experiences with the new information being learned.

Adults Are Goal Oriented

Adult students are motivated to learn something when it is connected to completing a real-life task or goal. As a fieldwork educator, you can facilitate the student's readiness for problem-based learning and increase his or her awareness of the need for a knowledge or skill as it relates to reaching a specific goal by doing the following:

- Provide meaningful learning experiences that are clearly linked to personal, client, and fieldwork goals as well as assessment and future life goals.

- Provide the student with case studies from which he or she can learn about theory and treatment methods and how they both relate to functional implications.
- Ask the student probing questions that motivate reflection, inquiry, and further research.

Adults Are Relevancy Oriented

Adult learners want to know the relevance of what they are learning to what they want to achieve. As a fieldwork educator, you can use the following to help the student see the value of his or her observations and practical experiences throughout the fieldwork experience:

- Ask the student before the fieldwork experience what he or she expects to learn and after the experience what was learned and how that information can be applied in the future or can help the student meet his or her learning goals.
- Provide two or more choices for fieldwork projects so that learning is more likely to reflect the student's interests.

Adults Are Practical

Through practical fieldwork experiences—interacting with real clients and their real-life situations—the student moves from classroom and textbook learning to hands-on problem solving, during which he or she can recognize first-hand how fieldwork learning applies to real life and work. As a fieldwork educator, you can facilitate practical learning by doing the following:

- Be explicit and think out loud when explaining to the student your clinical reasoning when choosing assessments and interventions and when prioritizing a client's clinical needs.
- Explain to the student how what he or she is learning is specifically useful and applicable to the job and the client group you are working with.
- Allow the student to actively participate in assessment, interview, and intervention processes, rather than only observe, to promote his or her skills, confidence, and competence.

Adult Learners Like to Be Respected

Respect goes a long way in establishing a positive relationship between you and your student. As a fieldwork educator, you can cultivate a good relationship with the student by doing the following:

- Take an interest in what the student says by using active listening strategies.
- Acknowledge the wealth of experiences that the student brings to the placement.
- Regard the student as a future colleague who is equal in life experience.
- Encourage the student to express ideas, ask questions, make suggestions, describe his or her clinical reasoning, and provide feedback at every opportunity.

Learning Theories

There are many dozens of learning theories, and it is beyond the scope of this chapter to describe them all. However, many educational resources are available both in print and online that describe these theories. Here, the major theories that relate to occupational therapy fieldwork education are discussed.

Transformative Learning

Transformative learning, a subset of adult learning, is considered to be a learning theory in development (Santalucia & Johnson, 2010). Mezirow (1997) is credited with introducing the theory of *transformative learning*, which he defines as the process of effecting change in the way people view themselves and their world. The process begins with a dilemma that the person confronts and ends with the person changing some of his or her existing assumptions that lead to a change in some aspect of his or her life.

For example, when students first enter fieldwork, they are armed with an arsenal of knowledge and have some classroom-learned skills. Then they encounter real patients, and it is not the same as being in the classroom. They have to change how they perform tasks. A student may have learned wheelchair transfer skills in the classroom, practicing on a non-disabled classmate. But then the student has to teach a patient who has had a spinal cord injury and is paralyzed how to transfer from bed to a wheelchair.

In addition, as a fieldwork educator about to get a student for a Level II fieldwork experience, you have certain assumptions about how the process will go, and it rarely goes as planned. Therefore, you adapt the strategies you use or adopt new ones to facilitate a successful experience for the student.

As the fieldwork educator, you are changed by the experience as much as the student. Mezirow (1991) describes this process of knowledge transformation or paradigm shift or perspective transformation as

> the process of becoming critically aware of how and why our assumptions have come to constrain the way we perceive, understand, and feel about our world; changing these structures of habitual expectation to make possible a more inclusive, discriminating, and integrating perspective; and finally, making choices or otherwise acting upon these new understandings. (p. 167)

Cognitive Theories

Several people, including Jean Piaget (1936), Jerome Bruner (1966), and Robert Gagné (1965), have developed cognitive theories emphasizing the process of how people think and how they search for meaning. Cognitive processes are at work throughout fieldwork education, and supervisors sequence learning activities in response to them.

Humanistic Theories

Carl Rogers (1951) and Abraham Maslow (1968) developed humanistic theories that emphasized how the learner searches for meaning and that learning involves an emotional and cognitive component. Fieldwork students can become emotional. They are under a lot of pressure to perform, and many have strong perfectionistic tendencies. Students want to know why they are learning something, and the learning becomes more relevant for them when there is meaning attached.

Behavioral Theories

Ivan Pavlov (1927) and B. F. Skinner (1953) focused their behavioral theory research on examining how learning occurs in response to a stimulus and is affected by the presence or absence of reinforcers. In fieldwork education, supervisors shape students' behaviors, providing feedback that the students view as positive (praise) or negative (correction).

Constructivism

Constructivism is frequently mentioned in the literature of fieldwork education. This learning theory emphasizes active rather than passive learning, and learners construct their own knowledge based on what they already know. This theory was influenced by the work of Lev Vygotsky (1978), Jean Piaget (1936), and John Dewey (1916).

Learning Styles

Learning styles refers to how people approach learning and differences in the way each person learns. Learning styles are influenced by a person's previous life experiences, the formal education he or she received, and work experiences. Each person may have a combination of learning styles and may use different styles when learning different things.

Experiential Learning Cycle

The experiential learning cycle, created by David Kolb (1984), is a cyclical process of learning that includes four phases: (1) concrete experiencing, (2) reflective observing, (3) abstract conceptualizing, and (4) active experimenting. Kolb developed the Learning Style Inventory to assess which of the four phases is most preferred by the learner.

Myers–Briggs Type Inventory

The Myers–Briggs Type Inventory (Briggs-Myers & Briggs, 1985) is based on Carl Jung's (1921) work and categorizes people on the basis of their focus of interest (introverted or extraverted), the way they gather information (sensing or intuiting), how they focus on subjective experiences (feeling or thinking), and how they manage information (judging or perceiving). This classification results in a configuration of specific personality type and is used in the clinical supervision field.

Dunn and Dunn Model

Educational researchers Rita and Kenneth Dunn (1985) examined different kinds of stimuli in the environment and created learning preferences based on the learner's ability to process new information. They included environmental stimuli (i.e., sound, light, temperature, seating design), emotional stimuli (i.e., motivation, persistence, responsibility, structure), sociological stimuli learning (i.e., alone or in teams, dyads, peers, varied groups), physical stimuli (i.e., perceptual stimuli, intake stimuli, peak energy levels, mobility), and psychological stimuli (i.e., global or analytical, right- or left-brained, impulsive or reflective).

Other Types of Learning

Some applications of learning theories and models are relevant to fieldwork education. Some are pedagogical approaches (i.e., problem-based learning), and others are an application of a learning theory (i.e., collaborative learning).

Clinical Skills Learning

Clinical skills learning involves, for example, teaching a student manual skills such as manual muscle testing or wheelchair transfers. These skills must be learned by hands-on practice.

Reflective Practice

Reflection about what has happened during fieldwork can often lead to deeper levels of learning. One of the commonly used learning activities in fieldwork to promote reflective practice and deeper learning is the use of journals. Whether students are given sentence prompts to guide their writing or spontaneously write, the result is usually an examination of assumptions, meanings, and feelings surrounding a particular issue (Hanson, Larsen, & Nielsen, 2011).

Problem-Based Learning

Problem-based learning is frequently adopted as a curricular theme within an academic program. It is based on constructivist theory and involves students working together in small groups to solve a clinical problem and construct knowledge together.

Collaborative Learning

A great deal of literature exists on collaborative learning, which is based on constructivist theory.

This type of learning generally occurs within a group where the teacher or fieldwork educator is more of a facilitator of learning than a teacher. The group members support each other as they construct their own knowledge.

Supervision Theories and Models

Theories and models of supervision help us use and organize information; they provide a framework to view and work with our supervisees. One of the items in the Self-Assessment Tool for Fieldwork Educator Competency (Chapter 27) addresses the need for the fieldwork educator to use "current supervision models and theories to facilitate student performance and professional behavior" (AOTA, 2009, p. 5). Bernard and Goodyear (2009) define *supervision* as

> an intervention provided by a more senior member of a profession to a more junior member or members of that same profession. This relationship is: evaluative and hierarchical, extends over time, has the simultaneous purposes of enhancing the professional functioning of the more junior person(s), monitoring the quality of professional services offered to the clients that she, he, or they see, and serving as a gatekeeper for those who are to enter that particular profession. (p. 7)

Supervision Theories

Psychotherapy-Based Theories

Psychotherapy-based theories are based on widely accepted psychotherapy models such as the Psychodynamic Model derived from Sigmund Freud's (1923) theories and the Person-Centered Model developed by Carl Rogers (Rogers, 1942, as cited in Bernard & Goodyear, 2009). In these approaches, traditionally used in the mental health fields, supervision often mimics personal psychotherapy.

Developmental Theories

The developmental theories category includes several models, such as Stoltenberg's Integrated Developmental Model (Stoltenberg, 1981, as cited in Bernard & Goodyear, 2009); the Ronnestad and Skovholt Model (Ronnestad & Skovholt, 1993, as cited in Bernard & Goodyear, 2009); and the Loganbill, Hardy, and Delworth Model (Loganbill, Hardy, & Delworth, 1982, as cited in Bernard & Goodyear, 2009). All of these models are process-oriented and describe stages that a supervisee goes through.

The Loganbill, Hardy, and Delworth Model has been mentioned often in the occupational therapy literature. In this model, the student moves through the three stages of stagnation, confusion, and integration and the fieldwork educator uses suggested strategies in each stage.

Social Role Models

Social role theories come out of the counseling field, and the role of supervisor is differentiated from that of teacher, counselor, or therapist.

Situational Leadership Model

The Situational Leadership Model emerged from the management approach of Paul Hersey and Ken Blanchard (Hersey, Blanchard, & Johnson, 2001). This model describes a dynamic rather than static supervision approach in which the type of supervision provided changes in response to the task being performed and the amount of confidence and motivation of the student. The model includes four distinct types of supervisory strategies:

1. *Directing Style.* The student does not appear ready for the task assigned and is insecure about how to proceed. The fieldwork educator responds by telling the student exactly what to do, providing clear instructions.
2. *Coaching Style.* The student appears more ready for assigned tasks but still lacks self-confidence. The fieldwork educator responds by explaining the rationale behind treatment decisions and gives the student opportunities to ask questions.
3. *Supporting Style.* The student feels able to perform the assigned task but is still insecure. The fieldwork educator responds by sharing ideas with the student and engaging in a collaborative process.
4. *Delegating Style.* The student is ready to perform and self-confident. The fieldwork educator

needs to respond by backing off and letting the student be as independent as possible (given the parameters of the practice setting).

Transformative Model

The Transformative Model is process oriented and based on transformative learning theory. It requires both the student and fieldwork educator to reflect on the assumptions they have in any given situation and then examine how those assumptions change as they emerge from an experience. It could be said that all fieldwork is reflective of this approach.

Supervision Formats

A variety of supervision formats are used in occupational therapy fieldwork education throughout the world. The one used depends on the nature of the fieldwork site and the theoretical orientation of the fieldwork educator.

1:1 or Traditional Apprenticeship Model

The 1:1 model is the most widely used and involves one fieldwork educator, who is viewed as the expert, supervising one student.

2:1 or Shared Clinical Placement Model

The 2:1 model involves two fieldwork educators supervising one student. This model is often used when both educators work part-time or when one is learning the role of being a fieldwork educator.

1:2 Model

The 1:2 model involves one fieldwork educator supervising two students.

Collaborative Approach

The collaborative approach is becoming increasingly popular because it promotes more active learning on the part of the student, with the fieldwork educator guiding the process rather than being the expert. This approach is usually used with a group of students, and it can be a combination of occupational therapy and occupational therapy assistant students.

Group Model

In the group model, one fieldwork educator, who is viewed as the expert, supervises a group of students.

Peer Model

The peer model involves students providing feedback to each other. However, in fieldwork, this type of management cannot be the only form of supervision. The Accreditation Council of Occupational Therapy Education standards (2012) require that an occupational therapist or occupational therapy assistant be the fieldwork educator and that students receive a specified amount of supervision.

Role-Emerging Model

The role-emerging model is used at fieldwork sites where occupational therapy services are being developed. The fieldwork educator might be employed by the fieldwork site or the academic program, but is generally present only for a portion of the time that the students are there. It requires that another staff member at the fieldwork site provides structure and support for the student when the fieldwork educator is not present.

Summary

This chapter has provided a brief overview of the many theories and models that exist for learning and for supervision. It is important for fieldwork educators to be aware of these theories and models and be able to articulate the approaches that they use with students. Theories and models provide the fieldwork educator with a lens through which to view the supervisory process.

References

American Occupational Therapy Association. (2009). *Self-Assessment Tool for Fieldwork Educator Competency*. Retrieved from http://www.aota.org/-/media/Corporate/Files/EducationCareers/Educators/Fieldwork/Supervisor/Forms/Self-Assessment%20Tool%20FW%20Ed%20Competency%20(2009).pdf

American Occupational Therapy Association. (2013). *Commission on Education guidelines for an occupational therapy fieldwork experience—Level II*. Retrieved from http://www.aota.org/-/media/Corporate/Files/EducationCareers/Educators/Fieldwork/LevelII/COE%20Guidelines%20for%20an%20Occupational%20Therapy%20Fieldwork%20Experience%20--%20Level%20II--Final.pdf

Accreditation Council for Occupational Therapy Education. (2012, December). Accreditation Council for Occupational Therapy Education (ACOTE) standards and interpretive guide. *American Journal of Occupational Therapy, 66*, S6–S74. http://dx.doi.org/10.5014/ajot.2012.6656

Bernard, J., & Goodyear, R. (2009). *Fundamentals of clinical supervision* (4th ed.). Upper Saddle River, NJ: Pearson.

Briggs-Myers, I., & Briggs, K. C. (1985). *Myers-Briggs Type Indicator (MBTI)*. Palo Alto, CA: Consulting Psychologists Press.

Bruner, J. S. (1966). *Toward a theory of instruction*. Cambridge, MA: Belkapp Press.

Cohn, E., Dooley, N., & Simmons, L. (2001). Collaborative learning applied to fieldwork education. *Occupational Therapy in Health Care, 15*(1/2), 69–83.

Costa, D. (2007). *Clinical supervision in occupational therapy: A guide for fieldwork and practice*. Bethesda, MD: AOTA Press.

Costa, D. (2014). Supervision module. In *Fieldwork educator certificate program*. Bethesda, MD: American Occupational Therapy Association.

Dewey, J. (1916). *Democracy and education*. New York: Macmillan.

Dunn, R., Dunn K., & Price, G. E. (1985). *Learning Styles Inventory (LSI): An inventory for the identification of how individuals in grades 3 through 12 prefer to learn*. Lawrence, KS: Price Systems.

Freud, S. (1923). *The ego and the id*. New York: W.W. Norton.

Gagné, R. M. (1965). *The conditions of learning and theory of instruction*. New York: Holt, Rinehart, & Winston.

Hanson, D. (2011a). Collaborative fieldwork education: Intraprofessional and interprofessional learning. *OT Practice, 16*(9), 16–23.

Hanson, D. (2011b). Collaborative supervision models: Are two (or more) students better than one? *OT Practice, 16*(1), 25–26.

Hanson, D., Larsen, J., & Nielsen, S. (2011). Reflective writing in Level II fieldwork: A tool to promote clinical reasoning. *OT Practice, 16*(7), 11–14

Hersey, P., Blanchard, K. H., & Johnson, D. E. (2001). *Management of organizational behavior: Leading human resources*. Englewood Cliffs, NJ: Prentice Hall.

Higgs, J., & Edwards, H. (Eds.). (1999). *Educating beginning practitioners: Challenges for health professional education*. Boston: Butterworth-Heinemann.

Johnson, C., Haynes, C., & Ames, J. (2007). Supervision competencies for fieldwork educators. *OT Practice, 12*(22), CE-1–CE-8.

Jung, C. G. (1921). *The collected works of C. G. Jung: Vol. 6. Psychological types.* Princeton, NJ: Princeton University Press.

Kolb, D. (1984). *Experiential learning as the science of learning and development.* Englewood Cliffs, NJ: Prentice Hall.

Knowles, M. (1980). *The modern practice of adult education: From pedagogy to androgogy.* New York: Cambridge University Press.

Knowles, M., Holton, E., & Swanson, R. (2005). *The adult learner: The definitive classic in adult education and human resource development* (6th ed.). New York: Taylor & Francis.

Loganbill, C., Hardy, E., & Delworth, U. (1982). Supervision: A conceptual model. *Counseling Psychologist, 10,* 3–42.

Martin, M., Morris, J., Moore, A., Sadlo, G., & Crouch, R. (2004). Evaluating practice education models in occupational therapy: Comparing 1:1, 2:1, and 3:1 placements. *British Journal of Occupational Therapy, 67*(5), 192–200.

Maslow, A. H. (1968). *Toward a psychology of being* (2nd ed.). New York: D. Van Nostrand.

McAllister, L., Paterson, M., Higgs, J., & Bithell, C. (Eds). (2010). *Innovations in allied health education: A critical appraisal.* Boston: Sense Publishing.

Mezirow, J. (1991). *Transformative dimensions of adult learning.* San Francisco, CA: Jossey-Bass.

Mezirow, J. (1997). Transformative learning: Theory to practice. *New Directions for Adult and Continuing Education, 74,* 5–12.

Pavlov, I. P. (1927). *Conditioned reflexes.* London: Oxford University Press.

Piaget, J. (1936). *Origins of intelligence in the child.* London: Routledge & Kegan Paul.

Polgase, T., & Treseder, R. (2012). *The occupational therapy handbook: Practice education.* Keswick, UK: M & K Publishing.

Provident, I., Dolhi, C., Leibold, M., & Jeffcoat, J. (2009). Education module. In C. Johnson & P. Stutz-Tanenbaum (Eds.), *Fieldwork educator certificate program manual.* Bethesda, MD: American Occupational Therapy Association.

Queensland Occupational Therapy Fieldwork Collaborative. (2007). *Clinical educator's resource kit: Adult learning theory and principles.* Victoria, Australia: Occupational Therapy Australia.

Rogers, C. R. (1942). *Counseling and psychotherapy: Newer concepts in practice.* Boston, MA: Houghton Mifflin.

Rogers, C. (1951). *Client-centered therapy: Its current practice, implications and theory.* London: Constable.

Ronnestad, M. H., & Skovolt, T. M. (1993). Supervision of beginning and advanced graduate students of counseling and psychotherapy. *Journal of Counseling and Development, 71,* 396–405.

Rose, M., & Best, D. (Eds.). (2005). *Transforming practice through clinical education, professional supervision and mentoring.* New York: Elsevier.

Santalucia, S., & Johnson, C. (2010). Transformative learning: Facilitating growth and change through fieldwork. *OT Practice, 15*(19), CE-1–CE-8.

Skinner, B. F. (1953). *Science and human behavior.* New York: Simon & Schuster.

Stoltenberg, C. D. (1981). Approaching supervision from a developmental perspective: The counselor complexity model. *Journal of Counseling Psychology, 28,* 59–65.

Thew, M., Edwards, M., Baptiste, S., & Molineux, M. (Eds.). (2011). *Role-emerging occupational therapy: Maximizing occupation-focused practice.* Ames, IA: Wiley-Blackwell.

Vygotsky, L. S. (1978). *Mind in society: The development of higher psychological processes.* Cambridge, MA: Harvard University Press.

Chapter 4.

TRANSFORMATIVE LEARNING: FACILITATING GROWTH AND CHANGE THROUGH FIELDWORK

Susan Santalucia, MS, OTR/L
Instructor and Assistant Academic Fieldwork Coordinator
Thomas Jefferson University, Philadelphia, PA

Caryn R. Johnson, MS, OTR/L, FAOTA
Assistant Professor and Academic Fieldwork Coordinator
Thomas Jefferson University, Philadelphia, PA

Abstract

Occupational therapy and occupational therapy assistant students enter into academic programs and fieldwork experiences with many ideas about various patient and client populations, how occupational therapy should be provided, what motivates individuals to engage in the therapeutic process, and so on. These preconceptions, which are influenced by an individual's worldview and sociocultural context, can result in assumptions that lead to actions. *Transformative learning* is a process that uses critical self-reflection to question those assumptions and facilitate new ways of thinking and acting in regard to individuals, challenges, and the therapeutic process. This article will present the reader with a background on transformative learning and methods for applying it to fieldwork education, though the content has broader application and will have us thinking about why we choose any given course of action.

Learning Objectives

After reading this article, you should be able to:

1. Identify the basic tenets of transformative learning and recognize its relationship to adult learning theory.
2. Recognize elements of an environment that are conducive to transformative learning in the fieldwork setting.
3. Select learning opportunities in the fieldwork setting that can facilitate the process of self-evaluation and reflection as it pertains to transformative learning.

According to Taylor, occupational therapists and occupational therapy assistants ". . . who are knowledgeable, curious, and motivated to embrace new behaviors and perspectives are more likely to relate effectively with a wider range of clients" (2008, p. 191). It is paramount that practitioners possess the cultural competence necessary to adjust their practices to manage the complexities introduced by diversity in the therapeutic relationship (Taylor, 2008). Becoming a competent entry-level practitioner requires the mastery of many different levels of knowledge and skills during the fieldwork experience, and a critical role for educators is to create learning environments in both the classroom and the clinic that challenge students to engage in critical and clinical reflection and to reach beyond their own beliefs, assumptions, and culture to fully understand the life circumstances of other individuals. While for some, constructive feedback and explanation from an authority figure will suffice, in a contemporary society individuals must learn to actively question and interpret their own beliefs, purposes, judgments, and feelings rather than rely on the interpretations of others (Imel, 1998).

Transformative Learning and Adult Education Theory

Jack Mezirow introduced the concept of transformative learning in a study based on 83 women returning to college in 12 different reentry programs (Mezirow, 1975). He initially described a process of personal perspective transformation that included 10 phases. Since that time, the concept of transformative learning has been a topic of continued theory development and research within the area of adult learning and education. Over the past 2 decades, transformative learning theory has developed "into a comprehensive and complex description of how learners construe, validate, and reformulate the meaning of their experience" (Cranton, 1994, p. 22). Although Mezirow is considered to be the "father" of transformative learning theory, other theorists with thoughts regarding transformative learning have emerged as well.

Transformative learning is considered to be a theory in progress and a subset of adult learning (Cranton, 2006). There are many theories, patterns, and classification systems found in the literature

for adult learning. Adult learners are frequently described as self-directed and voluntary learners (Cranton, 2006). Following his exploration of the literature related to self-direction, Candy (1991) developed a framework that includes four facets of self-direction: learner control (organizing and managing learning in formal education settings), autonomy (personal characteristics of self-directed learners), self-management (willingness and ability to conduct one's own education), and autodidaxy (pursuit of learning in the natural setting). Many have asserted that adult learning should be practical or experiential in nature, based on the assumption that adult learners have practical problems to solve, such as applying their learning to jobs or new career tracks. Knowles (1980) emphasized the importance of adult learners' life experiences and knowledge in learning.

Humanistic learning theories view adult education as collaborative and participatory. According to constructivist learning theories, learners share their experiences and resources with each other to create new knowledge. Transformative learning theory is largely based on constructivist assumptions that meaning is seen to exist within one's self and not in external forms (Cranton, 2006). Constructivism asserts that learning is contextual; that we do not learn isolated facts and theories in an abstract, ethereal land of the mind separate from the rest of our lives. Rather, we learn in relationship to what else we know, what we believe, our prejudices, and our fears. On reflection, it becomes clear that this point is actually a corollary of the idea that learning is active and social. We cannot divorce our learning from our lives (Hein, 1991). We develop or construct personal meaning from our experiences and validate it through interaction and communication with others (Cranton, 2006).

All of these tenets of adult learning may be viewed as inherent in the transformative learning experience. Learning is voluntary in that the student must be willing to engage in critical self-reflection. Students must also be self-directed in order to take the steps to examine their own beliefs, assumptions, and perspectives, as well as to actively participate in discussion related to self-examination. Transformative learning may also incorporate sharing experiences with others via discourse, which Mezirow (2000) saw as a necessary component of transformative learning.

Over the past decade, interest in the practice of transformative learning has been growing in the fields of adult and higher education. According to Mezirow, the goal of adult education and transformative learning is "to help adult learners become more critically reflective, participate more fully and freely in rational discourse and action, and advance developmentally by moving toward meaning perspectives that are more inclusive, discriminating, permeable, and integrative of experience" (1991, pp. 224–225). Transformative learning has become the dominant teaching paradigm discussed within the field of adult education and has become a standard of practice in a variety of disciplines and educational settings, including higher education, professional education, organizational development, international education, and community education (Taylor, 2009).

How We Make Meaning of Our World

To understand how individuals make meaning of the world and the events that they encounter, one must understand how people view the world and their experiences. How can two people watch the same scenario and have very different understandings or viewpoints as to what has transpired and why? This may occur because each individual views the world differently through his or her own unique "lens." This observation does not imply that one is right or wrong, but rather recognizes that differences exist and why. What shapes those lenses and what makes them different?

According to Mezirow (2000), we view the world through a web of assumptions and expectations described as a frame of reference that consists of two dimensions—habits of mind and the resulting points of view, or assumptions. Habits of mind include our ways of learning, sociocultural background and language, our psychological nature, moral and ethical views, religious doctrine or worldview, and how we view beauty (Mezirow, 2000). They are absorbed from our family, community, and culture (Cranton, 2006). Beliefs, assumptions, and expectations arise from an individual's habits of mind. Assumptions are personal and variable. They shape our expectations, perceptions, understandings, and feelings,

and therefore, our actions. Assumptions shape what practitioners see, influence how they interpret events, and guide which action they select to make (Hooper, 2008).

Assumptions play an influential role in actions by filtering and directing attention, guiding choices, and interpreting the meaning of an act or experience (Mezirow, 2000). A practitioner's assumptions may become a habituated way of viewing things, and attention may focus on specific elements and cues within the therapy environment (Hooper, 2008). Mezirow (1991) asserted that there is overwhelming evidence to support the idea that we tend to accept and integrate experiences that comfortably fit our frame of reference. This may limit our ability to understand and consider broader options and possibilities in our interactions and treatment planning with clients.

Ultimately, our unique points of view are a combination of interwoven beliefs, assumptions, values, feelings, and expectations that have arisen from our habits of mind. This process is what creates the lens through which we see the world and forms the basis for our actions. Habits of mind can contribute to prejudices, stereotypes, and unquestioned or unexamined beliefs and assumptions. They can create limitations and form subconscious barriers that we are unable to get beyond (Cranton, 2006).

The Transformative Learning Process

Transformative learning reflects a process as well as an outcome of adult learning. It aids in the adult's development and "moves the individual towards a more inclusive, differentiated permeable (open to other points of view), and integrated meaning perspective, the validity of which has been established through rational discourse" (Mezirow, 1991, p. 7).

Transformative learning can take place in many different environments and can be related to personal or professional life. The process of transformation "begins with a disorienting dilemma and concludes with a changed self-concept that enables a reintegration into one's life context" (Mezirow, 1991, p. 193). Transformative learning is not a linear process; therefore, the phases between the first and last are not necessarily sequential.

Mezirow (2000) identified 10 phases of learning that become clarified in the transformative process based on the findings from his 1978 study:

- Experiencing a disorienting dilemma
- Undergoing self-examination
- Critically assessing assumptions
- Recognizing a connection between one's discontent and the process of transformation
- Exploring options for new roles, relationships, and actions
- Planning or revising a course of action
- Acquiring knowledge and skills for implementing one's plan
- Trying new roles on a provisional basis
- Building competence and self-confidence in new roles and relationships
- Integrating the changes into one's life.

Key to transformative learning is a disorienting dilemma or triggering event that activates the process. This event is a catalyst, stimulating learners to undergo a process of critical self-reflection and self-examination in which they must closely examine their assumptions, beliefs, and underlying habits of mind. The triggering event may be a single dramatic event, a series of almost unnoticed cumulative events, a deliberate conscious effort to make a change in one's life, or a natural developmental progression (Cranton, 2006).

Mezirow maintained that reflection is an essential component of transformative learning, and that two distinctively adult learning capabilities are required: (1) the development of a capacity to be critically self-reflective and (2) the ability to exercise reflective judgment (2003). He also distinguished among three types of reflection. Content reflection examines the content, or description, of the problem, asking, "What is the problem?" Process reflection involves checking on the problem-solving strategies being used: "Did I miss something?" Premise reflection is an examination of the premise or basis of the problem: "Why is this important?"

Content and process reflection may lead to the transformation of a specific belief or assumption, but it is premise reflection that engages learners in seeing themselves and the world in a different way. It is premise reflection that has the potential to lead people to the transformation of a habit of mind.

Fieldwork Education

Students arrive for their fieldwork experiences with assumptions about many things, including occupational therapy, patients and clients, groups of people, supervision, the environment, and themselves. They are often unaware that their assumptions and beliefs are influenced by their own personal experiences and habits of mind, family values, religious beliefs, and educational and sociocultural backgrounds. They may also be unaware of how these assumptions and beliefs were formed and how strongly they influence their choice of actions with their clients and other individuals at the fieldwork setting, including the supervisor.

During fieldwork, the fieldwork educator may function in many roles: teacher, guide, mentor, and colleague. The fieldwork educator is charged with invoking as much learning as possible: teaching skills, providing knowledge, and fostering personal and professional growth (Velde, Wittman, & Mott, 2007). It is therefore important to provide carefully planned activities and opportunities for transformative learning and growth. Differences in learning contexts, students, and fieldwork educators all affect the potential for transformative learning experiences.

Barriers to Transformative Learning

Not all fieldwork educators and students feel comfortable with a goal of transformative learning. Based on findings from empirical studies, Taylor (1998) suggested that not all students are predisposed to engage in transformative learning. The same may be true for fieldwork educators. We are comfortable with our own beliefs and what we think we "know" (Cranton, 2002). When those beliefs are challenged, it can feel uncomfortable or be perceived as threatening, and many people may not want to consider alternatives and therefore do not engage in reflection or consideration of alternative points of view. Even if the fieldwork educator has created an environment that will support transformative learning, critical reflection on the part of the student is not ensured. Students themselves must willingly and actively engage in the process of critical self-reflection. Some students may even engage in the process and question, reflect, and discuss, but they may ultimately not undergo any significant change as a result of this process because of a deeply seated need to hold onto their "truths."

Establishing Environments Conducive to Transformative Learning

If transformative learning is your goal, how can it be fostered given the variables in contexts, students, and fieldwork educators? There is no one way to teach for transformation, but there are some general recommendations and fundamental principles to follow in order to foster a learning environment that will support transformative learning.

Role of the Fieldwork Educator

The fieldwork educator must serve as a role model and demonstrate a willingness to learn and change by expanding and deepening his or her understanding of perspectives about both subject matter and teaching (Cranton, 1994). It is the teacher's responsibility to create a "community of knowers"—individuals who are "united in a shared experience of trying to make meaning of their life experience" (Loughlin, 1993, pp. 320–321). As the teacher, the fieldwork educator is a member of this community and responsible for establishing an environment that builds trust and facilitates the development of sensitive relationships among all other members (Cranton, 1994).

Role of the Student

The student, as part of the fieldwork site community, shares the responsibility for developing and maintaining an environment that supports conditions under which transformative learning can occur. Unlike traditional learning environments, the role of the teacher in transformative learning should be de-emphasized and the responsibility of the students heightened. Although it can be difficult for transformative learning to take place without a facilitator or teacher, the student must accept responsibility to be an active participant in the process and an active member of the community of knowers.

Fostering Clinical Self-Reflection and Self-Knowledge

Fieldwork educators can provide opportunities and assist students in reflective learning activities that involve assessing or reassessing assumptions. According to Mezirow, "reflective learning becomes transformative whenever assumptions or premises are found to be distorting, inauthentic, or otherwise invalid" (1991, p. 6). Examining their biases and assumptions is an essential part of the transformative learning process that will help move students toward a new understanding of the information they encounter.

Providing students with an opportunity to think about and respond to well-designed questions yields opportunities for them to see things in new ways and consider different options. Wiessner and Mezirow (2000) discussed how questioning can serve as an effective process that fosters transformative learning. There are many guidelines for asking good questions in the adult learning literature. A few suggestions offered by Cranton (2006) include:

- Be specific—relate questions to specific events and situations.
- Move from the particular to the general.
- Be conversational.
- Avoid echoing students' responses to a question.
- Use follow-up questions or probes to encourage more specific responses.
- Avoid close-ended questions.
- Ask questions that draw on students' experiences and interests related to the topic.

Costa (2009) also suggested several strategies to foster transformative learning. We need to improve our skill at asking the right questions, and then patiently wait for the answers. We need to keep encouraging students to continue questioning their assumptions, and recognize that their confidence level will grow in time. Fieldwork educators also need to model these same skills for students, "thinking out loud" our own internal processes about the clients we serve (pp. 19–20).

Example of Fieldwork Activities

Although fieldwork experiences themselves can stimulate reflection, there are things that fieldwork educators can do to help facilitate reflection and help students to identify habits of mind, assumptions, beliefs, and expectations. Fieldwork educators can then provide opportunities for the students to openly dialogue and consider alternative viewpoints. Mentoring and learning opportunities should also be provided to assist students in gaining competence and confidence with new roles and ideas. Students can then plan a course of action to implement these actions and ideas. Ideally, students can experience opportunities to try out the new roles and actions during the fieldwork experience.

Additional strategies include setting a designated time aside for critical discourse about the students' experiences and suggesting that students write about experiences in a journal (Kolb, 1984). When journals are used to encourage reflection rather than log events, they can be a powerful strategy for initiating transformative learning. Students can be encouraged to share parts of the journal with the supervisor. Students should never be judged, and educators should not contradict how the student views him- or herself (Cranton, 2006). Rather, fieldwork educators can make comments and pose questions that are challenging and provocative in order to question the origin of the student's perceptions and the consequences of holding them. Uncomfortable questions can promote critical self-reflection if a student is willing and ready to consider them.

Fieldwork educators can provide structured, scheduled activities during the fieldwork experience so that students can have the opportunity to engage in the transformative learning process. The following are some examples that educators may choose to implement.

- **Have the student observe a treatment session.** After dividing a piece of paper in half vertically, ask the student to write down observations on one side. On the other side, ask him or her to write down thoughts, feelings, related experiences, or images provoked by watching the scene. Discuss the results and ask questions such as:
  - "Why do you think you felt that way?"
  - "What do you value and why?"
  - "What experiences in your past might have contributed to you thinking about it that way?"
  - "Why is that important to you?"

  These types of probing questions force the student to reflect on habits of mind, beliefs, and assumptions. Identifying and critically reflecting on habits of mind, beliefs, and assumptions are essential parts of the transformative learning process.
- **Schedule time for students to share and compare related experiences** with each other or with a group of practitioners. For example, share experiences following a therapy session that focused on teaching a new skill to a client with a high-level spinal cord injury.

- **Choose a topic or experience for discussion** among a group of students and practitioners. Ask members of the group to share both successful and unsuccessful experiences related to the topic. Open the discussion with questions about possible explanations for why the experiences were successful or not, and what alternative approaches might have worked. For example, discuss a successful (or unsuccessful) intervention session or activity that you implemented to motivate a client.
- **Use a written case example** that contains a controversial issue or an unresolved dilemma. The fieldwork educator and student, or a student pair, can brainstorm and generate a list of insights, thoughts, and feelings regarding how to solve the issue or dilemma. At the end of the discussion, highlight two or three very different endings to the case example that will continue to offer consideration and reflection on alternative viewpoints.
- **Instruct students to develop personal goals or plans** for change in regard to their performance during fieldwork.
- **Ask students to take a specific approach to intervention** for a case example. Assign another student a different approach. Have the students engage in a "critical debate," a discussion regarding the evidence supporting the assigned intervention approach. Ensure that students are open to and accepting of the alternative points of view. Have students discuss any new ideas or information they have learned about their own assumptions or habits of mind based on the dialogue.
- **Engage students in sharing their own personal experiences** as "storytelling." Fieldwork educators can prompt the sharing with open-ended questions, such as "What is the most compelling, rewarding, exciting, surprising, or disappointing experience you have had this week during fieldwork?"

A Transformative Learning Activity

The authors use a learning activity from the book *Clinical and Professional Reasoning in Occupational Therapy* (Schell & Schell, 2008) called "The Aha Moment." This activity helps students recognize that they hold assumptions, what those assumptions are, where the assumptions come from, and how assumptions influence their actions. Students are asked to identify a "triggering event" or a "disorientating dilemma" they experienced during fieldwork. They then reflect on their assumptions and underlying habits of mind and consider alternative options or viewpoints. This process can enable them to develop a broader, more open world view, which in turn may change their assumptions, allowing them to make more effective choices about their actions. Many of the students were able to build confidence and competence by applying these new ideas and techniques in practice during fieldwork. (Note: For this assignment, "habits of mind" was incorporated into the broad area of "sociocultural context/world view.")

Activity

"Aha" experiences can happen when we are unaware of a set of assumptions we hold; then something happens and those assumptions are brought into new light. Can you think of a similar experience that occurred during this fieldwork experience? It may have been assumptions you held about human nature, learning, a group of people, occupational therapy, patient treatment, therapeutic use of self, or supervision, to name a few. Hooper (2008) used a flower analogy to recapture the details of that experience.

Case Examples (Level I Students)

Aubrey

Aubrey's ideas about parenting and discipline were "based on my own experiences, education, and values." She assumed that "bad behavior" of children resulted from "poor parenting and living in unstructured environments where the child reigned supreme." Aubrey wrote,

> I grew up with two parents who enforced rules and chores. If one did not follow these expectations and directions, they were met with punishments. I feel this made me respect my parents and other adults, as well as teaching me manners and how to behave. Additionally, in today's schools students are rewarded and punished for their behaviors.... Furthermore, in American society adults expect their children to be well behaved and have

good manners because this enables the child and their family to make a good impression on others, as well as being a quality that is valuable in today's world. Therefore, I felt as though the parents of these out-of-control children were not instilling these values and beliefs in their children and letting them get away with their bad behavior.

Aubrey's actions were to "get frustrated easier and have less patience with these children. I would use a more authoritarian approach by talking loudly during my instructions with little to no inflection in my voice, as well as using a stern facial expression during most of the time spent with these children."

The triggering dilemma came while working with a 4-year-old girl with a possible diagnosis of bipolar disorder. Aubrey wrote,

> This little girl had a hard time transitioning from the waiting room to the treatment room and would throw a temper tantrum. Once in the treatment room, she would pound the floor with her fist, cry, scream, and try to run out of the room. However after approximately 5 minutes she stopped, walked over to me, and asked me politely what my name was. After this, she changed into a whole new individual. She was cheerful, pleasant, and followed instructions. But when it was time to leave, the little girl would again cry, kick, and scream. This was my "Aha" moment. I noticed how this little girl's disorder was playing a role in the way she behaves. After this I began to notice how many of the children's psychiatric disorders affected their behaviors and I started interacting with these children differently.

This transformational experience allowed Aubrey to change her actions, enabling her to "become more calm, patient, and understanding with these clients. I tried to collaborate with them during treatment to make the session more meaningful to them, hoping this would promote better behavior."

Aubrey's new point of view includes awareness that "Many parents of children with psychological disorders who I encountered read books on the disorders, read information online, and even attended educational classes to help them better understand their child and the disorder. Parents

Figure 4.1.   Chris's perceptions of differences between men and women.

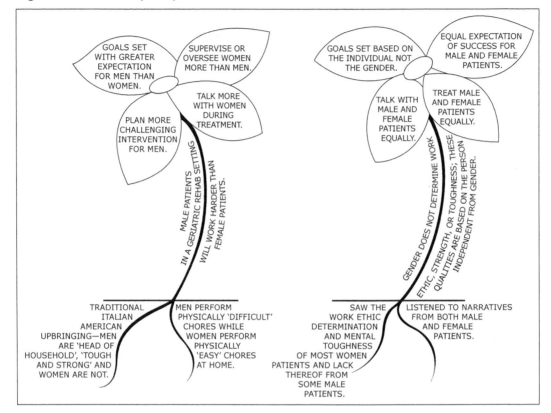

who do this would be considered good parents in American society and therefore, just because their child acts a certain way, it doesn't mean it's due to poor parenting." She stated that

> My new assumption is that if I can think outside of the box and take into consideration that there may be other reasons why the child is misbehaving, it will be easier to interact in a calmer manner and be more patient with these children . . . . Furthermore, I now better understand how to look at the whole individual, not just their behavior.

Chris

Chris had specific ideas about differences between men and women. Figure 4.1 illustrates his pre- and post-Aha perceptions. Chris wrote:

> This belief that men are physically and mentally stronger and tougher than women was

not directly taught to me by my parents or anyone else; rather, I believe it is something that I concluded based on my environment. The men in my family, as well as most others in the neighborhood, performed "strong and tough" household tasks such as chopping wood, landscaping, and shoveling snow, while the women performed "less strenuous" tasks such as laundry, cooking, and cleaning the house. Additionally, in my household, as well as in most other households in my neighborhood, the father was the head of the house and therefore took on a "strong and tough" role while the mother took on a more submissive role. Lastly, the mentality, physical appearance, and personality of most men in my neighborhood was one that projected strength and toughness to me while the mentality, physical appearance, and personality of most women in my neighborhood projected elegance and tenderness, but not strength and toughness.

At the end of his first week, Chris looked back over the treatment plans he had developed for his patients in a subacute facility. He noticed that

> My treatment plans for the male patients were much more thorough and challenging than they were for the females, and the goals for the male patients were much more ambitious than they were for the females. At that point I chalked it up to coincidence but kept it in the back of my head for the next week. When the next week arrived, I noticed that I was supervising the women much more than the men, thinking they may "slack off." Additionally, I noticed myself talking with the women more during treatment to make sure they were doing what they were supposed to, whereas I didn't feel a need to stay with the men the whole time, expecting that they wouldn't "slack off."

The triggering dilemma came when Chris observed that the two women were very motivated and willing to work while the men would often "slack off" when not supervised:

> After putting these pieces together I had my "Aha" moment. I was exercising a gender bias and expecting the male patients to be strong and tough and the female patients to be weak and frail. Whereas initially I assumed that the men would work hard independently and that the women would slack off if not supervised, I eventually realized that it is the individual who determines work ethic, strength, and toughness, and not the gender of the individual. I also realized that this is something I'll need to be careful of in myself moving forward.

Chris described a heightened self-awareness, and wrote how he changed his actions by changing [his] intervention plan, goals, and interaction with the patients and eliminating any gender biases:

> I began dealing with the individual patients without a preconceived expectation based on gender and was much more effective as a practitioner. I'm thankful that this "Aha" moment opened my eyes, not only to the fact that strength and toughness is not gender-based,

but also of my own tendency to revert back to that assumption.

Students have found this learning activity particularly meaningful. They often comment, months or semesters later, how it has affected their own way of looking at clients, challenges, and themselves, both in the fieldwork environment and in life.

Conclusion

Many factors influence an individual's readiness and capacity for a transformative learning experience, including differences in learning contexts and the receptiveness, insight, and capacity of both the student and fieldwork educator. Although fieldwork educators cannot teach transformation, they can approach the fieldwork experience as though the possibility that the student will have a transformative experience exists (Cranton, 2002). Fieldwork educators can provide a safe learning environment with stimulating and challenging learning opportunities where students can grow and transform.

"Like guides, we walk at times ahead of our students, at times beside them; at times, we follow their lead. In sensing where to walk lies our art, for as we support our students in their struggle, challenge them toward their best, and cast light on the road ahead, we do so in the name of our respect for their potential and our care for their growth." (Daloz, 1999, p. 245)

References

Candy, P. (1991). *Self-direction for lifelong learning.* San Francisco: Jossey-Bass.

Costa, D. (2009). Fieldwork Issues: Transformative learning in fieldwork. *OT Practice, 14*(1), 19–20.

Cranton, P. (1994). *Understanding and promoting transformative learning: A guide for educators of adults.* San Francisco: Jossey-Bass.

Cranton, P. (2002, Spring). Contemporary viewpoints on teaching adults effectively. *New Directions for Adult and Continuing Education, 96,* 93.

Cranton, P. (2006). *Understanding and promoting transformative learning: A guide for educators of adults.* San Francisco: Jossey-Bass.

Daloz, L. (1999). *Mentor: Guiding the journey of adult learners.* San Francisco: Jossey-Bass.

Imel, S. (1998). *Transformative learning in adulthood.* (ERIC Document Reproduction Service No. ED423426).

Hein, G. (1991, October). *Constructivist learning theory.* Presentation at the International Committee of Museum Educators Conference, Jerusalem, Israel. Retrieved August 30, 2010, from http://www.exploratorium.edu/IFI/resources/constructivistlearning.html

Hooper, B. (2008). Therapists' assumptions as a dimension of professional reasoning. In B. B. Schell & J. W. Schell (Eds.), *Clinical and professional reasoning in occupational therapy* (pp. 13–35). Philadelphia: Lippincott Williams & Wilkins.

Knowles, M. (1980). *Self-directed learning: A guide for learners and teachers.* Chicago: Follett.

Kolb, D. (1984). *Experiential learning: Experience as the source of learning and development.* Upper Saddle River, NJ: Prentice Hall.

Loughlin, K. A. (1993). *Women's perceptions of transformative learning experiences within consciousness-raising.* San Francisco: Mellen Research University Press.

Mezirow, J. (1975). *Education for perspective transformation: Women's reentry programs in community colleges.* New York: Center for Adult Education, Teachers College, Columbia University.

Mezirow, J. (1991). *Transformative dimensions of adult learning.* San Francisco: Jossey-Bass.

Mezirow, J. (2000). Learning to think like an adult. In J. Mezirow & Associates (Eds.), *Learning as a transformation: Critical perspectives on a theory in progress* (pp. 3–35). San Francisco: Jossey-Bass.

Mezirow, J. (2003). Transformative learning as discourse. *Journal of Transformative Education, 1*(1), 58–63.

Schell, B. B., & Schell, J. W. (2008). *Clinical and professional reasoning in occupational therapy.* Baltimore: Lippincott Williams and Wilkins.

Taylor, E. W. (1998). The theory and practice of transformative learning: A critical review. *ERIC Clearinghouse on Adult, Career, and Vocational Education, Center on Education and Training for Employment, 374.* Columbus: College of Education, The Ohio State University.

Taylor, E. W. (2009). Fostering transformative learning. In J. Mezirow, E. W. Taylor, & Associates (Eds.), *Transformative learning in practice: Insights from community, workplace and higher education* (pp. 3–17). San Francisco: John Wiley & Sons.

Taylor, R. R. (2008). *The intentional relationship, occupational therapy and use of self.* Philadelphia: F. A. Davis.

Velde, B., Wittman, P., & Mott, V. (2007). Hands on learning in Tillery. *Journal of Transformative Education, 5*(1), 79–82.

Wiessner, C. A., & Mezirow, J. (2000). Theory building and the search for common ground. In J. Mezirow & Associates (Eds.), *Learning as transformation: Critical perspectives on a theory in progress* (pp. 329–358). San Francisco: Jossey-Bass.

Chapter 5.

THE *OCCUPATIONAL THERAPY PRACTICE FRAMEWORK,* *3rd Edition,* AND FIELDWORK

Donna Costa, DHS, OTR/L, FAOTA

The *Occupational Therapy Practice Framework: Domain and Process* (3rd ed.; hereafter referred to as the *Framework;* American Occupational Therapy Association [AOTA], 2014) is an AOTA official document that was originally written in 2002. This replaced *Uniform Terminology for Occupational Therapy,* which was used from 1979 until 2002. The intent of the document is to articulate the domain and process of the delivery of occupational therapy services to its intended audiences of occupational therapy practitioners, students, and the public. Its language reflects current practice in the profession and defines the areas of occupational performance that occupational therapy practitioners address with those to whom they deliver services.

As an official document, the *Framework* is revised every 5 years to keep it current with practice. Because it contains the language and process that is taught to occupational therapy and occupational therapy assistant students in all education programs, it is important for fieldwork educators to be familiar with its terminology.

Some of the newer terms used in the *Framework* (AOTA, 2014) are as follows:

- *Occupational therapy practitioner.* This term refers to both occupational therapists and occupational therapy assistants (p. S1).
- *Achieving health, well-being, and participation in life through engagement in occupation.* This phrase is the overarching theme of the document and captures the essence of the domain and process of occupational therapy (p. S4).
- *Clients.* The term includes people, groups, or populations (p. S2).
- *Self-advocacy.* This term refers to the process of advocating for oneself, which can include making decisions, developing a support system, learning about rights and responsibilities, acquiring self-determination, and learning how to access information needed for everyday life (p. S30).
- *Domain.* This first section of the *Framework* (AOTA, 2014, p. S4) describes the depth and breadth of occupational therapy practice and

includes occupations, client factors, performance skills, performance patterns, and contexts and environments.

- *Occupations.* They are defined as the life activities that people engage in on a daily basis and that are influenced by the interaction among client factors, performance patterns, and performance skills (p. S5). Occupations include activities of daily living, instrumental activities of daily living, rest and sleep, education, work, play, leisure, and social participation (pp. S19–S21).
- *Client factors.* This term refers to what makes each person unique—his or her capacities, characteristics, and beliefs. The first category under client factors is values, beliefs, and spirituality. The second category is body functions and includes mental functions; sensory functions; neuromuscular and movement-related functions; cardiovascular, hematological, integumentary, and respiratory functions; voice and speech functions; digestive, metabolic, and endocrine functions; genitourinary and reproductive functions; skin and related structure functions; and body structures (pp. S22–S24).
- *Performance skills.* These skills are defined as the goal-directed actions that can be observed in people as they engage in daily life activities. These skills are a way of classifying actions and affect a person's ability to engage in occupations. Included in this category are motor skills (e.g., reaches, bends, walks, manipulates), process skills (e.g., attends, chooses, initiates, sequences), and social interaction skills (e.g., empathizes, thanks, discloses, questions; pp. S25–S26).
- *Performance patterns.* They are defined as the habits, routines, roles, and rituals that a person uses when engaging in an occupation or activity. They can either support or interfere with a person's occupational performance. Performance patterns can be observed in individual people, groups, or populations (p. S27).
- *Context and environment. Context* refers to those elements and conditions within and around people that affect their occupational performance. Contexts can be cultural (customs, beliefs, activity patterns, behavioral expectations), personal (age, gender, socioeconomic status, education level), temporal (stage of life, time of day or year, history), and virtual (use of computer- or airwave-based communication). *Environment* refers to the physical and social settings in which people engage in their chosen occupations. Physical environments include buildings, furniture, tools, and devices. Social environments are relational in nature and include both the availability and expectations of the people in a person's life (p. S28).

- *Process.* The second section of the *Framework* (AOTA, 2014) focuses on the process of the delivery of occupational therapy to the clients being served. It is divided into four sections: (1) an overview of the process of the delivery of client-centered occupational therapy, (2) evaluation, (3) intervention, and (4) outcomes (pp. S9–S10).
  - *Process overview.* Although many professions use a similar process of evaluating and treating clients, the distinct and unique focus of occupational therapy lies in its use of occupations to promote health, well-being, and participation in life. The process overview section includes service delivery models (where practitioners provide services to clients), clinical reasoning used throughout the process, therapeutic use of self, and activity analysis (pp. S10–S13).
  - *Evaluation.* Determining what a client needs and wants to do in his or her life and what he or she can and cannot do is the starting point for the evaluation process. Evaluation is composed of two parts: (1) the occupational profile and (2) the analysis of occupational performance. The occupational profile summarizes a client's occupational history; previous life experiences; what he or she does every day; and his or her interests, needs, and values. The analysis of occupational performance looks more in detail at how a client performs his or her chosen occupations. The occupational therapy practitioner may use observation and standardized or nonstandardized assessments, or both, to measure performance and identify the client's strengths and problem areas. Evaluation includes the collaborative goal-setting process that occurs between the client and the occupational therapy practitioner (pp. S13–S14).
  - *Intervention.* This section discusses the services that occupational therapy practitioners provide collaboratively to a client that will lead to his or her engagement in occupation.

The intervention process has three steps: (1) the intervention plan, (2) the intervention implementation, and (3) the intervention review. This section specifies the types of interventions to be provided and the approaches to use. The types of interventions are divided into occupations and activities, preparatory methods or tasks, education and training, advocacy, and group interventions. The approaches to intervention are divided into the categories of create and promote (aimed at health promotion), establish and restore (aimed at remediation, restoration, or both), maintain, modify (through compensation, adaptation, or both), and prevent (further disability; pp. S14–S16).

- *Outcomes.* Outcomes focus on the end results of the occupational therapy process, or what a client has been able to accomplish through the occupational therapy intervention. They can be reflected in a description of the client's occupational performance, specifying improvement or enhancement of skills, or in a description of the client's prevention efforts, movement toward health and wellness, improved quality of life, increased participation, role competence, increased sense of well-being, and occupational justice (p. S16).

Summary

This overview of the *Framework* attempts to describe to the fieldwork educator what students are learning in the classroom. For occupational therapy practitioners not familiar with the document, a suggested learning activity for fieldwork students is to have them do an in-service presentation on it. Fieldwork educators are encouraged to read the *Framework* (AOTA, 2014) and include a copy of it in their fieldwork site manuals.

References

American Occupational Therapy Association. (1979). *Occupational therapy product output reporting system and uniform terminology for reporting occupational therapy services.* (Available from American Occupational Therapy Association, 4720 Montgomery Lane, PO Box 31220, Bethesda, MD 20824-1220; pracdept@aota.org)

American Occupational Therapy Association. (1989). *Uniform terminology for occupational therapy* (2nd ed.). (Available from American Occupational Therapy Association, 4720 Montgomery Lane, PO Box 31220, Bethesda, MD 20824-1220; pracdept@aota.org)

American Occupational Therapy Association. (1994). Uniform terminology for occupational therapy (3rd ed.). *American Journal of Occupational Therapy, 48,* 1047–1054. http://dx.doi.org/10.5014/ajot.48.11.1047

American Occupational Therapy Association. (2014). Occupational therapy practice framework: Domain and process (3rd ed.). *American Journal of Occupational Therapy, 68*(Suppl. 1), S1–S48. http://dx.doi.org/10.5014/ajot.2014.682006

Chapter 6.

A DESCRIPTIVE REVIEW OF OCCUPATIONAL THERAPY EDUCATION

American Occupational Therapy Association

Introduction

In an August 2002 Commission on Education (COE) meeting, COE members decided to design and write a *Guide to Occupational Therapy Education*. With the advent and passing of Resolution J—which became Resolution 670-99 at the 1999 Representative Assembly meeting of the American Occupational Therapy Association (Accreditation Council for Occupational Therapy Education [ACOTE®], 1999b)—and new degree structures within the profession (i.e., professional or clinical doctorate), a guide to occupational therapy education is warranted. This guide, retitled *A Descriptive Review of Occupational Therapy Education,* is intended for practitioners, academicians, and potential occupational therapy program applicants to augment their understanding of occupational therapy education.

Organization of Review

The review is organized into eight sections. The first, the introductory section, describes the process of the development of the Descriptive Review. The second section distinguishes between professional and graduate education. This information provides the background and foundational groundwork for the Review. The next section includes the underpinning information that describes the levels of education in the United States as used by most colleges and universities. It is the common language used in all degree majors and programs and should be the guide for occupational therapy education language so that degrees in occupational therapy can be recognized and understood by fields other than occupational therapy.

The fourth section delineates the levels of education in occupational therapy in the United States from the technical level of education to the doctoral level, using the previous foundational information as the basis of the descriptions. The Review then lists suggested factors that should be considered when choosing an occupational therapy program.

The Review was written to describe the present state of occupational therapy education within the U.S. educational system and is limited to this perspective only. It is purposefully written in a factual format and does not intend to promote one occupational therapy degree over any other, nor is it intended to resolve the multiple issues regarding the various degree levels or entry-level competencies. Those issues need to be addressed by a broad-based consensus group or other professional bodies.

Professional and Graduate Education

The terms *professional education* and *graduate education* are often used synonymously. Educational institutions have the prerogative to house degree programs in any appropriate organizational structure. For example, some master's-degree programs award the degree under the auspices of the graduate school, whereas others offer the degree from a professional school. However, a distinction between *graduate* and *professional* education is needed to understand the nature of the organizational context of occupational therapy educational programs within colleges and universities. Although there is a paucity of literature distinguishing the two types of education, Mayhew and Ford's (1974) *Reform in Graduate and Professional Education* was a welcomed resource to higher educational planners. Mayhew and Ford eloquently articulated the purposes and problems of both graduate and professional education.

Professional Education

Professional education is a term used to describe educational programs in which students are enrolled to study service delivery of a particular profession (e.g., dentistry, medicine, nursing, pharmacy, veterinary science). Studying a profession is different from studying a discipline (e.g., physics, theology, mathematics, biology, sociology; Mayhew & Ford, 1971). A discipline has its own "unique epistemology" that serves as its foundation for autonomy (Knowles, 1977, p. 2209). Professional programs are highly influenced by the professions they serve. The professional standards are at a minimally acceptable level, and governance from the institution often requires higher and different standards (e.g., requirement of thesis, capstone project, electives, additional coursework, interdisciplinary classes).

The purpose of professional education is to admit and educate a sufficient number of students who meet minimum theoretical knowledge and practice skill competencies to practice a profession (Mayhew & Ford, 1974). "Professional education should be directed toward significant objectives, including professional competence, understanding of society, ethical behavior, and scholarly concern" (Mayhew & Ford, 1974, p. 3).

Graduate Education

Graduate education comprises the master's (e.g., MA, MS) degree and doctor of philosophy (PhD) degree (Carmichael, 1961). The graduate school is the organizational authority within colleges and universities that houses graduate educational programs. Traditionally, graduate education focused on advanced study and scholarship within a discipline; however, more recently, some graduate programs in professional fields have emerged (e.g., master's degree in nursing, PhD in rehabilitation).

Historically, graduate education was intended for four purposes (Mayhew & Ford, 1974). The first purpose of graduate education was character formation—to produce broadly learned graduates. The second purpose, preparation of college teachers, was traditionally the primary purpose of PhD programs. The paradox of this intent was that traditional PhD graduate education focused primarily on producing independent researchers and rarely addressed preparation for college teaching. A third purpose of graduate education was "to prepare people for research and scholarship in a specialized field" (Mayhew & Ford, 1974, p. 94). The fourth purpose of graduate education was to have graduates enter the work force and apply their research competencies in professional fields.

Levels of Education in the United States

One of the hallmarks of higher education in the United States is the diversity of institutions, degrees, and programs available. Levels of education are represented by the academic degree conferred to graduates. A degree is a credential or title "conferred by a college or university as official recognition for the completion of a program of studies" (Shafritz, Koeppe, & Soper, 1988, p. 145). Academic degree levels include associate, baccalaureate, master's, and doctoral.

Associate Degree

According to the National Center for Education Statistics, an *associate degree* is "an award that requires the completion of at least 2 but less than 4 full-time equivalent academic years of college-level work in an academic or occupationally specified field of study, and which meets institutional standards for otherwise satisfying the requirements for this degree level" (U.S. Department of Education [USDE], 2002, p. A-63).

Baccalaureate

A *baccalaureate degree* is an award requiring completion of 4 to 5 full-time equivalent academic years of college-level work in an academic or occupationally specific field of study, and which satisfies institutional standards of the requirement of the degree level (USDE, 2002, p. A-63). Two common baccalaureate degrees are the bachelor of arts (BA or AB, for the Latin *atrium baccalareus*) for programs in the humanities and the bachelor of science (BS) for programs in the sciences. Some institutions offer baccalaureate degrees in specialized areas, for example, bachelor of music (BMus) or bachelor of education (BEd; Unger, 1996).

Master's

A *master's degree* typically requires approximately 36 credits of postbaccalaureate education in a subject field. Three master's degrees are commonly awarded. One type includes both the master of arts (MA) and the master of science (MS). MA and MS degrees are "awarded in liberal arts and sciences for advanced scholarship in a subject field or discipline and demonstrated ability to perform scholarly research" (USDE, 2002, p. 298). A second type of master's degree is conferred for completion of a professional entry-level program; for example, an MEd in education, an MBA in business administration, or an MFA in fine arts. In occupational therapy, the MOT, or master of occupational therapy, degree is awarded by some institutions. The third type of master's degree includes the award in professional fields for study beyond the first-professional (entry-level) degree, such as the master of laws (LLM) and the master of science (MS) in various medical professions. Occupational therapy

has typically referred to this level of degree as a postprofessional master's degree.

Various classifications of master's degrees exist, including *academic, professional,* and *experiential* (Glazer, 1988). Curricular requirements for master's degrees vary from institution to institution and from state to state. The diversity in master's degree curricula makes comparison of degree programs, fields, and credentials difficult (Glazer, 1988). For example, some master's-degree programs require a thesis, whereas others do not. The master's degree must be approached "as a class of degrees rather than as a generic model, and as a credential sought increasingly for its own merits rather than in relation to the bachelor's or doctoral degree" (Glazer, 1988, p. 1).

Historically, the purpose of a master's degree was to produce graduates with beginning research or inquiry skills. Not all professions offer a degree at the doctoral level, and thus the master's degree may be the *terminal degree* (highest degree conferred) for some professions.

During the 1980s, master's-degree programs were challenged by more convenient educational alternatives that were shorter in duration and less expensive (e.g., certificate programs). Such certificate alternatives typically did not result in the conferral of a graduate degree. To compete with certificate programs, some master's-degree programs were oriented toward practice rather than research. Currently, approximately 85% of all master's-degree programs in the United States are considered to be practice-oriented or professional degrees (LaPidus, 2000). These programs are specialized in their focus, applied in terms of their content, and decentralized in that they are frequently not housed under the auspices of a graduate school (LaPidus, 2000).

Doctorate: Professional and Research

A *doctoral degree* is the highest degree conferred by an institution of higher education. Most doctoral degrees require the equivalent of 3 years of full-time postbaccalaureate study (Kapel, Gifford, & Kapel, 1991). Commonly, universities require a minimum of 72 hours of postbaccalaureate study plus a residence requirement. "Doctorate entitles bearers to be addressed as 'Doctor' and to append their names with the appropriate letters of their degrees—that is, PhD (doctor of philosophy) or MD (doctor of medicine)" (Unger, 1996, p. 305).

There are two types of doctoral degrees: the *research doctorate* and the *professional doctorate* (Shafritz et al., 1988; Unger, 1996). The professional doctorate is also referred to as a *clinical doctorate* in many health professions (Pierce & Peyton, 1999).

The *research doctorate* (also called the *academic doctorate*), or PhD, was originally awarded for the study of philosophy in the mid to late 19th century. However, the degree was extended to include many disciplines of the humanities and sciences, with each PhD simply modified to indicate the field of study; for example, PhD in engineering, PhD in history, or PhD in chemistry. The purpose of the PhD degree is to develop graduates who are independent researchers and are knowledgeable in a specific area of study. Requirements for the PhD degree usually include a course of didactic study, followed by written or oral comprehensive examinations (upon passing, one applies for candidacy), and the completion of a dissertation in some area of new knowledge as deemed appropriate by a committee of senior faculty after an oral defense of the research (Shafritz et al., 1988)

The *Doctor of Science* (ScD) is an alternative doctoral degree similar to the PhD. Its curriculum is focused on the study of an applied science, such as audiology, occupational therapy, and so forth. ScD degree programs commonly include didactic coursework focused on the study of an applied science, an advanced clinical practicum, and a supervised clinical research project (Kidd, Cox, & Matthies, 2003). Other alternative doctoral degrees include the doctor of education (EdD) and the doctor of public health (DPH).

The professional doctorate reflects academic attainment and seldom requires a master's degree or dissertation (Unger, 1996). Unlike the PhD's focus on developing independent researchers, "sophisticated practice competencies" (Pierce & Peyton, 1999, p. 64) are emphasized in the professional doctorate degree. A person with a professional doctorate, such as an MD or doctor of jurisprudence (JD), must pass state or national qualifying examinations to obtain a license to practice (Unger, 1996). In the health sciences, the term *clinical doctorate* is synonymous with the term *professional doctorate* and the program of study typically requires "mentored advanced clinical experiences for autonomous practice competencies" (Edens & Labadie, 1987; Faut-Callahan,

1992; Hummer, Hunt, & Figuers, 1994; Pierce & Peyton, 1999; Watson, 1988).

Postdoctoral Education

With the growing complexity of knowledge and the need for scholars trained to high, creative levels, postdoctoral education has become increasingly popular to meet work demands in universities, industries, and government (Carmichael, 1961). However, postdoctoral education is widely misunderstood because there is little uniformity.

The adjective *postdoctoral* is frequently used to describe the variety of postdoctoral educational experiences. For example, terms such as *postdoctoral fellow, postdoctoral research associate,* and *postdoctoral trainee* are typically used. Despite the lack of uniformity among terms, postdoctoral is used to denote a *research* appointment after a doctoral degree has been awarded within a discipline or profession (Knowles, 1977).

Residencies

Although residencies are not common practice in occupational therapy, they are a form of postdoctoral education. "The purpose of postprofessional residency education is to advance the resident's preparation as a provider of patient care services in a defined (specialized) area of clinical practice" (DiFabio, 1999, p. 81). Residency training activities are designed to promote the integration of practice, research, and scholarly inquiry (Medeiros, 1998). Professions such as medicine, pharmacy (American Society of Health-System Pharmacists, 2001; Miller & Clarke, 2002), and physical therapy (DiFabio, 1999; Farrell, 1996; Medeiros, 2000) offer postdoctoral specialty residencies to qualified practitioners.

Levels of Education in Occupational Therapy Within the United States

Technical Level

OTA

Occupational therapy assistant (OTA) programs are classified as technical and obtain accreditation from the Accreditation Council for Occupational

Therapy Education (ACOTE®). OTA programs are commonly offered at community colleges, private junior colleges, and some 4-year colleges and universities. All OTA programs must adhere to the *Standards for an Accredited Educational Program for the Occupational Therapy Assistant* (ACOTE, 1999b). As articulated in the Preamble of the Standards, an entry-level OTA must

- Have acquired an educational foundation in the liberal arts and sciences, including a focus on issues related to diversity;
- Be educated as a generalist, with a broad exposure to the delivery models and systems utilized in settings where occupational therapy is currently practiced and where it is emerging as a service;
- Have achieved entry-level competence through a combination of academic and fieldwork education;
- Be prepared to work under the supervision of and in cooperation with the occupational therapist;
- Be prepared to articulate and apply occupational therapy principles, intervention approaches and rationales, and expected outcomes as these relate to occupation;
- Be prepared to be a lifelong learner and keep current with best practice;
- Uphold the ethical standards, values, and attitudes of the occupational therapy profession (ACOTE, 1999b, p. 583).

After completing the OTA didactic and fieldwork requirements, the OTA graduate is eligible to sit for the national certification examination for OTAs. On successful completion, the certified occupational therapy assistant (COTA) may apply for the appropriate state credential and, under specified supervision, render occupational therapy services at the technical level of practice.

Professional Level

Master's: Entry-Level and Postprofessional

As of January 2007 the master's degree is the lowest degree level at which one can enter the profession as an occupational therapist. In occupational therapy education, there are entry-level (sometimes referred to as the *first professional degree*) and postprofessional master's-degree programs. Distinguishing between entry-level and postprofessional master's-degree programs is not typical in other professions and disciplines (Rogers, 1980a, 1980b). Entry-level master's-degree programs are the entrance into the profession of occupational therapy and are accredited by ACOTE. Some entry-level programs may require students to earn a baccalaureate degree in a related field before entering the master's-degree program in occupational therapy. Other entry-level programs may require extensive prerequisite coursework but not mandate a baccalaureate degree. For example, the course of study may be a 5-year program leading to a master's degree; or, in other programs, the study comprises two semesters beyond an undergraduate degree in a major such as occupational science. Coursework that may be considered remedial or prerequisite is not generally included in the total credits required for the master's degree. On successful completion of the academic and fieldwork requirements, the graduate is eligible to take the national certification examination, then apply for state licensure and provide occupational therapy services at the professional level.

Postprofessional master's-degree programs are available to individuals who have a professional degree in occupational therapy (e.g., baccalaureate, entry-level master's, entry-level doctorate degree). Such postprofessional degrees are typical of master's-degree programs in other disciplines with a range of 30 to 36 credits. Postprofessional programs are developed to enhance occupational therapy skills in a specific area (e.g., pediatrics, assistive technology, gerontology). Other master's-degree programs may provide a general program with a curricular emphasis (e.g., leadership or research).

Doctorate: Professional and Research

Currently, doctoral-level occupational therapy offerings include the professional (or clinical) and research doctorates. Some programs offer the PhD degree in occupational therapy. Other doctoral-degree programs related to occupational therapy exist, such as the PhD degree in rehabilitation sciences or occupational science or the ScD. Although many of these programs focus on the application of occupational therapy, it is beyond the scope of this document to describe the variations of doctoral programs closely aligned with occupational therapy.

The professional or clinical doctorate degree in occupational therapy confers the degree of *doctor of occupational therapy* (OTD) or *doctor of occupational therapy* (DrOT) degree to graduates. Two pathways exist for pursuing the clinical doctorate degree. The first is available to postprofessional students, that is, students who have an entry-level degree in occupational therapy. The second pathway leading to the clinical doctorate degree is an entry-level program. Entry-level clinical doctorate degree programs are available for individuals who do not have an entry-level degree in occupational therapy but who have completed specified prerequisite coursework and, as of 2010, a baccalaureate degree.

Although the clinical-doctorate-degree programs vary in philosophy and curriculum, typically the postprofessional clinical-doctorate programs are shorter in duration than the entry-level clinical-doctorate programs. The rationale for the difference in program length is that postprofessional clinical-doctorate students have previously completed an entry-level occupational therapy degree.

Several occupational therapy programs offer the PhD degree in occupational therapy. These doctoral programs focus on preparing graduates who are independent researchers and who will develop original knowledge pertinent to occupational therapy.

Accreditation

There are two types of accreditation: institutional (or regional) accreditation and program (or specialized) accreditation (Kaplin & Lee, 1995). Accreditation of occupational therapy programs is completed by ACOTE, which is part of a larger accreditation context (Kramer & Graves, 2005).

Institutional Accreditation

Regional or national accrediting bodies do not accredit programs but rather accredit institutions. "Institutional accreditation applies to the entire institution and all its programs, departments, and schools" (Kaplin & Lee, 1995, p. 873). There are 6 regional agencies that accredit institutions located in distinct

geographical areas. Accreditation standards from regional or national accrediting bodies influence ACOTE in that their standards must be aligned with requirements from the USDE and the Council for Higher Education Accreditation (CHEA; Kramer & Graves, 2005). In postprofessional OT programs, there is no specialized accrediting body. However, institutional accrediting bodies can require a focus visit of a particular program. A focus visit does not result in the accrediting of a specific program.

Program or Specialized Accreditation

Program or specialized accreditation "applies to a particular school, department or program within the institution" and "may also apply to an entire institution if it is a free-standing, specialized institution…whose curriculum is all in the same program area" (Kaplin & Lee, 1995, p. 873). The USDE and the CHEA afford ACOTE "the distinction of being reflected as a national recognized accrediting agency that is seen as a reliable authority about the quality of education offered by the occupational therapy and occupational therapy assistant programs it accredits" (Kramer & Graves, 2005, p. 1). Currently, ACOTE accredits OTA and entry-level or first professional-degree programs in occupational therapy. Such accreditation endeavors are considered specialized, because the accrediting body, ACOTE, reviews occupational therapy and OTA programs to ensure quality and that educational standards are met. The educational standards are developed through ACOTE with input from stakeholders.

Suggested Considerations When Choosing an Occupational Therapy Educational Program

When choosing an occupational therapy educational program, important factors must be considered (see Table 6.1).

A variety of resources can help one to obtain information about specific education programs. Institutional websites can be helpful in acquiring information about the program's curriculum and faculty. Brochures, catalogs, and bulletin

Table 6.1. Considerations for Occupational Therapy Entry-Level and Postprofessional Education

- Location of program
- Tuition
- Length of program
- Availability of student scholarships
- Full- or part-time programs
- On-campus or distance-formatted programs
- Admission requirements
  - Interview
  - Entrance exams (e.g., Miller's Analogy, Graduate Record Exam)
  - Letters of recommendation, essays
  - Prerequisite classes or degree
  - Observation hours in occupational therapy
- Type of program
  - Degree awarded (e.g., AA, MS, MA, MOT, PhD, ScD, OTD)
  - Thesis requirement
  - Dissertation requirement
  - Curriculum (e.g., courses offered, course descriptions printed in catalog)
  - Program mission and philosophical grounding
  - Specialization (e.g., gerontology, pediatrics, entrepreneurialism)
  - Experiential components
    - Fieldwork, internships, rotations, etc.
    - Length of clinical preparation
    - Opportunities for postdegree experiences (e.g., residencies, fellowships)
- Institutional variables
  - Carnegie classification
  - Library resources
  - Information technology or computer support
  - Stability of program
  - Graduate or professional school
  - Ratings and rankings of programs
- Graduate and alumni accomplishments
  - Graduation rate
  - Employment rates, sites
  - Employer satisfaction with graduates
  - Consumer satisfaction with graduate performance
- Faculty
  - Faculty credentials (e.g., doctorally prepared, specialty certified)
  - Faculty-to-student ratios
  - Faculty accessibility
  - Faculty projects (e.g., grants, publications)
  - Faculty clinical practice

In addition, it is important to answer the following questions:
- What are my future career goals?
- Does the degree offered contribute to accomplishing my short-term and long-term goals?
- If considering an online program, do I have the necessary skills to be successful (e.g., motivation, self-initiative, technical skills)?

descriptions often present the program's mission, philosophy, curriculum, or policies. These materials can be requested from the admissions office of each institution. Contacting faculty within the program is frequently useful to answer specific questions. Prospective students may request contact with a current student or alumni to gain a consumer's perspective of the program.

References and Resources

Accreditation Council for Occupational Therapy Education. (1999a, August). *ACOTE Motion* and *Resolution J* [Minutes at the meeting of the Accreditation Council for Occupational Therapy Education]. Bethesda, MD: Author.

Accreditation Council for Occupational Therapy Education. (1999b). Standards for an accredited educational program for the occupational therapy assistant. *American Journal of Occupational Therapy, 53,* 583–589.

American Occupational Therapy Association. (2001). *ACOTE sets timeline for post baccalaureate degree programs.* Retrieved June 19, 2001, from http://www.aota.org/nonmembers/area13/links/LINK16.asp

American Society of Health-System Pharmacists. (2001). *The residency learning system (RLS) model* (2nd ed.). Bethesda, MD: Author.

Carmichael, O. C. (1961). *Graduate education: A critique and a program.* New York: Harper & Brothers.

DiFabio, R. P. (1999). Clinical expertise and the DPT: A need for residency training. *Journal of Orthopaedic and Sports Physical Therapy, 29,* 80–82.

Edens, G. E., & Labadie, G. C. (1987). Opinions about the professional doctorate in nursing. *Nursing Outlook, 35,* 136–140.

Farrell, J. P. (1996). In search of clinical excellence. *Journal of Orthopaedic and Sports Physical Therapy, 24,* 115–121.

Faut-Callahan, M. (1992). Graduate education for nurse anesthetists: Master's versus a clinical doctorate. *Journal of the American Association of Nurse Anesthetists, 60,* 98–103.

Glazer, J. S. (1988). *The master's degree* (Report No. EDO-HE-88-3). Washington, DC: Office of Educational Research and Improvement. (ERIC Document Reproduction Service No. ED301140)

Hummer, L. A., Hunt, K. S., & Figuers, C. C. (1994). Predominant thought regarding entry-level doctor of physical therapy programs. *Journal of Physical Therapy Education, 8,* 60–66.

Kapel, D. E., Gifford, C. S., & Kapel, M. B. (1991). *American educators' encyclopedia* (rev. ed.). Westport, CT: Greenwood.

Kaplin, W. A., & Lee, B. A. (1995). *The law of higher education* (3rd ed.). San Francisco: Jossey-Bass.

Kidd, G. D., Cox, C. C., & Matthies, M. L. (2003). Boston University doctor of science degree program: Clinical doctorate in audiology. *American Journal of Audiology, 12,* 3–6.

Knowles, A. S. (1977). Postdoctoral education. In *The international encyclopedia of higher education* (Vol. 5, pp. 1923–1928). San Francisco: Jossey-Bass.

Kramer, P., & Graves, S. (2005, March). Accreditation 101: Understanding the broad world of accreditation. *Education Special Interest Section Quarterly, 15,* 1–2.

LaPidus, J. B. (2000). Postbaccalaureate and graduate education: A dynamic balance. In K. Kohl & J. LaPidus (Eds.) *Postbaccalaureate futures* (pp. 3–9). Phoenix, AZ: Oryx.

Mayhew, L. B., & Ford, P. J. (1971). *Changing the curriculum.* San Francisco: Jossey-Bass.

Mayhew, L. B., & Ford, P. J. (1974). *Reform in graduate and professional education.* San Francisco: Jossey-Bass.

Medeiros, J. M. (1998). Post professional clinical residency programs. *Journal of Manual and Manipulative Therapy, 6,* 10.

Medeiros, J. M. (2000). Educational standards for residency education. *Journal of Manual and Manipulative Therapy, 8,* 50.

Miller, S., & Clarke, A. (2002). Impact of postdoctoral specialty residencies in drug information on graduates' career paths. *American Journal of Health-System Pharmacy, 59,* 961–963.

Pierce, D., & Peyton, C. (1999). A historical cross-disciplinary perspective on the professional doctorate in occupational therapy. *American Journal of Occupational Therapy, 53,* 64–71.

Rogers, J. C. (1980a). Design of the master's degree in occupational therapy, part 1. A logical approach. *American Journal of Occupational Therapy, 34,* 113–118.

Rogers, J. C. (1980b). Design of the master 's degree in occupational therapy, part 2. An empirical approach. *American Journal of Occupational Therapy, 34,* 176–184.

Shafritz, J. M., Koeppe, R. P., & Soper, E. W. (1988). *American educators' encyclopedia.* Westport, CT: Greenwood Press.

Unger, H. G. (1996). *Encyclopedia of American education.* New York: Facts on File.

U.S. Department of Education. (2002). *Classification of instructional programs: 2000 edition.* Washington, DC: Office of Educational Research and Improvement.

Watson, J. (1988). *The professional doctorate as an entry level into practice. Perspectives in nursing—1987–1989.* New York: National League for Nursing.

Authors
Brenda M. Coppard, PhD, OTR/L
*Creighton University, Omaha, NE
Member, AOTA Commission on Education,
2002–2007*
Anne Dickerson, PhD, OTR/L, FAOTA
*East Carolina University, Greenville, NC
Member, AOTA Commission on Education,
2000–2006*

for

The Commission on Education
Linda Fazio, PhD, OTR/L, FAOTA, *Chairperson*
Brenda M. Coppard, PhD, OTR/L, *Postprofessional Academic Educator*
Donna Costa, MS, OTR/L, *Academic Fieldwork Educator*
Linda Musselman, PhD, OTR, FAOTA, *Professional Program Director*
David Haynes, MBA, OTR/L, *OTA Program Director*
Kelly Fischer, OTR/L, *Fieldwork Educator*
Terrianne Jones, MA, OTR/L, *OTA Academic Educator*
Marc Freedman, *ASD Liaison*
Shirley Marino, COTA, AP, *OTA Educator*
Jaime Muñoz, PhD, OTR/L, FAOTA, *Professional Academic Educator*
René Padilla, PhD, OTR/L, FAOTA, *Chair-Elect*
Jyothi Gupta, PhD, OTR/L, *EDSIS Liaison*

Adopted by the Representative Assembly 2007C11

Chapter 7.

EVIDENCE-BASED PRACTICE AND HOW IT RELATES TO FIELDWORK

Donna Costa, DHS, OTR/L, FAOTA

Evidence-based practice has become an integral part of practice and education in occupational therapy. Students at both the occupational therapist and occupational therapy assistant levels are learning about research in their respective curricula and are expected to become effective consumers of research. Current Accreditation Council for Occupational Therapy Education (ACOTE®) standards for doctoral, master's, and associate's degrees specify that students must be able to locate evidence found in journals and other sources to make evidence-based practice decisions (ACOTE, 2012).

Sometimes fieldwork educators express concern about taking a student from a higher educational level than their own. As a fieldwork educator, you may work with students who have had more research-related classroom education than you, which should not be a concern. This chapter discusses basic information about evidence-based practice and how to integrate evidence-based practice into the fieldwork site.

What Is Evidence-Based Practice?

David Sackett, a British physician, has written extensively about evidence-based practice and provides the following definition: "The conscientious, explicit, and judicious use of the current best evidence in making decisions about the care of individual patients. The practice of evidence-based medicine means integrating individual clinical expertise with the best available external clinical evidence from systematic research" (Sackett, Rosenberg, Gray, Haynes, & Richardson, 1996, pp. 71–72).

Two competencies that reference the use of evidence in fieldwork are listed under "Education Competencies" in the Self-Assessment Tool for Fieldwork Educator Competency (American Occupational Therapy Association [AOTA], 2009; Chapter 27). The first is Number 13: "Provides reference materials to promote student and fieldwork educator professional development and use of evidence-based practice (e.g., publications, texts, videos, Internet)." Students are accustomed to producing assignments in the classroom in which they have to find articles that support the assessment or intervention they are proposing. As a fieldwork educator, you can encourage them to continue to do the same. The fieldwork site may have a medical library where students can search the literature for evidence-based practice resources. In addition, you might form a journal club and keep copies of all the articles read in a binder or electronic file.

The second competency is Number 14: "Uses evidence-based research to guide student performance and learning for effective teaching strategies" (AOTA, 2009). This competency focuses on the fieldwork educator using evidence about fieldwork education. What approaches or models of supervision work best with which students? What are the most important characteristics that students value in fieldwork educators? What contributes to a quality fieldwork placement? This is an emerging area of research within education, and more studies are needed to grow a body of evidence for fieldwork education. Readers are referred to a recently published article (Roberts, Hooper, Wood, & King, 2015) for an excellent review of the research done thus far in fieldwork education and what still needs to be done.

Three items that address the use of evidence-based practice in fieldwork are in the AOTA (2002a, 2002b) Fieldwork Performance Evaluation for the Occupational Therapy and Occupational Therapy Assistant Student forms (Chapters 58 and 59). The first is Number 16 on the occupational therapist form: "Establishes an accurate and appropriate plan based on the evaluation results, through integrating multiple factors such as client's priorities, context(s), theories, and evidence-based practice" (AOTA, 2002b). The second is Number 19 on the occupational therapist form: "Uses evidence from published research and relevant resources to make informed intervention decisions" (AOTA, 2002b). The third is Number 6 from the occupational therapy assistant form: "Makes informed practice decisions based on published research and relevant informational resources" (AOTA, 2002a).

Levels of Evidence

Research articles are categorized into levels of evidence according to the type of research design. Multiple levels of evidence are used in clinical decision making, and higher levels of evidence typically mean stronger evidence for decision making. As a fieldwork educator, it is important to understand the different, hierarchical levels of evidence and be able to help your students analyze and apply evidence appropriately. Table 7.1 lists the most widely used categorization of levels of evidence within occupational therapy.

Table 7.1. Levels of Evidence

Level	Type of Study
I	Randomized controlled trial, meta-analysis, and systematic review
II	Two groups, nonrandomized study (e.g., cohort, case-control)
III	One group, nonrandomized study (e.g., before and after, pretest–posttest design)
IV	Descriptive study that includes analysis of outcomes (e.g., nonexperimental studies, observational studies, single-subject design)
V	Case report and expert opinion that include narrative literature reviews and consensus statements (e.g., descriptive case studies, surveys, qualitative studies)

Note. Adapted from "Using AOTA's Critically Appraised Topic (CAT) and Critically Appraised Paper (CAP) Series to Link Evidence to Practice," by M. Arbesman, J. Scheer, and D. Lieberman, 2008, *OT Practice, 13*(5), p. 19. Copyright © 2008 by the American Occupational Therapy Association. Used with permission.

Level I: Randomized Controlled Trial

Randomized controlled trials (RCTs) include two groups of participants. One group (control) does not get the treatment being studied, and the other group (experimental) receives the treatment being studied. Participants are randomly assigned to one of the groups. One of the disadvantages to this type of study is that the researchers may believe it is unethical to withhold treatment from a group of people. This type of research is also expensive to conduct because of the number of participants, recruitment efforts, and data analysis.

Clark et al. (1997) conducted one of the most well-known studies within occupational therapy in this category. It was conducted in Los Angeles over a 3-year period from 1994 to 1997. The sample included 361 participants from diverse backgrounds and were men and women 60 years and older who resided in or frequented federally subsidized apartments for independent seniors. The participants were randomly assigned to one of three groups for a 9-month period. One experimental group of 122 participants received preventive occupational therapy, the second experimental group of 120 participants engaged in a nonprofessionally led social activities program, and the third group of 119 participants served as the control group with no treatment provided.

The occupational therapy experimental group received 2 hours a week of group treatment and 1 hour per month of individual occupational therapy, with an emphasis on preventing health risks of older adulthood and on lifestyle redesign. Participants were encouraged to creatively use occupation in a personalized way to adapt to challenges of aging. The nonprofessionally led social activities group participated in diversional activities: viewing films, playing games, and going on outings. The outcome at the end of the 9 months was that the experimental group that received occupational therapy had greater gains in physical health, fewer declines in overall functioning, increased vitality, and improved life satisfaction compared with the nonprofessionally led group and the control group, which had similar outcomes.

Level I: Meta-Analysis

Meta-analysis is a type of study that combines several RCTs, comparing the statistical evidence across studies. This design allows for a synthesis of various findings in an objective manner. The disadvantage is that if the individual studies have design flaws, then the quality of a meta-analysis is diminished. Also, there may not be enough published studies to review in a particular area.

An example of a meta-analysis in occupational therapy is an article by Maitra et al. (2014) in which 40 different articles were reviewed. The results showed that low-birthweight children exhibit difficulty in mental, neuromusculoskeletal, and movement-related tasks compared with children born at normal birthweight. Combining numerous studies increased the sample size, allowing the researchers to conclude that "deficits in mental and motor functions in children born low birthweight or preterm have significant effects on school readiness and academic achievement" (p. 140).

Level I: Systematic Review

Systematic reviews are similar to meta-analyses because several studies are reviewed and synthesized. However, the statistical outcome measures are not analyzed.

An example of this kind of study in occupational therapy is Golisz (2014), which reviewed 29 articles related to driving interventions for older adults. The results yielded a low to moderate effect for interventions used by occupational therapy practitioners to improve the driving performance of older adults, and the researcher recommended more research in this area.

Level II: Two Groups, Nonrandomized

Level II studies include two nonrandomized groups of participants. The researcher may be studying two different interventions and provide one intervention to one group of participants and another intervention to the other group. In addition, the researcher may test the intervention more than once in the two groups of participants. Usually, participants in both groups have the same diagnosis or condition.

An example of this kind of study is Legoff and Sherman (2006), in which one group of children with autism was observed playing with LEGO® and another group of children with autism was observed playing with other materials over a 3-year period. The results showed that the LEGO therapy group had a higher level of social interaction with their peers than the non–LEGO group. The main limitation of this type of research study is that it does not have a control group.

Level III: One Group, Nonrandomized

Level III studies include one nonrandomized group of participants. The researcher objectively measures the participants' condition before the study starts to establish baseline performance. These measures are compared with outcome measures taken at the end of the intervention. The disadvantage of this category of research is that because it involves only one group and no randomization, the researcher cannot be sure what caused the change, if any, in the participants' condition.

An example of a Level III study is one I am conducting on the effectiveness of mindfulness-based chronic pain management (MBCPM). Because of the small sample size of recruited participants, the study does not have a control group. Participants with a variety of chronic pain conditions are assessed before the start of the intervention using several well-known outcome measures. These assessments are repeated again at the end of the intervention and at a 3-month follow-up. Although the results have been encouraging, the lack of a control group precludes me from saying that the participants' improvements are due to MBCPM.

Level IV: Descriptive Study

In this type of research, a single-subject design involves one or a small number of participants followed over time or evaluated on the basis of interest; each participant acts as his or her own control using baseline information. The participants can come from more than one facility. The disadvantage of this type of study is similar to the Level II studies: It is difficult to conclude that the treatment alone is responsible for change over time.

An example of this type of study is Wilkes-Gillan, Bundy, Cordier, and Lincoln (2014), in which five children with attention deficit hyperactivity disorder participated in a parent-led home intervention addressing social behaviors during play. Outcome measures were administered before the 7-week intervention, immediately after the intervention, and at 1-month follow-up. The results demonstrated that children's social play outcomes greatly improved from pretest to 1-month follow-up.

Level V: Case Report and Expert Opinion

Studies in the category are generally narrative articles containing the opinions of respected authorities on the basis of clinical evidence. This level of evidence also includes descriptive studies, surveys or reports of expert committees, and qualitative studies. A disadvantage of these studies is that bias may be possible as a result of returned surveys or patients behaving a certain way because they have knowledge of being studied. Bias also may be present because the evidence presented is based only on what the researcher has been exposed to rather than all evidence. An example of Level V research is a 2007 article by Turner et al. in which the authors interviewed 54 people with first-episode psychosis to examine their purpose in life.

Introducing Evidence-Based Assignments Into Fieldwork

Fieldwork educators can introduce several assignments to increase students' focus on evidence-based practice. Students can perform literature searches to find evidence relevant to the fieldwork setting and present it as part of the treatment-planning process. A popular assignment is to have students conduct in-service presentations to staff, which provides them with an opportunity to share search strategies with clinicians or give general updates on the importance of using and analyzing evidence. Students can also implement a journal club at the fieldwork site (see http://www.aota.org/practice/researchers/journal-club-toolkit.aspx for the AOTA Journal Club Toolkit).

References

Accreditation Council for Occupational Therapy Education. (2012). *2011 Accreditation Council for Occupational Therapy Education (ACOTE®) standards and interpretive guide*. Retrieved from http://www.aota.org/-/media/Corporate/Files/EducationCareers/Accredit/Standards/2011-Standards-and-Interpretive-Guide-August-2013.pdf

American Occupational Therapy Association (2002a). *Fieldwork performance evaluation for the occupational therapy assistant student*. Bethesda, MD: AOTA Press.

American Occupational Therapy Association. (2002b). *Fieldwork performance evaluation for the occupational therapy student*. Bethesda, MD: AOTA Press.

American Occupational Therapy Association. (2009). *Self-Assessment Tool for Fieldwork Educator Competency*. Bethesda, MD: AOTA Press. Available at http://www.aota.org/-/media/Corporate/Files/Education/Careers/Accredit/FEATCHART Midterm.pdf

Arbesman, M., Scheer, J., & Lieberman, D. (2008). Using AOTA's Critically Appraised Topic (CAT) and Critically Appraised Paper (CAP) Series to link evidence to practice. *OT Practice, 13*(5), 18–22.

Clark, F., Azen, S., Zemke, R., Jackson, J., Carlson, M., Mandel, . . . Lipson, L. (1997). Occupational therapy for independent-living older adults: A randomized controlled trial. *Journal of the American Medical Association, 278,* 1321–1326.

Golisz, K. (2014). Occupational therapy interventions to improve driving performance in older adults: A systematic review. *American Journal of Occupational Therapy, 68,* 662–669. http://dx.doi.org/10.5014/ajot.2014.011247

Legoff, D., & Sherman, M. (2006). Long-term outcome of social skills interaction based on interactive LEGO play. *Autism, 1,* 317–329.

Maitra, K., Park, H. Y., Eggenberger, J., Matthiessen, A., Knight, E., & Ng, B. (2014). Difficulty in mental, neuromusculoskeletal, and movement-related school functions associated with low birthweight or preterm birth: A meta-analysis. *American Journal of Occupational Therapy, 68,* 140–148. http://dx.doi.org/10.5014/ajot.2014.009985

Roberts, M., Hooper, B., Wood, W., & King, R. (2015). An international systematic mapping review of fieldwork education in occupational therapy. *Canadian Journal of Occupational Therapy, 82,* 106–118.

Sackett, D., Rosenberg, W., Gray, J., Haynes, R. B., & Richardson, W. S. (1996). Evidence-based medicine: What it is and what it isn't. *British Medical Journal, 312,* 71–72.

Turner, N., Jackson, D., Renwick, L., Sutton, M., Foley, S., McWilliams, S., . . . O'Callaghan, E. (2007). What influences purpose in life in first-episode psychosis? *British Journal of Occupational Therapy, 70,* 401–406.

Wilkes-Gillan, S., Bundy, A., Cordier, R., & Lincoln, M. (2014). Evaluation of a pilot parent-delivered play-based intervention for children with attention deficit hyperactivity disorder. *American Journal of Occupational Therapy, 68,* 700–709. http://dx.doi.org/10.5014/ajot.2014.012450

Part 2.

LEVEL I FIELDWORK

OVERVIEW OF PART 2

Donna Costa, DHS, OTR/L, FAOTA

Part 2 focuses on Level I fieldwork education, which differs widely across occupational therapy educational programs in its length, placement in the curriculum, focus, and evaluation of student performance. The purpose of Level I fieldwork is to introduce students to fieldwork, provide them with an opportunity to work with clients, and help them understand some of the processes they have been learning in the classroom.

It is the purview of each academic program to design Level I fieldwork to be consistent with its curriculum and to develop the sequence of Level I rotations, rotation length, assignments, and the mechanisms used to evaluate students. Chapter 8 contains the "Level I Fieldwork Guidelines," which describe the focus and intent of the fieldwork experience. Chapter 9, "Sample Level I Fieldwork Assignments," contains a few sample Level I fieldwork assignments used in occupational therapy programs. In addition, because no nationally prescribed evaluation format exists for the Level I fieldwork experience, the reader may find the sample Level I fieldwork evaluation forms in Chapter 10, "Sample Level I Fieldwork Evaluation Forms," helpful.

Chapter 8.

LEVEL I FIELDWORK GUIDELINES

American Occupational Therapy Association

I. Definition and Purpose

The American Occupational Therapy Association (AOTA) *Standards of Practice for Occupational Therapy* (AOTA, 2005) describe the goal of Level I Fieldwork as "to introduce students to the fieldwork experience, and develop a basic comfort level with an understanding of the needs of clients." Level I Fieldwork is not intended to develop independent performance, but to "include experiences designed to enrich didactic coursework through directed observation and participation in selected aspects of the occupational therapy process."

Services may be provided to a variety of populations through a variety of settings. Experiences may include those directly related to occupational therapy, as well as other situations to enhance an understanding of the developmental stages, tasks, and roles of individuals throughout the life span. Day care centers, schools, neighborhood centers, hospice, homeless shelters, community mental health centers, and therapeutic activity or work centers are among the many possible sites. Level I Fieldwork may also include services management and administrative experiences in occupational therapy settings, community agencies, or environmental analysis experiences. Populations may include

disabled or well populations and age-specific or diagnosis-specific clients.

Qualified personnel for supervision of Level I Fieldwork may include, but are not limited to, academic or fieldwork educators, occupational therapy practitioners initially certified nationally, psychologists, physician assistants, teachers, social workers, nurses, physical therapists, and social workers, among others. The supervisors must be knowledgeable about occupational therapy and cognizant of the goals and objectives of the Level I Fieldwork experience.

II. Objectives

Objectives of Level I Fieldwork may vary significantly from one academic institution to another. These variations occur as a result of differences in individual academic institutional missions, programmatic philosophical base, curriculum design and resources, and so forth. As a result, the individual academic institutions should provide information regarding the specific didactic relationship and should provide objectives for the experience. Fieldwork educators should determine if the resources of their facilities are adequate to meet the objectives of the educational institution, and then apply the objectives to the fieldwork setting.

Fieldwork objectives should reflect role delineation between professional and technical level students as specified by "The Guide to OT Practice" (Moyers, 1999). In the event that a facility provides Level I Fieldwork experiences to both levels of students, separate objectives and learning experiences should be used, as developed by the academic program faculty. Students should be evaluated using these objectives.

In instances where students will have a prolonged or consecutive fieldwork experience in the same facility, the objectives should also reflect a sequential orientation and move from concrete to conceptual or from simple to more complex learning activities. In the event that the student will rotate through a variety of settings, it is recommended that a master list of objectives be developed that demonstrates a developmental learning continuum and indicates which objectives and learning experiences have been provided in previous experiences.

Schedule design of Level I Fieldwork will depend on the type of setting and the curriculum of the academic institution. Options include, but are not limited to, full days for one-half a term, full days in alternating weeks for one term, half days for one term, or 1 week.

Academic Institution

- Identify course content areas to be enhanced by Level I Fieldwork experiences.
- Develop general goals that clearly reflect the purpose of the experience and level of performance to be achieved.
- Ensure that objectives reflect the appropriate role of an occupational therapy (OT) or occupational therapy assistant (OTA) student.
- Sequence the objectives from concrete to conceptual or from simple to increasing complexity.
- Identify facilities that may be able to provide the necessary learning experiences.
- Share the objectives with the fieldwork educators and ask them to identify those objectives that could be met in their facility.
- Discuss and coordinate fieldwork administration issues, such as scheduling, work load, report deadlines, and so forth.

- Collaborate with fieldwork educators to clearly identify the skill levels necessary for successful completion of Level I Fieldwork experience.
- Develop an evaluation form and protocol.

Fieldwork Education Center

- Evaluate administrative aspects of the program to determine the feasibility of providing education experiences of high quality while maintaining the effectiveness of services.
- Consider providing the necessary supervision, scheduling learning experiences, and discussing staff attitudes toward fieldwork.
- Review objectives and learning experiences with academic representatives to assure that they address the Level I Fieldwork objectives of the program.
- Review the evaluation form and associated protocols and seek any necessary clarification prior to its implementation.
- Review the Level I Fieldwork objectives and the evaluation form to determine if the learning experiences can be provided at your fieldwork agency and if they are compatible with the philosophy of the program.
- Collaborate with the academic program faculty to identify and design, if possible, specific learning activities that will meet Level I objectives.
- Ensure that agencies providing fieldwork for both the professional and technical level student have different learning experiences designed to clearly reflect role delineation.

References

American Occupational Therapy Association. (2005). Standards of practice for occupational therapy. *American Journal of Occupational Therapy, 59,* 663–665. http://dx.doi.org/10.5014/ajot.59.6.663

Moyers, P. A. (1999). The guide to occupational therapy practice. *American Journal of Occupational Therapy, 53*(3), 247–322. http://dx.doi.org/10.5014/ajot.53.3.247

AOTA Commission on Education (COE) and Fieldwork Issues Committee (FWIC)

Amended and Approved by FWIC 11/99 and COE 12/99

Reprinted from http://www.aota.org/Education-Careers/Fieldwork/LevelI.aspx

Chapter 9.

SAMPLE LEVEL I FIELDWORK ASSIGNMENTS

Donna Costa, DHS, OTR/L, FAOTA; University of Utah Division of Occupational Therapy

Level I fieldwork for occupational therapy and occupational therapy assistant students is designed to be an introduction to a particular practice setting. The length of the placement and the learning objectives vary widely across educational institutions. It is generally up to the academic program to develop the learning objectives and create the learning activities for the placement. The following are some of the more typically used assignments:

- *Evaluation and assessment.* Depending on the academic institution and the clinical site, students may be expected to administer an evaluation or assessment or a portion of an evaluation or assessment that they learned in the classroom. As an alternative, they may be able to participate in the screening or assessment that is routinely done at the fieldwork site.
- *Occupational profile.* This assignment is frequently used in a Level I placement. The student interviews a patient or client to complete an occupational profile by following the format listed in the *Occupational Therapy Practice Framework: Domain and Process* (3rd ed., American Occupational Therapy Association, 2014).
- *Progress notes.* Students may be asked to write a progress note using a Subjective, Objective, Assessment, and Plan (SOAP) format if they learned

that in school, or a more narrative note. If students are participating in a group treatment session, they may be asked to write a group progress note.

- *Intervention plans.* Students are often asked to write up a sample treatment plan for a particular patient or client they have seen. The format they use may be different than or the same as the format your fieldwork site uses.
- *Journal entries.* Some academic institutions and fieldwork sites require students to write daily or weekly journal entries. The aim of this assignment is to promote reflective practice, so they should not be superficial in content.

This chapter includes sample instructions for a Level I fieldwork project and an activity scorecard from the University of Utah. Chapter 10 includes sample feedback and evaluation forms for Level I fieldwork from the University of Southern California and Colorado State University.

Reference

American Occupational Therapy Association. (2014). Occupational therapy practice framework: Domain and process (3rd ed.). *American Journal of Occupational Therapy, 68*(Suppl. 1). http://dx.doi.org/10.5014/ajot.2014.682006

University of Utah

Division of Occupational Therapy

Project or Presentation for Fieldwork

You will complete a project or presentation that benefits the clients or professionals of your fieldwork site. Some examples are a literature review on a pertinent topic, development of a group activity that includes directions and resources necessary to carry it out after you leave, and fabrication of a needed piece of equipment to increase occupation-based practice. It should be something tangible you can leave behind. Discuss your idea with your fieldwork supervisor and review your idea with your fieldwork coordinator to make sure you are on the right track before you complete it. The project will probably take between 2 and 4 hours to complete.

After your project is completed, submit a one-page summary that includes the following headings.

- Your name and name of the fieldwork placement.
- Description of the clients served and the work that is carried out there, in your own words. (2 points)
- Explanation about how your project supports the work of the agency. (3 points)
- A thorough description and picture or copy of the project itself. Be sure to give enough information so it can be graded. (10 points)
- Comments from your fieldwork supervisor. Ask him or her to write a sentence or two on the bottom of your one-page summary about the project and comment on its quality, usefulness, or creativity. (2 points)
- Explanation of what went well and what could be done better next time? (3 points)

Submitted by Jeanette Koski, OTD, OTR/L, Academic Fieldwork Coordinator, University of Utah, Division of Occupational Therapy. Used with permission.

University of Utah

Division of Occupational Therapy

Level I Fieldwork Activity Score Card

Observation Activities—With the therapist's and client's permission

_____ Watch a treatment from start to finish and discuss with the therapist how it relates to the client's goals.

_____ Watch an intervention by another professional and discuss how it relates to the client's overall treatment program.

_____ Observe an evaluation and discuss how it will shape the client's future participation.

_____ Review a client's record.

Equipment Activities—With the therapist's permission

_____ Investigate what resources are available for treatment activities in the various storage areas of your placement.

_____ Read through some of the handouts and client education materials available and choose one to summarize to your supervisor.

_____ Practice using one piece of equipment on yourself or another staff member.

What was the piece of equipment? _____

Feedback:

_____ Request feedback from a therapist on your therapeutic use of self.

Handling Activities—With the therapist's permission and immediate supervision

_____ Feel how a limb with high tone moves.

_____ Feel how a limb with low tone moves.

_____ Assist in or perform a transfer.

_____ Assist in or perform bed mobility.

_____ Use a piece of equipment with a patient, such as a dynamometer, goniometer, or an evaluation tool.

What was the piece of equipment? _____

_____ Perform passive range of motion on a client.

Treatment Activities—With the therapist's permission and immediate supervision

_____ Devise one activity to be used in a treatment session and do that activity with the client.

Briefly describe the activity: _____

_____ Instruct a client in one activity as part of his or her home program.

_____ After an intervention by the therapist, discuss with the therapist how the same activity could have been graded up or down if the client's performance had been different.

_____ Other: _____

Have the therapist initial each activity completed.

_____

Activity submitted by Jeanette Koski, OTD, OTR/L, Academic Fieldwork Coordinator at the University of Utah, Division of Occupational Therapy. Used with permission.

Chapter 10.

SAMPLE LEVEL I FIELDWORK EVALUATION FORMS

Compiled by Donna Costa, DHS, OTR/L, FAOTA; Colorado State University; University of Southern California, Mrs. T.H. Chan Division of Occupational Science and Occupational Therapy

To be completed by FIELDWORK EDUCATOR

USC Division of Occupational Science
and Occupational Therapy

LEVEL I FIELDWORK PROFESSIONAL DEVELOPMENT FEEDBACK FORM

STUDENT (Please print): _____

RATER (Please print with credentials): _____

Name of Facility: _____ Practice Setting: _____

The purpose of this form is to provide the student with feedback regarding his or her performance in professional behavior development.

Unsatisfactory:	The student does not demonstrate the required level of professional skill (U)
Needs Improvement:	The student has a beginning level of professional skill, but needs improvement in either quality or quantity (S-)
Satisfactory:	The student demonstrates the appropriate level of professionalism (S)
Exceeds Expectations:	The student demonstrates refinement of additional qualities beyond that required by the curriculum (S+)

* Please circle rating (U, S-, S, S+)

	U	S-	S	S+
Time Management Skills & Organization Prompt, arrives on time; completes assignments and documentation on time; manages time and materials to meet program requirements; flexible in coping with change in routine; sets priorities; follows through with responsibilities.	◯	◯	◯	◯
Comments:				

	U	S-	S	S+
Engagement in the Fieldwork Experience Demonstrates active participation, positive attitude, and motivation to learn; invested in individuals and treatment outcomes; able to anticipate potential challenges and act proactively to address it.	◯	◯	◯	◯
Comments:				

	U	S-	S	S+
Professionalism Assumes professional role with confidence; manages personal and professional boundaries, responsibilities, and frustrations; respects confidentiality; takes responsibility for personal choices; dresses appropriately for context.	◯	◯	◯	◯
Comments:				

	U	S-	S	S+
Initiation & Self-Directed Learning Independently seeks and acquires information from a variety of sources; asks relevant questions; takes responsibility for own behavior and learning.	◯	◯	◯	◯
Comments:				

	U	S-	S	S+
Cultural Sensitivity Demonstrates sensitivity to diverse views and opinions; open to individual and cultural differences; respects dignity, values, and beliefs of each individual.	◯	◯	◯	◯
Comments:				

	U	S-	S	S+
Interpersonal Communication Interacts cooperatively and effectively with clients, families, and professionals; establishes rapport; responsive to social cues, including body language and nonverbal communication; handles conflict constructively; demonstrates empathy and support of others.	◯	◯	◯	◯
Comments:				

Professional Reasoning/Problem Solving Uses self-reflection; analyzes, synthesizes, and interprets information; understands the occupational therapy process; uses appropriate judgment and safety awareness.	U ◯	S- ◯	S ◯	S+ ◯
Comments:				

Participation in the Supervisory Process Seeks and provides feedback using it to modify actions and behavior; seeks guidance when necessary; follows proper channels for line of authority.	U ◯	S- ◯	S ◯	S+ ◯
Comments:				

Written Communication Attention to grammar, spelling, and legibility in written assignments and documentation; applies professional terminology (such as the *Occupational Therapy Practice Framework*, acronyms, abbreviations, etc.) in written and oral communication.	U ◯	S- ◯	S ◯	S+ ◯
Comments:				

Additional comments:

Student comments:

Prepared by:

Signature: _____ Date: _____

Title of rater: _____

Reviewed with:

Student signature: _____ Date: _____

PLEASE HAVE THE STUDENT RETURN THE COMPLETED FORM TO HIS/HER COURSE INSTRUCTOR.

**Adapted from Philadelphia Region Fieldwork Consortium & Colorado State University Occupational Therapy. Reprinted with permission.

USC Division of Occupational Science
and Occupational Therapy

LEVEL I FIELDWORK

Student Evaluation of Level I Fieldwork Experience

Student Name (Please print): _____

Facility Name: _____

Type of Fieldwork (practice area/specialty): _____

Name of FW Educator(s) with <u>credentials</u>: _____

Age Range of Population: _____

Fieldwork Educator/Student ratio: _____
(e.g., 1 FW Educator to 2 students)

Rate each item below:	Very Poor	Poor	Fair	Good	Excellent
Overall Level I fieldwork experience (choose one):	◯1	◯2	◯3	◯4	◯5
Environment supported my learning (choose rating):	◯1	◯2	◯3	◯4	◯5
Supervision/staff met your needs as a Level I student: (choose one and comment below)	◯1	◯2	◯3	◯4	◯5

Describe your experience in terms of:

Directed Observation:

Hands-on Participation:

(Continued)

Describe assessments and interventions in which you observed and/or participated:

Educational experiences and resources I found helpful:

Changes I recommend to this site to enhance the learning experience for Level I fieldwork:

Any additional comments:

Evaluation completed by:

(PRINT NAME of Student): _____

Student Signature and Date: _____

PLEASE RETURN COMPLETED FORM TO COURSE INSTRUCTOR.

Reprinted with permission of the University of Southern California, Mrs. T.H. Chan Division of Occupational Science & Occupational Therapy.

COLORADO STATE UNIVERSITY OCCUPATIONAL THERAPY DEPARTMENT
LEVEL IA FIELDWORK EVALUATION OF STUDENT

STUDENT: _____

_____ FIELDWORK DATES: _____ to _____

FIELDWORK EDUCATOR: _____ TOTAL CONTACT HOURS COMPLETED: _____

FACILITY: _____ PRACTICE AREA: _____

CLIENT AGE RANGE: _____ EVALUATION COMPLETED BY FIELDWORK EDUCATOR _____

STUDENT _____

Indicate the student's level of performance using the following scale:

3 = Meets Standards: Student carries out required tasks and activities as expected. This rating
                                 represents good, solid performance expected from a Level I fieldwork
                                 student, ready to progress to additional Level I fieldwork in a practice
                                 setting with adults and older adults.

2 = Needs Improvement: Student performance is progressing but still needs improvement.

1 = Unsatisfactory: Student performance is inadequate and requires more experience before
                                 progressing to additional Level I fieldwork. This rating is given when there
                                 is a concern about performance.

LEVEL IA FIELDWORK STUDENT EVALUATION

1. Acceptance of Responsibility. The student . . .			
1a. Upholds the OT Code of Ethics and policies and procedures of fieldwork site.	1	2	3
1b. Evaluates his or her professional behavior as needed, modifying behavior based on self-evaluation and feedback from others.	1	2	3
1c. Seeks and uses a variety of resources to solve problems related to fieldwork performance and professional behavior.	1	2	3
1d. Accepts consequences of his or her actions or lack of action.	1	2	3
Specific observations:			

2. Commitment to Learning. The student . . .			
2a. Comes to fieldwork experiences fully prepared.	1	2	3
2b. Identifies own learning needs, then initiates action, including the pursuit and use of resources as needed.	1	2	3
2c. Persists in learning and mastering challenging concepts and skills.	1	2	3
2d. Applies full attention to available learning opportunities, without distracting behaviors or inappropriate multitasking (e.g., emailing or texting during fieldwork; holding "side bar" conversations with other individuals during sessions; engaging in personal cell phone use during fieldwork).	1	2	3
2e. Independently initiates and completes any missed work or activities in a timely manner or as negotiated with the fieldwork educator.	1	2	3
Specific observations:			

3. Communication Style: Written, Verbal, and Nonverbal. The student . . .			
3a. Communicates verbally, in writing, and through actions with respect for alternative viewpoints and individual differences.	1	2	3
3b. Uses professional terminology: able to apply professional terminology, such as *Occupational Therapy Practice Framework* terminology, acronyms, and abbreviations, in written and oral communication.	1	2	3
3c. Demonstrates awareness of own and others' nonverbal communication (affect, body language, voice) and can modify as needed to improve communication and understanding.	1	2	3
3d. Listens attentively in order to accurately understand others' viewpoints and perspectives.	1	2	3
3e. Respects email etiquette by (a) personally addressing emails; (b) keeping emails concise and to the point, (c) not overusing "reply all," (d) avoiding profanity or offensive language, and (d) using email to convey information rather than strong emotions.	1	2	3
3f. Speaks only for him- or herself, using "I" language.	1	2	3
3g. Uses eye contact during communication with others.	1	2	3
Specific observations:			

4. Interaction With Others. The student . . .			
4a. Addresses interpersonal conflicts and frustrations directly (face to face) with the involved person or persons in a respectful and constructive manner.	1	2	3
4b. Is a reliable team member who meets deadlines and contributes actively and substantively to team activities and projects.	1	2	3
4c. Considers the impact of his or her words and actions on others and modifies words or actions as needed.	1	2	3
4d. Demonstrates concern and takes action to support the physical or emotional safety and well-being of clients and others.	1	2	3
4e. Maintains confidentiality whenever appropriate.	1	2	3
Specific observations:			

5. Participation in the Supervisory Process. The student . . .			
5a. Respectfully and tactfully gives, receives, and responds to feedback from fieldwork educator and team members.	1	2	3
5b. Proactively seeks assistance or guidance when necessary.	1	2	3
5c. Follows proper authority channels to communicate or address concerns.	1	2	3
5d. Seeks support or training when needed.	1	2	3
5e. Respectfully advocates for self and others as needed.	1	2	3
5f. Collaborates with fieldwork educator to maximize learning (asks appropriate questions, asks for clarification, asks for particular learning experiences as appropriate, uses fieldwork educator and others as learning resources, and also explores resources independently).	1	2	3
Specific observations:			

6. Time Management and Organization. The student . . .			
6a. Attends—and is on time for—fieldwork, appointments, and meetings.	1	2	3
6b. Communicates unexpected emergencies or schedule conflicts with involved others in a timely and direct fashion.	1	2	3
6c. Manages personal, family, and job-related demands so that obligations to fieldwork are consistently met.	1	2	3
6d. Follows through with responsibilities and commitments.	1	2	3
6e. Manages multiple time and task demands.	1	2	3
6f. Meets deadlines for all assigned fieldwork, assignments, and activities.	1	2	3

Specific observations:

7. Assumes the student therapist role. The student . . .			
7a. Actively engages with clients and staff within the therapeutic context (i.e., interview client/caregiver/staff, fetch equipment, assist FW educator with therapeutic activities, organize equipment in preparation for interventions, focused attention to therapeutic activity, practice documentation, client chart review).	1	2	3
7b. Initiates engagement to appropriately support the fieldwork educator during the therapeutic process.	1	2	3
7c. Assumes the role as student therapist with confidence.	1	2	3
7d. Handles personal/professional frustrations appropriately.	1	2	3
7e. Discusses and shares hypotheses about the impact of client's *physical factors* on occupational engagement.	1	2	3
7f. Discusses and shares hypotheses about the impact of client's *psychological and social factors* on occupational engagement.	1	2	3
7g. Discusses and shares hypotheses about the impact of *environmental factors* on client's occupational engagement.	1	2	3
7h. Responds to client interaction professionally as appropriate for Level I student role.	1	2	3
7i. Wears student OT name tag and dresses professionally for the fieldwork context.	1	2	3

Specific observations:

Comments:

Based on the above ratings and comments:

☐ The student's performance is **Satisfactory**   ☐ The student's performance is **Unsatisfactory,** additional Level IA fieldwork is necessary.

Summary comments related to the student progressing with additional Level I Fieldwork:

• The student is *performing at or above expectations* for progressing to Level IB fieldwork in the following areas:

• The student is *not performing* at or above expectations for progressing to Level IB fieldwork in the following areas:

_____   _____

Student Signature   Date   *Fieldwork Educator Signature   Date

Please attach additional pages with comments if needed.

*Fieldwork educator: If student needs more than typical support, please notify the academic fieldwork coordinator.

Courtesy of Colorado State University. Used with permission.

Part 3.

LEVEL II FIELDWORK

OVERVIEW OF PART 3

Donna Costa, DHS, OTR/L, FAOTA

Level II fieldwork is the focus of Part 3. This section includes two American Occupational Therapy Association (AOTA) official documents. The first, presented in Chapter 11, is the "COE Guidelines for an Occupational Therapy Fieldwork Experience—Level II," which describes the desired characteristics of the Level II fieldwork experience. It is not a recap of the Accreditation Council for Occupational Therapy Education standards but rather a document outlining best practice. The guidelines describe various fieldwork models, preparation of the fieldwork educator, fieldwork site development, and approaches to learning during fieldwork. "Fieldwork Level II and Occupational Therapy Students: A Position Paper," presented in Chapter 12, articulates that students delivering services to clients during Level II fieldwork are considered skilled services providers under the supervision of a credentialed occupational therapy practitioner.

Chapter 13 contains the Fieldwork Experience Assessment Tool, which aids fieldwork educators in discussing with students whether the fieldwork experience is providing the just-right challenge to maximize student learning. Chapter 14, "Suggestions for Level II Fieldwork Assignments," includes sample Level II fieldwork assignments that help readers plan a fieldwork experience for students. Chapter 15, "Sample 12-Week Assignment Outlines for Level II Fieldwork," contains 12-week outlines of how to structure and sequence learning at the fieldwork site.

The importance of timely feedback to students cannot be overemphasized because it positively influences student learning outcomes. Therefore, Chapter 16, "Sample Weekly Supervisor–Student Feedback Forms," contains examples of weekly feedback forms that can be used to provide students with structured feedback and create the all-important paper trail. Chapter 17, "Infusing 'Occupation' in Fieldwork Assignments," contains an updated article that originally appeared in *OT Practice* in which the authors described ways to make assignments more occupation-focused during Level II fieldwork.

Chapter 11.

COE GUIDELINES FOR AN OCCUPATIONAL THERAPY FIELDWORK EXPERIENCE— LEVEL II

American Occupational Therapy Association Commission on Education

History and Purpose

The intent of this document is to describe the desired characteristics of a fieldwork placement for occupational therapy (OT) and occupational therapy assistant (OTA) students in Level II Fieldwork Education. It is intended to be a reference document that articulates the desired attributes of a fieldwork setting to maximize students' learning in context. It is not a document of standards for fieldwork education, and programs are not mandated to follow these guidelines.

This document was originally prepared by the Loma Linda Fieldwork Council at the request of the Commission on Education (COE) and approved by the COE on April 15, 1985. The document was revised by the American Occupational Therapy Association (AOTA) Fieldwork Issues Committee in 1992, and by the COE in 2000 and 2012.

Definition

The *Accreditation Council for Occupational Therapy Education (ACOTE®) Standards* describe fieldwork as "a crucial part of professional preparation." (ACOTE, 2012). The goal of Level II Fieldwork is to develop competent, entry-level, generalist occupational therapists and occupational therapy assistants (ACOTE, 2012).

I. The Fieldwork Experience

A. Description and Purpose:

The Level II Fieldwork experience, an integral part of OT education, should be designed to promote clinical reasoning and reflective practice, to support ethical practice through transmission of the values and beliefs of the profession, to communicate and model professionalism as a developmental process and a career responsibility, and to expand knowledge and application of a repertoire of occupational therapy assessments and interventions related to human occupation and performance. Through the fieldwork experience, students learn to apply theoretical and scientific principles learned in the didactic portion of the academic program to address actual client needs and develop a professional identity as an occupational therapy practitioner within an interdisciplinary context. The fieldwork experience shall meet requirements in accordance with the Standards for an Accredited Educational Program for the Occupational Therapist and/or the Standards for an Accredited Educational Program for the Occupational Therapy Assistant (ACOTE, 2012).

i. Level II Fieldwork must be integral to the program's curriculum design and must include an in-depth experience in delivering occupational therapy services to clients, focusing on the application of purposeful and meaningful occupations. Throughout the fieldwork experience, the fieldwork educator should structure opportunities for informal and formal reflection with the student regarding the OT process in action with the client population.

ii. The OT and OTA student should have the opportunity to develop increased knowledge, attitudes, and skills in advocacy, administration, management, and scholarship.

1. Skills in administration and management may be attained through the actual supervision of support staff, volunteers, or Level I Fieldwork students in certain tasks or work assignments and involvement in administrative/staff/team meetings.

2. Scholarship may be enhanced as students learn to use evidence to inform their professional decision making and to generate new evidence through independent or collaborative research at the fieldwork site. This may be accomplished through investigation of the effectiveness of an intervention; the reliability, validity or utility of assessment tools; and publication or presentation of scholarly work.

iii. Interprofessional practice competencies should be encouraged throughout the fieldwork experience through engagement of OT and OTA students in interactive learning with students of different professions.

B. Outcomes Desired

The fieldwork placements should provide the student with experience with various groups across the life span, persons with various psychosocial and physical performance challenges, and various service delivery models reflective of current practice in the profession.

i. Within the required total of 16 weeks for the occupational therapy assistant student and 24 weeks for the occupational therapy student, there should be exposure to a variety of traditional and emerging practice settings and a variety of client ages and conditions. In all settings, psychosocial factors influencing engagement in occupation must be understood and integrated for the development of client-centered, occupation-based outcomes. What this means is that even if this is not a mental health placement, the fieldwork educator should assist the student in addressing any psychosocial issues the client may have. This will help to ensure that the student will have developed some entry-level competencies in mental health practice even if they do not complete a fieldwork experience in a mental health setting. See link: http://tinyurl.com/FWMentalHealth

C. Expectations of Fieldwork Students

Students are responsible for compliance with site requirements as specified in the fieldwork site student handbook developed by the fieldwork site and the affiliation agreement between the fieldwork site and the academic program. This typically includes completion of prerequisite requirements (health requirements, background checks, HIPAA training, orientation to site documentation system, etc.) and attention to state regulations affecting student provision of client services. In addition to providing the required occupational therapy services to clients, students are also responsible for active participation in the supervision process, which includes the creation, review, and completion of learning objectives; completion of assigned learning activities and assignments; proactive and ongoing communication with the assigned fieldwork educator; continual self-assessment and reflection; and participation in formal and informal assessments directed by the fieldwork educator. By the end of the fieldwork experience, the student should demonstrate the attitudes and skills of an entry-level practitioner, including assumption of responsibility for independent learning.

D. Fieldwork Educator Preparation

Fieldwork educators responsible for supervising Level II Fieldwork occupational therapy students shall meet state and federal regulations governing practice, have a minimum of 1 year of practice experience subsequent to initial certification, and be adequately prepared to serve as a fieldwork educator. If supervising in a role-emerging site where there is no on-site occupational therapy practitioner, the fieldwork educator should have a minimum of 3 years of practice experience after initial certification (see II.H for more specific detail).

i. Initial and ongoing education supporting the fieldwork educator role should include attention to the following:
1. Principles and theories of adult education models, knowledge of learning styles, and diverse teaching approaches.
2. Administrative aspects, including relevant regulations and content for development and management of the fieldwork program.
3. The design of educational experiences supporting student development as an OT practitioner.
4. Adaptation of supervisor strategies in response to individual student learning style.
5. Enhancement of student clinical and professional reasoning through guided learning experiences.
6. Provision of formal and informal evaluation of student performance.
ii. Methods for becoming adequately prepared to serve as a fieldwork educator include, but are not limited to, the following:
1. Attendance at an AOTA Fieldwork Educator Certificate Program (preferred).

2. Completion of the Self-Assessment Tool for Fieldwork Educator Competency (SAFECOM).
3. Attendance at continuing education events on the topic of practice education.
4. Mentorship by an experienced fieldwork educator.
5. Completion of online training modules.
6. Documented readings of texts or papers on clinical or fieldwork education.

E. Fieldwork Models

A variety of fieldwork models can be used, depending on the preferences of the fieldwork educator, the nature of the fieldwork site, and the learning needs of the students. Fieldwork models exist on a continuum from the traditional apprenticeship model in which one fieldwork educator has one student to a more collaborative approach in which a group of students work with one fieldwork educator. Each fieldwork model has an inherent theoretical approach to learning. The more collaborative the fieldwork model, the more active student learning occurs. Fieldwork models can also be classified as either role-established, which is a more traditional fieldwork site, or role-emerging, where occupational therapy services are being introduced or developed.

i. *1:1*—this is the traditional model of one student to one fieldwork educator, also known as the apprenticeship model.
ii. *1:2*—one fieldwork educator to two students.
iii. *2:1*—two fieldwork educators sharing one student.
iv. *Multiple sites*—a model in which one fieldwork educator has a group of students spread out at several fieldwork sites, usually all the same type of setting.
v. *Group*—a model in which one fieldwork educator has a group of students, but maintains the traditional "fieldwork educator as expert" role.
vi. *Peer*—a model in which students provide feedback to each other; this cannot be the sole form of supervision provided to students, because there must be an OT or OTA identified as the fieldwork educator.

vii. *Off-site or role-emerging*—a fieldwork model in which occupational therapy services are in the process of being developed; the occupational therapy practitioner setting this up may be employed by the agency or the educational program.

viii. *Collaborative*—a specific model of fieldwork education used with a group of students in which knowledge is constructed jointly between the fieldwork educator and the students. This is an active model of student learning that places more responsibility on the student for his or her own learning. The fieldwork educator does not function as the "expert" but more in the role of facilitator of learning.

ix. *Role-emerging fieldwork sites* are those at which the provision of occupational therapy services is being developed. The occupational therapy practitioner developing the services may be employed by the agency as a consultant, or may be employed by the academic program. When fieldwork placements occur in role-emerging practice settings, the occupational therapy fieldwork educator is typically only present on site for a limited amount of time. The ACOTE Standards require that the fieldwork educator provide a minimum of 8 hours per week at the site (ACOTE, 2012). In addition, the fieldwork educator must be easily accessible by a variety of means during the hours a student is at the site. Furthermore, the person serving as the fieldwork educator must have a minimum of 3 years' experience after initial certification, because this is considered advanced supervision.

x. *International fieldwork* occurs in another country and requires a great deal of advance planning from the academic program, student, and fieldwork educator because there are multiple issues involved. The Academic Fieldwork Coordinator should ensure that the fieldwork educator and fieldwork site staff are conversant with and in compliance with current ACOTE standards and that regular formal and informal communication is maintained during the fieldwork experience. The

ACOTE Standards require that the individual serving as the fieldwork educator must be a graduate of a World Federation of Occupational Therapists (WFOT)–approved educational program. Students cannot complete more than 12 weeks in an international placement. The reader is referred to the section of the AOTA website where there are multiple documents describing policies, procedures, and other issues related to international fieldwork.

II. Fieldwork Site Development

When developing a fieldwork experience for a new site, the preferred way to begin is by reaching out to the academic programs in the immediate area. The establishment of a contract between the fieldwork site and the academic program can take a very long time and so it is best to start with that process early. Students cannot be accepted until the contract has been signed by both parties. If there are several academic programs in the area, there is no reason why contracts cannot be initiated with all of them at once.

During the contract development and approval process, the fieldwork educator can begin doing some of the other activities that will need to be in place before students are accepted. The reader is referred to the AOTA website for additional fieldwork educator resources, including "Steps to Starting a Fieldwork Program," located at the following link: http://www.aota.org/en/Education-Careers/Fieldwork/NewPrograms/Steps.aspx

A. **The fieldwork site should meet all existing local, state, and federal safety and health requirements, and should provide adequate and efficient working conditions. The occupational therapy practitioner should comply with state regulations governing the scope of practice for OT services.**

i. Adherence to standards of quality in regard to safety, health requirements, and working conditions may be verified through a review process by the university or program using the center as a fieldwork site or by an established body such as the Joint

Commission, the Commission on Accreditation of Rehabilitation Facilities, or a state regulatory board.

ii. Adequate time should be available to supervising staff for student supervision activities.

iii. Space for client-related consultation, preparation, writing, in-service education, and research activities by occupational therapists, practitioners, and students should be provided.

iv. The fieldwork educator and student should have access to current professional information, publications, texts, and Internet resources related to occupational therapy education and practice.

v. Client records should be available to the staff and students for intervention planning and practice.

B. **Ideally, the fieldwork site will have a stated philosophy regarding service delivery that serves as a guide for the delivery of service, scholarly activities, and education for individuals and groups. Where occupational therapy services are already established, the occupational therapy philosophy, mission, or vision regarding practice and education programs should be stated in writing, and should reflect the specific contribution occupational therapy makes to the overall agency. Where established, the occupational therapy philosophy, mission, or vision guides the development of learning objectives for the fieldwork experience. Ideally, the established occupational therapy program will articulate a philosophy, mission, or vision of service delivery reflective of best practices in the profession. Best practices in the profession result in services that are client-centered, occupation-based, and supported by research evidence. The partnering academic institution will work with the fieldwork site to provide resources to support best practice ideals.**

i. Client-centered practice is evident when there are regular intervention planning and review meetings between the client and occupational therapy practitioner to ensure client participation in the evaluation and intervention process (Mortenson & Dyck, 2006).

1. In situations where there is limited possibility for client participation in intervention planning and review meetings due to the nature or severity of the client's impairment, the occupational therapy practitioner should seek the perspectives of family members or significant others who would act in the client's best interest.

ii. Occupation-based practice is client-centered and requires an understanding of the client's needs, wants, and expectations. Interventions are meaningful to the client and include participation in occupations that are reflective of the client's lifestyle and context (Chisholm, Dolhi, & Schreiber, 2000).

iii. Evidence-based intervention includes the creation of "strategies and tools for practitioners to access, understand, and use the latest research knowledge to improve services for clients" (Law & MacDermid, 2008, p. 6).

C. **The administrators of the fieldwork setting should articulate support for the fieldwork education program.**

i. Since the occupational therapy fieldwork education experience exists within the philosophy and policies of the fieldwork agency, it is essential that the administration as well as the occupational therapy staff accept and support the education of future practitioners.

D. **At fieldwork sites where occupational therapy services are already established, there should be occupational therapy representation in planning programs and formulating policies that would affect occupational therapy practice and services delivery or involvement.**

i. The occupational therapy perspective should be represented at program-related conferences, in quality review processes, and in planning for occupational therapy services delivery. The profession of occupational therapy should be represented in policy-making groups at the fieldwork site.

ii. Consideration should be given to the occupational therapy department philosophy of service delivery in planning programs and forming of policies influencing occupational therapists' service delivery at the fieldwork site.

E. **The fieldwork agency should recognize that the primary objective of the fieldwork experience is to benefit the student's education.**

   i. The educational value of the student fieldwork experience should be of primary importance, and the placement should not be used to extend services offered by the fieldwork agency.

F. **Opportunities for continuing education and professional development of the occupational therapy staff and students should be encouraged to support life-long learning.**

   i. Attendance at workshops, institutes, conferences, courses, in-services, and professional meetings should be encouraged.
   ii. Financial support should be given for professional development whenever feasible within the budget of the fieldwork agency.
   iii. Fieldwork students should be encouraged to participate in continuing education and be provided time to do so, when content is relevant to the fieldwork experience.
   iv. State and National Association membership is encouraged.

G. **Collaboration with academic program—Both the ACOTE Standards (ACOTE, 2012) and the Model Curriculum documents (OT Model Curriculum Ad Hoc Committee, 2008a and 2008b) address the need for collaboration between the fieldwork site or fieldwork educator and the academic program. The ACOTE Standards require that the Academic Fieldwork Coordinator and the fieldwork educator collaborate when establishing fieldwork objectives, identifying fieldwork site requirements, and when communicating students' performance and progress during fieldwork (ACOTE, 2012). The OT Model Curriculum documents describe how fieldwork experiences need to be planned in such a way that they are integrated into the academic program's mission and curriculum design. The reader is referred**
to the OT Model Curriculum, the OTA Model Curriculum, and the ACOTE Standards for more information.

H. **Supervision guidelines—Multiple sources of supervision guidelines are applicable to Level II fieldwork. The first source is state laws and state practice acts that govern the practice of occupational therapy. These documents will specify if there are any specific requirements for supervision that need to be upheld in that state. Another source of supervision guidelines is federal regulations such as Medicare that specify what type of supervision must be provided to fieldwork students in certain health care settings and with certain types of Medicare coverage. The AOTA website is a good source for the most up-to-date information on Medicare regulations for student supervision. The ACOTE Standards specify that during Level II fieldwork, students must be supervised by a licensed or credentialed occupational therapy practitioner with at least 1 year of experience who is adequately prepared to serve as a fieldwork educator. Further, the Standards state that supervision should initially be direct, and then progress to less direct supervision as is possible given the demands of the fieldwork site, the complexity of the client's condition being treated, and the abilities of the fieldwork student. The COE and Commission on Practice (COP) Fieldwork Level II position paper (COE/COP, 2012) additionally recommends that supervision of occupational therapy and occupational therapy assistant students in Fieldwork Level II settings will be of the quality and scope to ensure protection of consumers and provide opportunities for appropriate role modeling of occupational therapy practice, and that the supervising occupational therapist or occupational therapy assistant must recognize when direct versus indirect supervision is needed and ensure that supervision supports the student's current and developing levels of competence (COE/COP, 2012).**

Specific to the role-emerging fieldwork placement, where the site does not employ an occupational therapist on staff and the fieldwork is designed to promote the development of occupational therapy services, supervision guidelines specify that students be supervised daily on site by another professional familiar with the role of occupational therapy and 8 hours of direct supervision should be provided weekly by an occupational therapist or occupational therapy assistant with at least 3 years of experience. It is recommended that the Academic Fieldwork Coordinator (AFWC), fieldwork educator (FWEd), the on-site coordinator (if identified) and student maintain regular formal and informal communication during the fieldwork experience (AOTA, 2001).

III. Student Engagement in the Learning Process

A. It is recommended that students collaborate with their fieldwork educator to develop learning objectives that stem from the site-specific learning objectives for the individual fieldwork site. This may be accomplished through the use of learning contracts, which are both a teaching strategy and an assessment tool used to encourage self-directed learning. Learning contracts allow for shared responsibility in the planning of learning experiences offered in fieldwork. Proactive learning contracts are an effective teaching strategy and encourage students to become intrinsically motivated to attain competence in the fieldwork experience.

  i. The use of learning contracts is highly recommended. If used, learning contracts should be developed within 2 weeks of initiating the fieldwork experience. They should address individual student learning styles, needs, and interests, and should include specific learning objectives, resources and strategies, assessment, and target dates for completion. Learning contracts should be reviewed and updated regularly to reflect and communicate student progress toward the attainment of objectives.

  ii. The student shall be evaluated and kept informed on an ongoing basis of his or her performance status.

1. The student will collaborate with the fieldwork educator to determine the most effective supervision style and feedback methods.

2. Formative assessment shall be provided to students on a weekly basis and recorded in written format, providing specific recommendations addressing observable behaviors.

3. Supervision and feedback are intended to empower the student to change performance, facilitate student self-reflection and self-assessment, and guide the student regarding strengths and opportunities for growth based on site-specific objectives.

4. AOTA's COE recommends the use of the AOTA Fieldwork Performance Evaluation for the Occupational Therapy Student (AOTA, 2002a; Chapter 59) and the AOTA Fieldwork Performance Evaluation for the Occupational Therapy Assistant Student (AOTA, 2002b; Chapter 58) as rating tools. The student's performance should be evaluated formally at midterm and at the completion of the fieldwork experience.

5. The student should self-assess performance at midterm using a copy of the AOTA Fieldwork Performance Evaluation (FWPE), and student evaluation and fieldwork educator evaluation scores should be compared and differences discussed.

6. Weekly supervision logs are a good way for both the supervisor and student to keep track of what was discussed in supervision sessions. It is important for both the fieldwork educator and student to sign and date each log to verify the supervision process.

7. When there are multiple supervisors, care should be taken to ensure that communication regarding student progress is shared among all supervisors and that all contribute to evaluation of the student's progress.

B. Learning Challenges on Fieldwork

  i. Fieldwork educators should monitor student progress, and match students' abilities with the demands of the setting by providing the just-right challenges designed to maximize each student's individual learning needs.

ii. Structured forms of feedback, such as the Fieldwork Experience Assessment Tool (FEAT; AOTA, 2001; Chapter 13), should be used to promote fieldwork educator and student communication.

iii. If the student's performance is not satisfactory at midterm or any point in the fieldwork experience, both the student and academic institution must be notified immediately, and documentation concerning the student's progress and outcomes of interventions should be maintained.

iv. Fieldwork educators should initiate written remedial learning contracts with clear expectations and specific time frames for all students who are struggling to meet site-specific objectives.

IV. Continued Assessment and Refinement of the Fieldwork Program

A. Fieldwork experiences should be implemented and evaluated for their effectiveness by the educational institution and the fieldwork agency.

i. The Academic Fieldwork Coordinator representing the educational institution should regularly evaluate learning opportunities offered during fieldwork to ensure that settings are equipped to meet curricular goals and ensure student exposure to psychosocial factors, occupation-based outcomes, and evidence-based practice.

1. This may be accomplished through regular communication (e.g., emails, phone calls, written correspondence) between the AFWC and faculty and ongoing communication regarding the academic program's curriculum design to the fieldwork site. In addition, the fieldwork site should have opportunity to inform the didactic program preparation.

ii. The fieldwork site should regularly evaluate the effectiveness of its fieldwork program to ensure that students are able to meet learning objectives and deliver ethical, evidence-based, and occupation-centered intervention to clients. The learning objectives should be reviewed regularly to maximize the effectiveness of the fieldwork experience and create new opportunities. Supervisors are encouraged to participate in routine evaluations of their effectiveness in the supervisory role.

1. Fieldwork site evaluation may occur through:
   a. AOTA Student Evaluation of Fieldwork Experience (SEFWE; Chapter 30)
   b. Cumulative review of AOTA Fieldwork Performance Evaluations (FWPE) to determine student patterns of strength and weaknesses
   c. Fieldwork Experience Assessment Tool (FEAT)
   d. Review of the Self-Assessment Tool for Fieldwork Educator Competency (SAFECOM)

Resources

Accreditation Council for Occupational Therapy Education. (2012). 2011 Accreditation Council for Occupational Therapy Education (ACOTE®) standards. *American Journal of Occupational Therapy, 66*(Suppl.), S6–S74. http://dx.doi.org/10.5014/ajot.2012.66S6

American Occupational Therapy Association. (n.d.). *Fieldwork educator's certificate workshop.* Retrieved from http://www.aota.org/Education-Careers/Fieldwork/Workshop.aspx

American Occupational Therapy Association. (1997). *Self-assessment tool for fieldwork educator competency (SAFECOM).* Retrieved from http://www.health.utah.edu/occupational-therapy/fieldwork/fwfiles/selfassessmentfwedcompetency.pdf

American Occupational Therapy Association. (2001). *Fieldwork experience assessment tool (FEAT).* Retrieved from http://www.aota.org/-/media/Corporate/Files/EducationCareers/Accredit/FEATCHARTMidterm.pdf

American Occupational Therapy Association. (2002a). *AOTA fieldwork performance evaluation for the occupational therapy student.* Bethesda, MD: Author.

American Occupational Therapy Association. (2002b). *AOTA fieldwork performance evaluation for the occupational therapy assistant student.* Bethesda, MD: Author.

American Occupational Therapy Association. (2009a). *Occupational therapy fieldwork education: Value and purpose. American Journal of Occupational Therapy, 63,* 393–394.

American Occupational Therapy Association. (2009b). Specialized knowledge and skills of occupational therapy educators of the future. *American Journal of Occupational Therapy, 63,* 804–818.

American Occupational Therapy Association, Commission on Education. (2009). *Recommendations for occupational therapy fieldwork experiences.* Retrieved from http://www.jefferson.edu/content/dam/tju/jshp/occupational_therapy/recommendationsforFWexperiences.pdf

American Occupational Therapy Association, Commission on Education/Commission on Practice. (2012). *Fieldwork level II and occupational therapy students: A position paper.* Retrieved from https://www.aota.org/-/media/Corporate/Files/AboutAOTA/OfficialDocs/Position/Fieldwork-Level-II-2012.PDF

Chisholm, D., Dolhi, C., & Schreiber, J. (2000). Creating occupation-based opportunities in a medical model clinical practice setting. *OT Practice, 5*(1), CE-1–CE-8.

International Fieldwork Ad Hoc Committee for the Commission on Education. (2009). *General guide to planning international fieldwork.* Retrieved from https://www.aota.org/-/media/Corporate/Files/EducationCareers/Educators/International/Guide%20for%20planning%20international%20FW.pdf

Law, M., & MacDermid, J. (2008). *Evidence-based rehabilitation* (2nd ed.). Thorofare, NJ: Slack.

Mortenson, W. B., & Dyck, I. (2006). Power and client-centred practice: An insider exploration of occupational therapists' experiences. *Canadian Journal of Occupational Therapy, 73,* 261–271.

OT Model Curriculum Ad Hoc Committee. (2008a). *Occupational therapy model curriculum.* Retrieved from https://www.aota.org/-/media/Corporate/Files/EducationCareers/Educators/FINAL%20Copy%20Edit%20OT%20Model%20Curriculum%20Guide%2012-08.pdf

OT Model Curriculum Ad Hoc Committee (2008b). *Occupational therapy assistant model curriculum.* Retrieved from https://www.aota.org/-/media/Corporate/Files/EducationCareers/Educators/Model%20OTA%20Curriculum%20-%20October%202008.pdf

AOTA Commission on Education and Fieldwork Issues Committee (FWIC). Amended and Approved by FWIC June 2000 and COE August 2000.

Last updated: January 2013.

Chapter 12.

FIELDWORK LEVEL II AND OCCUPATIONAL THERAPY STUDENTS: A POSITION PAPER

American Occupational Therapy Association

The purpose of this paper is to define the Level II fieldwork experience and to clarify the appropriate conditions and principles that must exist to ensure that interventions completed by Level II fieldwork students are of the quality and sophistication necessary to be clinically beneficial to the client. When appropriately supervised, adhering to professional and practice principles, and in conjunction with other regulatory and payer requirements, the American Occupational Therapy Association (AOTA) considers that students at this level of education are providing occupational therapy interventions that are skilled according to their professional education level of practice.

AOTA asserts that Level II occupational therapy fieldwork students may provide occupational therapy services under the supervision of a qualified occupational therapist in compliance with state and federal regulations. Occupational therapy assistant fieldwork students may provide occupational therapy services under the supervision of a qualified occupational therapist or occupational therapy assistant under the supervision of an occupational therapist in compliance with state and federal regulations.

Occupational therapy Level II fieldwork students are those individuals who are currently enrolled in an occupational therapy or occupational therapy assistant program accredited, approved, or pending accreditation by the Accreditation Council for Occupational Therapy Education (ACOTE®; 2012). At this point in their professional education, students have completed necessary and relevant didactic coursework that has prepared them for the field experience.

The fieldwork Level II experience is an integral and crucial part of the overall educational experience that allows the student an opportunity to apply theory and techniques acquired through the classroom and Level I fieldwork learning. Level II fieldwork provides an in-depth experience in delivering occupational therapy services to clients, focusing on the application of evidence-based purposeful and meaningful occupations, administration, and management of occupational therapy services. The experience provides the student with the opportunity to carry out professional responsibilities under supervision and to observe professional role models in the field (ACOTE, 2012).

The academic program and the supervising occupational therapy practitioner[1] are responsible for ensuring that the type and amount of supervision meet the needs of the student and ensure the safety of all stakeholders. The following General Principles represent the minimum criteria that must be present during a Level II fieldwork experience to ensure the quality of services being provided by the Level II student practitioner:

- The student is supervised by a currently licensed or credentialed occupational therapy practitioner who has a minimum of 1 year of practice experience subsequent to initial certification and is adequately prepared to serve as a fieldwork educator.
- Occupational therapy students will be supervised by an occupational therapist. Occupational therapy assistant students will be supervised by an occupational therapist or an occupational therapy assistant in partnership with the occupational therapist who is supervising the occupational therapy assistant (AOTA, 2009).
- Occupational therapy services provided by students under the supervision of a qualified practitioner will be billed as services provided by the supervising licensed occupational therapy practitioner.
- Supervision of occupational therapy and occupational therapy assistant students in fieldwork Level II settings will be of the quality and scope to ensure protection of consumers and provide opportunities for appropriate role modeling of occupational therapy practice.
- The supervising occupational therapist or occupational therapy assistant must recognize when direct versus indirect supervision is needed and ensure that supervision supports the student's current and developing levels of competence with the occupational therapy process.
- Supervision should initially be direct and in line of sight and gradually decrease to less direct supervision as is appropriate depending on the
  - Competence and confidence of the student,
  - Complexity of client needs,

- Number and diversity of clients,
- Role of occupational therapy and related services,
- Type of practice setting,
- Requirements of the practice setting, and
- Other regulatory requirements (ACOTE, 2012).
- In all cases, the occupational therapist assumes ultimate responsibility for all aspects of occupational therapy service delivery and is accountable for the safety and effectiveness of the occupational therapy service delivery process involving the student. This also includes provision of services provided by an occupational therapy assistant student under the supervision of an occupational therapy assistant (AOTA, 2009).
- In settings where occupational therapy practitioners are not employed,
  - Students should be supervised daily on site by another professional familiar with the role of occupational therapy in collaboration with an occupational therapy practitioner (see b. above).
  - Occupational therapy practitioners must provide direct supervision for a minimum of 8 hours per week and be available through a variety of other contact measures throughout the workday. The occupational therapist or occupational therapy assistant (under the supervision of an occupational therapist) must have 3 years of practice experience to provide this type of supervision (ACOTE, 2012).
- All state licensure policies and regulations regarding student supervision will be followed, including the ability of the occupational therapy assistant to serve as fieldwork educator.
- Student supervision and reimbursement policies and regulations set forth by third-party payers will be followed.

It is the professional and ethical responsibility of occupational therapy practitioners to be knowledgeable of and adhere to applicable state and federal laws and payer rules and regulations related to fieldwork education.

---

[1]When the term *occupational therapy practitioner* is used in this document, it refers to both occupational therapists and occupational therapy assistants (AOTA, 2006).

References

Accreditation Council for Occupational Therapy Education. (2012). 2011 Accreditation Council for Occupational Therapy Education (ACOTE®) standards. *American Journal of Occupational Therapy, 66*(Suppl.), S4– S74. http://dx.doi.org/10.5014/ajot.2012.66S4

American Occupational Therapy Association. (2006). Policy 1.44: Categories of occupational therapy personnel. In *Policy manual* (2011 ed., pp. 33–34). Bethesda, MD: Author.

American Occupational Therapy Association. (2009). Guidelines for supervision, roles, and responsibilities during the delivery of occupational therapy services. *American Journal of Occupational Therapy, 63,* 797–803. http://dx.doi.org/10.5014/ajot.63.6.797

Authors

Debbie Amini, EdD, OTR/L, CHT, C/NDT
Chairperson, Commission on Practice
Jyothi Gupta, PhD, OTR/L, OT, *Chairperson, Commission on Education*

for

The Commission on Practice
Debbie Amini, EdD, OTR/L, CHT, *Chairperson*

and

The Commission on Education
Jyothi Gupta, PhD, OTR/L, OT, *Chairperson*

Adopted by the Representative Assembly Coordinating Council (RACC) for the Representative Assembly, 2012 in response to RA Charge # 2011AprC26.

Note. This document is based on a 2010 Practice Advisory, "Services Provided by Students in Fieldwork Level II Settings." Prepared by a Commission on Practice and Commission on Education Joint Task Force:
Debbie Amini, EdD, OTR/L, CHT, C/NDT
Janet V. DeLany, DEd, OTR/L, FAOTA
Debra J. Hanson, PhD, OTR
Susan M. Higgins, MA, OTR/L
Jeanette M. Justice, COTA/L
Linda Orr, MPA, OTR/L

Chapter 13.

FIELDWORK EXPERIENCE ASSESSMENT TOOL (FEAT)

Fieldwork Research Team

Student name:		Supervisor(s) names:	
Facility name:			
Type of fieldwork experience (setting, population, level):		Date:	Week #:

Context:

The Fieldwork Experience Assessment Tool (FEAT) is the result of an American Occupational Therapy Foundation qualitative study completed by six occupational therapy programs across the United States and Puerto Rico. Data were collected from fieldwork students and fieldwork educators. In their interviews, students and fieldwork educators described fieldwork education in terms of a dynamic triad of interaction among the environment, the fieldwork educator, and the student. Interviewees indicated that a positive educational experience occurred when a balance existed among these three key components.

Purpose:

The FEAT identifies essential characteristics of the three key components. By providing a framework to explore the fieldwork experience,

the FEAT can help students and fieldwork educators consider how to promote the best possible learning experience.

The purpose of the FEAT is to contribute to student and fieldwork educator discussions, so that reflection and problem solving can occur to enhance the fieldwork experience. The tool is designed both to assess the balance of the three key components and to facilitate discussion about student and fieldwork educator behaviors and attitudes, and environmental resources and challenges. By mutually identifying issues present during fieldwork, the fieldwork educator and student can use the FEAT as a tool to promote dialogue and foster the identification of strategies to facilitate the just-right challenge. The FEAT may be used early in fieldwork as a tool to promote dialogue, or at anytime throughout fieldwork as the need for problem solving emerges.

Directions:

In the Assessment Section, the FEAT is organized according to the three key components: environment, fieldwork educator, and student. Under each component, essential characteristics and examples are listed. These examples are not all-inclusive; new descriptors may be added to individualize the tool for different settings. The fieldwork educator and student, either individually or together, should complete the FEAT by describing each component using the continuum provided at the top of each section (limited → just right challenge → excessive).

Following the assessment portion of the FEAT, questions are provided to guide student and fieldwork educator discussion and problem solving. Collaboratively reflect upon the student and fieldwork educator descriptions on the FEAT to identify commonalities and differences between the two perspectives, and identify patterns across the key components. Based on these discussions, develop strategies for a more balanced fieldwork experience. Consider environmental experiences and resources; fieldwork educator attitudes, behaviors, and professional attributes; and student attitudes or behaviors that could enhance the experience. The examples listed within each section are intended to guide discussion between the fieldwork educator and student in an effort to create a successful fieldwork experience. Additional elements may be identified and included according to the nature of the setting or the fieldwork process.

Use of the FEAT at the end of the fieldwork experience is different than at midterm. At the end of the fieldwork, the FEAT is completed exclusively by the student to provide "student-to-student" feedback based upon what characteristics the ideal student in this setting should possess to make the most of this fieldwork experience. This final FEAT is sent directly to the university by the student.

A. Assessment Section

ENVIRONMENT	
I. VARIETY OF EXPERIENCES	**Descriptions** (Limited → Just right challenge → Excessive)
A. Patients/Clients/Diagnoses – Different diagnoses – Range of abilities for given diagnosis (complexity, function-dysfunction) – Diversity of clients, including socioeconomic and lifestyle	
B. Therapy Approaches – Engage in the entire therapy process (evaluation, planning, intervention, documentation) – Learn about different roles of therapist (direct service, consultation, education, and administration) – Use variety of activities with clients – Observe and use different frames of reference/theoretical approaches – Use occupation vs. exercise	
C. Setting Characteristics – Pace (setting demands; caseload quantity) – Delivery system	

II. RESOURCES	**Descriptions** (Limited → Just right challenge → Excessive)
A. OT Staff – See others' strengths and styles – Have multiple role models, resources, and support	
B. Professional Staff – Observe and hear a different perspective on clients – See/experience co-treatments and team work to get whole person perspective – Have others with whom to share ideas and frustrations	
C. OT Students – Able to compare observations and experiences – Exchange ideas	
<td colspan="1" align="center">**FIELDWORK**</td>	
I. ATTITUDE	**Descriptions** (Limited → Just right challenge → Excessive)
A. Likes Teaching/Supervising Students – Devote time, invest in students – Enjoy mental workout, student enthusiasm	
B. Available/Accessible – Take time	
C. Supportive – Patient – Positive and caring – Encourages questions – Encourages development of individual style	
D. Open – Accepting – Alternative methods – To student requests – Communication	
E. Mutual Respect	

II. TEACHING STRATEGIES	**Descriptions** (Limited → Just right challenge → Excessive)
A. Structure – Organize information (set learning objectives, regular meetings) – Introduce treatment (dialogue, observation, treatment, dialogue) – Base structure on student need – Identify strategies for adjusting to treatment environment	
B. Graded Learning – Expose to practice (observe, model) – Challenge student gradually (reduce direction, probing questions, independence) – Base approach on student learning style – Individualize based on student's needs – Promote independence (trial and error)	
C. Feedback/Processing – Timely, confirming – Positive and constructive (balance) – Guide thinking – Promote clinical reasoning	
D. Teaching – Share resources and knowledge	
E. Team Skills – Include student as part of team	
III. PROFESSIONAL ATTRIBUTES	**Descriptions** (Limited → Just right challenge → Excessive)
A. Role Model – Set good example – Enthusiasm for occupational therapy – Real person – Lifelong learning	
B. Teacher – Able to share resources and knowledge	

FIELDWORK STUDENT	
I. ATTITUDE	**Descriptions** (Limited → Just right challenge → Excessive)
A. Responsible for Learning – Active learner (ask questions, consult) – Prepare (review, read, and research materials) – Self-direct (show initiative, assertive) – Learn from mistakes (self-correct and grow)	
B. Open/Flexible – Sensitive to diversity (nonjudgmental) – Responsive to client/consumer needs – Flexible in thinking (make adjustments, try alternate approaches)	
C. Confident – Comfort in knowledge and abilities – Comfort with making and learning from mistakes (take risks, branch out) – Comfort with independent practice (take responsibility) – Comfort in receiving feedback	
D. Responsive to Supervision – Receptive to feedback (open-minded, accept criticism) – Open communication (two-way)	
II. LEARNING BEHAVIORS	**Descriptions** (Limited → Just right challenge → Excessive)
A. Independent – Have and use knowledge and skills – Assume responsibility of OT without needing direction – Incorporate feedback into behavioral changes – Use "down time" productively – Become part of team	
B. Reflection – Self (processes feelings, actions, and feedback) – With others (supervisor, peers, others)	
C. Active in Supervision – Communicate needs to supervisor (seek supervision for guidance and processing; express needs) – Ask questions	

B. Discussion Section: Questions to Facilitate Dialogue and Problem Solving

1. A positive fieldwork experience includes a balance among the environment, fieldwork educator, and student components. Collaboratively reflect upon the descriptions outlined by the student and fieldwork educator and identify perceptions below.

Common Perspectives Between Student and Fieldwork Educator	Different Perspectives Between Student and Fieldwork Educator
Environment Fieldwork Educator Student	

2. What patterns are emerging across the three key components?

3. What strategies or changes can be implemented to promote a successful fieldwork experience? Describe below:

Components of a Successful Fieldwork	Environment, Fieldwork Educator, and/or Student Strategies and Changes to Promote Successful Fieldwork Experience at This Setting
Environment Experiences Resources	
Fieldwork Educator Attitudes Behaviors Professional attributes	

Student Attitudes Behaviors	

© [April 1998] [Revised August 2001] FEAT 13.doc This Fieldwork Assessment Tool (FEAT) was developed by The Fieldwork Research Team: Karen Atler, Karmen Brown, Lou Ann Griswold, Wendy Krupnick, Luz Muniz de Melendez, and Patricia Stutz-Tanenbaum; project funded by The American Occupational Therapy Foundation.

Chapter 14.

SUGGESTIONS FOR LEVEL II FIELDWORK ASSIGNMENTS

Donna Costa, DHS, OTR/L, FAOTA

When creating an outline for an 8- to 12-week Level II fieldwork experience, the fieldwork educator may consider many different kinds of learning activities and assignments for a student.

Case Study

Some of the more traditional assignments include a case study that is both written and presented to staff and an in-service presentation on a topic either assigned to or chosen by the student. If the student does a case study, it should be in an occupational profile and analysis of occupational performance format, following the *Occupational Therapy Practice Framework: Domain and Process* (3rd ed.; American Occupational Therapy Association [AOTA], 2014).

Research

If an in-service is assigned to the student, the student should include all of the relevant research evidence on the topic being presented. An idea for an in-service is to have the student demonstrate the use of a new assessment or treatment not being used at the fieldwork facility.

Fieldwork Manual

If the fieldwork site is a new one in development, consider having the student create the fieldwork manual for future students. The AOTA website has a suggested outline for the manual content (http://www.aota.org/Education-Careers/Fieldwork/NewPrograms/Content.aspx; see also Chapter 38, Suggested Content for Fieldwork Site Manuals). The student can add additional sections such as sample documentation or a copy of the in-service he or she presented.

Equipment Use and Inventory

To introduce the student to the fieldwork site, have him or her locate all of the equipment and supplies in the occupational therapy department as part of his or her orientation. The student can categorize equipment and supplies by type (e.g., assessments, treatment supplies, exercise equipment) or by location (e.g., cabinets, drawers). Alternatively, if the department has an inventory list, the student can find the items on the list and check them off.

Visits to Other Units

Visits to other units or other facilities in the community can be a great way to broaden the student's knowledge about other services. The visit could be related to aftercare locations for patients being discharged from a hospital or community resources available for follow-up services. If the fieldwork site is a large health care system or hospital, the student could visit other departments or units identified by the student as areas of interest or suggested by the fieldwork educator.

Sample Job Descriptions

Fieldwork educators working at sites that do not employ both occupational therapy assistants and occupational therapists may be particularly challenged with scoring items on the AOTA Fieldwork Performance Evaluation form (see Chapters 58 and 59) that address the student's ability to work collaboratively with the occupational therapy assistant or aide. Therefore, a useful assignment is to have the student research and write a sample job description for an occupational therapy assistant, including the duties and activities he or she would be responsible for in the program. The fieldwork educator could also assign the student to go on a site visit to a facility similar to the fieldwork site that employs an occupational therapy assistant. Another idea is to conduct a role-play scenario of the weekly meeting, with the fieldwork educator playing the role of the occupational therapy assistant and the student playing the role of the occupational therapist. This assignment can help the student understand the concepts of role delineation and delegation.

Assigned Readings and Journal Clubs

Assign readings from journals and textbooks to expand the student's knowledge about a particular condition or intervention approach. These materials can be incorporated into a journal club, or have the student start a journal club during his or her rotation (see http://www.aota.org/practice/researchers/journal-club-toolkit.aspx for AOTA journal club resources). Students can discuss the articles they read during the weekly meetings.

Resources and Kits

Another frequently assigned learning activity is to have a student design and fabricate a useful project for the occupational therapy department, such as a piece of equipment, resource binder, group activity, or occupation-based kit. The kit is a collection of materials that an occupational therapy practitioner could use to provide an occupation-based treatment intervention for clients. Some ideas are kits for pet care, games, car care, knitting or crocheting, child care, gardening, or medication management.

Patient Education

Students could focus on patient education for assignments. For example, they could create a handout on a treatment or resource or a resource binder of community resources for patients to use during the discharge planning process. In addition, they could develop and lead a patient education session on a particular topic for clients or caregivers. When developing patient education materials, students should remember health literacy concepts and take into account the intended population and their learning needs, for example, using larger print for older adults, supplying pictures and captions that are culturally relevant, and considering the language needs of clients.

Mentoring

If fieldwork students have overlapping schedules, consider having Level II students supervise Level I students or mentor new Level II students. This experience boosts self-confidence as they demonstrate to others how much they have learned. It is likely that fieldwork students will be supervising others shortly after they graduate, so it is helpful to give them an opportunity to learn supervisory skills while doing fieldwork.

Program Planners

Students could be involved in the planning process of developing a new program, service, or group by researching background information or completing a needs assessment. In addition, they could assist in a presentation to management about or create promotional materials for this new initiative.

Office Organization

Organizational activities might be turned into valuable learning assignments. Students could develop a new form or a new filing system or clean and organize closets, cabinets, and drawers and then update the department inventory list.

Conclusion

None of these learning activities and assignments should be busywork for the students. Rather, they should be presented in the context of meeting learning objectives for the fieldwork experience. Students are creative and have a lot of energy and ideas; therefore, activities and assignments should reflect these traits and include tasks that students will undertake with their first job.

Reference

American Occupational Therapy Association. (2014). Occupational therapy practice framework: Domain and process (3rd ed.). *American Journal of Occupational Therapy, 68* (Suppl. 1). http://dx.doi.org/10.5014/ajot.2014.682006

Chapter 15.

SAMPLE 12-WEEK ASSIGNMENT OUTLINES FOR LEVEL II FIELDWORK

Compiled by Donna Costa, DHS, OTR/L, FAOTA; University of North Dakota Occupational Therapy Department; Central Nassau Guidance and Counseling Services, Inc.,; Stony Brook University

University of North Dakota Occupational Therapy Department
Template: Weekly Learning Activities for Level II Fieldwork

The learning activities below represent suggestions that may be appropriate to support student learning across the continuum of the 12-week Level II experience. It is NOT meant to be used in its entirety, but to use as a resource to stimulate ideas as you construct a weekly schedule suitable to your site and your learning objectives.

Week 1	**Suggested Learning Activities** **Note:** Suggested activities in *italics* are sequential and can be used over a number of weeks.	Mark chosen activities in this column
	Student will tour facility and attend orientation sessions, or view department videos on select topics to review policies and procedures. Student will then review manual contents with fieldwork educator and is expected to refer and utilize manual throughout fieldwork.	
	Student will review facility objectives and assignments and clarify expectations with supervisor as needed.	
	Student will review security protocol, codes, and environmental care information. (This may include attention to sharps safety, transfer protocol, confidentiality, etc.)	
	Student will demonstrate competency in use of hospital communication systems including pager, telephone, Dictaphone, etc.	

(Continued)

	Student will become familiar with electronic documentation and billing protocol including therapy codes, charges, attendance record and care maps. May meet with facility representative regarding insurance authorization.	
	Observe intake process of one new client.	
	Student will shadow assigned staff therapist as scheduled and a. observe initial evaluation (specific evaluation names may be appropriate here) b. observe intervention procedures (specific types of intervention may be assigned such as dressing program, homemaking, leisure skills group, etc.) c. write two progress notes on assigned clients following the facility documentation format.	
	Student will demonstrate competency in administering two to three selected assessment tools. (Others may be assigned throughout the fieldwork experience.) To obtain competency, the student may observe the supervisor administering assessment twice with different clients, then the supervisor and student administer the assessment together, then the supervisor observes the student administering the assessment twice with different clients. The student will be expected to take responsibility to study assessment materials as needed and will be responsible for clarifying with the supervisor any areas of assessment protocol not understood.	
	Student will become familiar with facility records and files through chart/history review of one client, including review of evaluation, intervention, and documentation of client plus other assigned areas. Student will ask for clarification of all terminology, language, and processes not understood.	
	Student will complete scavenger hunt to become familiar with facility resources for therapy (supplies, assessment tools, reference books/ videos, equipment, etc.)	
	Student will attend treatment/team meetings as scheduled. Student will begin interviews of selected disciplines to understand their role on the treatment team (complete 3 interviews of student choice). Student and supervisor will determine possible observation sites.	
	Student will review theories/models/frames of reference used at facility and prepare summary for week 2 meeting.	
	Student will brainstorm with supervisor his/her ideas for independent study project. See next page for suggested final project ideas.	

End of Week 1
Student will meet with supervisor and discuss student performance in regard to facility expectations, student learning style, and goals/objectives for upcoming week. Professional readings, journaling, or reflective learning assignments for the coming week may be given. For a format and description of weekly meeting guidelines and suggested reflective learning assignments, go to www.ot.und.edu. Look for the fieldwork link, and the link for fieldwork resources.

The final project may include but is not limited to:

- Present an in-service to OT staff on the *Occupational Therapy Practice Framework.*
- Present a case study completing each section of the *Framework* with information obtained/observed about the specific patient.
- Have students develop patient education materials on specific diseases, symptoms, and/or treatments.
- Perform literature searches on assessment and intervention techniques to support evidence-based practice.
- Develop documentation formats for staff supervision, treatment consultation, and/or monitoring.
- Design a needs assessment for a given population.
- Perform background research for a potential new program (e.g., driving program, teen parenting program).
- Compile resources for staff that are reflective of occupation-based practice.
- Fabricate a treatment medium to leave at the facility.
- Present a research/educational project that would benefit staff and/or patients.
- Present articles of interest or conference proceedings to staff.
- Construct adaptive equipment to benefit client participation in a desired occupation.
- Create a notebook/brochure of available community resources, such as self-help groups, crisis hotlines, social service agencies, and other community service providers.

- Organize an OT month display/celebration/event for the entire facility.
- Develop a new group, program, or protocol. Organize materials and documents to support program implementation.
- Make a presentation to a support group on a topic of interest to that group's participants such as crisis hotlines for members of a depression support group, or energy conservation techniques for an arthritis or fibromyalgia support group.
- Conduct a practice analysis examining the population, assessments, or interventions commonly seen in the fieldwork setting. Through study of the typical diagnoses or conditions seen, the gender distribution, age distribution, typical occupational roles, average duration of services, average frequency of services, typical disposition destination, and common reimbursement sources of the fieldwork site, strategic plans might be developed to provide occupation-based services to the populations served.
- Students could develop and implement a group for the population served at the facility. The student must provide a protocol for the group, occupations addressed by the group, and objectives and goals for the group. Step-by-step instructions, along with a list of necessary equipment and supplies and time frames for each step, would assist in a successful implementation of the group in the future. The headings included in the Activity Demands category of the *Framework* can serve as an excellent guide for completing this assignment.

Beginning of Week 2

Student is assigned *two clients* and will shadow therapist in evaluation, treatment, and documentation process; this may be supervising therapist or another assigned therapist. *(If therapy is provided in a group context, student may be assigned one–two groups initially.)*

Week 2	**Suggested Learning Activities** **Note:** Suggested activities in *italics* are sequential and can be used over a number of weeks.	Mark chosen activities in this column
	Student will determine, with supervisor, appropriate assessment protocol for assigned clients and will complete and document assessment results (within facility timeline), specifically indicating the need/rationale for OT services.	
	Student will determine, with supervisor input, appropriate intervention methods and will carry out interventions with supervisor assistance.	
	For one client diagnosis, student completes literature search to determine research evidence for one intervention method and reports to supervisor at the end of the week.	
	Student will demonstrate competence in selected interventions (e.g., one-handed dressing techniques, adaptive cooking procedures, general wheelchair positioning, demonstration of relaxation techniques [*you may list expected competencies here*])	
	Student will demonstrate use of adaptive equipment or adapted procedure as needed for therapy intervention with supervisor assistance.	
	Student continues to gain familiarity with facility programs, observing treatment protocols in occupational therapy with a diverse client group.	
	Student continues to gain competency in selected assessment instruments and protocol as assigned (facility determines list).	
	Student completes all interviews/observations of other disciplines as assigned from week 1.	
	Student narrows down ideas for final project to three options.	

End of Week 2

Student meets with supervisor at end of the week to review assignment for research evidence and theory/model review; applications are made to existing clientele at facility. Student strengths and weaknesses in performance are discussed and a goal focus is determined for corning week.

Beginning of Week 3

Student is assigned *three to four clients* and will shadow assigned therapist in evaluation, treatment, and documentation process for one–two of assigned clients, treating the other one to two assigned clients independently once competence is determined by supervising therapist. *(If therapy is provided in a group context, student may be assigned primary responsibility in planning and leading one to two groups while co-leading two additional groups or individual therapy sessions.)*

Week 3	**Suggested Learning Activities** **Note:** Suggested activities in *italics* are sequential and can be used over a number of weeks.	Mark chosen activities in this column
	Student will work independently to determine appropriate assessment protocol for one to two assigned clients (obtaining approval from supervisor before implementation) and will complete and document assessment results with minimal assistance from supervisor (within facility timeline), specifically indicating the need/rationale for OT services.	
	Student will construct treatment plans for one to two assigned clients independently, identifying the appropriate theory, model, or frame of reference for intervention and choosing intervention methods appropriate for theoretical orientation. Student will gain approval of plan before carrying out intervention with minimal supervisor assistance.	
	For assigned client, student will demonstrate the ability to grade intervention from simple to more advanced and will identify a balance of preparatory, purposeful, and occupation-based activities for intervention.	
	Student will develop one occupation kit that contains all of the supplies needed for completing a meaningful activity for use with assigned client or group. Activities such as hand sewing, cutting coupons, caring for nails, shaving, applying make-up, wrapping packages, doing carpentry, plumbing, mechanical skills, paying bills, and working on crossword or word search puzzles are some examples that lend themselves to inclusion in occupation-based intervention kits.	
	Student will demonstrate use of adaptive equipment or adapted procedure as needed for therapy intervention with minimal supervisor assistance.	
	Student will set up therapy room and clean up after session.	
	Student will complete documentation with supervisor feedback as needed.	
	Student will initiate the completion of managerial tasks related to assigned clients/groups, with minimal supervisor assistance.	
	Student will meet with patient and family to review assessment results/treatment plan as assigned, with assistance from supervisor.	

(Continued)

	Student will report in team meeting the progress of assigned clients (those whom he/she is treating independently).	
	Student will demonstrate competency in administration of safety procedures pertinent to facility (following transfer and transportation guidelines, sharps precautions, etc.)	
	Student continues to gain competency in assessment instruments as assigned (facility determines list).	
	Student will continue to demonstrate competence in selected interventions focusing on application to more complex client populations. Specific intervention methods to be reviewed include: (facility determines list).	
	Student will determine focus of final project and present outline of project scope.	

End of Week 3

Student meets with supervisor to address strengths and weaknesses of performance, with particular focus on performance in relation to client assessment and treatment as well as documentation of therapy progress and outcomes. A goal focus is determined for the coming week. At this point, a learning contract format may be introduced to involve the student in identifying goals and learning experiences or resources/supports that the fieldwork educator might provide to support student learning. The intention is to involve the student in taking more ownership for his or her learning experience. See UND OT department website, www.ot.und.edu. Look for the fieldwork link, and then look under "fieldwork resources" to find an overview of the use of learning contracts and a sample format for use.

Beginning of Week 4

Student is assigned *four to five clients* and will shadow assigned therapist in evaluation, treatment, and documentation process for one–two of assigned clients, treating the other three to four assigned clients independently once competence is determined by supervising therapist. *(If therapy is provided in a group context, student may be assigned primary responsibility in planning and leading two to three groups while co-leading in two additional groups or individual therapy session.)*

Week 4	**Suggested Learning Activities** **Note:** Suggested activities in *italics* are sequential and can be used over a number of weeks.	Mark chosen activities in this column
	Student will work independently to determine appropriate assessment protocol for three to four assigned clients (obtaining approval from supervisor before implementation) and will complete and document assessment results with minimal assistance from supervisor (within facility timeline), specifically indicating the need/rationale for OT services.	
	Student will construct treatment plans for three to four assigned clients independently, identifying the appropriate theory, model, or frame of reference for intervention and choosing intervention methods appropriate for theoretical orientation. In addition, student will investigate research evidence for intervention chosen and will include evidence in justification of therapy plan. Student will gain approval of plan before carrying out intervention with initial supervisor assistance.	
	For assigned clients, student will demonstrate the ability to grade appropriate interventions from simple to more advanced and will identify a balance of preparatory, purposeful, and occupation-based activities for intervention.	
	Student will develop one occupation kit that contains all of the supplies needed for completion of a meaningful activity for use with assigned client or group.	
	Student will demonstrate use of adaptive equipment or adapted procedure as needed for therapy intervention.	
	Student will set up therapy room and clean up after session.	
	Student will complete appropriate documentation with supervisor feedback as needed.	
	Student will initiate the completion of managerial tasks related to assigned clients/groups, with initial supervisor assistance.	
	Student will meet with patient and family to review assessment results/treatment plan as assigned, with minimal assistance from supervisor.	
	Student will report in team meeting the progress of assigned clients (those whom he/she is treating independently).	

(Continued)

	Student continues to gain competency in assessment instruments as assigned. Specific assessments to be reviewed this week include: (facility determines list).	
	Student will continue to demonstrate competence in selected interventions focusing on application to more complex client populations. Specific intervention methods to be reviewed include: (facility determines list).	
	Student will update supervisor on progress of final project.	

End of Week 4
Student meets with supervisor at end of the week to discuss strengths and weaknesses of performance, with particular focus on performance in relation to client assessment, intervention, and documentation of therapy progress and outcomes. A goal focus is determined for the coming week to include progressively more complex clientele, broader focus of assessment experience, and wider scope of interventions.

Beginning of Week 5

Student is assigned *five to six clients* and will shadow assigned therapist in evaluation, treatment, and documentation process for one to two more complex clients, treating the other four to five assigned clients independently once competence is determined by supervising therapist. *(If therapy is provided in a group context, student may be assigned primary responsibility in planning and leading three to four groups while co-leading in two additional groups or individual therapy session, which are more complex in nature.)*

Students will begin to demonstrate ability to ration out caseload and participate in choosing and prioritizing the treatment level of all patients in the caseload.

Week 5	**Suggested Learning Activities** **Note:** Suggested activities in *italics* are sequential and can be used over a number of weeks.	Mark chosen activities in this column
	Student will work independently to determine appropriate assessment protocol for three to four assigned clients (obtaining approval from supervisor before implementation) and will complete and document assessment results with occasional and minimal assistance from supervisor (within facility timeline), specifically indicating the need/rationale for OT services.	
	Student will construct treatment plans for four to five assigned clients independently, identifying the appropriate theory, model, or frame of reference for intervention and choosing intervention methods appropriate for theoretical orientation. In addition, student will investigate research evidence for intervention chosen and will include evidence in justification of therapy plan. Student will gain approval of plan before carrying out intervention with occasional minimal supervisor assistance.	
	For assigned clients, student will demonstrate the ability to grade appropriate interventions from simple to more advanced, and will identify a balance of preparatory, purposeful, and occupation-based activities for intervention.	
	Student will develop two to three occupation kits that contain all of the supplies needed for completing a meaningful activity for use with assigned client or group.	
	Student will construct adaptive equipment as needed for therapy intervention.	
	Student will set up therapy room and clean up after session.	
	Student will co-treat with a COTA or COTA student if available for at least one client or group, and work cooperatively to accomplish therapy objectives.	
	Student will complete documentation with supervisor feedback as needed.	
	Student will initiate the completion of managerial tasks related to assigned clients/groups, with minimal supervisor assistance.	

(Continued)

	Student will meet with patient and family to review assessment results/treatment plan as assigned, with occasional minimal assistance from supervisor.	
	Student will report in team meeting the progress of assigned clients (those whom he/she is treating independently) and will initiate communication with team members as needed throughout the week.	
	Student continues to gain competency in assessment instruments as assigned.	
	Specific assessments to be reviewed this week include: (facility determines list).	
	Student will continue to demonstrate competence in selected interventions focusing on application to more complex client populations. Specific intervention methods to be reviewed include: (facility determines list).	
	Student will update supervisor of progress of final project.	

End of Week 5

Student meets with supervisor at end of the week to address strengths and weaknesses of performance, with particular focus on performance in relation to client assessment, intervention, and documentation of therapy progress and outcomes. Goals for the coming week should include progressively more complex clientele, broader focus of assessment experience, and wider scope of interventions.

In addition, the student and fieldwork educator will complete the AOTA Fieldwork Evaluation Form (FEW) for review at the next weekly meeting. The student may also complete the Student Evaluation of Fieldwork (SEFW) form to give feedback to the site on supervision provided.

Beginning of Week 6

Student is assigned *six to eight clients* (or whatever is considered to be 90% of entry-level therapist caseload) and will shadow assigned therapist in evaluation, treatment, and documentation process for one–two complex clients, treating the other five to six assigned clients independently once competence is determined by supervising therapist. *(If therapy is provided in a group context, student may be assigned primary responsibility in planning and leading three to four groups and 2–3 individual sessions while co-leading in two additional groups or individual therapy sessions, which are more complex in nature.)*

Student will begin to demonstrate ability to ration out caseload and participate in choosing and prioritizing the treatment level of all patients on the caseload.

Week 6	**Suggested Learning Activities** **Note:** Suggested activities in *italics* are sequential and can be used over a number of weeks.	Mark chosen activities in this column
	Student will demonstrate the ability to assist other therapists with their caseload as needed; e.g., to start therapy following established treatment plan as needed.	
	Student will demonstrate the ability to orient Level I fieldwork students and volunteers, and communicate the scope of occupational therapy services accurately.	
	Student will determine appropriate assessment protocol for 6–8 assigned clients (obtaining approval from supervisor before implementation) and will complete and document assessment results with occasional and minimal assistance from supervisor (within facility timeline), specifically indicating the need/rationale for OT services.	
	Student will construct treatment plans for six to eight assigned clients independently, identifying the appropriate theory, model, or frame of reference for intervention and choosing intervention methods appropriate for theoretical orientation. In addition, student will investigate research evidence for key interventions chosen and will include evidence in justification of therapy plan. Student will gain approval of plan before carrying out intervention with occasional minimal supervisor assistance.	
	For assigned clients, student will demonstrate the ability to grade appropriate interventions from simple to more advanced and will identify a balance of preparatory, purposeful, and occupation-based activities for intervention.	
	During the course of the week, student will develop two to three occupation kits that contain all of the supplies needed for completion of a meaningful activity for use with assigned client or group.	
	Student will set up therapy room and clean up after session.	

(Continued)

	Student will co-treat with a COTA or COTA student if available for at least one client or group, and work cooperatively to accomplish therapy objectives.
	Student will complete appropriate documentation with supervisor feedback as needed.
	Student will initiate the completion of managerial tasks related to assigned clients/groups, with minimal supervisor assistance.
	Student will meet with patient and family to review assessment results/treatment plan as assigned, with occasional minimal assistance from supervisor.
	Student will report in team meeting the progress of assigned clients (those whom he/she is treating independently) and will initiate communication with team members as needed throughout the week.
	Student continues to gain competency in assessment instruments as assigned. Specific assessments to be reviewed this week include: (facility determines list).
	Student will continue to demonstrate competence in selected interventions focusing on application to more complex client populations. Specific intervention methods to be reviewed include: (facility determines list).
	Student will update supervisor on progress of final project.

End of Week 6
Student meets with supervisor at end of the week to complete midterm evaluation (FWE), which will include assessment of performance across all areas. Goals for the coming week should include progressively more complex clientele, broader focus of assessment experience, and wider scope of interventions. The student evaluation of fieldwork (SEFW) form can be reviewed to provide fieldwork educator with feedback to adjust student caseload and learning supports provided as needed. In addition, other tools such as the Fieldwork Experience Assessment Tool (FEAT) may be used to gather data regarding student perception of the learning experience.

Weeks 7–10

The student continues to treat patients as assigned, gradually assuming the entire caseload of the supervising therapist. With those clients who are more complex, the supervising therapist acts as consultant, providing direction and assistance as requested by the student. Ultimately, the student should achieve competency in all primary treatment and documentation responsibilities and demonstrate the ability to work progressively more independently the last 4 weeks of the fieldwork experience. The continuation of weekly meetings to summarize student strengths and weaknesses in all areas will serve to focus student efforts toward independence and ensure that the student is progressing satisfactorily.

Weeks 7–10	**Suggested Learning Activities** Note: Suggested activities in *italics* are sequential and can be used over a number of weeks.	Mark chosen activities in this column
	Specific assignments are phased out as student demonstrates competency in entry-level therapist skills. Learning contracts constructed cooperatively between student and supervising therapist are encouraged as a means for students to take initiative to develop targeted skills and to ensure continued accountability in student learning.	
	Student demonstrates increased competency in specific assessments assigned and researches one–two additional assessments that would be appropriate in the facility, presenting an overview of assessment instruments chosen in an appropriate format.	
	The student demonstrates increased competency in specific interventions provided within the facility. Based on literature searches conducted throughout the fieldwork, the student provides presentation to the faculty on research evidence to support existing interventions used, or provides in-service introducing intervention procedure/method that is new to the facility but supported by existing research evidence.	

The student will present a final project of his or her choice to a selected audience.

End of Weeks 7–10

Weekly meetings to summarize student strengths and weaknesses in all areas will serve to focus student efforts toward independence and ensure that the student is progressing satisfactorily.

Weeks 11–12

The student continues to treat patients as assigned, assuming the entire caseload of the supervising therapist. With those clients who are more complex, the supervising therapist acts as consultant, providing direction and assistance as requested by the student. The student has achieved competency in all primary treatment and documentation responsibilities and demonstrates the ability to work independently, requiring only indirect supervision by the supervising therapist.

Weeks 11–12	**Suggested Learning Activities** **Note:** Suggested activities in *italics* are sequential and can be used over a number of weeks.	Mark chosen activities in this column
	Student will participate in additional learning experiences as initiated by the student. This might include shadowing therapists in other areas of the facility, participating in treatment areas not originally assigned, or any learning experience deemed appropriate by supervising therapist.	
	Student will plan and prepare for closure with clients, demonstrating the ability to re-assign patient to other therapists or groups as indicated and to construct a clear and concise treatment plan that can be carried out by other therapists as needed.	
Required Activity	Student will complete the AOTA Student Evaluation of the Fieldwork Experience, providing feedback to the supervising therapist in a professional manner.	

End of Weeks 11–12

Final meetings with supervising therapist. At Week 11, the fieldwork educator begins to gather data to fill out the AOTA fieldwork evaluation form (FWE), gathering supporting information from other therapists and staff as needed. The student gathers data to fill out the student evaluation of fieldwork form (SEFW). At the final meeting at the conclusion of Week 12, the student first reviews with the site the SEFW; this is followed by fieldwork educator evaluation of the student using the FWE.

Reprinted with permission of the University of North Dakota.

Central Nassau Guidance and Counseling Services, Inc.
Level II Occupational Therapy Fieldwork—Mental Health
Weekly Schedule of Assignments

Week 1:
➤ Orientation to facility, staff, safety procedures, expectations.
➤ Program philosophy, supervisory structure, frames of reference.
➤ Review of weekly assignments, group process, occupation-based practice, evidence-based practice.
➤ Review of psychiatric diagnoses and symptoms.
➤ Attend groups and staff meetings.
➤ Write 1 behavioral observation note daily on 1 patient in 1 activity or in 1 work unit daily.
➤ Reflective journal entry once daily for duration of fieldwork.
➤ Weekly supervision log due on each Friday for duration of fieldwork.
➤ Read all assigned journal articles and/or reference material and be prepared to discuss.
➤ Review as many charts as possible.

Week 2:
➤ Lead and/or co-lead as many groups as possible for duration of fieldwork.
➤ Administer 1st occupational therapy assessment—written evaluation and treatment plan due by Friday of Week 3. (There will be 6 assessments with written evaluations and treatment plans; Week 2–Week 8.)
➤ Complete group process sheets for each group that is run.
➤ Actively participate in staff and member meetings.

Week 3:
➤ Administer 2nd occupational therapy assessment, with written evaluation and treatment plan due by Friday of Week 4.
➤ Begin to identify 1 journal article per week relevant to this fieldwork to be discussed on Monday of Week 4.

Week 4:
➤ Administer 3rd occupational therapy assessment, with written evaluation and treatment plan due by Friday of Week 5.
➤ Plan and write up group protocol for 4-session group. (To be approved by supervisor.)

Week 5:
➤ Administer 4th occupational therapy assessment, with written evaluation and treatment plan due by Friday of Week 6.
➤ Select in-service topic and associated research.
➤ Start writing 6 progress notes weekly for remainder of fieldwork—document on 2 members from each work unit. To be reviewed by supervisor prior to being placed in chart.
➤ Discuss role of COTA with fieldwork supervisor.

Week 6:
➤ Administer 5th occupational therapy assessment, with written evaluation and treatment plan due by Friday of Week 7.
➤ Conduct first of 4 group protocol sessions.
➤ Schedule midterm evaluation with supervisor.
➤ Complete fieldwork performance evaluation on self using standard rating.

Week 7:
➤ Administer 6th occupational therapy assessment, with written evaluation and treatment plan due by Friday of Week 8.
➤ Conduct second of 4 group protocol sessions.
➤ Attempt to observe transitional employment specialist with a member in the field.
➤ Begin to identify special project to be presented in Week 11.

Week 8:
- ➢ Conduct 3rd of 4 group protocol sessions.
- ➢ Schedule fieldtrip to visit mental health agency, preferably another clubhouse (Fountain House, The Gathering Place, etc.).

Week 9:
- ➢ Conduct fourth of 4 group protocol sessions.
- ➢ Write up evaluation of group protocol (What went well? Were outcome measures positive? What did you learn? etc.).

Week 10:
- ➢ Begin termination process with members and staff.
- ➢ Present in-service to staff.

Week 11:
- ➢ Begin to complete student evaluation of fieldwork experience.
- ➢ Finish special project.

Week 12:
- ➢ Complete termination with members and staff.
- ➢ Submit student evaluation of fieldwork experience to supervisor at time of final evaluation.
- ➢ Review fieldwork performance evaluation with supervisor and sign, indicating that you have read it.
- ➢ Turn in identification badges and keys.

Occupational Therapy Assessments Used in Mental Health Practice:

- Canadian Occupational Performance Measure (COPM)*
- Adolescent/Adult Sensory Profile*
- Barth Time Construct*
- The Kohlman Evaluation of Living Skills (KELS)*
- Self Assessment Questionnaire*
- Volitional Sentence Completion*
- Comprehensive Occupational Therapy Evaluation (COTE)*
- Lifestyle Inventory*
- Occupational Performance History Interview II (OPHI II)*
- Interest Checklist*
- Roles Checklist*
- Recreation Interest Checklist*
- Worker Role Interview *
- Vocational Readiness Checklist*
- Activity Card Sort
- Bay Area Functional Performance Evaluation (BAFPE)
- Mini-Mental Status Examination (MMSE)

---

* = Present at Connections (if no *, assessment can be obtained)

CONNECTIONS CLUBHOUSE
PREVOCATIONAL PROGRAM WEEKLY SCHEDULE

	MONDAY	TUESDAY	WEDNESDAY	THURSDAY	FRIDAY
9:00 am	Sensory Room	Sensory Room	Sensory Room	Sensory Room	Sensory Room
9:00 am – 9:30 am 9:30 am – 9:45 am	Breakfast and Socialization Daily Forum	Breakfast and Socialization Daily Forum	Breakfast and Socialization Daily Forum	Breakfast and Socialization Daily Forum	Breakfast and Socialization Community (Events Planning—last Friday of each month)
9:45 am – 10:45 am	Work Units & Writing Group	Work Units & Current Events Group	Work Units & Education Mentoring	Work Units & Swellness	Work Units & Education Mentoring Group
10:45 am – 11:00 am	Rest Break	Rest Break	Rest Break	Rest Break	Rest Break
11:00 am – 11:45 am	Coping Skills Group	Recovery Group	Advocacy Group and Arts & Crafts	Anger Management Group	Women's Group & Men's Group
11:45 am – 12:30 pm	Lunch and Relaxation	Lunch and Relaxation	Lunch and Relaxation	Lunch and Relaxation	Lunch and Relaxation
12:30 pm – 12:45 pm	Chores	Chores	Chores	Chores	Chores
12:30 pm – 1:00 pm	Health & Fitness Group and Sensory Room	Health & Fitness Group and Sensory Room	Health & Fitness Group and Sensory Room	Health & Fitness Group and Sensory Room	Health & Fitness Group and Sensory Room
1:00 pm – 1:45 pm	Living Well With Disability Group	Socialization Skills Group and Art Group	Advocacy Group and Brain Games Group	Arts & Crafts and Budget Assistance With Kathy	Transitional Employment Group
1:45 pm	Metro Cards & Car Fare	Metro Cards & Car Fare	Metro Cards & Car Fare	Metro Cards & Car Fare	Metro Cards & Car Fare
2:00 pm	Van Ride to RR Station	Van Ride to RR Station	Van Ride to RR Station	Van Ride to RR Station	Van Ride to RR Station

Reprinted with permission of Stony Brook University.

Chapter 16.

SAMPLE WEEKLY SUPERVISOR–STUDENT FEEDBACK FORMS

Compiled by Donna Costa, DHS, OTR/L, FAOTA; Washington University School of Medicine; University of North Dakota; University of Southern California Division of Occupational Science and Occupational Therapy

Washington University School of Medicine
Program in Occupational Therapy

STUDENT/SUPERVISOR WEEKLY REVIEW

Week #: _____ Student: _____ Fieldwork Instructor: _____

STRENGTHS

GROWTH AREAS

GOALS FOR NEXT WEEK

MEETINGS, ASSIGNMENTS DUE, ETC.

Reprinted with permission of the Washington University School of Medicine.

University of North Dakota
Occupational Therapy Student Weekly Review Form

Student Name: _____

Fieldwork Educator Name: _____

Date: _____ Week #: _____

FUNDAMENTALS/BASIC TENETS OF PRACTICE	
Areas of Strength	Areas of Need

EVALUATION AND SCREENING	
Areas of Strength	Areas of Need

INTERVENTION	
Areas of Strength	Areas of Need

MANAGEMENT OF OT SERVICES	
Areas of Strength	Areas of Need

COMMUNICATION/PROFESSIONAL BEHAVIORS	
Areas of Strength	Areas of Need

PROGRESS SUMMARY

Fieldwork Schedule Revisions
Additional Student Support Needed

STUDENT LEARNING GOALS		
Student-Initiated Objectives	**Activities to Achieve Goals**	**Desired Supervisor Support**
1.		
2.		
3.		

Student Signature: _____ Date: _____

Fieldwork Educator Signature: _____ Date: _____

Reprinted with permission of the University of North Dakota.

Level II Fieldwork Weekly Review Meeting

Student Name:

Week of:

What went well this week that you feel good about?

What things did you struggle with in the past week?

What did you learn this week that you did not know before?

What are you able to do now that you couldn't do last week?

What aspects of supervision were helpful to you this week?

What do you need more of from our supervision next week?

What are your goals for next week?

Courtesy of D. Costa.

USC Division of Occupational Science
and Occupational Therapy

Level II Fieldwork 4-Week Evaluation

Student's name: _____

Supervisor's name: _____

Fieldwork site: _____

Date: _____

*Form to be filled out by both student and supervisor
and shared at 4 weeks of the Level II
fieldwork experience.*

1. What is the student *(are you)* doing well in this Level II fieldwork experience (e.g., accurate observations, creative treatment ideas, reliable and prompt, enthusiastic, establishes rapport with both clients and staff)?

2. What aspects of the student's *(your)* performance and/or behavior need to be improved to gain entry-level competency in this setting (e.g., adjust behaviors to match situations, show consistent listening skills, prioritize treatment alternatives, contribute to meetings and supervision, accuracy of assessment skills)?

3. What strategies do you recommend for this student (for *yourself*)?

Reprinted with permission of the University of Southern California.

Chapter 17.

INFUSING "OCCUPATION" IN FIELDWORK ASSIGNMENTS

Denise Chisholm, PhD, OTR/L, FAOTA, and Cathy Dolhi, OTD, OTR/L, FAOTA

Clients are not the only ones who benefit from an occupation-based approach. Try some of these ideas to enhance your students' fieldwork experiences.

Think back. Are the assignments you have your fieldwork students complete the same ones you did as a fieldwork student? Do all fieldwork students at your facility do the same assignments? Is the sole purpose of the assignments to meet the students' learning needs? Do the assignments need to be revised to focus on occupation? If you answered "yes" to any of these questions, read on! We want to stimulate your creative thinking to maximize the use of *occupation* in your students' fieldwork assignments not only to meet the students' learning needs, but also to contribute to your professional needs and your practice.

Baum and Baptiste (2002) defined *occupation-based practice* as "a client-centered approach that makes the individual's need for occupation central to the treatment process and has participation as the outcome" (p. 3). Fisher (2013) further defined *occupation-based interventions* as "those where the occupational therapist uses engagement in occupation as the therapeutic agent of change ..." (p. 164). As occupational therapy practitioners, we recognize the importance of engaging clients in meaningful and relevant occupations to support their achieving health, well-being, and participation in life situations. We need to take that same principle and apply it to fieldwork education. We need to engage our students in meaningful and relevant occupations that facilitate their capacity for professional health, well-being, and participation. In doing so, we also have the potential to contribute to our own professional health as fieldwork educators. Creating student assignments that focus on occupation can help us gain a different perspective and greater appreciation for the unique feature of occupational therapy. Occupation-based fieldwork assignments can enhance our awareness of opportunities for capitalizing on occupation in the services we provide our clients.

Over the past decade, occupation-based practice has resurfaced as a priority in occupational therapy (Aiken, Fourt, Cheng, & Polatajko, 2011; Baum, 2000; Chisholm, Dolhi, & Schreiber, 2000, 2004; Crist, 2003; Dolhi & Chisholm, 2004; Fisher, 2013; Hildenbrand & Lamb, 2013; Piersol, 2002). The *Occupational Therapy Practice Framework: Domain and Process* (3rd ed.; the *Framework;* American Occupational Therapy Association [AOTA], 2014) emphasizes occupational participation and its applications for practitioners and students when providing occupational therapy services. Academicians value and emphasize occupation-based practice for students in the classroom setting. At the same time, we are acutely aware that practitioners are often challenged to provide occupation-based services in settings that are less conducive or supportive of this process. In addition, fieldwork educators are challenged to provide students with an experience that supports occupation-based practice and includes assignments that are meaningful to the student, staff, fieldwork site, and clients.

We know that we are more motivated to succeed and maximize our learning capacity when an experience is meaningful to us. The same is true for our clients and our students. When students are engaged in occupation-based assignments during their fieldwork experiences, the connection between classroom and practice is strengthened. Additionally, the students' contributions can help you develop and provide interventions grounded in occupation.

Intervention Continuum

To put occupation into fieldwork assignments, we first need a foundation that defines and establishes a structure for occupation-based practice. The *Framework* (AOTA, 2014) describes occupational therapy interventions as including, but not limited to, occupations, activities, preparatory methods and tasks, and education and training. The types of interventions outlined in the *Framework* can be ordered similarly to the intervention continuum introduced by Pedretti (1996) and expanded by Chisholm, Dolhi, and Schreiber (2000) for use with people across the lifespan, across health conditions, and across practice settings (Table 17.1).

Although intervention categories are presented sequentially, interventions do not need to be provided in this order, and for some clients, it may be appropriate to omit, skip, or repeat categories. It may not be appropriate or realistic to address each of the categories of the continuum within one intervention session or even within the client's intervention program. The decision of which intervention to include should be made by the practitioner and the client based on an analysis of the client's occupational performance and desired occupations.

"Centering" Fieldwork Assignments

Fisher (2013) suggested that to *be centered* means to put an idea in a central position where it is of primary importance. Fieldwork assignments can be thought of as being either site-centered or student-centered (Dolhi & Chisholm, 2004). Although assignments in both categories present learning opportunities for the student, each has a unique focus.

Site-centered assignments address the needs and specific characteristics of the practice setting. Consequently, they can assist in the student's orientation to the site or may result in information, ideas, or products that can support quality occupational therapy services at that particular site. However, site-centered assignments still benefit the student and directly contribute to his or her knowledge, skills, and clinical reasoning. For example, having the student identify and categorize the assessment tools used in the practice setting within the categories of the intervention continuum provides the facility with a current inventory of tools and gives the student the opportunity to familiarize him- or herself with the tools and to consider which features of occupational performance they address.

Student-centered assignments are more narrowly defined and focus on developing students' skills, knowledge, and clinical reasoning as they relate to the individual clients with whom the student is working. These assignments systematically build on students' academic training with the aim of direct application in preparation for entry-level practice. As a byproduct, you and the other fieldwork site staff may benefit from the student-centered assignment. Examples of site-centered and student-centered assignments are presented later in the chapter.

There is no magic formula to determine whether the student should have more of one type of assignment than another. Most certainly, it is critical to include student-centered assignments that will facilitate the student's focus on learning objectives that relate directly to the clients who have been assigned to the student's caseload. The degree to which site-centered assignments are used is associated with the needs of the site and the occupational therapy staff. For instance, you may find it helpful to use the site-centered approach

Table 17.1. Intervention Continuum

	Description	Examples
Education and Training Interventions	Imparting knowledge and information and facilitating of the acquisition of concrete skills	Being given verbal instruction Reading written materials
Preparatory Method Interventions	Modalities, devices, techniques, products, and technology used to prepare the client for occupational performance	Using physical agent modalities, splints, wheeled mobility, and a weighted vest
Preparatory Task Interventions	Actions used to target specific client factors or performance skills	Performing hand exercises using therapy putty to increase strength Practicing stress management techniques to improve emotion regulation Participating in a sensory diet to regulate attention to tasks
Activity Interventions	Actions that support the development of performance skills and performance patterns necessary to engage in occupations by facilitating practice and problem solving	Practicing dressing using hospital garments Completing a desired craft to improve fine motor skills and sequencing Developing a transportation plan using local bus schedules
Occupation Interventions	Daily life activities that are perceived as desirable, match individualized goals, and occur in appropriate context	Doing own laundry Caring for hair with own supplies Writing a letter to a friend

Note: Categorization of interventions is client specific. For example, an intervention categorized as an activity for one client may be categorized as an occupation for another client.

Adapted from *Occupational Therapy Intervention Resource Manual: A Guide for Occupation-Based Practice* by D. Chisholm, C. Dolhi, & J. Schreiber, 2004, Clifton Park, NY: Thomson Delmar, and "Occupational Therapy Practice Framework: Domain and Process (3rd ed.)," by the American Occupational Therapy Association, 2014, *American Journal of Occupational Therapy, 68,* pp. S1–S48. Adapted with permission.

to supplement or replace direct staff time spent in student orientation. Likewise, you may use these types of assignments to assist you in completing a materials inventory or to identify new options for your evaluation and intervention supplies.

Make a list of the assignments your fieldwork students complete. Are they site-centered or student-centered? As you consider each assignment, a key question for consideration is, does the assignment include an occupation-based component? If not, the majority of fieldwork assignments can be redirected to support occupation-based practice. The list of fieldwork assignments presented in Exhibit 17.1 can be a starting point for reworking your current assignments or creating new ones. Although we have categorized the assignments as either site-centered or student-centered, the majority can be modified to reflect either category.

Exhibit 17.1. *Focusing on Occupation: Site-Centered and Student-Centered Fieldwork Assignments*

Site-Centered Assignments	Student-Centered Assignments
• Practice analysis (population, assessments, and interventions) • Equipment and supplies • Group intervention resources • Intervention kits • Public awareness • Occupation-based library • Research • Advocacy activities	• Recommended readings • Real-life clinical scenarios • Consumer education • Literature review • Journal article leader • Practice analysis (population, assessments, and interventions)

Site-Centered Assignments

A practice analysis can be used to help orient the student to the fieldwork site. In a practice analysis, the student examines the population, assessments, or interventions commonly seen in the practice setting. This assignment helps to familiarize the student with the setting and provides you and your staff with a fresh look at your clients and the evaluation and intervention tools you use in daily practice.

To analyze your client population, have the student identify characteristics such as those listed in Exhibit 17.2. Understanding the demographics of the clients served by your site is critical for implementing occupation-based services. Students also can be asked to categorize the assessment tools and interventions that they observe in practice to determine

Exhibit 17.2. Practice Analysis: Population

- Typical diagnoses or conditions
- Gender distribution
- Age distribution
- Typical occupational roles
- Average duration of services
- Average frequency of services
- Typical disposition destination
- Common reimbursement sources

their relationship to occupation (see Exhibit 17.3). This assignment can help identify possible ways to enhance occupation-based services. A practice analysis template is provided in Appendix 17.A to be copied and used as a worksheet.

Exhibit 17.3. Practice Analysis: Examples of Assessments and Interventions

Examples of Assessments				
Occupations	**Performance Skills**	**Performance Patterns**	**Context and Environment**	**Client Factors**
Performance Assessment of Self-care Skills (Rogers & Holm, 1989)	Motor-Free Visual Perception Test, 3rd edition (Colarusso & Hammill, 2003)	Occupational Role History (Florey & Michelman, 1982)	Accessibility Checklist (Goltsman, Gilbert, & Wohlford, 1992)	Jebsen Hand Function Test (Jebsen et al., 1969)
Canadian Occupational Performance Measure (Law et al., 1998)	Pediatric Evaluation of Disability Inventory (Haley et al., 1992)	Vineland Adaptive Behavior Scales, 2nd edition (Sparrow, Cicchetti, & Balla, 2005)	Work Environment Impact Scale (Moore-Corner, Kielhofner, & Olson, 1998)	Montreal Cognitive Assessment (Nasreddine et al., 2005)

Examples of Interventions				
Education and Training Interventions	**Preparatory Method Interventions**	**Preparatory Task Interventions**	**Activity Interventions**	**Occupation Interventions**
Education materials	Passive range of motion	Upper-extremity exercises	Playing checkers	Preparing cookies for family visitors
Home exercise program handout	Splints	Cognitive worksheets	Role-playing activities	Going on community outing
		Pegboards		Purchasing items from the gift shop

Exhibit 17.4. Group Intervention Template

- Name of group:
- Group topic:
- Purpose:
- Evidence to support the group intervention:
- Goals of intervention:
- Inclusion criteria for participating in the group:
- Condition/criteria that are contraindicated for participating in the group:
- List/description of the specific tasks:
- Materials, supplies, and equipment needed:
- Time-of-day restrictions for conducting the group:
- Duration of the group:
- Location, space, and environmental considerations required for the group:
- Leader responsibilities of the group intervention:
- Other related information:

Another assignment is to have the students conduct an inventory of your equipment and supplies. All equipment and supplies can then be categorized using the intervention continuum—similar to the strategy for the practice analysis assignment. This task offers the student an active role in the orientation to your site, and the completed inventory will help you determine whether you have the necessary items to provide occupation-based services to your specific client population.

Given the required skill of the entry-level practitioner to manage more than one client at a time, requiring students to develop and implement a group is a common fieldwork assignment. However, group interventions developed by students frequently are not implemented by staff because often no tangible record of the session exists—only our recall of what occurred—and we know that re-creating even a good idea takes time. Capitalize on students' creative thinking by having them contribute to your group intervention resources. In addition to being asked to identify an idea, students should establish a protocol that clearly identifies inclusion and exclusion criteria for members; the occupations addressed by the group; and objective, measurable goals for the group. To maximize the potential for the group intervention to be used in the future, students should prepare a list of necessary equipment and supplies, step-by-step instructions with an estimated time frame for completing each step, and any environmental considerations that will contribute to successfully implementing the group intervention.

The specific features included in the "Activity and Occupational Demands" of the *Framework* (AOTA, 2014, p. S32) can serve as an excellent resource for this fieldwork assignment. Having this information in an organized, structured format in a readily accessible location will facilitate the use of occupation-based group intervention that addresses the needs of your clients. Exhibit 17.4 provides items that are beneficial to include in a group intervention template (Chisholm et al., 2004).

After students have completed a thorough demographic analysis of your clients, give them the opportunity to develop intervention kits, which will facilitate efficient implementation of meaningful occupation-based interventions. Having labeled boxes containing all the materials needed for each activity eliminates the need to spend time locating and assembling the items. Activities such as hand sewing, cutting coupons, caring for nails, shaving, applying make-up, wrapping packages, doing carpentry, doing crossword or word search puzzles, and paying bills all lend themselves to being included in intervention kits.

Enhancing public awareness of the value of occupation and the benefit of occupational therapy services is the responsibility of every practitioner. With new ideas and a fresh perspective, your fieldwork students are in an excellent position to create short, memorable phrases that relate to the occupational therapy services provided in your clinic setting. Think about how well "Skills for the job of living" or "Living life to its fullest" sticks with you! This type of tag line or sound bite can be included on all of your printed materials (e.g., handouts, business and appointment cards, letterhead, fax cover sheets, posters, informational materials), computer screen savers, and at the beginning or end of your emails. Regardless of when students participate in fieldwork at your site, use their energy to help you plan activities that you can implement during Occupational Therapy Month in April. Events that focus on occupation and its use as a therapeutic modality will help to enhance others' understanding of the benefits of occupational therapy.

Have students develop an occupation-based library that addresses the occupational needs and profiles of your clients. The library can include a variety of occupation-based resources that will benefit practitioners and students. Students can retrieve, review, and catalog articles, books, videos, and other electronic media that focus on the use of occupation as a therapeutic tool. Students can also use the faculty from their academic program and contacts from other fieldwork experiences to establish a list of people with expertise in a specific area of practice or with a specific population. This assignment will enable students to use their skills in evidence-based practice in combination with what they have learned about your clients to provide you, your staff, and future students with meaningful, readily accessible resources.

Have you and your colleagues wondered about the effectiveness of one particular intervention versus another intervention or been challenged to provide evidence that supports the occupational therapy interventions you provide? Fieldwork students can use their evidence-based practice skills to develop a clinical question relevant to your practice. After the question has been identified, students can be instrumental in establishing a research plan to address it. The project does not have to be completed during a single student's fieldwork experience. After the plan has been outlined, a series of students can contribute to the various aspects of the project (e.g., literature search, study design, study implementation, data collection, data analysis, publication, presentation) with practitioners who are responsible for overseeing it. Work with the faculty of the institutions from which you accept students—they are a great resource and typically welcome these opportunities for collaboration.

It is important for everyone—students, practitioners, and our clients—to develop skills in advocacy. Include advocacy activities in your fieldwork assignment toolbox. Have students identify efforts that promote occupational justice (e.g., collaborating with a community agency to ensure accessibility for their clients; collaborating with clients who have mental illness in the development of materials to raise public awareness of the effect of stigma; participating in an AOTA Hill Day event or writing to their elected official about an issue affecting their clients, fieldwork setting, or profession). Advocacy activities also include promoting and supporting clients' abilities to seek and obtain resources to fully participate in their daily life occupations. Students can develop a group intervention on self-advocacy and empowerment for the clients at their fieldwork setting.

Student-Centered Assignments

Although student-centered assignments may have value for occupational therapy practitioners, they are designed primarily to promote student learning and growth. These assignments provide students with the opportunity to expand their knowledge base within the context of the occupational therapy process through evaluating, planning treatment, and implementing programs for clients assigned to their caseloads.

You, your staff, and the student can identify key readings that will help to facilitate the student's growth and development as an entry-level practitioner and gain knowledge relevant to your practice setting. Recommended readings may be related to the types of clients on the student's caseload or interventions being used or considered. As they read the articles, students should identify critical points that are applicable to a specific client or practice setting. They should then discuss these points and the practice implications with their fieldwork educator and identify an audience or forum in which to present their findings.

Rather than doing a typical case study, which often is descriptive in nature and tends to be formatted following a medical model approach, have the student create a real-life clinical scenario (Chisholm et al., 2004) that incorporates the occupational therapy process outlined in the *Framework* (AOTA, 2014). Have the student review the client's records and gather information relevant to the occupational profile (AOTA, 2014; Crist, 2003). This information is needed to outline a client-centered evaluation and intervention planning process.

Based on knowledge of the client's condition and review of the record, the student can begin to identify assessments to include in the evaluation process. These tools can be categorized using the structure of the *Framework* (AOTA, 2014) so the student gains a greater understanding of what the assessments are designed to measure. For example, range-of-motion and manual muscle testing primarily measure client factors, as does the Jebsen Hand Function Test (Jebsen, Taylor, Trieschmann, Trotter, & Howard, 1969) and the Montreal Cognitive Assessment (Nasreddine et al., 2005). The Motor-Free Visual Perception Test (Colarusso & Hammill, 2003) and Pediatric Evaluation of Disability Inventory (Haley, Coster, Ludlow, Haltiwanger, & Andrellos, 1992) measure performance skills. Client factor and performance skill assessments often overlap, that is, an assessment may measure client factors and performance skills. Additionally, these assessments tend to be associated with the preparatory methods and tasks of the intervention continuum.

In contrast, the Performance Assessment of Self-Care Skills (Rogers & Holm, 1989) and the Canadian Occupational Performance Measure (Law et al., 1998) target occupations that are consistent with the occupation intervention category. As the student gathers information to understand the client's occupational history and experiences, patterns of daily living, interests, values, and needs and administers assessment tools and interprets the data, he or she should be able to develop the client's occupational profile and analysis of occupational performance. The student should then be challenged to identify the client's strengths and problem areas, using *Framework* (AOTA, 2014) terminology. To do so, the student must determine whether the problems are related to occupations, performance skills, performance patterns, contexts and environments, or client factors.

At this point, it is critical to ensure that the client's perspective has been considered and included in the evaluation process. At a minimum, the student should ask the client what occupations he or she needs, wants, and is expected to do in the context of day-to-day life. This information must be considered in combination with other evaluation data, what the client has reported, and what the student knows about the client's condition (e.g., typical course, associated occupational performance deficits, prognosis).

After completing these pieces, the student should have a working knowledge of the client's needs from an occupation perspective and from the client's point of view. The next step is for the student to brainstorm a list of potential interventions that will address the client's concerns and problems while capitalizing on the client's strengths. The list may include interventions that will remediate, restore, maintain, compensate, adapt, or prevent occupational performance problems and that promote health. The student should then critically consider each possible intervention and categorize it in the intervention continuum. Next, the student should organize selected interventions into a realistic, time-defined intervention session, including how much time each intervention will take during the session. A series of sessions can be developed for the client's occupational therapy intervention program. Exhibit 17.5 provides a checklist of the steps for completing a real-life clinical scenario, and a clinical scenario worksheet is provided in Appendix 17.B.

As noted earlier, all occupational therapy practitioners are responsible for enhancing public awareness of the distinct value and benefits of occupation and occupational therapy services. Students should be challenged to develop this skill early on in their careers and can start by providing consumer education to their clients. Having students formulate a definition and explanation of occupational therapy that is relevant to the individual client will help prepare them to articulate this information clearly and concisely throughout their careers.

In her Eleanor Clarke Slagle Lecture, Holm (2000) explored the status of evidence in occupational therapy and the challenges associated with providing intervention that lacks sufficient research. Holm challenged practitioners to search for, read, analyze, and use the evidence in their day-to-day practice. Let your students assist you in pursuing the path of evidence while practicing and refining their skills by completing a literature review. To make the assignment more meaningful,

---

Exhibit 17.5. *Clinical Scenario Checklist*

- Review client records.
- Identify and categorize possible assessment tools using the *Framework.*
- Administer appropriate assessments.
- Develop the occupational profile and analysis of occupational performance.
- Generate a list of the client's strengths and problem areas.
- Identify a list of the occupations, performance skills, client factors, performance patterns, and contexts and environments you anticipate addressing in the client's occupational therapy intervention plan.
- Identify the occupations the client needs, wants, and is expected to perform.
- Brainstorm a list of possible interventions that will address the client's occupational performance deficits and maximize his or her strengths.
- Consider the evidence that supports your intervention list.
- Consider each intervention on your brainstorm list and categorize it in the intervention continuum.
- Plan an occupational therapy intervention session that incorporates selected strategies from your brainstorm list (remember to consider how long the session will run and include an occupation-based component).
- Plan a series of sessions to include in the client's occupational therapy program.

---

have your students identify a clinical question that is related to a specific client or client group on their caseload. Then send the students to explore the literature. They should search, identify relevant studies reflecting the highest levels of evidence, read and analyze the most relevant studies, and present and discuss the findings.

This process can take on the form of a Journal Club, with your fieldwork students taking the role of journal article leader. The student can use the AOTA Journal Club Toolkit as a resource (see http://www.aota.org/practice/researchers/journal-club-toolkit.aspx). The toolkit consists of resources for planning and implementing a journal club, including sample fliers, worksheets, references, critical appraisal guides, a statistical reference sheet, and continuing education documentation. This is a great way to promote lifelong learning for your student and for your staff and to infuse evidence into your practice setting.

The assessment and intervention sections of the site-centered practice analysis can easily be modified to become student centered. Have students analyze the assessments they administer with a specific client. Have them reflect upon the data collected through the evaluation process related to the client's occupations, performance patterns, performance skills, client factors, and contexts and environments. Did the data cluster in one or two areas? Were any areas omitted? Was the focus on occupations, performance patterns, and contexts and environments? If not, how could the focus of the evaluation be on the client's occupations?

Students should then think critically about the interventions they use with a select client, during a day's worth of client sessions or over the course of a week. Have them categorize the interventions using the continuum and assess the degree to which they address their client's desired occupations.

Summary

Our aim has been to provide a starting point for adapting existing or creating new assignments that are focused on occupation for fieldwork students. Have your students read this chapter and identify assignments they feel would be relevant and meaningful for them and your facility or have them create an occupation-based assignment. The goal is to ensure that each student's experience includes meaningful and pertinent assignments focused on occupation. The inclusion of occupation-based assignments in occupational therapy fieldwork can increase the relevance of fieldwork education and, ultimately, enhance the quality of occupational therapy services.

References

Aiken, F. E., Fourt, A. M., Cheng, I. K. S., & Polatajko, H. J. (2011). The meaning gap in occupational therapy: Finding meaning in our own occupation. *Canadian Journal of Occupational Therapy, 78,* 294–302. http://dx.doi.org/10.2182/cjot.2011.78.5.4

American Occupational Therapy Association. (2014). Occupational therapy practice framework: Domain and process (3rd ed.). *American Journal of Occupational Therapy, 68*(Suppl. 1), S1–S48. http://dx.doi.org/10.5014/ajot.2014.682006

Baum, C. (2000, January 3). Occupation-based practice: Reinventing ourselves for the new millennium. *OT Practice, 5*(1), 12–15.

Baum, C., & Baptiste, S. (2002). Reframing occupational therapy practice. In M. Law, C. M. Baum, & S. Baptiste (Eds.), *Occupation-based practice: Fostering performance and participation* (pp. 3–15). Thorofare, NJ: Slack.

Chisholm, D., Dolhi, C., & Schreiber, J. (2000, January 3). Creating occupation-based opportunities in a medical model clinical practice setting. *OT Practice, 5*(1), CE-1–CE-8.

Chisholm, D., Dolhi, C., & Schreiber, J. (2004). *Occupational therapy intervention resource manual: A guide for occupation-based practice.* Clifton Park, NY: Thomson Delmar.

Colarusso, R. P., & Hammill, D. D. (2003). *Motor-Free Visual Perception Test* (3rd ed.). Torrance, CA: Western Psychological Services.

Crist, P. (2003, October 20). Teaching the occupational profile in FW [issues in fieldwork]. *Advance for Occupational Therapy Practitioners, 19*(21), 13.

Dolhi, C., & Chisholm, D. (2004). Putting "occupation" in fieldwork assignments. In D. M. Costa (Ed.), *Essential guide to occupational therapy fieldwork education: Resources for today's educators and practitioners* (pp. 42–47). Bethesda, MD: AOTA Press.

Fisher, A. G. (2013). Occupation-centred, occupation-based, occupation-focused: Same, same or different? *Scandinavian Journal of Occupational Therapy, 20,* 162–173. http://dx.doi.org/10.3109/11038128.2012.754492

Florey, L., & Michelman, S. M. (1982). The Occupational Role History: A screening tool for psychiatric occupational therapy. *American Journal of Occupational Therapy, 36,* 301–308.

Goltsman, S., Gilbert, T., & Wohlford, S. (1992). *The accessibility checklist: An evaluation system for building and outdoor settings.* Berkeley, CA: M.I.G. Communications.

Haley, S. M., Coster, W. J., Ludlow, L. H., Haltiwanger, J. T., & Andrellos, P. J. (1992). *Pediatric Evaluation of Disability Inventory.* San Antonio: Pearson.

Hildenbrand, W. C., & Lamb, A. J. (2013). Health Policy Perspectives—Occupational therapy in prevention and wellness: Retaining relevance in a new health care world. *American Journal of Occupational Therapy, 67,* 266–271. http://dx.doi.org/10.5014/ajot.2013.673001

Holm, M. B. (2000). Our mandate for the new millennium: Evidence-based practice (Eleanor Clarke Slagle Lecture). *American Journal of Occupational Therapy, 54,* 575–585.

Jebsen, R. H., Taylor, N., Trieschmann, R. B., Trotter, M. J., & Howard, L. A. (1969, June). An objective and standardized test of hand function. *Archives of Physical Medicine and Rehabilitation, 50,* 311–319.

Law, M., Baptiste, S., Carswell, A., McColl, M. A., Polatajko, H., & Pollack, N. (1998). *Canadian Occupational Performance Measure* (3rd ed.). Ottawa, Ontario: CAOT Publications.

Moore-Corner, R. A., Kielhofner, G., & Olson, L. (1998). *Work Environment Impact Scale.* University of Illinois at Chicago: Model of Human Occupational Clearinghouse.

Nasreddine, A., Phillips, N., Bédirian, V., Charbonneau, S., Whitehead, V., Collin, I., . . . Chertkow, H. (2005). The Montreal Cognitive Assessment, MoCA: A brief screening test for mild cognitive impairment. *Journal of the American Geriatrics Society, 53,* 695–699.

Pedretti, L. W. (1996). Use of adjunctive modalities in occupational therapy. In R. P. Fleming-Cottrell (Ed.), *Perspectives on purposeful activity: Foundations and future of occupational therapy* (pp. 451–453). Bethesda, MD: American Occupational Therapy Association.

Piersol, C. V. (2002). Weaving occupation into the classroom and fieldwork. *OT Practice, 7*(15), 15–20.

Rogers, J. C., & Holm, M. B. (1989). *Performance Assessment of Self-Care Skills.* Unpublished performance test, University of Pittsburgh [contact OTpitt@shrs.pitt.edu].

Sparrow, S. S., Cicchetti, D. V., & Balla, D. A. (2005). *Vineland Adaptive Behavior Scales* (2nd ed.). San Antonio: Pearson.

Appendix 17.A. Practice Analysis—Population

Consider your primary practice setting and answer the following.

Describe your occupational therapy practice setting.

Identify the typical diagnoses or conditions of your clients.

Identify whether your clients are primarily males or females.

Identify the age range of your clients.

List the typical occupational roles of your clients.

Identify the frequency your clients receive occupational therapy services.

Identify the average duration your clients receive occupational therapy services.

List the typical discharge plans and destinations of your clients.

List the common reimbursement sources for your occupational therapy services.

Practice Analysis: Assessment Tools and Evaluation Strategies

Consider your practice setting. Identify the assessment tools and evaluation strategies you typically use. Categorize each tool and strategy by the area(s) it measures (see following page).

Occupations	Performance Skills	Performance Patterns	Client Factors	Contexts and Environments

Occupations

- Activities of Daily Living

    Bathing, showering, toileting and toilet hygiene, dressing, swallowing/eating, feeding, functional mobility, personal care device, personal hygiene and grooming, sexual activity

- Instrumental Activities of Daily Living

    Care of others (including selecting and supervising caregivers), care of pets, child rearing, communication management, driving and community mobility, financial management, health management and maintenance, home establishment and management, meal preparation and cleanup, religious and spiritual activities and expression, safety procedures and emergency responses, shopping

- Rest and Sleep

    Rest, sleep preparation, sleep participation

- Education

    Formal educational participation, informal personal education needs or interests exploration (beyond formal education), informal personal education participation

- Work

    Employment interests and pursuits, employment seeking and acquisition, job performance, retirement preparation and adjustment, volunteer exploration, volunteer participation

- Play

    Play exploration, play participation

- Leisure

    Leisure exploration, leisure participation

- Social Participation

    Community, family, peer, friend

Performance Skills

- Motor Skills

    Aligns, stabilizes, positions, reaches, bends, grips, manipulates, coordinates, moves, lifts, walks, transports, calibrates, flows, endures, paces

- Process

    Paces, attends, heeds, chooses, uses, handles, inquires, initiates, continues, sequences, terminates, searches/locates, gathers, organizes, restores, navigates, notices/responds, adjusts, accommodates, benefits

- Communication/Interaction Skills

    Approaches/starts, concludes/disengages, produces speech, gesticulates, speaks fluently, turns toward, looks, places self, touches, regulates, questions, replies, discloses, expresses emotion, disagrees, thanks, transitions, times response, times duration, takes turns, matches language, clarifies, acknowledges and encourages, empathizes, heeds, accommodates, benefits

Performance Patterns

- Habits, Routines, Rituals, Roles

Client Factors

- Values, Beliefs, and Spirituality
- Body Functions

    Mental functions; specific mental functions; global mental functions; sensory functions; neuromusculoskeletal and movement-related functions; muscle functions; movement functions; cardiovascular, hematological, immunological, and respiratory system functions; voice and speech functions; digestive, metabolic, and endocrine system functions; genitourinary and reproductive functions; skin and related structure functions

- Body Structures

    Structures of the nervous system; eye, ear, and related structures; structures involved in voice and speech; structures of the cardiovascular, immunological, and respiratory systems; structures of the cardiovascular, immunological, and respiratory systems; structures related to the digestive, metabolic, and endocrine systems; structures related to the genitourinary and reproductive systems; structures related to movement; skin and related structures

Contexts and Environments
- Contexts
- Cultural, personal, temporal, virtual
- Environments
- Physical, social

From "Occupational Therapy Practice Framework: Domain and Process (3rd ed.)," by the American Occupational Therapy Association, 2014, *American Journal of Occupational Therapy, 68,* pp. S1–S48. Copyright © 2014 American Occupational Therapy Association. Reprinted with permission.

Practice Analysis: Interventions

Consider your practice setting. Identify the intervention you typically use. Categorize each intervention by the area(s) it addresses.

Education and Training Interventions	Preparatory Method Interventions	Preparatory Task Interventions	Activity Interventions	Occupation Interventions

Appendix 17.B "Real-Life" Clinical Scenario

Client's name:

Setting:

Diagnosis/condition:

Estimated length of occupational therapy services:

Anticipated discharge plans:

Evaluation:

List information from the client's occupational profile (needs, problems, and concerns about performance in occupations).

Helpful Hint: Use the Client-Centered Interview/Questionnaire on the next page to assist in developing your client's occupational profile.

```



```

List information from the client's analysis of occupational performance (assets and problems or potential problems that support or hinder occupational performance).

```



```

Client-Centered Interview/Questionnaire

Think about the daily activities (occupations) you perform on a typical day and provide 3 to 5 responses to the following:

Daily activities (occupations) I *need* to do:

1.

2.

3.

4.

5.

Daily activities (occupations) I *want* to do:

1.

2.

3.

4.

5.

Daily activities (occupations) I am *expected* to do:

1.

2.

3.

4.

5.

Circle the 5 *most important* daily activities (occupations).

Based on the client's occupational profile and analysis of occupational performance, list occupations, performance skills, performance patterns, client factors, and contexts and environments you plan to address with the client.

Occupations	Performance Skills	Performance Patterns	Client Factors	Contexts and Environments

Intervention Planning

List specific interventions that you plan to include in the client's intervention plan.

Categorize the interventions you identified in the intervention continuum below.

Education and Training Interventions	Preparatory Method Interventions	Preparatory Task Interventions	Activity Interventions	Occupation Interventions

Using the list of interventions you identified, develop a plan for an occupational therapy session for the client.

Helpful Hint: It is not necessary to address all categories of the intervention continuum during a single session; however, the session should facilitate movement toward the occupation intervention category.

Helpful Hint: Identify which of the client's priority daily activities (occupations) will be addressed in the session.

Education and Training Interventions	Preparatory Method Interventions	Preparatory Task Interventions	Activity Interventions	Occupation Interventions

Develop another occupational therapy session for the client. Consider progressing to the next session or to a session that is closer to discharge of occupational therapy services.

Education and Training Interventions	Preparatory Method Interventions	Preparatory Task Interventions	Activity Interventions	Occupation Interventions

Adapted from *Occupational Therapy Intervention Resource Manual: A Guide for Occupation-Based Practice* by D. Chisholm, C. Dolhi, & J. Schreiber, 2004, Clifton Park, NY: Thomson Delmar, and "Occupational Therapy Practice Framework: Domain and Process (3rd ed.)," by the American Occupational Therapy Association, 2014, *American Journal of Occupational Therapy, 68,* pp. S1–S48. Adapted with permission.

Part 4.

POLICIES AFFECTING FIELDWORK

OVERVIEW OF PART 4

Donna Costa, DHS, OTR/L, FAOTA

Many policies affect fieldwork education, and academic fieldwork coordinators and fieldwork educators must be familiar with them and have a way of tracking any changes that occur in these policies.

Chapter 18 is of critical importance, as it contains the "OT/OTA Student Supervision and Medicare Requirements." Fieldwork sites that bill Medicare for patient care services need to pay close attention to this document because it limits the services that students can provide. The limits on student services differ based on the type of Medicare reimbursement (Part A or B) and the type of setting (e.g., skilled nursing facility, hospice, inpatient, outpatient). Because Medicare reimbursement guidelines change, fieldwork educators and academic fieldwork coordinators should check the AOTA website frequently to stay updated.

Chapter 19 contains an official AOTA document, "Practice Advisory: Services Provided by Students in Fieldwork Level II Settings," which states that the American Occupational Therapy Association (AOTA) considers Level II fieldwork students as providing skilled therapy intervention when they provide services under the supervision of a qualified occupational therapist or occupational therapy assistant, provided they follow certain principles.

Each state has established its own regulatory board and regulations governing the practice of occupational therapy. Chapter 20 contains the "State Occupational Therapy Statutes, Regulations, and Board Guidance: Occupational Therapy Students," compiled by AOTA state policy staff. Because changes frequently occur in each state regarding licensure, fieldwork educators and academic fieldwork coordinators need to frequently check the AOTA website and their own states' regulatory boards for up-to-date information.

Policies regarding confidentiality for both clients and students are vital in the health care environment in which we work. Chapter 21 contains information on both the Healthcare Insurance Portability and Accountability Act (HIPAA) and the Family Educational Rights and Privacy Act (FERPA). The last chapter in this section contains the *2011 Accreditation Council for Occupational Therapy Education (ACOTE®) Standards*. These standards are divided into sections for both OT and OTA programs and cover the educational requirements at the associate-degree, master's-degree, and doctoral-degree levels.

Chapter 18.

OT/OTA STUDENT SUPERVISION AND MEDICARE REQUIREMENTS

American Occupational Therapy Association

Historically, occupational therapy (OT) and occupational therapy assistant (OTA) students have participated in the delivery of occupational therapy services under the supervision of occupational therapy personnel in a variety of fieldwork sites. The following provides information about the way in which the Centers for Medicare and Medicaid Services (CMS) interpret how and whether the Medicare program should provide payment for services provided by students.

In the article "Strategies for Creative Fieldwork Opportunities," the American Occupational Therapy Association's (AOTA's) Academic Affairs, Federal Affairs, Practice, and Reimbursement and Regulatory Policy staff provide guidance for occupational therapy programs, fieldwork sites, and facilities (AOTA, n.d.).

For those settings that serve Medicare patients, it is important to be aware of both new and existing Medicare payment policies. CMS has published specific criteria regarding how and when the program will pay for services when students participate in service delivery. When developing fieldwork plans for sites that serve Medicare patients, two issues must be considered:

1. Whether Medicare payment rules specifically allow students to participate in the delivery of services to Medicare beneficiaries, and
2. What type and level of supervision are required by the Medicare program.

All relevant Medicare coverage criteria must be reviewed if reimbursement is sought for services when the student participates in service delivery. In addition, many state practice acts and regulations address occupational therapy services provided by students. You can find the regulatory board contact information on the State-by-State OT Law Database located in the Licensure section of the AOTA website. For details regarding AOTA's position on Level II fieldwork, please see the document Practice Advisory: Services

The following chart sets out for each Medicare setting whether Medicare payment rules specifically allow or restrict coverage of services provided by students and what type and level of supervision Medicare requires to raise the services provided by students to the level of covered "skilled" occupational therapy. Practitioners should take care to ensure an appropriate level of supervision, whether or not a specific CMS rule regarding students has been issued.

Medicare Coverage of Services When a Student Participates in Service Delivery

- Medicare Part A—*Hospital and inpatient rehabilitation*
  Type and Level of Student Supervision Required:
  CMS has not issued specific rules, but in the excerpt here referencing skilled nursing facilities (SNFs), CMS mentions other inpatient settings. In the Final SNF PPS Rule for FY 2012 (76 Fed. Reg. 48510-48511), CMS stated: *"We are hereby discontinuing the policy announced in the FY 2000 final rule's preamble requiring line-of-sight supervision of therapy students in SNFs, as set forth in the FY 2012 proposed rule. Instead, effective October 1, 2011,* **as with other inpatient settings, each SNF/provider will determine for itself the appropriate manner of supervision of therapy students consistent with state and local laws and practice standards."** See relevant state law for further guidance on supervision for the services to be considered occupational therapy.

- Medicare Part A—*SNF*
  Type and Level of Student Supervision Required:
  The minutes of therapy services provided by OT and OTA students may be recorded on the MDS as minutes of therapy received by the beneficiary. Before October 1, 2011, services of OT and OTA students had to be provided in the "line of sight" of the OT. OTAs could provide clinical supervision to OTA students; however, if the services were to be recorded for payment purposes, they had to be performed in "line of sight" of an OT.

  CURRENT POLICY: Effective October 1, 2011, line-of-sight supervision is no longer required in the SNF setting (76 Fed. Reg. 48510-48511). The time the student spends with a patient will continue to be billed as if it were the supervising therapist alone providing the therapy, meaning that a therapy student's time is not separately reimbursable. See the *RAI Manual for the Minimum Data Set, Version 3.0 (MDS 3.0 RAI Manual),* Chapter 3, Section O Therapies for more details and examples (http://www.cms.gov/Medicare/Quality-Initiatives-Patient-Assessment-Instruments/NursingHomeQuality-

Inits/MDS30RAIManual.html). According to the *MDS 3.0 RAI Manual,* supervising therapists and therapy assistants within individual facilities must determine whether or not a student is ready to treat patients without line-of-sight supervision. The supervising therapist or assistant may not be engaged in any other activity or treatment, with the exception of documenting. It is AOTA's policy that OTAs may supervise OTA students, not OT students.

  - **Because of advocacy by AOTA, CMS has posted Recommended Guidelines by AOTA, APTA, and ASHA on its SNF PPS website:** https://www.cms.gov/Medicare/Medicare-Fee-for-Service-Payment/SNFPPS/Spotlight.html (see "Student Supervision Guidelines" under "Downloads"). AOTA, APTA, and ASHA worked together to develop suggested guidelines for CMS to incorporate into its guidance on student supervision. CMS recognized the guidelines and posted them on its website. In the final rule, CMS stated, "we appreciate the detailed supervision guidelines that several of the trade associations have developed, which we recognize as playing a significant role in helping to define the applicable standards of practice on which providers rely in this context."

Recommended Skilled Nursing Facility Therapy Student Supervision Guidelines Submitted to CMS by the American Occupational Therapy Association (AOTA) During the Comment Period for the FY 2012 SNF PPS Final Rule

Please note, these suggested guidelines would be in addition to the student supervision guidelines outlined in the *RAI MDS 3.0 Manual* and All Relevant Federal Regulations

- The amount and type of supervision as determined by the supervising therapist/assistant must be appropriate to the student's documented level of knowledge, experience, and competence.
- Students who have been approved by the supervising therapist or assistant to practice independently in selected patient/client situations can perform those selected patient/client services without line-of-sight supervision by the supervising therapist/assistant.

- The supervising therapist/assistant must be physically present in the facility and immediately available to provide observation, guidance, and feedback as needed when the student is providing services at all levels of supervision.
- When the supervising therapist has approved the student to perform medically necessary patient/client services and the student provides the appropriate services, the services will be counted on the MDS as skilled therapy minutes.
- The supervising therapist/assistant is required to review and sign all students' patient/client documentation for all levels of clinical experience and retains full responsibility of care of the patient/client.
- The supervising therapist/assistant is required to have 1 year of practice experience prior to supervising any students.
- Students who have not been approved by the supervising therapist/assistant to practice independently require line-of-sight supervision by the qualified therapist/assistant during all services. In addition, under these circumstances the supervising therapist/assistant will have direct contact with the patient/client during each visit.

- **Medicare Part A—*Hospice***
  Type and Level of Student Supervision Required: CMS has not issued specific rules. AOTA is recommending that the approach for Part A inpatient settings be followed for hospice providers. See relevant state law for further guidance on supervision for the services to be considered occupational therapy.

- **Medicare Part A—*Home health***
  Type and Level of Student Supervision Required: Regulations (§484.115) specifically cite definitions for "qualified personnel," which do not include students. However, CMS has not issued specific restrictions regarding students providing services in conjunction with a qualified OT or OTA. Services by students can be provided (as allowed by state law) as part of a home health visit, when the student is supervised by an OT or OTA in the home. AOTA is recommending that the approach for Part A inpatient settings be followed for home health agencies. See relevant state law for further guidance on supervision for the services to be considered occupational therapy.

- **Medicare Part B—*Private practice, hospital outpatient, SNF, CORF, ORF, rehabilitation agency, and other Part B providers including home health agencies when providing Part B services***
  Type and Level of Student Supervision Required: Under the Medicare Part B outpatient benefit, the services of students directly assisting a qualified practitioner (OT) are covered when the type and level of supervision requirements are met as follows: Students can participate in the delivery of services when the qualified practitioner (OT) is directing the service, making the skilled judgment, responsible for the assessment and treatment in the same room as the student, and not simultaneously treating another patient. The qualified practitioner is solely responsible and must sign all documentation.

For details about current student supervision guidelines that affect Part B in SNFs in particular, see http://aota.org/News/AdvocacyNews/SNF-Students.aspx?FT=.pdf.

Following is guidance to the entities that pay for Medicare benefits contained in the *Medicare Benefit Policy Manual, Chapter 15*—see Section 230B:

1. General
Only the services of the therapist can be billed and paid under Medicare Part B. The services performed by a student are not reimbursed even if provided under "line of sight" supervision of the therapist; however, the presence of the student "in the room" does not make the service unbillable. Pay for the direct (one-to-one) patient contact services of the physician or therapist provided to Medicare Part B patients. Group therapy services performed by a therapist or physician may be billed when a student is also present "in the room."

EXAMPLES:
Therapists may bill and be paid for the provision of services in the following scenarios:
- The qualified practitioner is present and in the room for the entire session. The student participates in the delivery of services when the qualified practitioner is directing the service,

making the skilled judgment, and is responsible for the assessment and treatment.

- The qualified practitioner is present in the room guiding the student in service delivery when the therapy student and the therapy assistant student are participating in the provision of services, and the practitioner is not engaged in treating another patient or doing other tasks at the same time.

- The qualified practitioner is responsible for the services and as such, signs all documentation. (A student may, of course, also sign, but it is not necessary because the Part B payment is for the clinician's service, not for the student's services.)

AOTA continues to work with a coalition of practitioner organizations to advocate for additional government support for education of allied health providers and to develop long-term solutions to the problems caused by Medicare's limitations on reimbursement when students participate in service delivery.

Reference

American Occupational Therapy Association. (n.d.) *Strategies for creative fieldwork opportunities*. Retrieved from http://www .aota.org/education-careers/fieldwork/newprograms/strate gies.aspx

Reprinted from http://www.aota.org/-/media/Corporate/Files/ Secure/Advocacy/Reimb/Coverage/ot-ota-student-medicare-requirements.pdf

Chapter 19.

PRACTICE ADVISORY: SERVICES PROVIDED BY STUDENTS IN FIELDWORK LEVEL II SETTINGS

American Occupational Therapy Association

Level II fieldwork students may provide occupational therapy services under the supervision of a qualified occupational therapist or occupational therapy assistant in compliance with state and federal regulations. When adhering to the principles stated below, along with other regulatory and payer requirements, the American Occupational Therapy Association (AOTA) considers that students at this level of education are providing skilled occupational therapy intervention.

General Principles

a. Supervision of occupational therapy and occupational therapy assistant students in fieldwork Level II settings should ensure protection of consumers and provide opportunities for appropriate role modeling of occupational therapy practice.

b. To ensure safe and effective occupational therapy services, it is the responsibility of the supervising occupational therapist and occupational therapy assistant to recognize when supervision is needed and ensure that supervision supports the student's current and developing levels of competence with the occupational therapy process.

c. In all cases the occupational therapist is ultimately responsible for all aspects of occupational therapy service delivery and is accountable for the safety and effectiveness of the occupational therapy service delivery process. This would include provision of services provided by an occupational therapy assistant student under the supervision of an occupational therapy assistant (see Addendum 1).

d. Initially, supervision should be in line of sight and gradually decrease to less direct supervision as is appropriate depending on the (Accreditation Council for Occupational Therapy Education [ACOTE®], 2007a, b, & c):
- Competence and confidence of the student,
- Complexity of client needs,
- Number and diversity of clients,
- Role of occupational therapy and related services,
- Type of practice setting,
- Requirements of the practice setting, and
- Other regulatory requirements.

In settings where occupational therapy practitioners[1] are employed:

- Occupational therapy students should be supervised by an occupational therapist.
- Occupational therapy assistant students should be supervised by an occupational therapist or occupational therapy assistant in partnership with an occupational therapist.

In settings where occupational therapy practitioners are not employed:

- Students should be supervised by another professional familiar with the role of occupational therapy in collaboration with an occupational therapy practitioner.

References

Accreditation Council for Occupational Therapy Education. (2007a). Accreditation standards for a doctoral-degree-level educational program for the occupational therapist. *American Journal of Occupational Therapy, 61,* 641–651. http://dx.doi.org/10.5014/ajot.61.6.641

Accreditation Council for Occupational Therapy Education. (2007b). Accreditation standards for a master's-degree-level educational program for the occupational therapist. *American Journal of Occupational Therapy, 61,* 652–661. http://dx.doi.org/10.5014/ajot.61.6.652

Accreditation Council for Occupational Therapy Education. (2007c). Accreditation standards for an educational program for the occupational therapy assistant. *American Journal of Occupational Therapy, 61,* 662–671. http://dx.doi.org/10.5014/ajot.61.6.662

American Occupational Therapy Association. (2006). Policy 1.44: Categories of occupational therapy personnel. In *Policy manual* (2009 ed., pp. 33–34). Bethesda, MD: Author

American Occupational Therapy Association. (2009). Guidelines for supervision, roles, and responsibilities during the delivery of occupational therapy services. *American Journal of Occupational Therapy, 63,* 797–803. http://dx.doi.org/10.5014/ajot.63.6.797

Prepared by:

Commission on Practice and Commission on Education Joint Task Force
September, 2010.

Deborah Ann Amini, EdD, OTR/L, CHT
Janet V. DeLany, DEd, OTR/L, FAOTA
Debra J. Hanson, PhD, OTR
Susan M. Higgins, MA, OTR/L
Jeanette M. Justice, COTA/L
Linda Orr, MPA, OTR/L

Addendum 1: Supervision Requirements and Responsibilities for Occupational Therapy Assistant Students During the Delivery of Occupational Therapy Services.

The American Occupational Therapy Association (AOTA) asserts that occupational therapy assistants can provide supervision to occupational therapy assistant students completing Level II fieldwork experiences. The following recommendations have been developed to ensure the delivery of safe and effective occupation therapy services and appropriate supervisory requirements:

- ACOTE Standards (ACOTE, 2007) indicate that an occupational therapy assistant with a minimum of 1-year professional experience is qualified to be the fieldwork educator in order to teach and assess the skills of the occupational therapy assistant student.

And,

- The purpose of the Level II fieldwork experience is to provide the student with the opportunity to enact the occupational therapy skills that they have been taught during the didactic portion of their occupational therapy assistant training program.

And,

- The occupational therapy assistant is equipped to role model the skills and behaviors of his or her level of practice while interacting with the occupational therapy assistant student in the clinic setting.

And,

- The occupational therapy assistant possesses skills and knowledge of practice fundamentals that include: professional behaviors, interpersonal skills, safety, ethics, documentation, occupational therapist/occupational therapy assistant collaborative relationship, implementing a treatment plan, and delegated assessments.

---

[1]When the term *occupational therapy practitioner* is used in this document, it refers to both occupational therapists and occupational therapy assistants (AOTA, 2006).

And,

- The licensure laws governing the practice of occupational therapy of many states allow the occupational therapy assistant to supervise the occupational therapy assistant student as a fieldwork educator.

And,

- In all cases the occupational therapist is ultimately responsible for all aspects of occupational therapy service delivery and is accountable for the safety and effectiveness of the occupational therapy service delivery process. This would include provision of services provided by an occupational therapy assistant student under the supervision of an occupational therapy assistant.

And,

- The level of supervision including the need for "line of sight" should be at the discretion of the occupational therapist and occupational therapy assistant consulting together to determine the student's competence, needs of the client, setting, and other variables delineated above.

And,

- Co-signatures of the supervising occupational therapy assistant and/or occupational therapist on documentation indicates that the occupational therapy assistant student is provided with the appropriate level of supervision and is deemed competent to perform documented therapeutic intervention.

And,

- When a student provides skilled occupational therapy services under the supervision of a qualified practitioner, those services are billed as services provided by the supervising licensed occupational therapy practitioner.

And,

- An occupational therapist would offer the occupational therapy assistant student the opportunity to observe the process of client evaluation, development and modification of a treatment plan, and specific interventions that are within the scope of practice for an occupational therapist, or in which an occupational therapist has specialty training. These additional learning opportunities are beneficial but may not be representative of entry level occupational therapy assistant practice.

Therefore,

- An occupational therapy assistant, under the appropriate supervision of an occupational therapist, and in accordance with applicable state and federal regulations, who has a minimum of 1-year clinical experience and who has demonstrated competence as a practitioner and a fieldwork educator should be allowed to supervise an occupational therapy assistant student during Level II fieldwork.

Reference

Accreditation Council for Occupational Therapy Education. (2007). Accreditation standards for an educational program for the occupational therapy assistant. *American Journal of Occupational Therapy, 61,* 662–671. http://dx.doi.org/10.5014/ajot.61.6.662

Reprinted from http://www.aota.org/-/media/Corporate/Files/EducationCareers/Educators/Fieldwork/StuSuprvsn/Practice%20Advisory%20Services%20provided%20by%20students%20in%20FW%20Level%20II%20final.pdf

Chapter 20.

STATE OCCUPATIONAL THERAPY STATUTES, REGULATIONS, AND BOARD GUIDANCE: OCCUPATIONAL THERAPY STUDENTS

American Occupational Therapy Association

State	Statute	Regulation (plus Board Guidance[1] if applicable)	URL
Alabama	Section 34-39-5 Exceptions. Nothing in this chapter shall be construed as preventing or restricting the practice, services, or activities of any of the following persons: (3) Any person pursuing a course of study leading to a degree or certificate in occupational therapy at an accredited or approved educational program if the activities and services constitute a part of a supervised course of study, if the person is designated by a title that clearly indicates his or her status as a student or trainee. (4) Any person fulfilling the supervised fieldwork experience requirements of subdivision (2) of Section 34-39-8. (Acts 1990, No. 90-383, p. 515, §5; Acts 1995, No. 95-279, p. 502, §3.)	625-X-2-.01 Exemptions Code of Alabama 1975, §34-39-5 provides that certain persons may be exempt from the licensure requirements of the Alabama State Occupational Therapy Practice Act. In determining whether a person is exempt from obtaining a license, the following shall apply: 625-X-2-.01 Exemptions. The requirement for a license as an Occupational Therapist or an Occupational Therapy Assistant does not apply to a person who is: (c) Pursuing a course of study leading to a degree or certificate in occupational therapy at an accredited or approved educational program, provided that any occupational therapy activities and services are part of the supervised course of study and the person is wearing a badge or other emblem designating by title the fact that such person is a student or trainee and not a licensed Occupational Therapist or Occupational Therapy Assistant. (d) Fulfilling the supervised fieldwork experience requirements provided that such activities and services constitute a part of the experience necessary to meet the requirements of the educational program.	**Statute** http://www.ot.alabama.gov/code.htm **Regulation** http://www.ot.alabama.gov/rules.htm#CHAPTER_625-X-2

---

[1]A number of state occupational therapy entities address student issues through policy statements and/or guidance posted on state websites. These provisions are included after regulatory text if applicable.

Note: This chart reflects statutory, regulatory, and other board provisions that specifically provide guidance on the supervision or license exempt status of students. States that do not specifically mention students in the statutory or regulatory definition of supervision are not included in the chart, as it is unclear as to whether these states apply supervision definitions to students.
Website addresses and other information included in this chapter may be out of date.

State	Statute	Regulation (plus Board Guidance if applicable)	URL
Alaska	Sec. 08.84.150. Exceptions to license requirements. (b) A person may not provide services that the person describes as occupational therapy without being licensed under this chapter unless the person is (1) a student in an accredited occupational therapy program or in a super-vised fieldwork program; (2) a graduate of a foreign school of occupational therapy fulfilling the internship requirement of AS 08.84.032, and then only unless under the continuous direction and immediate supervision of an occupational therapist.	12 AAC 54.620. SUPERVISED FIELD WORK. As used in AS 08.84.030(b)(2), "supervised fieldwork" means experience that is part of the educational program completed by the applicant under the supervision of a licensed occupational therapist. If the training occurred in a state that does not require licensure, the supervising occupational therapist must be certified by the National Board for Certification in Occupational Therapy (NBCOT). Supervised fieldwork must include, (1) for occupational therapists, at least two three-month internships and shall provide for the development of skills in data col-lection, treatment planning, and treatment implementation; and (2) for occupational therapy assistants, at least one two-month internship.	**Statute and Regulation** http://www. commerce. state.ak.us/ occ/pub/ PT-OTStat utes.pdf
Arizona	32-3422. Persons and practices not required to be licensed. This chapter does not prevent or restrict the practice, services, or activities of: (4) A person pursuing a super-vised course of study leading to a degree or certificate in occupational therapy at an accredited or approved educa-tional program pursuant to section 32-3404, if the person is designated by a title that clearly indicates the person's status as a student or trainee. (5) A person fulfilling the supervised fieldwork experi-ence requirements of section 32-3423, if the experience constitutes a part of the fieldwork experience nec-essary to meet the require-ments of section 32-3423.	Not Available	**Statute** http://www. azleg.gov/ FormatDocu ment.asp?in Doc=/ars/32/ 03422. htm&Ti tle=32&Doc Type=ARSh **Regulation** http://www.az sos.gov/public services/ Title_ 04/4-43. htm
Arkansas	17-88-103. Exceptions. Nothing in this chapter shall be construed as preventing or restricting the practice, services, or activities of: (3) Any person pursuing a course of study leading to a degree or certificate in occupational therapy at an	Not Available	**Statute** http://www. armedical board.org/ professionals/ pdf/MPA.pdf

State	Statute	Regulation (plus Board Guidance if applicable)	URL
	accredited or approved educational program, if such activities and services constitute a part of a supervised course of study and if such a person is designated by a title that clearly indicates his or her status as a student or trainee.		
California	Nothing in this chapter shall be construed as preventing or restricting the practice, services, or activities of any of the following persons: (a) Any person licensed or otherwise recognized in this state by any other law or regulation when that person is engaged in the profession or occupation for which he or she is licensed or otherwise recognized. (b) Any person pursuing a supervised course of study leading to a degree or certificate in occupational therapy at an accredited educational program, if the person is designated by a title that clearly indicates his or her status as a student or trainee. (c) Any person fulfilling the supervised fieldwork experience requirements of subdivision (c) of Section 2570.6, if the experience constitutes a part of the experience necessary to meet the requirement of that provision. (d) Any person performing occupational therapy services in the state if all of the following apply: (1) An application for licensure as an occupational therapist or an occupational therapy assistant has been filed with the board pursuant to Section 2570.6 and an application for a license in this state has not been previously denied. (2) The person possesses a current, active, and	§ 4180. Definitions In addition to the definitions found in Business and Professions Code sections 2570.2 and 2570.3, the following terms are used and defined herein: (b) "Level I student" means an occupational therapy or occupational therapy assistant student participating in activities designed to introduce him or her to fieldwork experiences and develop an understanding of the needs of clients. (c) "Level II student" means an occupational therapy or occupational therapy assistant student participating in delivering occupational therapy services to clients with the goal of developing competent, entry-level practitioners. § 4181. Supervision Parameters (a) Appropriate supervision of an occupational therapy assistant includes, at a minimum: (1) The weekly review of the occupational therapy plan and implementation and periodic onsite review by the supervising occupational therapist. The weekly review shall encompass all aspects of occupational therapy services and be completed by telecommunication or on site. (2) Documentation of the supervision, which shall include either documentation of direct client care by the supervising occupational therapist, documentation of review of the client's medical and/or treatment record and the occupational therapy services provided by the occupational therapy assistant, or co-signature of the occupational therapy assistant's documentation. (3) The supervising occupational therapist shall be readily available in person or by telecommunication to the occupational therapy assistant at all times while the occupational therapy assistant is providing occupational therapy services. (4) The supervising occupational therapist shall provide periodic on-site supervision and observation of client care rendered by the occupational therapy assistant.	**Statute** http://www. leginfo. ca.gov/cgi-bin/dis playcode?sec tion=bpc&g roup=0200 1-03000&fi le=2570-2571 **Regulation** http://www. bot.ca.gov/ board_activi ty/laws_regs/ cc_regula tions.shtml **CA Board of OT FAQs regarding students:** http://www. bot.ca.gov/ forms_pubs/ students_faqs. shtml

State	Statute	Regulation (plus Board Guidance if applicable)	URL
	nonrestricted license to practice occupational therapy under the laws of another state that the board determines has licensure requirements at least as stringent as the requirements of this chapter. (3) Occupational therapy services are performed in association with an occupational therapist licensed under this chapter, and for no more than 60 days from the date on which the application for licensure was filed with the board. (e) Any person employed as an aide subject to the supervision requirements of this section.	(b) The supervising occupational therapist shall at all times be responsible for all occupational therapy services provided by an occupational therapy assistant, a limited permit holder, a student, or an aide. The supervising occupational therapist has continuing responsibility to follow the progress of each client, provide direct care to the client, and ensure that the occupational therapy assistant, limited permit holder, student, or aide do not function autonomously. (c) The level of supervision for all personnel is determined by the supervising occupational therapist whose responsibility it is to ensure that the amount, degree, and pattern of supervision are consistent with the knowledge, skill, and ability of the person being supervised. (d) Occupational therapy assistants may supervise: (1) Level I occupational therapy students; (2) Level I and Level II occupational therapy assistant students; and (3) Aides providing non–client-related tasks. (e) The supervising occupational therapist shall determine that the occupational therapy practitioner possesses a current license, certificate, or permit to practice occupational therapy prior to allowing the person to provide occupational therapy services. § 4183. Treatments Performed by Occupational Therapy Limited Permit Holders and Students (a) Consistent with Code section 2570.4, subdivisions (b) and (c), a Level II student may, at the discretion of the supervising occupational therapy practitioner, be assigned duties or functions commensurate with his or her education and training. (c) All documented client-related services by the limited permit holder or student shall be reviewed and cosigned by the supervising occupational therapist. **CA Board of OT—FAQs regarding students:** **Q. What kind of services can I provide?** **A.** Title 16, Division 39, California Code of Regulations (CCR) Section 4183(a) allows Level II students to be assigned duties or functions commensurate with their education and training. NOTE: You and/or your supervisor should be aware of fiscal intermediary requirements regarding students.	

State	Statute	Regulation (plus Board Guidance if applicable)	URL
		Q. How often must the OT services I provide be reviewed by my supervising OT? **A.** Supervision may vary by practice setting and be dependent upon the: • Complexity of client needs, • Number and diversity of clients, • Competencies of the student, • Type of practice setting, • Requirements of the practice setting, and • Other regulatory requirements. Business and Professions Code (BPC) Section 2570.4(b) also requires that you be designated by a title that clearly indicates that you are a student or trainee. California Code of Regulations (CCR) Section 4183(b) also requires that "all documented client-related services by … a student shall be reviewed and cosigned by the supervising occupational therapist."	
Colorado	12-40.5-108. Scope of article—exclusions. (1) This article shall not prevent or restrict the practice, services, or activities of: (a) A person licensed or otherwise regulated in this state by any other law from engaging in his or her profession or occupation as defined in the article under which he or she is licensed; (b) A person pursuing a course of study leading to a degree in occupational therapy at an educational institution with an accredited occupational therapy program if that person is designated by a title that clearly indicates his or her status as a student and if he or she acts under appropriate instruction and supervision.	Not Available	**Statute** http://www.dora.state.co.us/occupational-therapists/index.htm

State	Statute	Regulation (plus Board Guidance if applicable)	URL
Connecticut	Sec. 20-74e. Exempt activities. (a) Nothing in this chapter shall be construed as preventing or restricting the practice, services, or activities of: (3) any person pursuing a course of study leading to a degree or certificate in occupational therapy at an accredited or approved educational program if such activities and services constitute part of a supervised course of study and if such person is designated by a title that clearly indicates his or her status as a student or trainee.	Not Available	**Statute** http://www. ct.gov/dph/ LIB/dph/pra ctitioner_lic ensing_and_ investigations/ plis/occupa tional_thera pist/ot_ota_ stats.pdf
Delaware	2009. Applicability of chapter. Nothing in this chapter shall be construed as preventing or restricting the practice, services, or activities of: (2) Any person pursuing a course of study leading to a degree or certificate in occu-pational therapy at an accred-ited or approved educational program if such activities and services constitute a part of a supervised course of study and if such a person is des-ignated by a title that clearly indicates that person's status as a student or trainee.	Not Available	**Statute** http:// delcode. delaware.gov/ title24/c020/ sc02/index. shtml **Regulation** http://regula tions.dela ware.gov/ AdminCode/ title24/2000. shtml
District of Columbia	Not Available	6309.6 An occupational therapist shall: (a) Directly supervise all students training to be occupational therapists or occupational therapy assistants; (b) Not permit a student to work independently with a client until such time as the student has demonstrated competency in practice under general supervision; and (c) Countersign all documentation drafted by students.	**Statute** http://hpla. doh.dc.gov/ hpla/frames. asp?doc=/ hpla/lib/hpla/ hora/hora_8- 5-09.pdf

State	Statute	Regulation (plus Board Guidance if applicable)	URL
		An occupational therapy assistant may directly supervise occupational therapy assistant students. An occupational therapist or occupational therapy assistant supervising a student shall be responsible for all of the actions performed by the student within the scope of practice during the time of supervision and shall be subject to disciplinary action for any violation of the Act or this chapter by the person supervised.	**Regulation** http://hpla. doh.dc.gov/ hpla/frames. asp?doc=/ hpla/lib/hpla/ occupational_ therapy/ot_ updated_ 03-14-08.pdf
Florida	468.225 Exemptions. (1) Nothing in this act shall be construed as preventing or restricting the practice, services, or activities of: (c) Any person pursuing a course of study leading to a degree or certificate in occupational therapy at an accredited or approved educational program, if such activities and services constitute a part of a supervised course of study and if such a person is designated by a title that clearly indicates his or her status as a student or trainee.	64B11-2.011 Definition of Supervised Fieldwork Experience. The term "supervised fieldwork experience" as provided for in Section 468.209(1)(c), F.S., shall mean experience at an occupational therapist level occurring in a clinical setting affiliated with an educational institution in occupational therapy for a minimum of at least 6 months, with the fieldwork experience supervised by a licensed occupational therapist. Supervision, for purposes of this rule, shall mean that the occupational therapist student has daily direct contact at the work site with his or her supervisor.	**Statute** http://www. leg.state.fl.us/ statutes/index. cfm?App_ mode=Disp lay_Statute& Search_String =&URL=Ch 0468/ SEC225. HTM&Title= -%3E2009- %3ECh0468- %3ESection %20225 #0468.225 **Regulation** https://www. flrules.org/ gateway/Rule No.asp?title =ADMISSI ON%20OF %20OCCUP ATIONALT HERAPISTS &ID=64B11- 2.011
Georgia	43-28-15. Exceptions to operation of chapter: Nothing in this chapter shall be construed as preventing or restricting the practice, services, or activities of: (3) Any person pursuing a course of study leading to a degree or certificate in occupational therapy in an	Not Available	**Statute** http://sos.geo rgia.gov/acro bat/PLB/ laws/ 14_Oc cupational_ Therapists_ 43-28.pdf

State	Statute	Regulation (plus Board Guidance if applicable)	URL
	educational program that is accredited by a recognized accrediting agency acceptable to the board and if such person is designated by a title that clearly indicates such person's status as a student or trainee; (5) Any person enrolled in a course of study designed to develop advanced occupational therapy skills when the occupational therapy activities are required as part of an educational program sponsored by an educational institution approved by the board and conducted under the supervision of an occupational therapist licensed under this chapter. If such person provides occupational therapy services outside the scope of the educational program, he shall then be required to be licensed in accordance with this chapter.		**Regulation** http://rules. sos.state.ga. us/docs/671/ 2/03.pdf
Hawaii	Not Available	Not Available	**Statute and Regulation** http://hawaii. gov/dcca/pvl/ pvl/hrs/hrs_ pvl_457g.pdf
Idaho	54-3704. Exemptions. Nothing in this chapter shall be construed as preventing or restricting the practice, services, or activities or requiring licensure pursuant to this chapter of: (3) Any person pursuing a supervised course of study leading to a degree or certificate in occupational therapy in an accredited or approved educational program, if the person is designated by a title that clearly indicates a student or trainee status.	011. Supervision. An occupational therapist shall supervise and be responsible for the patient care given by occupational therapy assistants, graduate occupational therapists, graduate occupational therapy assistants, student occupational therapists, student occupational therapy assistants, and aides. (3-29-10) 01. Skill Levels. The following skill levels apply to occupational therapy assistants, graduate occupational therapists, graduate occupational therapy assistants, student occupational therapists, student occupational therapy assistants and aides: (3-29-10) a. Entry Level-Working on initial skill development (zero to one (0–1)	**Statute** http://www. legislature. idaho.gov/ idstat/Title 54/T54CH3 7SECT54- 3704.htm **Regulation** http://adm. idaho.gov/ad minrules/ru les/idapa 24/0601.pdf

State	Statute	Regulation (plus Board Guidance if applicable)	URL
		year experience) or working in a new area of practice; (3-29-10) b. Intermediate Level—Increased independence and mastery of basic roles and functions. Demonstrates ability to respond to new situations based on previous experience (generally one to five (1–5) years' experience); (3-29-10) 1. Advanced Level—Refinement of skills with the ability to understand complex issues and respond accordingly. (3-29-10) Please click on the website link (Section 011).	
Illinois	(225 ILCS 75/3) (from Ch. 111, par. 3703) (Section scheduled to be repealed on January 1, 2014) Nothing in this Act shall be construed as preventing or restricting the practice, services, or activities of: (3) Any person pursuing a course of study leading to a degree or certificate in occupational therapy at an accredited or approved educational program if such activities and services constitute a part of a supervised course of study, and if such person is designated by a title that clearly indicates his or her status as a student or trainee.	Not Available	**Statute** http://ilga. gov/ legislation/ ilcs/ ilcs3.asp?Act ID=1314& ChapAct= 225%26nbsp; ILCS%26n bsp;75/& ChapterID =24&Chapter Name=PRO FESSIONS +AND+OCC UPATIONS &ActName =Illinois+Occ upational +Therapy +Practice +Act. **Regulation** http://www. ilga.gov/com mission/jcar/ admincode/ 068/068013 15 sections. html
Indiana	IC 25-23.5-0.5-2 Licensing exemption Sec. 2. The provisions of this article that require a license to engage in the practice of occupational therapy do not apply to the following: (1) The practice of occupational therapy by	Not Available	**Statute** http://www.in .gov/pla/files/ OTC.2009_ EDITION (1).pdf

State	Statute	Regulation (plus Board Guidance if applicable)	URL
	an individual who is practicing occupational therapy as part of a supervised course of study in an educational program approved by the board.		
Iowa	148B.3 Persons and practices not affected. This chapter does not prevent or restrict the practice, services, or activities of any of the following: (3) A person pursuing a course of study leading to a degree or certificate in occupational therapy in an accredited or approved educational program, if the activities and services constitute a part of a supervised course of study and the person is designated by a title which clearly indicates the person's status as a student or trainee.	Not Available	**Statute** http://search. legis.state.ia. us/nxt/gate way.dll/ic/ 2009codesup p/1/28203? f=templates &fn=default. htm
Kansas	65-5418. Construction of occupational therapy practice act and practice of occupational therapy. (a) Nothing in the occupational therapy practice act is intended to limit, preclude, or otherwise interfere with the practices of other health care providers formally trained and licensed, registered, credentialed or certified by appropriate agencies of the state of Kansas. (b) The practice of occupational therapy shall not be construed to include the following: (9) any person pursuing a supervised course of study leading to a degree or certificate in occupational therapy at an accredited or approved educational program, if the person is designated by the title that clearly indicates such person's status as a student or trainee.	Not Available	**Statute** http://www. ksbha.org/ statutes/book lets/occupa tionalthera pist.pdf

State	Statute	Regulation (plus Board Guidance if applicable)	URL
Kentucky	319A.090 Construction of chapter. (1) The provisions of this chapter shall not be construed as preventing or restricting the practices, services, or activities of: (c) A person pursuing a course of study leading to a degree or certificate in occupational therapy at an accredited or approved educational program, provided the activities and services are part of a supervised course of study and the person is designated by a title that clearly indicates the status of student or trainee and not licensed occupational therapist or occupational therapy assistant.	201 KAR 28:130. Supervision of occupational therapy assistants, occupational therapy aides, occupational therapy students, and temporary permit holders. Section 5. Occupational Therapy Students. (1) A person practicing occupational therapy and performing occupational therapy services under KRS 319A.090(1)(c) shall be enrolled in an ACOTE®-accredited occupational therapy or occupational therapy assistant educational program or its equivalent. (2) When an occupational therapy student is participating in supervised fieldwork education experiences, the student may, at the discretion of the supervising OT/L or OTA/L, be assigned duties or functions commensurate with his or her education and training. (3) A supervisor shall be responsible for ensuring the safe and effective delivery of OT services and for fostering the professional competence and development of the students under his or her supervision.	**Statute and Regulation** http://bot. ky.gov/NR/ rdonlyres/ 6B714ADD-3C38-4306-9A7F-E932F 3B0255F/0/ BOTLawsa ndRegula tions.pdf
Louisiana	3005. Persons and practices not affected: A. Nothing in this Chapter shall be construed as preventing or restricting the practice, services, or activities of: (3) Any person pursuing a course of study leading to a degree or certificate in occupational therapy at an institution whose program is accredited, recognized, or approved by an agency recognized by the United States Office of Education, if such activities and services constitute a part of a supervised course of study; or any person on a supervised fieldwork experience, if such activities and services constitute a part of the experience necessary to meet the requirements of certification and licensure, and if such a person is designated by a title which clearly indicates his or her status as a student or trainee.	Not Available	**Statute** http://www. lsbme.la.gov/ Laws/Prac tice%20 Acts%207% 2009%20 html/Occupa tional%20 Therapy% 20Practice% 20Act%207% 2009.htm **Regulation** http://www. lsbme.la.gov/ 46v45Med icalProfes sionsSeptem ber2009licen sure.htm#_Toc 243143611

State	Statute	Regulation (plus Board Guidance if applicable)	URL
Maine	2276. License required License required. [1997, c. 294, §3 (RP).] This subsection is not intended to prohibit occupational therapy students and occupational therapy assistant students completing fieldwork from using the letters "O.T.S." and "O.T.A.S." respectively. 2277. Persons and practices exempt. Nothing in this chapter may be construed as preventing or restricting the practice, services or activities of: [1983, c. 746, §2 (NEW).] 2. Students or trainees. Any person pursuing a supervised course of study leading to a degree or certificate in occupational therapy at a developing or an accredited or approved educational program, if the person is designated by a title that clearly indicates that person's status as a student or trainee. At the discretion of the supervising occupational therapist, the student or trainee may be assigned duties or functions commensurate with the student's or trainee's education and training. Occupational therapy students and occupational therapy assistant students completing fieldwork may use the letters "O.T.S." and "O.T.A.S." respectively.	Not Available	**Statute** http://www. mainelegisla ture.org/legis/ statutes/32/ title32ch32 sec0.html **Regulation** http://www. maine.gov/ sos/cec/rules/ 02/chaps02. htm#477
Maryland	10-301. License required; exceptions. (b) Exceptions.—This section does not apply to: (2) A student or trainee who is designated as a student or trainee, while: (i) Fulfilling a fieldwork requirement under §10-302 of this subtitle; or	10.46.01.04. 04 Supervision Requirements. A. Occupational Therapist. (1) A licensed occupational therapist may supervise the clinical practice of the following: (f) Occupational therapy student or occupational therapy assistant student. (4) An occupational therapy assistant, under the direction of the occupational therapist, is permitted to be the primary clinical supervisor for the following: (c) Level I fieldwork occupational therapy student; and	**Statute** http://www. mdotboard. org/legreg. htm

State	Statute	Regulation (plus Board Guidance if applicable)	URL
	(ii) Pursuing a supervised course of study in an accredited or approved educational program leading to a degree or certificate in: 1. Occupational therapy; or 2. Occupational therapy assistant.	(d) Level I and Level II fieldwork occupational therapy assistant student. (5) The occupational therapy assistant may be utilized to facilitate occupational therapy student and occupational therapy assistant student learning experiences in both Level I and Level II fieldwork under the direction of the occupational therapist. F. Occupational Therapy Students. An occupational therapist or occupational therapy assistant supervising a Level I or Level II fieldwork student shall have a minimum of 1 year of experience as a licensed occupational therapist or occupational therapy assistant, excluding temporary licensure.	**Regulation** http://www.dsd.state.md.us/comar/comarhtml/10/10.46.01.04.htm
Massachusetts	Not Available	3.02: Use of Supportive Personnel (3) Supervision by Occupational Therapists. (d) An occupational therapist must provide direct supervision to the following persons rendering occupational therapy services: 1. occupational therapist students; 2. occupational therapy assistant students; (5) Supervision by Occupational Therapy Assistants. (c) An occupational therapy assistant must provide direct supervision to the following persons providing occupational therapy services: 1. occupational therapy assistant students.	**Statute** http://www.mass.gov/legis/laws/mgl/gl-112-toc.htm **Regulation** http://www.mass.gov/?pageID=ocaterminal&L=6&L0=Home&L1=Licensee&L2=Division+of+Professional+Licensure+Boards&L3=Board+of+Registration+in+Allied+Health+Professionals&L4=Statutes+and+Regulations&L5=Rules+and+Regulations+Governing+Allied+Health+Professionals&sid=Eoca&b=terminalcontent&f=dpl_boards_ah_cmr_259cmr300&csid=Eoca#3.02

State	Statute	Regulation (plus Board Guidance if applicable)	URL
Michigan	Not Available	Not Available	**Statute** http://www. legislature. mi.gov/(S(m w3hlaemjk jeyv55rnblo tar))/mileg. aspx?page =getObject &objectName =mcl-368- 1978-15-183 **Regulation** http://www. state.mi.us/ orr/emi/ad mincode.asp? AdminCode =Single&Ad min_Num =33801191 &Dpt=CH &RngHigh=
Minnesota	148.6403 Licensure; protected titles and restrictions on use; exempt persons; sanctions. Subd. 5. Exempt persons. This section does not apply to: (2) a student participating in supervised fieldwork or supervised coursework that is necessary to meet the requirements of section 148.6408, subdivision 1, or 148.6410, subdivision 1, if the person is designated by a title that clearly indicates the person's status as a student trainee. Any use of the protected titles under these circumstances is allowed only while the person is performing the duties of the supervised fieldwork or supervised coursework.	Not Available	**Statute** http://www. health.state. mn.us/divs/ hpsc/hop/ otp/ms 148. 6401_09md hform.pdf

State	Statute	Regulation (plus Board Guidance if applicable)	URL
Mississippi	SEC. 73-24-9. Application of chapter; exceptions. Nothing in this chapter shall be construed as preventing or restricting the practice, services, or activities of: (a) Any person, licensed in this state by any other law, from engaging in the profession or occupation for which he or she is licensed; (b) Any person who is employed as an occupational therapist or occupational therapy assistant by the United States Armed Services, the United States Public Health Service, the Veterans Administration, or other federal agencies, if such person provides occupational therapy solely under the direction or control of the organization by which he is employed; (c) Any person pursuing a course of study leading to a degree or certificate in occupational therapy in an accredited, recognized, or approved educational program, or advanced training in a specialty area, if such activities and services constitute a part of the supervised course of study, and if such person is designated by a title that clearly indicates his status as a trainee or student; (d) Any person fulfilling the supervised fieldwork experience requirements of Section 73-24-19, if such activities and services constitute a part of the experience necessary to meet the requirements of that section; (e) Any person employed as an occupational therapy aide or who works under the supervision of a licensed occupational therapist; or	108 EXCEPTIONS AND EXEMPTIONS 108.01 Exceptions: Nothing in this chapter shall be construed as preventing or restricting the practice, services, or activities of: 3. Any person pursuing a course of study leading to a degree or certificate in occupational therapy in an accredited, recognized, or approved educational program, or advanced training in a specialty area, if such activities and services constitute a part of the supervised course of study, and if such person is designated by a title that clearly indicates his status as a trainee or student (revised 2/20/98).	**Statute** http://www. mscode.com/ free/stat utes/73/024 /0009.htm **Regulation** http://msdh. ms.gov/msd hsite/_static/ resources/ 138.pdf

State	Statute	Regulation (plus Board Guidance if applicable)	URL
	(f) Any person performing occupational therapy services in the state, if these services are performed for no more than thirty (30) days in a calendar year under the supervision of an occupational therapist licensed under this chapter, if: (i) The person is licensed under the law of another state that has licensure requirements at least as stringent as the requirements of this chapter, or (ii) The person is certified as an Occupational Therapist Registered (OTR) or a Certified Occupational Therapy Assistant (COTA), established by the National Board for Certification in Occupational Therapy, Inc. (NBCOT), or its successor organization. (g) Any person certified by the American Board of Certification in Orthotics and Prosthetics as a Certified Orthotist, C.O., Certified Prosthetist, C.P., Certified Prosthetist/Orthotist, C.P.O., or anyone working under their direct supervision.		
Missouri	Exceptions to licensing requirements. 324.059. If a person does not represent or hold himself or herself out as an occupational therapist or occupational therapy assistant as defined in section 324.050, nothing in sections 324.050 to 324.089 shall be construed to limit, preclude or otherwise interfere with: (3) Pursuing a supervised course of study leading to a degree or certificate in occupational therapy at an accredited or approved educational program,	Not Available	**Statute** http://www. moga. mo.gov/ statutes/ C300-399/ 3240000059 .HTM **Regulation** http://pr.mo. gov/octhera py-rules-statutes.asp

State	Statute	Regulation (plus Board Guidance if applicable)	URL
	if such person is designated by a title that clearly indicates the person's status as a student or trainee.		
Montana	37-24-104. Exemptions. Nothing in this chapter prevents or restricts the practice, services, or activities of: (4) a person pursuing a supervised course of study leading to a degree or certificate in occupational therapy at an accredited institution or under an approved educational program if the person is designated by a title that clearly indicates the person's status as a student or trainee.	Not Available	**Statute** http://data. opi.mt.gov/ bills/mca/37/ 24/37-24- 104.htm **Regulation** http://bsd.dli. mt.gov/ license/bsd_ boards/otp_ board/pdf/ otp_rules.pdf
Nebraska	38-2516. Occupational therapist; therapy assistant; licensure required; activities and services not prohibited. No person may represent himself or herself to be a licensed occupational therapist or occupational therapy assistant unless he or she is licensed in accordance with the Occupational Therapy Practice Act. Nothing in such act shall be construed to prevent: (1) Any person licensed in this state pursuant to the Uniform Credentialing Act from engaging in the profession or occupation for which he or she is licensed; (2) The activities and services of any person employed as an occupational therapist or occupational therapy assistant who serves in the armed forces of the United States or the United States Public Health Service or who is employed by the United States Department of Veterans Affairs, or other federal agencies, if their practice is limited to that service or employment;	Not Available	**Statute** http://www. dhhs.ne.gov/ crl/statutes/ Occupa tional%20 Therapy.pdf **Regulation** http://www. sos.state. ne.us/rules- and-regs/reg search/Rules/ Health_and_ Human_Ser vices_System/ Title-172/ Chapter-114. pdf

State	Statute	Regulation (plus Board Guidance if applicable)	URL
	(3) The activities and services of any person pursuing an accredited course of study leading to a degree or certificate in occupational therapy if such activities and services constitute a part of a supervised course of study and if such a person is designated by a title that clearly indicates his or her status as a student or trainee.		
Nevada	NRS 640A.070 Applicability of chapter. This chapter does not apply to a person: 3. Enrolled in an educational program approved by the Board that is designed to lead to a certificate or degree in occupational therapy, if the person is designated by a title that clearly indicates that he or she is a student.	NAC 640A.267 Delegation of duties to student or provisional licensee; limitations. (NRS 640A.110) An occupational therapist who is supervising a: (1) Student participating in the supervised experience required by NRS 640A.120; or (2) Provisional licensee, may delegate duties to the student or provisional licensee if the occupational therapist determines, before he delegates a duty, that the student or provisional licensee possesses the necessary knowledge, competence, training, and skills to perform the duty. (Added to NAC by Bd. of Occupational Therapy, eff. 5- 23-96; A by R179-01, 9-20-2002)	**Statute** http://www. leg.state. nv.us/NRS/ NRS-640A. html **Regulation** http://www. leg.state. nv.us/NAC/ NAC-640A. html# NAC640A Sec267
New Hampshire	326-C:3 Prohibition on Unauthorized Practice; Professional Identification. 1. No person shall practice or hold oneself out as being able to practice occupational therapy or assist in the practice of occupational therapy or provide occupational therapy services in this state unless the person is licensed under this chapter and RSA 328- F. Nothing in this paragraph shall be construed to prohibit students enrolled in board approved schools or courses in occupational therapy from performing occupational therapy that is incidental to their respective courses of study or supervised field work.	Occ 407.07 Direct Supervision of Fieldwork. Documentation of direct supervision of fieldwork shall be a memo signed by the supervisor of the facility where the fieldwork was supervised, specifying: (a) The name of the licensee; (b) The fieldwork student's school; and (c) The beginning and ending dates of the licensee's supervision of the student's fieldwork.	**Statute** http://www. gencourt. state.nh.us/ rsa/html/ XXX/326-C/326-C-3. htm **Regulation** http://www. gencourt. state.nh.us/ rules/state_ agencies/ occ100-500. html

State	Statute	Regulation (plus Board Guidance if applicable)	URL
New Jersey	45:9-37.60. Practices not requiring license in occupational therapy The provisions of this act shall not be construed to prevent the following provided that no word, letter, abbreviation, insignia, sign, card, or device is used to convey the impression that the person rendering the service is a licensed occupational therapist or occupational therapy assistant: (c) Any person pursuing a course of study leading to a degree or certificate in occupational therapy at an accredited or approved educational program if the pursuit is part of a supervised course of study and if the person is designated by a title that clearly indicates status as a student or trainee.	13:44K-5.3 Delegation of occupational therapy services (a) A licensed occupational therapist may delegate selected occupational therapy services to licensed occupational therapy assistants, temporary licensed occupational therapists, temporary licensed occupational therapy assistants, and to occupational therapy students fulfilling the required fieldwork component of their educational training, provided the services are within the scope of practice of the individual to whom they are delegated. 13:44K-7.2 Responsibilities of Designated Supervisor (b) A licensed occupational therapist may supervise five occupational therapy students who are fulfilling the required fieldwork component of their educational training.	**Statute** http://www. njconsum eraffairs. gov/occup/ ot_rules.htm **Regulation** http://www. njconsumer affairs.gov/ laws/OC Cregs.pdf
New Mexico	61-12A-7. Exemptions. (Repealed effective July 1, 2016.) Nothing in the Occupational Therapy Act [61-12A-1 to 61-12A-24 NMSA 1978] shall be construed as preventing or restricting the practice, services, or activities of: C. A person pursuing a course of study leading to a degree or certificate in occupational therapy in an educational program accredited or seeking accreditation by the Accreditation Council of Occupational Therapy Education if the activities and services constitute part of the supervised course of study and if that person is designated by a title that clearly indicates his status as a student or trainee;	Not Available	**Statute** http://www. conway greene.com/ nmsu/lpext. dll?f=tem plates&f n=main-h. htm&2.0

State	Statute	Regulation (plus Board Guidance if applicable)	URL
	D. A person fulfilling the supervised student fieldwork experience requirement pursuant to the Occupational Therapy Act [61-12A-1 to 61-12A-24 NMSA 1978] if the activities and services constitute part of the experience necessary to meet that requirement.		**Regulation** http://www.nmcpr.state.nm.us/nmac/_title16/T16C015.htm
New York	7906. Exempt persons. This article shall not be construed to affect or prevent the following, provided that no title, sign, card, or device shall be used in such manner as to tend to convey the impression that the person rendering such service is a licensed occupational therapist: 3. A student from engaging in clinical practice as part of an accredited program in occupational therapy, pursuant to subdivision 3 of section 794 of this article.	76.2 Supervised experience. The 6 months of full-time supervised experience in occupational therapy may be completed as part of the basic program described in section 76.1 of this Part. Full-time experience not completed as part of an approved program shall be under the supervision of a licensed occupational therapist. For candidates who have accumulated other than full-time supervised experience, part-time experience may be counted if it is obtained at the rate of at least two full days per week (minimum of 15 hours) and for continuous periods of not less than two months for an accumulated total of 6 months. **NY Office of the Professions, OT Practice Guidelines for Supervision:** Supervising students or applicants for licensure. When occupational therapists act as supervisors for persons gaining experience for licensure, the supervisee should not directly pay the supervisor. The supervisor should not accept payment directly from the supervisee for supervision that would lead to course credit in academic programs or licensure. When a supervisor accepts payment directly from the supervisee in these situations, it could be considered a conflict of interest and a dual relationship.	**Statute** http://www.op.nysed.gov/prof/ot/article156.htm **Regulation** http://www.op.nysed.gov/prof/ot/part76.htm **NY Office of the Professions, OT Practice Guidelines for Supervision:** http://www.op.nysed.gov/prof/ot/otsup.htm
North Carolina	90-270.81 Persons and practices not affected Nothing in this Article shall be construed to prevent or restrict: (3) Any person pursuing a course of study leading to a degree or certificate in occupational therapy at an accredited or approved educational program if the activities and services constitute a part of a supervised course of study and	0905 Delineation of clinical responsibilities Regardless of the setting in which occupational therapy services are delivered, the occupational therapist and the occupational therapy assistant have the following responsibilities during evaluation, intervention, and outcomes evaluation: (8) Supervision of occupational therapy students: (a) An occupational therapy practitioner shall comply with Accreditation Council for Occupational Therapy Education (ACOTE) requirements for experience when supervising Level II fieldwork	**Statute** http://www.ncbot.org/Downloads/practice%20act%20and%20rules/2009%20NCBOT%20Practice%20Act.pdf

State	Statute	Regulation (plus Board Guidance if applicable)	URL
	if the person is designated by a title that clearly indicates his or her status as a student or trainee. (4) Any person fulfilling the supervised fieldwork experience required for licensure under this Article if the person is designated by a title that clearly indicates his or her status as a student or trainee.	occupational therapist and occupational therapy assistant students, which ACOTE requirements, including subsequent amendments and editions, are incorporated by reference. Copies of the incorporated material are available for inspection at the Board office and are available for purchase for five dollars ($5.00); (b) The occupational therapist may supervise Level I and Level II fieldwork occupational therapist and occupational therapy assistant students; and (c) The occupational therapy assistant may: 　(i) Supervise Level I occupational therapist or occupational therapy assistant students; 　(ii) Supervise Level II occupational therapy assistant students; and 　(iii) Participate in the supervision of Level II occupational therapist students under the direction and guidance of the supervising occupational therapist. **NC BOARD OF OT** Roles and supervisory requirements of the occupational therapist and the occupational therapy assistant during the delivery of occupational therapy services: **STUDENT SUPERVISION** OT: Responsible for the supervision of OTA/S and Level I fieldwork OT/S. After 1 year of clinical experience, may supervise Level II OT/S. OTA: Supervise volunteers and ancillary staff under the supervision of an OT/L. Supervise Level I OT/S and OTA/S. After 1 year of clinical experience, may supervise Level II OTA/S under the direct supervision of an OT/L.	**Regulation** http://www. ncbot.org/ Downloads/ practice% 20act%20 and%20rules/ 2009% 20NCBOT% 20Rules.pdf **NC Board of OT Roles and Requirements for Supervision of OTs and OTAs:** http://www. ncbot.org/ Downloads/ Supervision %20and%20 Address%20 Change%20 Forms/Roles %20and%20 Req%20for% 20OT%20 and%20OTA. pdf
North Dakota	43-40-03.1. Occupational therapy students—Occupational therapy aides. 1. A person pursuing a supervised course of study leading to a degree or certificate in occupational therapy at an accredited or approved educational program may perform occupational therapy services if the services are a part of the student's supervised course of study, provided that the student	Not Available	**Statute** http://www. legis.nd.gov/ cencode/ t43c40.pdf **Regulation** http://www. ndotboard. com/law/ law.shtml

State	Statute	Regulation (plus Board Guidance if applicable)	URL
	is designated by a title that clearly indicates the student's status as a student or trainee. 2. Occupational therapy aides may assist in the practice of occupational therapy only under the direct supervision of an occupational therapist or occupational therapy assistant and in accordance with rules adopted by the board.		
Ohio	4755.13 Exemptions. (A) Nothing in sections 4755.04 to 4755.13 of the Revised Code shall be construed to prevent or restrict the practice, services, or activities of the following: (3) Any person pursuing a course of study leading to a degree or certificate in occupational therapy in an accredited or approved educational program if the activities and services constitute a part of a supervised course of study, if the person is designated by a title that clearly indicates the person's status as a student or trainee.	4755-7-04 Supervision. (A) Supervision must ensure consumer protection. The supervising occupational therapist is ultimately responsible for all clients and is accountable and responsible at all times for the actions of persons supervised, including the: (1) Occupational therapy assistant; (2) Student occupational therapist; (3) Student occupational therapy assistant; and (4) Unlicensed personnel. (D) Student occupational therapist. (1) A student occupational therapist shall be supervised by an occupational therapist who has completed at least 1 year of clinical practice as a fully licensed occupational therapist. (2) The student occupational therapist, who is being supervised in accordance with the laws and rules governing the practice of occupational therapy, may supervise unlicensed personnel. (E) Student occupational therapy assistant. (1) A student occupational therapy assistant shall be supervised by an occupational therapist or occupational therapy assistant who has completed at least 1 year of clinical practice as a fully licensed occupational therapist or occupational therapy assistant. (2) The student occupational therapy assistant, who is being supervised in accordance with the laws and rules governing the practice of occupational therapy, may supervise unlicensed personnel.	**Statute and Regulation** http://www.otptat.ohio.gov/LinkClick.aspx?filetick et=r9sSrd lhIKM%3d &tabid=100 &mid=609

State	Statute	Regulation (plus Board Guidance if applicable)	URL
Oklahoma	888.5. Practices, services, and activities not prohibited Nothing in this act shall be construed to prevent or restrict the practice, services, or activities of: 3. Any person pursuing a course of study leading to a degree or certificate in occupational therapy at an accredited educational program if such activities and services constitute a part of a supervised course of study, if such a person is designated by a title that clearly indicates his status as a student or trainee.	435:30-1-15. Supervision of students, new graduates, techs, and aides. The Occupational Therapist is responsible and accountable for the overall use and actions of unlicensed personnel under his/her supervision and control. (1) Students. Supervision of the student must occur by one of the following methods: (A) Direct, on-site supervision will be provided by the Oklahoma licensed Occupational Therapist for the Occupational Therapy student in models of health care or educational systems. Supervision of the Occupational Therapy Assistant student may be provided by an Oklahoma licensed Occupational Therapy Assistant working under supervision of an Oklahoma-licensed Occupational Therapist. (B) In emerging occupational therapy models, areas of innovative community-based and social systems-based occupational therapy practice where there is no occupational therapy practitioner on site, the occupational therapy practitioner must provide a minimum of 6 hours of weekly supervision. Supervision must include role modeling for the student, direct observation of client interaction, meeting with the student, review of student paperwork, and availability for communication and consultation. The supervisor must be readily available during all working hours. It is understood that supervision begins with more direct supervision and gradually decreases to a minimum of 6 hours weekly as the student demonstrates competence. The supervisor must be cognizant of the individual student's needs and must use judgment in determining when an individual student may need more of the supervisor's time. (2) New graduates. Direct on-site supervision will be provided by the Occupational Therapist for new Occupational Therapist and Occupational Therapist Assistant graduates.	**Statute** http://www. okmedical board.org/ download/ OTLAW.pdf **Regulation** http://www. okmedical board.org/ download/ OTLAW.pdf

State	Statute	Regulation (plus Board Guidance if applicable)	URL
Oregon	675.220 Representation as occupational therapist or therapy assistant prohibited without license; exception. (1) No person shall practice occupational therapy or purport to be an occupational therapist or occupational therapy assistant, or as being able to practice occupational therapy, or to render occupational therapy services, or use the abbreviations designated by the Occupational Therapy Licensing Board under ORS 675.320 unless the person is licensed in accordance with ORS 675.210 to 675.340. (2) ORS 675.210 to 675.340 do not apply to: (c) The practice of occupational therapy that is incidental to the planned program of study for students enrolled in an occupational therapist or occupational therapy assistant program approved by the board. [1977 c.858 §§2,3; 1981 c.250 §2]	39-010-0030 Supervised Fieldwork For purposes of ORS 675.240(1) and 675.250(4), applicants who have successfully completed training and experience in the practice of occupational therapy as part of a planned program of study in an occupational therapist or occupational therapy assistant educational program approved by the Board shall be considered to have received supervised field work. **OR OT Licensing Board Statement of Supervision: Supervision for Fieldwork Students** Fieldwork students must have supervision. In Oregon, Pacific University, School of OT has a fieldwork co-coordinator. Generally questions should go there first. The OT Licensing Board does get some questions on supervision, and often those questions come to the board because the question really deals with co-signing notes for reimbursement. Those questions deal with Medicare/Medicaid issues.	**Statute** http://www.leg.st ate.or.us/ors/675.html **Regulation** http://arcweb.sos.state.or.us/rules/OARs_300/OAR_339/339_010.ht ml **OR OT Licensing Board Statement of Supervision:** http://www.otlb.state.or.us/OTLB/Supervision.shtml
Pennsylvania	Section 7. Persons and practices not affected; exceptions. This act shall not be construed as preventing or restricting the practices, services, or activities of: (4) A person pursuing a course of study leading to the degree or certificate in occupational therapy at an accredited or approved educational program provided the activities and services are part of a supervised course of study and the person is designated by a title that clearly indicates the status of student or trainee and not licensed occupational therapist.	Not Available	**Statute** http://www.portal.state.pa.us/portal/server.pt?open=18&objID=487712&mode=2 **Regulation** http://www.pacode.com/secure/data/049/chapter42/chap42toc.html

State	Statute	Regulation (plus Board Guidance if applicable)	URL
Puerto Rico	Not Available	Not Available	**Statute and Regulation** http://www .michie.com/ puertorico/ lpext.dll? f=templates &fn=main-h. htm&cp =prcode
Rhode Island	§ 5-40.1-7 Persons and practices not affected. Nothing in this chapter shall be construed as preventing or restricting the practice, services, or activities of: (1) Any person licensed in this state by any other law from engaging in the profession or occupation for which he or she is licensed; (2) Any person employed as an occupational therapist or occupational therapy assistant by the government of the United States or any agency of it, if that person provides occupational therapy solely under the direction or control of the organization by which he or she is employed; (3) Any person pursuing a supervised course of study leading to a degree or certificate in occupational therapy at an accredited or approved educational program, if the person is designated by a title that clearly indicates his or her status as a student or trainee; or (4) Any person fulfilling the supervised fieldwork experience requirements of § 5-40.1-8(a)(3), if the experience constitutes a part of the experience necessary to meet the requirement of that section. http://www.rilin.state.ri.us/ Statutes/TITLE5/5-40.1/5-40.1-7.HTM	2.1.1 The Act shall not be construed as preventing or restricting the practice, services, or activities of the following: c) any individual pursuing a supervised course of study leading to a degree or certificate in occupational therapy at an accredited or approved educational program, if the person is designated by a title that clearly indicates his or her status as a student or trainee; 5.5 Supervision Occupational Therapists 5.5.1 A licensed occupational therapist shall exercise sound judgment and provide adequate care in the performance of duties. (a) A licensed occupational therapist is permitted to supervise the following: occupational therapists; occupational therapy assistants; occupational therapy aides; care extenders; occupational therapy students; and volunteers. Occupational Therapy Assistants 5.5.2 A licensed occupational therapy assistant shall exercise sound judgment and provide adequate care in the performance of duties. (a) A licensed occupational therapy assistant is permitted to supervise the following: occupational therapy aides; care extenders; students; and volunteers.	**Statute** http://www. rilin.state.ri .us/Statutes/ TITLE5/5-40.1/5-40.1-21.HTM **Regulation** http://www2. sec.state.ri.us/ dar_filing/ regdocs/ released/ pdf/DOH/ 4838.pdf

State	Statute	Regulation (plus Board Guidance if applicable)	URL
	§ 5-40.1-21 Supervision. (a) A licensed occupational therapist shall exercise sound judgment and shall provide adequate care in the performance of duties. A licensed occupational therapist shall be permitted to supervise the following: occupational therapists, occupational therapy assistants, occupational therapy aides, care extenders, occupational therapy students, and volunteers. (b) A licensed occupational therapy assistant shall exercise sound judgment and shall provide adequate care in the performance of duties. A licensed occupational therapy assistant shall be permitted to supervise the following: occupational therapy aides, care extenders, students, and volunteers.		
South Carolina	Section 40-36-280. Persons excepted from application of chapter. This chapter does not apply to a person: (2) Who is enrolled in a course of study leading to a degree or certificate in occupational therapy in a program approved by the board if the occupational therapy activities and services constitute a part of a supervised course of study and if the person is designated by a title that clearly indicates a student or trainee status including "Occupational Therapy Student," "Occupational Therapy Assistant Student," "O.T.S.," "O.T.A.S.," or other designation approved by the board	Not Available **SC Board of OT Position Statement on Fieldwork Supervision of Students:** The South Carolina Board recognizes two basic levels of fieldwork experience based on AOTA guidelines. I. Level I The Board expects Level I students to receive line of sight supervision in relation to any patient interactions. This supervision may or may not be provided by a licensed occupational therapist as is consistent with AOTA guidelines. Other health care providers may assist or be the primary supervisor of this student. "Line of sight" supervision is as it implies. Visual on-site contact is required at all times. Supervision through the use of telecommunication is not sufficient. When line of sight supervision cannot be provided, the occupational therapy student may no longer function in the role of a student. It is the determination of the facility and the academic institution to determine if credit will be granted for this form of learning experience.	**Statute** http://www.scstatehouse.gov/code/t40c036.htm **Regulation** http://www.scstatehouse.gov/coderegs/c094.htm **SC Board of OT Position Statement on Fieldwork Supervision of Students:** http://www.llr.state.sc.us/POL/OccupationalTherapy/index.asp?file=Student.htm

State	Statute	Regulation (plus Board Guidance if applicable)	URL
	SECTION 40-36-300. Responsibilities and duties of occupational therapy assistants and aides; restrictions. (D) An occupational therapy student may perform duties or functions commensurate with the student's training and experience under the direct on-site supervision of a licensed occupational therapist.	II. Level II The Board expects Level II students to receive on-site supervision, at a minimum, in relation to any patient interactions. The student must receive primary supervision from a licensed occupational therapy practitioner. In support of AOTA standards, "the student must receive a minimum of six (6) hours of supervision per week, including direct observation of client interaction." A supervisor must be readily available at all times when client interaction is possible. It is the responsibility of the licensed occupational therapy practitioner to maintain up-to-date knowledge of additional state, federal, and third-party reimbursement regulations as they relate to student supervision. "On-site supervision" means personal, daily supervision and specific delineation of tasks and responsibilities by a licensed occupational therapy practitioner and includes the responsibility for personally reviewing and interpreting the results of a supervisee on a daily basis. Telephone contact and other communication technologies may be used to supplement, but not to substitute, for face-to-face contact. "On-site" means the same premises where direct client treatment is being performed. When on-site supervision cannot be provided, the occupational therapy student may no longer function in the role of a student. They may only function in the role of an occupational therapy aide. This means that evaluations may not be performed. Skilled services that require the exercise of professional judgement of a licensed occupational therapy practitioner may not be provided. Billing of services should reflect the service provider level. It is the determination of the facility and the academic institution to determine if credit will be granted for this form of learning experience.	
South Dakota	36-31-4. Certain activities not proscribed or restricted. Nothing in this chapter may be construed as preventing or restricting the practice, services, or activities of: (3) Any person pursuing a supervised course of study leading to a degree or	Not Available	**Statute** http://legis.state.sd.us/statutes/DisplayStatute.aspx?Type=Statute&Statute=36-31-4

State	Statute	Regulation (plus Board Guidance if applicable)	URL
	certificate in occupational therapy at an accredited or approved educational program, if the person is designated by a title that clearly indicates his status as a student or trainee; or (7) Any person when providing therapy as related services as defined in a student's individualized educational plan, the therapy shall not be an activity that supplants or duplicates the educational instruction program provided by the teaching profession.		**Regulation** http://legis. state.sd.us/ rules/Display Rule.aspx? Rule=20% 3A64

Tennessee	63-13-208. Construction of part—Activities not prohibited. —
	(3) Any person pursuing a course of study leading to a degree or certificate in occupational therapy in an educational program accredited or granted developing program status by ACOTE, if:
	   (A) The activities and services constitute a part of a supervised course of study; and
	   (B) The person is designated by a title that clearly indicates the person's status as a student;
	(4) Any person fulfilling the supervised fieldwork experience requirements of § 63-13-202(3), if the activities and services constitute a part of the experience necessary to meet the requirements of § 63-13-202(3).
		1150-02-.02 Scope of Practice.
		Occupational therapy practice includes, but is not limited to:
		(f) Providing instruction in occupational therapy to students in an accredited occupational therapy or occupational therapy assistant educational program by persons who are trained as occupational therapists or occupational therapy assistants;
		
		TN Board of OT Policy Statement on Supervision of OT Doctoral Student Clinical Fieldwork:
		Concerning the clinical supervision of occupational therapy doctoral students in Tennessee, a licensed occupational therapist is not required for supervision of doctoral students in Level I fieldwork placements. However, supervision by a licensed occupational therapist of doctoral students in Level II fieldwork placements is required, pursuant to the Accreditation Council for Occupational Therapy Education (ACOTE).
			Statute http://www. michie.com/ tennessee/ lpext.dll?f =templates &fn=main-h. htm&cp =tncode
			
			Regulation http://tennes see.gov/sos/ rules/1150/ 1150-02. 20100119. pdf
			
			TN Board of OT Policy Statement on Supervision of OT Doctoral Student Clinical Fieldwork: http://health. state.tn.us/ Downloads/ OT_Supervi sion_Doct oral_Student_ Policy.pdf

State	Statute	Regulation (plus Board Guidance if applicable)	URL
Texas	454.005. Applicability. (a) This chapter does not apply to a holder of a license issued by another state agency who is performing health care services within the scope of the applicable licensing act. (b) The licensing provisions of this chapter do not apply to: (2) a person engaged in a course of study leading to a degree or certificate in occupational therapy at an accredited or approved educational program if: (A) the activities and services constitute a part of a supervised course of study; and (B) the person is designated by a title that clearly indicates the person's status as a student or trainee.	Not Available	**Statute** http://www.ecptote.state.tx.us/_private/2009_OT_Practice_Act.pdf **Regulation** http://www.ecptote.state.tx.us/_private/OT_Rules_2010_(3).pdf
Utah	58-1-307. Exemptions from licensure. (1) Except as otherwise provided by statute or rule, the following persons may engage in the practice of their occupation or profession, subject to the stated circumstances and limitations, without being licensed under this title: (b) A student engaged in activities constituting the practice of a regulated occupation or profession while in training in a recognized school approved by the division to the extent the activities are supervised by qualified faculty, staff, or designee and the activities are a defined part of the training program.	Not Available	**Statute** http://www.dopl.utah.gov/laws/58-1.pdf **Regulation** http://www.dopl.utah.gov/laws/R156-42a.pdf

State	Statute	Regulation (plus Board Guidance if applicable)	URL
Vermont	Not Available	Not Available	**Statute** http://www. leg.state.vt.us/ statutes/full chapter.cfm? Title=26& Chapter=071 **Regulation** http://www. vtprofes sionals.org/ opr1/o_ therapists/ rules/OT_ Rules.pdf
Virginia	Not Available	Not Available	**Statute** http://www. dhp.state.va. us/medicine/ leg/Chapter 29%20Medi cine.doc **Regulation** http://www. dhp.state.va. us/medicine/ leg/Occupa tional%20 Therapy%2 03-3-10.doc
Washington	18.59.040 Activities not regulated by chapter—Limited permits. This chapter shall not be construed as preventing or restricting the practice, services, or activities of: (3) A person pursuing a course of study leading to a degree or certificate in occupational therapy in an accredited or approved educational program if the activities and services constitute a part of a supervised course of study, if the person is designated by a title that clearly indicates the person's status as a student or trainee.	WAC 246-847-140 No agency filings affecting this section since 2003 Supervised fieldwork experience—Occupational therapists. "Supervised fieldwork experience" in RCW 18.59.050 (1)(c)(i) shall mean a minimum six months of Level II fieldwork conducted in settings approved by the applicant's academic program. Level II fieldwork is to provide an in-depth experience in delivering occupational therapy services to clients and to provide opportunities for supervised practice of occupational therapist entry-level roles. The minimum 6 months supervised fieldwork experience required by RCW 18.59.050 (1)(c)(i) shall not include Level I fieldwork experience as defined by the American Occupational Therapy Association.	**Statute** http://apps. leg.wa.gov/ RCW/default. aspx?cite =18.59.040 **Regulation** http://apps. leg.wa.gov/ WAC/default. aspx?cite =246-847

State	Statute	Regulation (plus Board Guidance if applicable)	URL

		The supervised fieldwork experience shall consist of a minimum of 6 months sustained fieldwork on a full-time basis. "Full-time basis" is as required by the fieldwork setting.
		    WAC 246-847-150 No agency filings affecting this section since 2003
		    Supervised fieldwork experience— Occupational therapy assistants.
		    "Supervised fieldwork experience" in RCW 18.59.050 (1)(c)(ii) shall mean a minimum two months of Level II fieldwork conducted in settings approved by the applicant's academic or training program. Level II fieldwork is to provide an in-depth experience in delivering occupational therapy services to clients and to provide opportunities for supervised practice of occupational therapy assistant entry-level roles. The minimum 2 months supervised fieldwork experience required by RCW 18.59.050. (1) (c) (ii) shall not include Level I fieldwork experience as defined by the American Occupational Therapy Association.
		
		    The supervised fieldwork experience shall consist of a minimum of two one-month sustained fieldwork placements not less than 40 full-time workdays. "Full-time workdays" is as required by the fieldwork setting.	

West Virginia	30-28-9. Persons and practices not affected. This article does not prevent or restrict the practice, services or activities of: (2) Any person pursuing a course of study leading to a degree in Occupational Therapy from an accredited educational program if the person acts under the supervision of a clinical supervisor or instructor of the accredited education program and is designated by a title that clearly indicates his or her status as a student.	§13-1-12. Responsibilities and Supervision Requirements of the Occupational Therapist, Occupational Therapy Assistant, or Limited Permit Holder. 12.5.c. A licensed supervising therapist must maintain direct continuous supervision over occupational therapy students. As the occupational therapy student demonstrates competency in performance, supervision can progress to direct close supervision at the discretion of the supervising occupational therapist; 12.5.d. A licensed supervising occupational therapist or occupational therapy assistant must maintain direct continuous supervision over occupational therapy assistant students. As the occupational therapy assistant student demonstrates competency in performance, supervision can progress to direct close supervision at the discretion of the supervising occupational therapist/occupational therapy assistant;	**Statute** http://wvbot. org/dharris/ legislative_ act/HB2309_ final.pdf **Regulation** http://wvbot. org/dharris/ legislative_ act/13-01 FIN.pdf

State	Statute	Regulation (plus Board Guidance if applicable)	URL
Wisconsin	48.962 Applicability. This subchapter does not do any of the following: (1) Require any of the following to be licensed as an occupational therapist: (b) Any person pursuing a supervised course of study, including internship, leading to a degree or certificate in occupational therapy under an accredited or approved educational program, if the person is designated by a title that clearly indicates his or her status as a student or trainee. (2) Require any of the following to be licensed as an occupational therapy assistant: (b) Any person pursuing a supervised course of study leading to a degree or certificate in occupational therapy assistantship under an approved educational program, if the person is designated by a title that clearly indicates his or her status as a student or trainee.	Not Available	**Statute** http://nxt.legis.state.wi.us/nxt/gateway.dll?f=templates&fn=default.htm&d=stats&jd=ch.%20448 **Regulation** http://nxt.legis.state.wi.us/nxt/gateway.dll?f=templates&fn=default.htm&d=code&jd=top
Wyoming	33 40 104. Persons and practices not affected. (a) Nothing in this act shall be construed as preventing or restricting the practice, services, or activities of: (ii) Any person pursuing a degree or certificate in occupational therapy at an accredited or board-approved program when the person is designated by title clearly indicating his status as a student or trainee.	Not Available	**Statute** http://legisweb.state.wy.us/statutes/compress/title33.doc **Regulation** http://soswy.state.wy.us/Rules/Rule_Search_Main.asp

Reprinted from http://www.aota.org/-/media/Corporate/Files/Secure/Advocacy/State/Students/Provisions%20related%20to%20students%20in%20state%20law.pdf

Chapter 21.

HIPAA AND FERPA GUIDELINES FOR FIELDWORK

Donna Costa, DHS, OTR/L, FAOTA, and the American Occupational Therapy Association

HIPAA Guidelines

The Healthcare Insurance Portability and Accountability Act of 1996 (HIPAA; Pub. L. 104–191) is a set of federal regulations administered by the U.S. Department of Health and Human Services (n.d.) and enforced by the U.S. Office of Civil Rights. The legislation was enacted to meet the following three broad needs:

- Make it easier for people to keep health insurance by allowing them to carry their health insurance from one job to another so that they do not have a lapse in coverage. It also restricts health plans from excluding people with preexisting conditions who switch from one health plan to another.
- Protect the confidentiality and security of all health care information—written and electronic—by providing for the protection of individually identifiable health information that is transmitted or maintained in any form or medium. The privacy rules affect the day-to-day business operations of all organizations that provide medical care and maintain personal health information.
- Help the health care industry control administrative costs.

HIPAA protects a person's health and demographic information. This information is called *protected health information (PHI)*. Information meets the definition of PHI if, even without the patient's name, it can reveal who the person is. The PHI can relate to the past, present, or future physical or mental health of the person. PHI describes a disease, diagnosis, procedure, prognosis, or condition of the person and can exist in any medium, for example, files, voicemail, email, fax, or verbal communications.

Per HIPAA guidelines, students cannot report any of the following information in any fieldwork assignments such as case study presentations:

- Name
- Location (includes anything smaller than a state, such as street address)
- Dates (all, including date of birth, admission and discharge dates, dates of medical treatment provided, and date of death)
- Telephone numbers
- Fax numbers
- Email addresses
- Social Security numbers
- Medical record numbers
- Health plan beneficiary numbers

- Account numbers
- Certificate or license numbers
- Vehicle identification numbers and license plate numbers
- Device identifiers and their serial numbers
- Web universal resource locators (or URLs)
- Internet protocol (or IP) address numbers
- Biometric identifiers, including finger and voice prints
- Full face photographic images and any comparable images
- Any other unique identifying number, characteristic, or code.

For written reports, the following information *can* be shared:

- Age (ages 90 years and over must be aggregated to prevent the identification of older people)
- Race
- Ethnicity
- Marital status
- Codes (a random code may be used to link cases as long as the code does not contain or is not a derivative of the person's Social Security number, date of birth, phone or fax numbers, or other personal information).

Students, as well as occupational therapy practitioners, often keep working files in their desk. This practice is allowed under HIPAA guidelines; however, this information must be locked in a file cabinet when not in use and must be shredded when no longer needed.

FERPA Guidelines for Fieldwork

The Family Educational Rights and Privacy Act of 1974 (FERPA; Pub. L. 93-380) is a federal law that was designed to protect the privacy of students' educational records. It is administered by the Family Policy Compliance Office in the U.S. Department of Education (n.d.). FERPA applies to all educational agencies and institutions (e.g., schools) that receive funding under any program administered by the department. According to FERPA, neither academic fieldwork coordinators or any other faculty or staff may release information about students to a fieldwork site without his or her expressed consent in writing. This information includes any of the following about a student:

- Medical information
- Immunization records
- Academic grades
- Fieldwork performance evaluations from prior fieldwork experiences
- Professional behavior monitoring forms
- Personal information known to school
- Disability status if disclosed to the school
- Accommodations provided for a disability if disclosed
- Any records regarding disciplinary action.

References

Family Educational Rights and Privacy Act of 1974, Pub. L. 93-380, 20 U.S.C. § 1232g, 34 CFR Part 99.

Health Insurance Portability and Accountability Act of 1996 (HIPAA), Pub. L. 104–191, 42 U.S.C. § 300gg, 29 U.S.C § 1181-1183, and 42 USC 1320d-1320d9.

U.S. Department of Education. (n.d.). *Family Educational Rights and Privacy Act.* Retrieved from http://www2.ed.gov/policy/gen/guid/fpco/ferpa/index.html

U.S. Department of Health and Human Services. (n.d). *Health information privacy.* Retrieved from http://www.hhs.gov/ocr/privacy/

Note. Part of the "HIPAA Guidelines" section is taken from "HIPAA Guidelines for Fieldwork," available at http://www.aota.org/Education-Careers/Fieldwork/Supervisor/HIPAA.aspx.

Chapter 22. 2011 Accreditation Council for Occupational Therapy Education (ACOTE®) Standards

(Adopted December 4, 2011; effective July 31, 2013)

Standard Number	Accreditation Standards for a Doctoral-Degree-Level Educational Program for the Occupational Therapist	Accreditation Standards for a Master's-Degree-Level Educational Program for the Occupational Therapist	Accreditation Standards for an Associate-Degree-Level Educational Program for the Occupational Therapy Assistant
PREAMBLE			
	The rapidly changing and dynamic nature of contemporary health and human services delivery systems provides challenging opportunities for the occupational therapist to use knowledge and skills in a practice area as a direct care provider, consultant, educator, manager, leader, researcher, and advocate for the profession and the consumer.	The rapidly changing and dynamic nature of contemporary health and human services delivery systems requires the occupational therapist to possess basic skills as a direct care provider, consultant, educator, manager, researcher, and advocate for the profession and the consumer.	The rapidly changing and dynamic nature of contemporary health and human services delivery systems requires the occupational therapy assistant to possess basic skills as a direct care provider, educator, and advocate for the profession and the consumer.
	A graduate from an ACOTE-accredited doctoral-degree-level occupational therapy program must • Have acquired, as a foundation for professional study, a breadth and depth of knowledge in the liberal arts and sciences and an understanding of issues related to diversity. • Be educated as a generalist with a broad exposure to the delivery models and systems used in settings where occupational therapy is currently practiced and where it is emerging as a service.	A graduate from an ACOTE-accredited master's-degree-level occupational therapy program must • Have acquired, as a foundation for professional study, a breadth and depth of knowledge in the liberal arts and sciences and an understanding of issues related to diversity. • Be educated as a generalist with a broad exposure to the delivery models and systems used in settings where occupational therapy is currently practiced and where it is emerging as a service.	A graduate from an ACOTE-accredited associate-degree-level occupational therapy assistant program must • Have acquired an educational foundation in the liberal arts and sciences, including a focus on issues related to diversity. • Be educated as a generalist with a broad exposure to the delivery models and systems used in settings where occupational therapy is currently practiced and where it is emerging as a service.

(Continued)

Standard Number	Accreditation Standards for a Doctoral-Degree-Level Educational Program for the Occupational Therapist	Accreditation Standards for a Master's-Degree-Level Educational Program for the Occupational Therapist	Accreditation Standards for an Associate-Degree-Level Educational Program for the Occupational Therapy Assistant
	• Have achieved entry-level competence through a combination of academic and field-work education.	• Have achieved entry-level competence through a combination of academic and field-work education.	• Have achieved entry-level competence through a combination of academic and field-work education.
	• Be prepared to articulate and apply occupational therapy theory and evidence-based evaluations and interventions to achieve expected outcomes as related to occupation.	• Be prepared to articulate and apply occupational therapy theory and evidence-based evaluations and interventions to achieve expected outcomes as related to occupation.	• Be prepared to articulate and apply occupational therapy principles and intervention tools to achieve expected outcomes as related to occupation.
	• Be prepared to articulate and apply therapeutic use of occupations with individuals or groups for the purpose of participation in roles and situations in home, school, workplace, community, and other settings.	• Be prepared to articulate and apply therapeutic use of occupations with individuals or groups for the purpose of participation in roles and situations in home, school, workplace, community, and other settings.	• Be prepared to articulate and apply therapeutic use of occupations with individuals or groups for the purpose of participation in roles and situations in home, school, work-place, community, and other settings.
	• Be able to plan and apply occupational therapy interventions to address the physical, cognitive, psychosocial, sensory, and other aspects of performance in a variety of contexts and environments to support engagement in everyday life activities that affect health, well-being, and quality of life.	• Be able to plan and apply occupational therapy interventions to address the physical, cognitive, psychosocial, sensory, and other aspects of performance in a variety of contexts and environments to support engagement in everyday life activities that affect health, well-being, and quality of life.	• Be able to apply occupational therapy interventions to address the physical, cognitive, psychosocial, sensory, and other aspects of performance in a variety of contexts and environments to support engagement in everyday life activities that affect health, well-being, and quality of life.
	• Be prepared to be a lifelong learner and keep current with evidence-based professional practice.	• Be prepared to be a lifelong learner and keep current with evidence-based professional practice.	• Be prepared to be a lifelong learner and keep current with the best practice.
	• Uphold the ethical standards, values, and attitudes of the occupational therapy profession.	• Uphold the ethical standards, values, and attitudes of the occupational therapy profession.	• Uphold the ethical standards, values, and attitudes of the occupational therapy profession.
	• Understand the distinct roles and responsibilities of the occupational therapist and occupational therapy assistant in the supervisory process.	• Understand the distinct roles and responsibilities of the occupational therapist and occupational therapy assistant in the supervisory process.	• Understand the distinct roles and responsibilities of the occupational therapist and occupational therapy assistant in the supervisory process.

(Continued)

Standard Number	Accreditation Standards for a Doctoral-Degree-Level Educational Program for the Occupational Therapist	Accreditation Standards for a Master's-Degree-Level Educational Program for the Occupational Therapist	Accreditation Standards for an Associate-Degree-Level Educational Program for the Occupational Therapy Assistant
	• Be prepared to effectively communicate and work interprofessionally with those who provide care for individuals and/or populations in order to clarify each member's responsibility in executing components of an intervention plan. • Be prepared to advocate as a professional for the occupational therapy services offered and for the recipients of those services. • Be prepared to be an effective consumer of the latest research and knowledge bases that support practice and contribute to the growth and dissemination of research and knowledge. • Demonstrate in-depth knowledge of delivery models, policies, and systems related to the area of practice in settings where occupational therapy is currently practiced and where it is emerging as a service. • Demonstrate thorough knowledge of evidence-based practice. • Demonstrate active involvement in professional development, leadership, and advocacy. • Relate theory to practice and demonstrate synthesis of advanced knowledge in a practice area through completion of a culminating project.	• Be prepared to effectively communicate and work interprofessionally with those who provide care for individuals and/or populations in order to clarify each member's responsibility in executing components of an intervention plan. • Be prepared to advocate as a professional for the occupational therapy services offered and for the recipients of those services. • Be prepared to be an effective consumer of the latest research and knowledge bases that support practice and contribute to the growth and dissemination of research and knowledge.	• Be prepared to effectively communicate and work interprofessionally with those who provide care for individuals and/or populations in order to clarify each member's responsibility in executing components of an intervention plan. • Be prepared to advocate as a professional for the occupational therapy services offered and for the recipients of those services.

(Continued)

Standard Number	Accreditation Standards for a Doctoral-Degree-Level Educational Program for the Occupational Therapist	Accreditation Standards for a Master's-Degree-Level Educational Program for the Occupational Therapist	Accreditation Standards for an Associate-Degree-Level Educational Program for the Occupational Therapy Assistant
	• Develop in-depth experience in one or more of the following areas through completion of a doctoral experiential component: clinical practice skills, research skills, administration, leadership, program and policy development, advocacy, education, and theory development.		

SECTION A: GENERAL REQUIREMENTS

A.1.0.   SPONSORSHIP AND ACCREDITATION

A.1.1.	The sponsoring institution(s) and affiliates, if any, must be accredited by the recognized regional accrediting authority. For programs in countries other than the United States, ACOTE will determine an alternative and equivalent external review process.	The sponsoring institution(s) and affiliates, if any, must be accredited by the recognized regional accrediting authority. For programs in countries other than the United States, ACOTE will determine an alternative and equivalent external review process.	The sponsoring institution(s) and affiliates, if any, must be accredited by a recognized regional or national accrediting authority.
A.1.2.	Sponsoring institution(s) must be authorized under applicable law or other acceptable authority to provide a program of postsecondary education and have appropriate doctoral degree–granting authority.	Sponsoring institution(s) must be authorized under applicable law or other acceptable authority to provide a program of postsecondary education and have appropriate degree-granting authority.	Sponsoring institution(s) must be authorized under applicable law or other acceptable authority to provide a program of postsecondary education and have appropriate degree-granting authority, or the institution must be a program offered within the military services.

(Continued)

Standard Number	Accreditation Standards for a Doctoral-Degree-Level Educational Program for the Occupational Therapist	Accreditation Standards for a Master's-Degree-Level Educational Program for the Occupational Therapist	Accreditation Standards for an Associate-Degree-Level Educational Program for the Occupational Therapy Assistant
A.1.3.	Accredited occupational therapy educational programs may be established only in senior colleges, universities, or medical schools.	Accredited occupational therapy educational programs may be established only in senior colleges, universities, or medical schools.	Accredited occupational therapy assistant educational programs may be established only in community, technical, junior, and senior colleges; universities; medical schools; vocational schools or institutions; or military services.
A.1.4.	The sponsoring institution(s) must assume primary responsibility for appointment of faculty, admission of students, and curriculum planning at all locations where the program is offered. This would include course content, satisfactory completion of the educational program, and granting of the degree. The sponsoring institution(s) must also be responsible for the coordination of classroom teaching and supervised fieldwork practice and for providing assurance that the practice activities assigned to students in a fieldwork setting are appropriate to the program.	The sponsoring institution(s) must assume primary responsibility for appointment of faculty, admission of students, and curriculum planning at all locations where the program is offered. This would include course content, satisfactory completion of the educational program, and granting of the degree. The sponsoring institution(s) must also be responsible for the coordination of classroom teaching and supervised fieldwork practice and for providing assurance that the practice activities assigned to students in a fieldwork setting are appropriate to the program.	The sponsoring institution(s) must assume primary responsibility for appointment of faculty, admission of students, and curriculum planning at all locations where the program is offered. This would include course content, satisfactory completion of the educational program, and granting of the degree. The sponsoring institution(s) must also be responsible for the coordination of classroom teaching and supervised fieldwork practice and for providing assurance that the practice activities assigned to students in a fieldwork setting are appropriate to the program.
A.1.5.	The program must • Inform ACOTE of the transfer of program sponsorship or change of the institution's name within 30 days of the transfer or change.	The program must • Inform ACOTE of the transfer of program sponsorship or change of the institution's name within 30 days of the transfer or change.	The program must • Inform ACOTE of the transfer of program sponsorship or change of the institution's name within 30 days of the transfer or change.

(Continued)

Standard Number	Accreditation Standards for a Doctoral-Degree-Level Educational Program for the Occupational Therapist	Accreditation Standards for a Master's-Degree-Level Educational Program for the Occupational Therapist	Accreditation Standards for an Associate-Degree-Level Educational Program for the Occupational Therapy Assistant
	• Inform ACOTE within 30 days of the date of notification of any adverse accreditation action taken to change the sponsoring institution's accreditation status to probation or withdrawal of accreditation. • Notify and receive ACOTE approval for any significant program changes prior to the admission of students into the new/changed program. • Inform ACOTE within 30 days of the resignation of the program director or appointment of a new or interim program director. • Pay accreditation fees within 90 days of the invoice date. • Submit a Report of Self-Study and other required reports (e.g., Interim Report, Plan of Correction, Progress Report) within the period of time designated by ACOTE. All reports must be complete and contain all requested information. • Agree to a site visit date before the end of the period for which accreditation was previously awarded. • Demonstrate honesty and integrity in all interactions with ACOTE.	• Inform ACOTE within 30 days of the date of notification of any adverse accreditation action taken to change the sponsoring institution's accreditation status to probation or withdrawal of accreditation. • Notify and receive ACOTE approval for any significant program changes prior to the admission of students into the new/changed program. • Inform ACOTE within 30 days of the resignation of the program director or appointment of a new or interim program director. • Pay accreditation fees within 90 days of the invoice date. • Submit a Report of Self-Study and other required reports (e.g., Interim Report, Plan of Correction, Progress Report) within the period of time designated by ACOTE. All reports must be complete and contain all requested information. • Agree to a site visit date before the end of the period for which accreditation was previously awarded. • Demonstrate honesty and integrity in all interactions with ACOTE.	• Inform ACOTE within 30 days of the date of notification of any adverse accreditation action taken to change the sponsoring institution's accreditation status to probation or withdrawal of accreditation. • Notify and receive ACOTE approval for any significant program changes prior to the admission of students into the new/changed program. • Inform ACOTE within 30 days of the resignation of the program director or appointment of a new or interim program director. • Pay accreditation fees within 90 days of the invoice date. • Submit a Report of Self-Study and other required reports (e.g., Interim Report, Plan of Correction, Progress Report) within the period of time designated by ACOTE. All reports must be complete and contain all requested information. • Agree to a site visit date before the end of the period for which accreditation was previously awarded. • Demonstrate honesty and integrity in all interactions with ACOTE.

(Continued)

Standard Number	Accreditation Standards for a Doctoral-Degree-Level Educational Program for the Occupational Therapist	Accreditation Standards for a Master's-Degree-Level Educational Program for the Occupational Therapist	Accreditation Standards for an Associate-Degree-Level Educational Program for the Occupational Therapy Assistant
A.2.0.	**ACADEMIC RESOURCES**		
A.2.1.	The program must identify an individual as the program director who is assigned to the occupational therapy educational program on a full-time basis. The director may be assigned other institutional duties that do not interfere with the management and administration of the program. The institution must document that the program director has sufficient release time to ensure that the needs of the program are being met.	The program must identify an individual as the program director who is assigned to the occupational therapy educational program on a full-time basis. The director may be assigned other institutional duties that do not interfere with the management and administration of the program. The institution must document that the program director has sufficient release time to ensure that the needs of the program are being met.	The program must identify an individual as the program director who is assigned to the occupational therapy educational program on a full-time basis. The director may be assigned other institutional duties that do not interfere with the management and administration of the program. The institution must document that the program director has sufficient release time to ensure that the needs of the program are being met.
A.2.2.	The program director must be an initially certified occupational therapist who is licensed or otherwise regulated according to regulations in the state(s) or jurisdiction(s) in which the program is located. The program director must hold a doctoral degree awarded by an institution that is accredited by a regional accrediting body recognized by the U.S. Department of Education (USDE). The doctoral degree is not limited to a doctorate in occupational therapy.	The program director must be an initially certified occupational therapist who is licensed or otherwise regulated according to regulations in the state(s) or jurisdiction(s) in which the program is located. The program director must hold a doctoral degree awarded by an institution that is accredited by a regional accrediting body recognized by the U.S. Department of Education (USDE). The doctoral degree is not limited to a doctorate in occupational therapy.	The program director must be an initially certified occupational therapist or occupational therapy assistant who is licensed or otherwise regulated according to regulations in the state(s) or jurisdiction(s) in which the program is located. The program director must hold a minimum of a master's degree awarded by an institution that is accredited by a regional or national accrediting body recognized by the U.S. Department of Education (USDE). The master's degree is not limited to a master's degree in occupational therapy.

(Continued)

Standard Number	Accreditation Standards for a Doctoral-Degree-Level Educational Program for the Occupational Therapist	Accreditation Standards for a Master's-Degree-Level Educational Program for the Occupational Therapist	Accreditation Standards for an Associate-Degree-Level Educational Program for the Occupational Therapy Assistant
A.2.3.	The program director must have a minimum of 8 years of documented experience in the field of occupational therapy. This experience must include • Clinical practice as an occupational therapist; • Administrative experience including, but not limited to, program planning and implementation, personnel management, evaluation, and budgeting; • Scholarship (e.g., scholarship of application, scholarship of teaching and learning); and • At least 3 years of experience in a full-time academic appointment with teaching responsibilities at the postbaccalaureate level.	The program director must have a minimum of 8 years of documented experience in the field of occupational therapy. This experience must include • Clinical practice as an occupational therapist; • Administrative experience including, but not limited to, program planning and implementation, personnel management, evaluation, and budgeting; • Scholarship (e.g., scholarship of application, scholarship of teaching and learning); and • At least 3 years of experience in a full-time academic appointment with teaching responsibilities at the postsecondary level.	The program director must have a minimum of 5 years of documented experience in the field of occupational therapy. This experience must include • Clinical practice as an occupational therapist or occupational therapy assistant; • Administrative experience including, but not limited to, program planning and implementation, personnel management, evaluation, and budgeting; • Understanding of and experience with occupational therapy assistants; and • At least 1 year of experience in a full-time academic appointment with teaching responsibilities at the postsecondary level.
A.2.4.	The program director must be responsible for the management and administration of the program, including planning, evaluation, budgeting, selection of faculty and staff, maintenance of accreditation, and commitment to strategies for professional development.	The program director must be responsible for the management and administration of the program, including planning, evaluation, budgeting, selection of faculty and staff, maintenance of accreditation, and commitment to strategies for professional development.	The program director must be responsible for the management and administration of the program, including planning, evaluation, budgeting, selection of faculty and staff, maintenance of accreditation, and commitment to strategies for professional development.

(Continued)

Standard Number	Accreditation Standards for a Doctoral-Degree-Level Educational Program for the Occupational Therapist	Accreditation Standards for a Master's-Degree-Level Educational Program for the Occupational Therapist	Accreditation Standards for an Associate-Degree-Level Educational Program for the Occupational Therapy Assistant
A.2.5.	(No related Standard)	(No related Standard)	In addition to the program director, the program must have at least one full-time equivalent (FTE) faculty position at each accredited location where the program is offered. This position may be shared by up to three individuals who teach as adjunct faculty. These individuals must have one or more additional responsibilities related to student advisement, supervision, committee work, program planning, evaluation, recruitment, and marketing activities.
A.2.6.	The program director and faculty must possess the academic and experiential qualifications and backgrounds (identified in documented descriptions of roles and responsibilities) that are necessary to meet program objectives and the mission of the institution.	The program director and faculty must possess the academic and experiential qualifications and backgrounds (identified in documented descriptions of roles and responsibilities) that are necessary to meet program objectives and the mission of the institution.	The program director and faculty must possess the academic and experiential qualifications and backgrounds (identified in documented descriptions of roles and responsibilities) that are necessary to meet program objectives and the mission of the institution.
A.2.7.	The program must identify an individual for the role of academic fieldwork coordinator who is specifically responsible for the program's compliance with the fieldwork requirements of Standards Section C.1.0 and is assigned to the occupational therapy educational program as a full-time faculty member as defined by ACOTE. The academic fieldwork coordinator may be assigned other institutional duties that do not interfere with the management and administration	The program must identify an individual for the role of academic fieldwork coordinator who is specifically responsible for the program's compliance with the fieldwork requirements of Standards Section C.1.0 and is assigned to the occupational therapy educational program as a full-time faculty member as defined by ACOTE. The academic fieldwork coordinator may be assigned other institutional duties that do not interfere with the management and administra-	The program must identify an individual for the role of academic fieldwork coordinator who is specifically responsible for the program's compliance with the fieldwork requirements of Standards Section C.1.0 and is assigned to the occupational therapy educational program as a full-time faculty member as defined by ACOTE. The academic fieldwork coordinator may be assigned other institutional duties that do not interfere with the management and administration

(Continued)

Standard Number	Accreditation Standards for a Doctoral-Degree-Level Educational Program for the Occupational Therapist	Accreditation Standards for a Master's-Degree-Level Educational Program for the Occupational Therapist	Accreditation Standards for an Associate-Degree-Level Educational Program for the Occupational Therapy Assistant
	of the fieldwork program. The institution must document that the academic fieldwork coordinator has sufficient release time to ensure that the needs of the fieldwork program are being met.	tion of the fieldwork program. The institution must document that the academic fieldwork coordinator has sufficient release time to ensure that the needs of the fieldwork program are being met.	of the fieldwork program. The institution must document that the academic fieldwork coordinator has sufficient release time to ensure that the needs of the fieldwork program are being met.
	This individual must be a licensed or otherwise regulated occupational therapist. Coordinators must hold a doctoral degree awarded by an institution that is accredited by a USDE-recognized regional accrediting body.	This individual must be a licensed or otherwise regulated occupational therapist. Coordinators must hold a minimum of a master's degree awarded by an institution that is accredited by a USDE-recognized regional accrediting body.	This individual must be a licensed or otherwise regulated occupational therapist or occupational therapy assistant. Coordinators must hold a minimum of a baccalaureate degree awarded by an institution that is accredited by a USDE-recognized regional or national accrediting body.
A.2.8.	Core faculty who are occupational therapists or occupational therapy assistants must be currently licensed or otherwise regulated according to regulations in the state or jurisdiction in which the program is located.	Core faculty who are occupational therapists or occupational therapy assistants must be currently licensed or otherwise regulated according to regulations in the state or jurisdiction in which the program is located.	Core faculty who are occupational therapists or occupational therapy assistants must be currently licensed or otherwise regulated according to regulations in the state or jurisdiction in which the program is located.
	Faculty in residence and teaching at additional locations must be currently licensed or otherwise regulated according to regulations in the state or jurisdiction in which the additional location is located.	Faculty in residence and teaching at additional locations must be currently licensed or otherwise regulated according to regulations in the state or jurisdiction in which the additional location is located.	Faculty in residence and teaching at additional locations must be currently licensed or otherwise regulated according to regulations in the state or jurisdiction in which the additional location is located.

(Continued)

Standard Number	Accreditation Standards for a Doctoral-Degree-Level Educational Program for the Occupational Therapist	Accreditation Standards for a Master's-Degree-Level Educational Program for the Occupational Therapist	Accreditation Standards for an Associate-Degree-Level Educational Program for the Occupational Therapy Assistant
A.2.9.	*(No related Standard)*	*(No related Standard)*	In programs where the program director is an occupational therapy assistant, an occupational therapist must be included on faculty and contribute to the functioning of the program through a variety of mechanisms including, but not limited to, teaching, advising, and committee work. In a program where there are only occupational therapists on faculty who have never practiced as an occupational therapy assistant, the program must demonstrate that an individual who is an occupational therapy assistant or an occupational therapist who has previously practiced as an occupational therapy assistant is involved in the program as an adjunct faculty or teaching assistant.
A.2.10.	All full-time faculty teaching in the program must hold a doctoral degree awarded by an institution that is accredited by a USDE-recognized regional accrediting body. The doctoral degree is not limited to a doctorate in occupational therapy.	The majority of full-time faculty who are occupational therapists or occupational therapy assistants must hold a doctoral degree. All full-time faculty must hold a minimum of a master's degree. All degrees must be awarded by an institution that is accredited by a USDE-recognized regional accrediting body. The degrees are not limited to occupational therapy. For an even number of full-time faculty, at least half must hold doctorates. The program director is counted as a faculty member.	All occupational therapy assistant faculty who are full-time must hold a minimum of a baccalaureate degree awarded by an institution that is accredited by a USDE-recognized regional or national accrediting body.

(Continued)

Standard Number	Accreditation Standards for a Doctoral-Degree-Level Educational Program for the Occupational Therapist	Accreditation Standards for a Master's-Degree-Level Educational Program for the Occupational Therapist	Accreditation Standards for an Associate-Degree-Level Educational Program for the Occupational Therapy Assistant
A.2.11.	The faculty must have documented expertise in their area(s) of teaching responsibility and knowledge of the content delivery method (e.g., distance learning).	The faculty must have documented expertise in their area(s) of teaching responsibility and knowledge of the content delivery method (e.g., distance learning).	The faculty must have documented expertise in their area(s) of teaching responsibility and knowledge of the content delivery method (e.g., distance learning).
A.2.12.	For programs with additional accredited location(s), the program must identify a faculty member who is an occupational therapist as site coordinator at each location who is responsible for ensuring uniform implementation of the program and ongoing communication with the program director.	For programs with additional accredited location(s), the program must identify a faculty member who is an occupational therapist as site coordinator at each location who is responsible for ensuring uniform implementation of the program and ongoing communication with the program director.	For programs with additional accredited location(s), the program must identify a faculty member who is an occupational therapist or occupational therapy assistant as site coordinator at each location who is responsible for ensuring uniform implementation of the program and ongoing communication with the program director.
A.2.13.	The occupational therapy faculty at each accredited location where the program is offered must be sufficient in number and must possess the expertise necessary to ensure appropriate curriculum design, content delivery, and program evaluation. The faculty must include individuals competent to ensure delivery of the broad scope of occupational therapy practice. Multiple adjuncts, part-time faculty, or full-time faculty may be configured to meet this goal. Each accredited additional location must have at least one full-time equivalent (FTE) faculty member.	The occupational therapy faculty at each accredited location where the program is offered must be sufficient in number and must possess the expertise necessary to ensure appropriate curriculum design, content delivery, and program evaluation. The faculty must include individuals competent to ensure delivery of the broad scope of occupational therapy practice. Multiple adjuncts, part-time faculty, or full-time faculty may be configured to meet this goal. Each accredited additional location must have at least one full-time equivalent (FTE) faculty member.	The occupational therapy assistant faculty at each accredited location where the program is offered must be sufficient in number and must possess the expertise necessary to ensure appropriate curriculum design, content delivery, and program evaluation. The faculty must include individuals competent to ensure delivery of the broad scope of occupational therapy practice. Multiple adjuncts, part-time faculty, or full-time faculty may be configured to meet this goal. Each accredited additional location must have at least one full-time equivalent (FTE) faculty member.

(Continued)

Standard Number	Accreditation Standards for a Doctoral-Degree-Level Educational Program for the Occupational Therapist	Accreditation Standards for a Master's-Degree-Level Educational Program for the Occupational Therapist	Accreditation Standards for an Associate-Degree-Level Educational Program for the Occupational Therapy Assistant
A.2.14.	Faculty responsibilities must be consistent with and supportive of the mission of the institution.	Faculty responsibilities must be consistent with and supportive of the mission of the institution.	Faculty responsibilities must be consistent with and supportive of the mission of the institution.
A.2.15.	The faculty–student ratio must permit the achievement of the purpose and stated objectives for laboratory and lecture courses, be compatible with accepted practices of the institution for similar programs, and ensure student and consumer safety.	The faculty–student ratio must permit the achievement of the purpose and stated objectives for laboratory and lecture courses, be compatible with accepted practices of the institution for similar programs, and ensure student and consumer safety.	The faculty–student ratio must permit the achievement of the purpose and stated objectives for laboratory and lecture courses, be compatible with accepted practices of the institution for similar programs, and ensure student and consumer safety.
A.2.16.	Clerical and support staff must be provided to the program, consistent with institutional practice, to meet programmatic and administrative requirements, including support for any portion of the program offered by distance education.	Clerical and support staff must be provided to the program, consistent with institutional practice, to meet programmatic and administrative requirements, including support for any portion of the program offered by distance education.	Clerical and support staff must be provided to the program, consistent with institutional practice, to meet programmatic and administrative requirements, including support for any portion of the program offered by distance education.
A.2.17.	The program must be allocated a budget of regular institutional funds, not including grants, gifts, and other restricted sources, sufficient to implement and maintain the objectives of the program and to fulfill the program's obligation to matriculated and entering students.	The program must be allocated a budget of regular institutional funds, not including grants, gifts, and other restricted sources, sufficient to implement and maintain the objectives of the program and to fulfill the program's obligation to matriculated and entering students.	The program must be allocated a budget of regular institutional funds, not including grants, gifts, and other restricted sources, sufficient to implement and maintain the objectives of the program and to fulfill the program's obligation to matriculated and entering students.
A.2.18.	Classrooms and laboratories must be provided that are consistent with the program's educational objectives, teaching methods, number of students, and safety and health standards of the	Classrooms and laboratories must be provided that are consistent with the program's educational objectives, teaching methods, number of students, and safety and health standards of the	Classrooms and laboratories must be provided that are consistent with the program's educational objectives, teaching methods, number of students, and safety and health standards of the

(Continued)

(Continued)

Standard Number	Accreditation Standards for a Doctoral-Degree-Level Educational Program for the Occupational Therapist	Accreditation Standards for a Master's-Degree-Level Educational Program for the Occupational Therapist	Accreditation Standards for an Associate-Degree-Level Educational Program for the Occupational Therapy Assistant
	institution, and they must allow for efficient operation of the program.	institution, and they must allow for efficient operation of the program.	institution, and they must allow for efficient operation of the program.
A.2.19.	If the program offers distance education, it must include • A process through which the program establishes that the student who registers in a distance education course or program is the same student who participates in and completes the program and receives academic credit, • Technology and resources that are adequate to support a distance-learning environment, and • A process to ensure that faculty are adequately trained and skilled to use distance education methodologies.	If the program offers distance education, it must include • A process through which the program establishes that the student who registers in a distance education course or program is the same student who participates in and completes the program and receives academic credit, • Technology and resources that are adequate to support a distance-learning environment, and • A process to ensure that faculty are adequately trained and skilled to use distance education methodologies.	If the program offers distance education, it must include • A process through which the program establishes that the student who registers in a distance education course or program is the same student who participates in and completes the program and receives academic credit, • Technology and resources that are adequate to support a distance-learning environment, and • A process to ensure that faculty are adequately trained and skilled to use distance education methodologies.
A.2.20.	Laboratory space provided by the institution must be assigned to the occupational therapy program on a priority basis. If laboratory space for occupational therapy lab classes is provided by another institution or agency, there must be a written and signed agreement to ensure assignment of space for program use.	Laboratory space provided by the institution must be assigned to the occupational therapy program on a priority basis. If laboratory space for occupational therapy lab classes is provided by another institution or agency, there must be a written and signed agreement to ensure assignment of space for program use.	Laboratory space provided by the institution must be assigned to the occupational therapy assistant program on a priority basis. If laboratory space for occupational therapy assistant lab classes is provided by another institution or agency, there must be a written and signed agreement to ensure assignment of space for program use.
A.2.21.	Adequate space must be provided to store and secure equipment and supplies.	Adequate space must be provided to store and secure equipment and supplies.	Adequate space must be provided to store and secure equipment and supplies.

Standard Number	Accreditation Standards for a Doctoral-Degree-Level Educational Program for the Occupational Therapist	Accreditation Standards for a Master's-Degree-Level Educational Program for the Occupational Therapist	Accreditation Standards for an Associate-Degree-Level Educational Program for the Occupational Therapy Assistant
A.2.22.	The program director and faculty must have office space consistent with institutional practice.	The program director and faculty must have office space consistent with institutional practice.	The program director and faculty must have office space consistent with institutional practice.
A.2.23.	Adequate space must be provided for the private advising of students.	Adequate space must be provided for the private advising of students.	Adequate space must be provided for the private advising of students.
A.2.24.	Appropriate and sufficient equipment and supplies must be provided by the institution for student use and for the didactic, supervised fieldwork, and experiential components of the curriculum.	Appropriate and sufficient equipment and supplies must be provided by the institution for student use and for the didactic and supervised fieldwork components of the curriculum.	Appropriate and sufficient equipment and supplies must be provided by the institution for student use and for the didactic and supervised fieldwork components of the curriculum.
A.2.25.	Students must be given access to and have the opportunity to use the evaluative and treatment methodologies that reflect both current practice and practice in the geographic area served by the program.	Students must be given access to and have the opportunity to use the evaluative and treatment methodologies that reflect both current practice and practice in the geographic area served by the program.	Students must be given access to and have the opportunity to use the evaluative and treatment methodologies that reflect both current practice and practice in the geographic area served by the program.
A.2.26.	Students must have ready access to a supply of current and relevant books, journals, periodicals, computers, software, and other reference materials needed for the practice areas and to meet the requirements of the curriculum. This may include, but is not limited to, libraries, online services, interlibrary loan, and resource centers.	Students must have ready access to a supply of current and relevant books, journals, periodicals, computers, software, and other reference materials needed to meet the requirements of the curriculum. This may include, but is not limited to, libraries, online services, interlibrary loan, and resource centers.	Students must have ready access to a supply of current and relevant books, journals, periodicals, computers, software, and other reference materials needed to meet the requirements of the curriculum. This may include, but is not limited to, libraries, online services, interlibrary loan, and resource centers.

(Continued)

Standard Number	Accreditation Standards for a Doctoral-Degree-Level Educational Program for the Occupational Therapist	Accreditation Standards for a Master's-Degree-Level Educational Program for the Occupational Therapist	Accreditation Standards for an Associate-Degree-Level Educational Program for the Occupational Therapy Assistant
A.2.27.	Instructional aids and technology must be available in sufficient quantity and quality to be consistent with the program objectives and teaching methods.	Instructional aids and technology must be available in sufficient quantity and quality to be consistent with the program objectives and teaching methods.	Instructional aids and technology must be available in sufficient quantity and quality to be consistent with the program objectives and teaching methods.
A.3.0. STUDENTS			
A.3.1.	Admission of students to the occupational therapy program must be made in accordance with the practices of the institution. There must be stated admission criteria that are clearly defined and published and reflective of the demands of the program.	Admission of students to the occupational therapy program must be made in accordance with the practices of the institution. There must be stated admission criteria that are clearly defined and published and reflective of the demands of the program.	Admission of students to the occupational therapy assistant program must be made in accordance with the practices of the institution. There must be stated admission criteria that are clearly defined and published and reflective of the demands of the program.
A.3.2.	Institutions must require that program applicants hold a baccalaureate degree or higher prior to admission to the program.	*(No related Standard)*	*(No related Standard)*
A.3.3.	Policies pertaining to standards for admission, advanced placement, transfer of credit, credit for experiential learning (if applicable), and prerequisite educational or work experience requirements must be readily accessible to prospective students and the public.	Policies pertaining to standards for admission, advanced placement, transfer of credit, credit for experiential learning (if applicable), and prerequisite educational or work experience requirements must be readily accessible to prospective students and the public.	Policies pertaining to standards for admission, advanced placement, transfer of credit, credit for experiential learning (if applicable), and prerequisite educational or work experience requirements must be readily accessible to prospective students and the public.
A.3.4.	Programs must document implementation of a mechanism to ensure that students receiving	Programs must document implementation of a mechanism to ensure that students receiving	Programs must document implementation of a mechanism to ensure that students receiving

(Continued)

Standard Number	Accreditation Standards for a Doctoral-Degree-Level Educational Program for the Occupational Therapist	Accreditation Standards for a Master's-Degree-Level Educational Program for the Occupational Therapist	Accreditation Standards for an Associate-Degree-Level Educational Program for the Occupational Therapy Assistant
	credit for previous courses and/or work experience have met the content requirements of the appropriate doctoral Standards.	credit for previous courses and/or work experience have met the content requirements of the appropriate master's Standards.	credit for previous courses and/or work experience have met the content requirements of the appropriate occupational therapy assistant Standards.
A.3.5.	Criteria for successful completion of each segment of the educational program and for graduation must be given in advance to each student.	Criteria for successful completion of each segment of the educational program and for graduation must be given in advance to each student.	Criteria for successful completion of each segment of the educational program and for graduation must be given in advance to each student.
A.3.6.	Evaluation content and methods must be consistent with the curriculum design, objectives, competencies of the didactic, fieldwork, and experiential components of the program.	Evaluation content and methods must be consistent with the curriculum design, objectives, and competencies of the didactic and fieldwork components of the program.	Evaluation content and methods must be consistent with the curriculum design, objectives, and competencies of the didactic and fieldwork components of the program.
A.3.7.	Evaluation must be conducted on a regular basis to provide students and program officials with timely indications of the students' progress and academic standing.	Evaluation must be conducted on a regular basis to provide students and program officials with timely indications of the students' progress and academic standing.	Evaluation must be conducted on a regular basis to provide students and program officials with timely indications of the students' progress and academic standing.
A.3.8.	Students must be informed of and have access to the student support services that are provided to other students in the institution.	Students must be informed of and have access to the student support services that are provided to other students in the institution.	Students must be informed of and have access to the student support services that are provided to other students in the institution.
A.3.9.	Advising related to professional coursework, fieldwork education, and the experiential component of the program must be the responsibility of the occupational therapy faculty.	Advising related to professional coursework and fieldwork education must be the responsibility of the occupational therapy faculty.	Advising related to coursework in the occupational therapy assistant program and fieldwork education must be the responsibility of the occupational therapy assistant faculty.

(Continued)

Standard Number	Accreditation Standards for a Doctoral-Degree-Level Educational Program for the Occupational Therapist	Accreditation Standards for a Master's-Degree-Level Educational Program for the Occupational Therapist	Accreditation Standards for an Associate-Degree-Level Educational Program for the Occupational Therapy Assistant
A.4.0.	**OPERATIONAL POLICIES**		
A.4.1.	All program publications and advertising—including, but not limited to, academic calendars, announcements, catalogs, handbooks, and Web sites—must accurately reflect the program offered.	All program publications and advertising—including, but not limited to, academic calendars, announcements, catalogs, handbooks, and Web sites—must accurately reflect the program offered.	All program publications and advertising—including, but not limited to, academic calendars, announcements, catalogs, handbooks, and Web sites—must accurately reflect the program offered.
A.4.2.	Accurate and current information regarding student and program outcomes must be readily available to the public on the program's Web page. At a minimum, the following data must be reported for the previous 3 years: • Total number of program graduates • Graduation rates. The program must provide the direct link to the National Board for Certification in Occupational Therapy (NBCOT) program data results on the program's home page.	Accurate and current information regarding student and program outcomes must be readily available to the public on the program's Web page. At a minimum, the following data must be reported for the previous 3 years: • Total number of program graduates • Graduation rates. The program must provide the direct link to the National Board for Certification in Occupational Therapy (NBCOT) program data results on the program's home page.	Accurate and current information regarding student and program outcomes must be readily available to the public on the program's Web page. At a minimum, the following data must be reported for the previous 3 years: • Total number of program graduates • Graduation rates. The program must provide the direct link to the National Board for Certification in Occupational Therapy (NBCOT) program data results on the program's home page.
A.4.3.	The program's accreditation status and the name, address, and telephone number of ACOTE must be published in all of the following materials used by the institution: catalog, Web site, and program-related brochures or flyers available to prospective students. A link to www.acoteonline.org must be provided on the program's home page.	The program's accreditation status and the name, address, and telephone number of ACOTE must be published in all of the following materials used by the institution: catalog, Web site, and program-related brochures or flyers available to prospective students. A link to www.acoteonline.org must be provided on the program's home page.	The program's accreditation status and the name, address, and telephone number of ACOTE must be published in all of the following materials used by the institution: catalog, Web site, and program-related brochures or flyers available to prospective students. A link to www.acoteonline.org must be provided on the program's home page.

(Continued)

Standard Number	Accreditation Standards for a Doctoral-Degree-Level Educational Program for the Occupational Therapist	Accreditation Standards for a Master's-Degree-Level Educational Program for the Occupational Therapist	Accreditation Standards for an Associate-Degree-Level Educational Program for the Occupational Therapy Assistant
A.4.4.	All practices within the institution related to faculty, staff, applicants, and students must be nondiscriminatory.	All practices within the institution related to faculty, staff, applicants, and students must be nondiscriminatory.	All practices within the institution related to faculty, staff, applicants, and students must be nondiscriminatory.
A.4.5.	Graduation requirements, tuition, and fees must be accurately stated, published, and made known to all applicants. When published fees are subject to change, a statement to that effect must be included.	Graduation requirements, tuition, and fees must be accurately stated, published, and made known to all applicants. When published fees are subject to change, a statement to that effect must be included.	Graduation requirements, tuition, and fees must be accurately stated, published, and made known to all applicants. When published fees are subject to change, a statement to that effect must be included.
A.4.6.	The program or sponsoring institution must have a defined and published policy and procedure for processing student and faculty grievances.	The program or sponsoring institution must have a defined and published policy and procedure for processing student and faculty grievances.	The program or sponsoring institution must have a defined and published policy and procedure for processing student and faculty grievances.
A.4.7.	Policies and procedures for handling complaints against the program must be published and made known. The program must maintain a record of student complaints that includes the nature and disposition of each complaint.	Policies and procedures for handling complaints against the program must be published and made known. The program must maintain a record of student complaints that includes the nature and disposition of each complaint.	Policies and procedures for handling complaints against the program must be published and made known. The program must maintain a record of student complaints that includes the nature and disposition of each complaint.
A.4.8.	Policies and processes for student withdrawal and for refunds of tuition and fees must be published and made known to all applicants.	Policies and processes for student withdrawal and for refunds of tuition and fees must be published and made known to all applicants.	Policies and processes for student withdrawal and for refunds of tuition and fees must be published and made known to all applicants.
A.4.9.	Policies and procedures for student probation, suspension, and dismissal must be published and made known.	Policies and procedures for student probation, suspension, and dismissal must be published and made known.	Policies and procedures for student probation, suspension, and dismissal must be published and made known.

(Continued)

Standard Number	Accreditation Standards for a Doctoral-Degree-Level Educational Program for the Occupational Therapist	Accreditation Standards for a Master's-Degree-Level Educational Program for the Occupational Therapist	Accreditation Standards for an Associate-Degree-Level Educational Program for the Occupational Therapy Assistant
A.4.10.	Policies and procedures for human-subject research protocol must be published and made known.	Policies and procedures for human-subject research protocol must be published and made known.	Policies and procedures for human-subject research protocol must be published and made known (if applicable to the program).
A.4.11.	Programs must make available to students written policies and procedures regarding appropriate use of equipment and supplies and for all educational activities that have implications for the health and safety of clients, students, and faculty (including infection control and evacuation procedures).	Programs must make available to students written policies and procedures regarding appropriate use of equipment and supplies and for all educational activities that have implications for the health and safety of clients, students, and faculty (including infection control and evacuation procedures).	Programs must make available to students written policies and procedures regarding appropriate use of equipment and supplies and for all educational activities that have implications for the health and safety of clients, students, and faculty (including infection control and evacuation procedures).
A.4.12.	A program admitting students on the basis of ability to benefit (defined by the USDE as admitting students who do not have either a high school diploma or its equivalent) must publicize its objectives, assessment measures, and means of evaluating the student's ability to benefit.	A program admitting students on the basis of ability to benefit (defined by the USDE as admitting students who do not have either a high school diploma or its equivalent) must publicize its objectives, assessment measures, and means of evaluating the student's ability to benefit.	A program admitting students on the basis of ability to benefit (defined by the USDE as admitting students who do not have either a high school diploma or its equivalent) must publicize its objectives, assessment measures, and means of evaluating the student's ability to benefit.
A.4.13.	Documentation of all progression, retention, graduation, certification, and credentialing requirements must be published and made known to applicants. A statement on the program's Web site about the potential impact of a felony conviction on a graduate's eligibility for certification and credentialing must be provided.	Documentation of all progression, retention, graduation, certification, and credentialing requirements must be published and made known to applicants. A statement on the program's Web site about the potential impact of a felony conviction on a graduate's eligibility for certification and credentialing must be provided.	Documentation of all progression, retention, graduation, certification, and credentialing requirements must be published and made known to applicants. A statement on the program's Web site about the potential impact of a felony conviction on a graduate's eligibility for certification and credentialing must be provided.
A.4.14.	The program must have a documented and published policy to ensure that students complete all	The program must have a documented and published policy to ensure that students complete all	The program must have a documented and published policy to ensure that students

(Continued)

(Continued)

Standard Number	Accreditation Standards for a Doctoral-Degree-Level Educational Program for the Occupational Therapist	Accreditation Standards for a Master's-Degree-Level Educational Program for the Occupational Therapist	Accreditation Standards for an Associate-Degree-Level Educational Program for the Occupational Therapy Assistant
	graduation, fieldwork, and experiential component requirements in a timely manner. This policy must include a statement that all Level II fieldwork and the experiential component of the program must be completed within a time frame established by the program.	graduation and fieldwork requirements in a timely manner. This policy must include a statement that all Level II fieldwork must be completed within a time frame established by the program.	complete all graduation and fieldwork requirements in a timely manner. This policy must include a statement that all Level II fieldwork must be completed within a time frame established by the program.
A.4.15.	Records regarding student admission, enrollment, fieldwork, and achievement must be maintained and kept in a secure setting. Grades and credits for courses must be recorded on students' transcripts and permanently maintained by the sponsoring institution.	Records regarding student admission, enrollment, fieldwork, and achievement must be maintained and kept in a secure setting. Grades and credits for courses must be recorded on students' transcripts and permanently maintained by the sponsoring institution.	Records regarding student admission, enrollment, fieldwork, and achievement must be maintained and kept in a secure setting. Grades and credits for courses must be recorded on students' transcripts and permanently maintained by the sponsoring institution.

A.5.0.   STRATEGIC PLAN AND PROGRAM ASSESSMENT

For programs that are offered at more than one location, the program's strategic plan, evaluation plan, and results of ongoing evaluation must address each program location as a component of the overall plan.

Standard Number	Doctoral	Master's	Associate
A.5.1.	The program must document a current strategic plan that articulates the program's future vision and guides the program development (e.g., faculty recruitment and professional growth, scholarship, changes in the curriculum design, priorities in academic resources, procurement of fieldwork and experiential component sites). A program program strategic plan must be for a minimum	The program must document a current strategic plan that articulates the program's future vision and guides the program development (e.g., faculty recruitment and professional growth, scholarship, changes in the curriculum design, priorities in academic resources, procurement of fieldwork sites). A program strategic plan must be for a minimum of a	The program must document a current strategic plan that articulates the program's future vision and guides the program development (e.g., faculty recruitment and professional growth, scholarship, changes in the curriculum design, priorities in academic resources, procurement of fieldwork sites). A program strategic plan must be for a minimum of a

Standard Number	Accreditation Standards for a Doctoral-Degree-Level Educational Program for the Occupational Therapist	Accreditation Standards for a Master's-Degree-Level Educational Program for the Occupational Therapist	Accreditation Standards for an Associate-Degree-Level Educational Program for the Occupational Therapy Assistant
	of a 3-year period and include, but need not be limited to, • Evidence that the plan is based on program evaluation and an analysis of external and internal environments. • Long-term goals that address the vision and mission of both the institution and the program, as well as specific needs of the program. • Specific measurable action steps with expected timelines by which the program will reach its long-term goals. • Person(s) responsible for action steps. • Evidence of periodic updating of action steps and long-term goals as they are met or as circumstances change.	3-year period and include, but need not be limited to, • Evidence that the plan is based on program evaluation and an analysis of external and internal environments. • Long-term goals that address the vision and mission of both the institution and the program, as well as specific needs of the program. • Specific measurable action steps with expected timelines by which the program will reach its long-term goals. • Person(s) responsible for action steps. • Evidence of periodic updating of action steps and long-term goals as they are met or as circumstances change.	3-year period and include, but need not be limited to, • Evidence that the plan is based on program evaluation and an analysis of external and internal environments. • Long-term goals that address the vision and mission of both the institution and the program, as well as specific needs of the program. • Specific measurable action steps with expected timelines by which the program will reach its long-term goals. • Person(s) responsible for action steps. • Evidence of periodic updating of action steps and long-term goals as they are met or as circumstances change.
A.5.2.	The program director and each faculty member who teaches two or more courses must have a current written professional growth and development plan. Each plan must contain the signature of the faculty member and supervisor. At a minimum, the plan must include, but need not be limited to, • Goals to enhance the faculty member's ability to fulfill designated responsibilities (e.g., goals related to currency in areas of teaching responsibility, teaching effectiveness, research, scholarly activity).	The program director and each faculty member who teaches two or more courses must have a current written professional growth and development plan. Each plan must contain the signature of the faculty member and supervisor. At a minimum, the plan must include, but need not be limited to, • Goals to enhance the faculty member's ability to fulfill designated responsibilities (e.g., goals related to currency in areas of teaching responsibility, teaching effectiveness, research, scholarly activity).	The program director and each faculty member who teaches two or more courses must have a current written professional growth and development plan. Each plan must contain the signature of the faculty member and supervisor. At a minimum, the plan must include, but need not be limited to, • Goals to enhance the faculty member's ability to fulfill designated responsibilities (e.g., goals related to currency in areas of teaching responsibility, teaching effectiveness, research, scholarly activity).

(Continued)

Standard Number	Accreditation Standards for a Doctoral-Degree-Level Educational Program for the Occupational Therapist	Accreditation Standards for a Master's-Degree-Level Educational Program for the Occupational Therapist	Accreditation Standards for an Associate-Degree-Level Educational Program for the Occupational Therapy Assistant
	• Specific measurable action steps with expected timelines by which the faculty member will achieve the goals. • Evidence of annual updates of action steps and goals as they are met or as circumstances change. • Identification of the ways in which the faculty member's professional development plan will contribute to attaining the program's strategic goals.	• Specific measurable action steps with expected timelines by which the faculty member will achieve the goals. • Evidence of annual updates of action steps and goals as they are met or as circumstances change. • Identification of the ways in which the faculty member's professional development plan will contribute to attaining the program's strategic goals.	• Specific measurable action steps with expected timelines by which the faculty member will achieve the goals. • Evidence of annual updates of action steps and goals as they are met or as circumstances change. • Identification of the ways in which the faculty member's professional development plan will contribute to attaining the program's strategic goals.
A.5.3.	Programs must routinely secure and document sufficient qualitative and quantitative information to allow for meaningful analysis about the extent to which the program is meeting its stated goals and objectives. This must include, but need not be limited to, • Faculty effectiveness in their assigned teaching responsibilities. • Students' progression through the program. • Student retention rates. • Fieldwork and experiential component performance evaluation. • Student evaluation of fieldwork and the experiential component experience. • Student satisfaction with the program. • Graduates' performance on the NBCOT certification exam.	Programs must routinely secure and document sufficient qualitative and quantitative information to allow for meaningful analysis about the extent to which the program is meeting its stated goals and objectives. This must include, but need not be limited to, • Faculty effectiveness in their assigned teaching responsibilities. • Students' progression through the program. • Student retention rates. • Fieldwork performance evaluation. • Student evaluation of fieldwork experience. • Student satisfaction with the program. • Graduates' performance on the NBCOT certification exam. • Graduates' job placement and performance as determined by employer satisfaction.	Programs must routinely secure and document sufficient qualitative and quantitative information to allow for meaningful analysis about the extent to which the program is meeting its stated goals and objectives. This must include, but need not be limited to, • Faculty effectiveness in their assigned teaching responsibilities. • Students' progression through the program. • Student retention rates. • Fieldwork performance evaluation. • Student evaluation of fieldwork experience. • Student satisfaction with the program. • Graduates' performance on the NBCOT certification exam. • Graduates' job placement and performance as determined by employer satisfaction.

(Continued)

(Continued)

Standard Number	Accreditation Standards for a Doctoral-Degree-Level Educational Program for the Occupational Therapist	Accreditation Standards for a Master's-Degree-Level Educational Program for the Occupational Therapist	Accreditation Standards for an Associate-Degree-Level Educational Program for the Occupational Therapy Assistant
	• Graduates' job placement and performance as determined by employer satisfaction. • Graduates' scholarly activity (e.g., presentations, publications, grants obtained, state and national leadership positions, awards).		
A.5.4.	Programs must routinely and systematically analyze data to determine the extent to which the program is meeting its stated goals and objectives. An annual report summarizing analysis of data and planned action responses must be maintained.	Programs must routinely and systematically analyze data to determine the extent to which the program is meeting its stated goals and objectives. An annual report summarizing analysis of data and planned action responses must be maintained.	Programs must routinely and systematically analyze data to determine the extent to which the program is meeting its stated goals and objectives. An annual report summarizing analysis of data and planned action responses must be maintained.
A.5.5.	The results of ongoing evaluation must be appropriately reflected in the program's strategic plan, curriculum, and other dimensions of the program.	The results of ongoing evaluation must be appropriately reflected in the program's strategic plan, curriculum, and other dimensions of the program.	The results of ongoing evaluation must be appropriately reflected in the program's strategic plan, curriculum, and other dimensions of the program.
A.5.6.	The average pass rate over the 3 most recent calendar years for graduates attempting the national certification exam within 12 months of graduation from the program must be 80% or higher (regardless of the number of attempts). If a program has less than 25 test takers in the 3 3 most recent calendar years, the program may include test takers from additional years until it reaches 25 or until the 5 most recent calendar years are included in the total.	The average pass rate over the 3 most recent calendar years for graduates attempting the national certification exam within 12 months of graduation from the program must be 80% or higher (regardless of the number of attempts). If a program has less than 25 test takers in the 3 most recent calendar years, the program may include test takers from additional years until it reaches 25 or until the 5 most recent calendar years are included in the total.	The average pass rate over the 3 most recent calendar years for graduates attempting the national certification exam within 12 months of graduation from the program must be 80% or higher (regardless of the number of attempts). If a program has less than 25 test takers in the 3 most recent calendar years, the program may include test takers from additional years until it reaches 25 or until the 5 most recent calendar years are included in the total.

A.6.0. CURRICULUM FRAMEWORK
The curriculum framework is a description of the program that includes the program's mission, philosophy, and curriculum design.

Standard Number	Accreditation Standards for a Doctoral-Degree-Level Educational Program for the Occupational Therapist	Accreditation Standards for a Master's-Degree-Level Educational Program for the Occupational Therapist	Accreditation Standards for an Associate-Degree-Level Educational Program for the Occupational Therapy Assistant
A.6.1.	The curriculum must ensure preparation to practice as a generalist with a broad exposure to current practice settings (e.g., school, hospital, community, long-term care) and emerging practice areas (as defined by the program). The curriculum must prepare students to work with a variety of populations including, but not limited to, children, adolescents, adults, and elderly persons in areas of physical and mental health.	The curriculum must include preparation for practice as a generalist with a broad exposure to current practice settings (e.g., school, hospital, community, long-term care) and emerging practice areas (as defined by the program). The curriculum must prepare students to work with a variety of populations including, but not limited to, children, adolescents, adults, and elderly persons in areas of physical and mental health.	The curriculum must include preparation for practice as a generalist with a broad exposure to current practice settings (e.g., school, hospital, community, long-term care) and emerging practice areas (as defined by the program). The curriculum must prepare students to work with a variety of populations including, but not limited to, children, adolescents, adults, and elderly persons in areas of physical and mental health.
A.6.2.	The curriculum must include course objectives and learning activities demonstrating preparation beyond a generalist level in, but not limited to, practice skills, research skills, administration, professional development, leadership, advocacy, and theory.	*(No related Standard)*	*(No related Standard)*
A.6.3.	The occupational therapy doctoral degree must be awarded after a period of study such that the total time to the degree, including both preprofessional and professional preparation, equals at least 6 FTE academic years. The program must document a system and rationale for ensuring that the length of study of the program is appropriate to the expected learning and competence of the graduate.	The program must document a system and rationale for ensuring that the length of study of the program is appropriate to the expected learning and competence of the graduate.	The program must document a system and rationale for ensuring that the length of study of the program is appropriate to the expected learning and competence of the graduate.

(Continued)

Standard Number	Accreditation Standards for a Doctoral-Degree-Level Educational Program for the Occupational Therapist	Accreditation Standards for a Master's-Degree-Level Educational Program for the Occupational Therapist	Accreditation Standards for an Associate-Degree-Level Educational Program for the Occupational Therapy Assistant
A.6.4.	The curriculum must include application of advanced knowledge to practice through a combination of experiential activities and a culminating project.	*(No related Standard)*	*(No related Standard)*
A.6.5.	The statement of philosophy of the occupational therapy program must reflect the current published philosophy of the profession and must include a statement of the program's fundamental beliefs about human beings and how they learn.	The statement of philosophy of the occupational therapy program must reflect the current published philosophy of the profession and must include a statement of the program's fundamental beliefs about human beings and how they learn.	The statement of philosophy of the occupational therapy assistant program must reflect the current published philosophy of the profession and must include a statement of the program's fundamental beliefs about human beings and how they learn.
A.6.6.	The statement of the mission of the occupational therapy program must be consistent with and supportive of the mission of the sponsoring institution. The program's mission statement should explain the unique nature of the program and how it helps fulfill or advance the mission of the sponsoring institution, including religious missions.	The statement of the mission of the occupational therapy program must be consistent with and supportive of the mission of the sponsoring institution. The program's mission statement should explain the unique nature of the program and how it helps fulfill or advance the mission of the sponsoring institution, including religious missions.	The statement of the mission of the occupational therapy assistant program must be consistent with and supportive of the mission of the sponsoring institution. The program's mission statement should explain the unique nature of the program and how it helps fulfill or advance the mission of the sponsoring institution, including religious missions.
A.6.7.	The curriculum design must reflect the mission and philosophy of both the occupational therapy program and the institution and must provide the basis for program planning, implementation, and evaluation. The design must identify curricular threads and educational goals and describe the selection of the content, scope, and sequencing of coursework.	The curriculum design must reflect the mission and philosophy of both the occupational therapy program and the institution and must provide the basis for program planning, implementation, and evaluation. The design must identify curricular threads and educational goals and describe the selection of the content, scope, and sequencing of coursework.	The curriculum design must reflect the mission and philosophy of both the occupational therapy assistant program and the institution and must provide the basis for program planning, implementation, and evaluation. The design must identify curricular threads and educational goals and describe the selection of the content, scope, and sequencing of coursework.

(Continued)

Standard Number	Accreditation Standards for a Doctoral-Degree-Level Educational Program for the Occupational Therapist	Accreditation Standards for a Master's-Degree-Level Educational Program for the Occupational Therapist	Accreditation Standards for an Associate-Degree-Level Educational Program for the Occupational Therapy Assistant
A.6.8.	The program must have clearly documented assessment measures by which students are regularly evaluated on their acquisition of knowledge, skills, attitudes, and competencies required for graduation.	The program must have clearly documented assessment measures by which students are regularly evaluated on their acquisition of knowledge, skills, attitudes, and competencies required for graduation.	The program must have clearly documented assessment measures by which students are regularly evaluated on their acquisition of knowledge, skills, attitudes, and competencies required for graduation.
A.6.9.	The program must have written syllabi for each course that include course objectives and learning activities that, in total, reflect all course content required by the Standards. Instructional methods (e.g., presentations, demonstrations, discussion) and materials used to accomplish course objectives must be documented. Programs must also demonstrate the consistency between course syllabi and the curriculum design.	The program must have written syllabi for each course that include course objectives and learning activities that, in total, reflect all course content required by the Standards. Instructional methods (e.g., presentations, demonstrations, discussion) and materials used to accomplish course objectives must be documented. Programs must also demonstrate the consistency between course syllabi and the curriculum design.	The program must have written syllabi for each course that include course objectives and learning activities that, in total, reflect all course content required by the Standards. Instructional methods (e.g., presentations, demonstrations, discussion) and materials used to accomplish course objectives must be documented. Programs must also demonstrate the consistency between course syllabi and the curriculum design.

Section B: CONTENT REQUIREMENTS

The content requirements are written as expected student outcomes. Faculty are responsible for developing learning activities and evaluation methods to document that students meet these outcomes.

B.1.0.	**FOUNDATIONAL CONTENT REQUIREMENTS** Program content must be based on a broad foundation in the liberal arts and sciences. A strong foundation in the biological, physical, social, and behavioral sciences supports an understanding of occupation across the lifespan. If the content of the Standard is met through prerequisite coursework, the application of foundational content in sciences must also be evident in professional coursework. The student will be able to		**FOUNDATIONAL CONTENT REQUIREMENTS** Program content must be based on a broad foundation in the liberal arts and sciences. A strong foundation in the biological, physical, social, and behavioral sciences supports an understanding of occupation across the

(Continued)

Standard Number	Accreditation Standards for a Doctoral-Degree-Level Educational Program for the Occupational Therapist	Accreditation Standards for a Master's-Degree-Level Educational Program for the Occupational Therapist	Accreditation Standards for an Associate-Degree-Level Educational Program for the Occupational Therapy Assistant
			lifespan. **If the content of the Standard is met through prerequisite coursework, the application of foundational content in sciences must also be evident in professional coursework. The student will be able to**
B.1.1.	Demonstrate knowledge and understanding of the structure and function of the human body to include the biological and physical sciences. Course content must include, but is not limited to, biology, anatomy, physiology, neuroscience, and kinesiology or biomechanics.	Demonstrate knowledge and understanding of the structure and function of the human body to include the biological and physical sciences. Course content must include, but is not limited to, biology, anatomy, physiology, neuroscience, and kinesiology or biomechanics.	Demonstrate knowledge and understanding of the structure and function of the human body to include the biological and physical sciences. Course content must include, but is not limited to, anatomy, physiology, and biomechanics.
B.1.2.	Demonstrate knowledge and understanding of human development throughout the lifespan (infants, children, adolescents, adults, and older adults). Course content must include, but is not limited to, developmental psychology.	Demonstrate knowledge and understanding of human development throughout the lifespan (infants, children, adolescents, adults, and older adults). Course content must include, but is not limited to, developmental psychology.	Demonstrate knowledge and understanding of human development throughout the lifespan (infants, children, adolescents, adults, and older adults). Course content must include, but is not limited to, developmental psychology.
B.1.3.	Demonstrate knowledge and understanding of the concepts of human behavior to include the behavioral sciences, social sciences, and occupational science. Course content must include, but is not limited to, introductory psychology, abnormal psychology, and introductory sociology or introductory anthropology.	Demonstrate knowledge and understanding of the concepts of human behavior to include the behavioral sciences, social sciences, and occupational science. Course content must include, but is not limited to, introductory psychology, abnormal psychology, and introductory sociology or introductory anthropology.	Demonstrate knowledge and understanding of the concepts of human behavior to include the behavioral and social sciences (e.g., principles of psychology, sociology, abnormal psychology) and occupational science.

(Continued)

Standard Number	Accreditation Standards for a Doctoral-Degree-Level Educational Program for the Occupational Therapist	Accreditation Standards for a Master's-Degree-Level Educational Program for the Occupational Therapist	Accreditation Standards for an Associate-Degree-Level Educational Program for the Occupational Therapy Assistant
B.1.4.	Apply knowledge of the role of sociocultural, socioeconomic, and diversity factors and lifestyle choices in contemporary society to meet the needs of individuals and communities. Course content must include, but is not limited to, introductory psychology, abnormal psychology, and introductory sociology or introductory anthropology.	Demonstrate knowledge and appreciation of the role of sociocultural, socioeconomic, and diversity factors and lifestyle choices in contemporary society. Course content must include, but is not limited to, introductory psychology, abnormal psychology, and introductory sociology or introductory anthropology.	Demonstrate knowledge and appreciation of the role of sociocultural, socioeconomic, and diversity factors and lifestyle choices in contemporary society (e.g., principles of psychology, sociology, and abnormal psychology).
B.1.5.	Demonstrate an understanding of the ethical and practical considerations that affect the health and wellness needs of those who are experiencing or are at risk for social injustice, occupational deprivation, and disparity in the receipt of services.	Demonstrate an understanding of the ethical and practical considerations that affect the health and wellness needs of those who are experiencing or are at risk for social injustice, occupational deprivation, and disparity in the receipt of services.	Articulate the ethical and practical considerations that affect the health and wellness needs of those who are experiencing or are at risk for social injustice, occupational deprivation, and disparity in the receipt of services.
B.1.6.	Demonstrate knowledge of global social issues and prevailing health and welfare needs of populations with or at risk for disabilities and chronic health conditions.	Demonstrate knowledge of global social issues and prevailing health and welfare needs of populations with or at risk for disabilities and chronic health conditions.	Demonstrate knowledge of global social issues and prevailing health and welfare needs of populations with or at risk for disabilities and chronic health conditions.
B.1.7.	Apply quantitative statistics and qualitative analysis to interpret tests, measurements, and other data for the purpose of establishing and/or delivering evidence-based practice.	Demonstrate the ability to use statistics to interpret tests and measurements for the purpose of delivering evidence-based practice.	Articulate the importance of using statistics, tests, and measurements for the purpose of delivering evidence-based practice.
B.1.8.	Demonstrate an understanding of the use of technology to support performance, participation, health and well-being. This technology may	Demonstrate an understanding of the use of technology to support performance, participation, health and well-being. This technology may	Demonstrate an understanding of the use of technology to support performance, participation, health and well-being. This technology may

(Continued)

Standard Number	Accreditation Standards for a Doctoral-Degree-Level Educational Program for the Occupational Therapist	Accreditation Standards for a Master's-Degree-Level Educational Program for the Occupational Therapist	Accreditation Standards for an Associate-Degree-Level Educational Program for the Occupational Therapy Assistant
	include, but is not limited to, electronic documentation systems, distance communication, virtual environments, and telehealth technology.	include, but is not limited to, electronic documentation systems, distance communication, virtual environments, and telehealth technology.	include, but is not limited to, electronic documentation systems, distance communication, virtual environments, and telehealth technology.

B.2.0. BASIC TENETS OF OCCUPATIONAL THERAPY
Coursework must facilitate development of the performance criteria listed below. The student will be able to

Standard Number	Accreditation Standards for a Doctoral-Degree-Level Educational Program for the Occupational Therapist	Accreditation Standards for a Master's-Degree-Level Educational Program for the Occupational Therapist	Accreditation Standards for an Associate-Degree-Level Educational Program for the Occupational Therapy Assistant
B.2.1.	Explain the history and philosophical base of the profession of occupational therapy and its importance in meeting society's current and future occupational needs.	Articulate an understanding of the importance of the history and philosophical base of the profession of occupational therapy.	Articulate an understanding of the importance of the history and philosophical base of the profession of occupational therapy.
B.2.2.	Explain the meaning and dynamics of occupation and activity, including the interaction of areas of occupation, performance skills, performance patterns, activity demands, context(s) and environments, and client factors.	Explain the meaning and dynamics of occupation and activity, including the interaction of areas of occupation, performance skills, performance patterns, activity demands, context(s) and environments, and client factors.	Describe the meaning and dynamics of occupation and activity, including the interaction of areas of occupation, performance skills, performance patterns, activity demands, context(s) and environments, and client factors.
B.2.3.	Articulate to consumers, potential employers, colleagues, third-party payers, regulatory boards, policymakers, other audiences, and the general public both the unique nature of occupation as viewed by the profession of occupational therapy and the value of occupation to support performance, participation, health, and well-being.	Articulate to consumers, potential employers, colleagues, third-party payers, regulatory boards, policymakers, other audiences, and the general public both the unique nature of occupation as viewed by the profession of occupational therapy and the value of occupation to support performance, participation, health, and well-being.	Articulate to consumers, potential employers, colleagues, third-party payers, regulatory boards, policymakers, other audiences, and the general public both the unique nature of occupation as viewed by the profession of occupational therapy and the value of occupation support performance, participation, health, and well-being.

(Continued)

Standard Number	Accreditation Standards for a Doctoral-Degree-Level Educational Program for the Occupational Therapist	Accreditation Standards for a Master's-Degree-Level Educational Program for the Occupational Therapist	Accreditation Standards for an Associate-Degree-Level Educational Program for the Occupational Therapy Assistant
B.2.4.	Articulate the importance of balancing areas of occupation with the achievement of health and wellness for the clients.	Articulate the importance of balancing areas of occupation with the achievement of health and wellness for the clients.	Articulate the importance of balancing areas of occupation with the achievement of health and wellness for the clients.
B.2.5.	Explain the role of occupation in the promotion of health and the prevention of disease and disability for the individual, family, and society.	Explain the role of occupation in the promotion of health and the prevention of disease and disability for the individual, family, and society.	Explain the role of occupation in the promotion of health and the prevention of disease and disability for the individual, family, and society.
B.2.6.	Analyze the effects of heritable diseases, genetic conditions, disability, trauma, and injury to the physical and mental health and occupational performance of the individual.	Analyze the effects of heritable diseases, genetic conditions, disability, trauma, and injury to the physical and mental health and occupational performance of the individual.	Understand the effects of heritable diseases, genetic conditions, disability, trauma, and injury to the physical and mental health and occupational performance of the individual.
B.2.7.	Demonstrate task analysis in areas of occupation, performance skills, performance patterns, activity demands, context(s) and environments, and client factors to formulate an intervention plan.	Demonstrate task analysis in areas of occupation, performance skills, performance patterns, activity demands, context(s) and environments, and client factors to formulate an intervention plan.	Demonstrate task analysis in areas of occupation, performance skills, performance patterns, activity demands, context(s) and environments, and client factors to implement the intervention plan.
B.2.8.	Use sound judgment in regard to safety of self and others and adhere to safety regulations throughout the occupational therapy process as appropriate to the setting and scope of practice.	Use sound judgment in regard to safety of self and others and adhere to safety regulations throughout the occupational therapy process as appropriate to the setting and scope of practice.	Use sound judgment in regard to safety of self and others and adhere to safety regulations throughout the occupational therapy process as appropriate to the setting and scope of practice.
B.2.9.	Express support for the quality of life, well-being, and occupation of the individual, group, or population to promote physical and mental health and	Express support for the quality of life, well-being, and occupation of the individual, group, or population to promote physical and mental health and	Express support for the quality of life, well-being, and occupation of the individual, group, or population to promote physical and mental

(Continued)

Standard Number	Accreditation Standards for a Doctoral-Degree-Level Educational Program for the Occupational Therapist	Accreditation Standards for a Master's-Degree-Level Educational Program for the Occupational Therapist	Accreditation Standards for an Associate-Degree-Level Educational Program for the Occupational Therapy Assistant
	prevention of injury and disease considering the context (e.g., cultural, personal, temporal, virtual) and environment.	prevention of injury and disease considering the context (e.g., cultural, personal, temporal, virtual) and environment.	health and prevention of injury and disease considering the context (e.g., cultural, personal, temporal, virtual) and environment.
B.2.10.	Use clinical reasoning to explain the rationale for and use of compensatory strategies when desired life tasks cannot be performed.	Use clinical reasoning to explain the rationale for and use of compensatory strategies when desired life tasks cannot be performed.	Explain the need for and use of compensatory strategies when desired life tasks cannot be performed.
B.2.11.	Analyze, synthesize, evaluate, and apply models of occupational performance.	Analyze, synthesize, and apply models of occupational performance.	Identify interventions consistent with models of occupational performance.

B.3.0. OCCUPATIONAL THERAPY THEORETICAL PERSPECTIVES
The program must facilitate the development of the performance criteria listed below. The student will be able to

Standard Number	Accreditation Standards for a Doctoral-Degree-Level Educational Program for the Occupational Therapist	Accreditation Standards for a Master's-Degree-Level Educational Program for the Occupational Therapist	Accreditation Standards for an Associate-Degree-Level Educational Program for the Occupational Therapy Assistant
B.3.1.	Evaluate and apply theories that underlie the practice of occupational therapy.	Apply theories that underlie the practice of occupational therapy.	Describe basic features of the theories that underlie the practice of occupational therapy.
B.3.2.	Compare, contrast, and integrate a variety of models of practice and frames of reference that are used in occupational therapy.	Compare and contrast models of practice and frames of reference that are used in occupational therapy.	Describe basic features of models of practice and frames of reference that are used in occupational therapy.
B.3.3.	Use theories, models of practice, and frames of reference to guide and inform evaluation and intervention.	Use theories, models of practice, and frames of reference to guide and inform evaluation and intervention.	Discuss how occupational therapy history, occupational therapy theory, and the sociopolitical climate influence practice.

(Continued)

Standard Number	Accreditation Standards for a Doctoral-Degree-Level Educational Program for the Occupational Therapist	Accreditation Standards for a Master's-Degree-Level Educational Program for the Occupational Therapist	Accreditation Standards for an Associate-Degree-Level Educational Program for the Occupational Therapy Assistant
B.3.4.	Analyze and discuss how occupational therapy history, occupational therapy theory, and the sociopolitical climate influence and are influenced by practice.	Analyze and discuss how occupational therapy history, occupational therapy theory, and the sociopolitical climate influence practice.	(No related Standard)
B.3.5.	Apply theoretical constructs to evaluation and intervention with various types of clients in a variety of practice contexts and environments, including population-based approaches, to analyze and effect meaningful occupation outcomes.	Apply theoretical constructs to evaluation and intervention with various types of clients in a variety of practice contexts and environments to analyze and effect meaningful occupation outcomes.	(No related Standard)
B.3.6.	Articulate the process of theory development in occupational therapy and its desired impact and influence on society.	Discuss the process of theory development and its importance to occupational therapy.	(No related Standard)
B.4.0.	SCREENING, EVALUATION, AND REFERRAL The process of screening, evaluation, referral, and diagnosis as related to occupational performance and participation must be culturally relevant and based on theoretical perspectives, models of practice, frames of reference, and available evidence. In addition, this process must consider the continuum of need from individuals to populations. The program must facilitate development of the performance criteria listed below. The student will be able to	SCREENING, EVALUATION, AND REFERRAL The process of screening, evaluation, and referral as related to occupational performance and participation must be culturally relevant and based on theoretical perspectives, models of practice, frames of reference, and available evidence. In addition, this process must consider the continuum of need from individuals to populations. The program must facilitate development of the performance criteria listed below. The student will be able to	SCREENING AND EVALUATION The process of screening and evaluation as related to occupational performance and participation must be conducted under the supervision of and in cooperation with the occupational therapist and must be culturally relevant and based on theoretical perspectives, models of practice, frames of reference, and available evidence. The program must facilitate development of the performance criteria listed below. The student will be able to

(Continued)

Standard Number	Accreditation Standards for a Doctoral-Degree-Level Educational Program for the Occupational Therapist	Accreditation Standards for a Master's-Degree-Level Educational Program for the Occupational Therapist	Accreditation Standards for an Associate-Degree-Level Educational Program for the Occupational Therapy Assistant
B.4.1.	Use standardized and nonstandardized screening and assessment tools to determine the need for occupational therapy intervention. These tools include, but are not limited to, specified screening tools; assessments; skilled observations; occupational histories; consultations with other professionals; and interviews with the client, family, significant others, and community.	Use standardized and nonstandardized screening and assessment tools to determine the need for occupational therapy intervention. These tools include, but are not limited to, specified screening tools; assessments; skilled observations; occupational histories; consultations with other professionals; and interviews with the client, family, significant others, and community.	Gather and share data for the purpose of screening and evaluation using methods including, but not limited to, specified screening tools; assessments; skilled observations; occupational histories; consultations with other professionals; and interviews with the client, family, and significant others.
B.4.2.	Select appropriate assessment tools on the basis of client needs, contextual factors, and psychometric properties of tests. These must be culturally relevant, based on available evidence, and incorporate use of occupation in the assessment process.	Select appropriate assessment tools on the basis of client needs, contextual factors, and psychometric properties of tests. These must be culturally relevant, based on available evidence, and incorporate use of occupation in the assessment process.	Administer selected assessments using appropriate procedures and protocols (including standardized formats) and use occupation for the purpose of assessment.
B.4.3.	Use appropriate procedures and protocols (including standardized formats) when administering assessments.	Use appropriate procedures and protocols (including standardized formats) when administering assessments.	(No related Standard)
B.4.4.	Evaluate client(s)' occupational performance in activities of daily living (ADLs), instrumental activities of daily living (IADLs), education, work, play, rest, sleep, leisure, and social participation. Evaluation of occupational performance using	Evaluate client(s)' occupational performance in activities of daily living (ADLs), instrumental activities of daily living (IADLs), education, work, play, rest, sleep, leisure, and social participation. Evaluation of occupational performance using	Gather and share data for the purpose of evaluating client(s)' occupational performance in activities of daily living (ADLs), instrumental activities of daily living (IADLs), education, activities of daily living (IADLs), education, work, play, rest, sleep, leisure, and social

(Continued)

Standard Number	Accreditation Standards for a Doctoral-Degree-Level Educational Program for the Occupational Therapist	Accreditation Standards for a Master's-Degree-Level Educational Program for the Occupational Therapist	Accreditation Standards for an Associate-Degree-Level Educational Program for the Occupational Therapy Assistant
	standardized and nonstandardized assessment tools includes • The occupational profile, including participation in activities that are meaningful and necessary for the client to carry out roles in home, work, and community environments. • Client factors, including values, beliefs, spirituality, body functions (e.g., neuromuscular, sensory and pain, visual, perceptual, cognitive, mental) and body structures (e.g., cardiovascular, digestive, nervous, genitourinary, integumentary systems). • Performance patterns (e.g., habits, routines, rituals, roles). • Context (e.g., cultural, personal, temporal, virtual) and environment (e.g., physical, social). • Performance skills, including motor and praxis skills, sensory–perceptual skills, emotional regulation skills, cognitive skills, and communication and social skills.	standardized and nonstandardized assessment tools includes • The occupational profile, including participation in activities that are meaningful and necessary for the client to carry out roles in home, work, and community environments. • Client factors, including values, beliefs, spirituality, body functions (e.g., neuromuscular, sensory and pain, visual, perceptual, cognitive, mental) and body structures (e.g., cardiovascular, digestive, nervous, genitourinary, integumentary systems). • Performance patterns (e.g., habits, routines, rituals, roles). • Context (e.g., cultural, personal, temporal, virtual) and environment (e.g., physical, social). • Performance skills, including motor and praxis skills, sensory–perceptual skills, emotional regulation skills, cognitive skills, and communication and social skills.	participation. Evaluation of occupational performance includes • The occupational profile, including participation in activities that are meaningful and necessary for the client to carry out roles in home, work, and community environments. • Client factors, including values, beliefs, spirituality, body functions (e.g., neuromuscular, sensory and pain, visual, perceptual, cognitive, mental) and body structures (e.g., cardiovascular, digestive, nervous, genitourinary, integumentary systems). • Performance patterns (e.g., habits, routines, rituals, roles). • Context (e.g., cultural, personal, temporal, virtual) and environment (e.g., physical, social). • Performance skills, including motor and praxis skills, sensory–perceptual skills, emotional regulation skills, cognitive skills, and communication and social skills.
B.4.5	Compare and contrast the role of the occupational therapist and occupational therapy assistant in the screening and evaluation process along with the importance of and rationale for supervision and collaborative work between the occupational therapist and occupational therapy assistant in that process.	Compare and contrast the role of the occupational therapist and occupational therapy assistant in the screening and evaluation process along with the importance of and rationale for supervision and collaborative work between the occupational therapist and occupational therapy assistant in that process.	Articulate the role of the occupational therapy assistant and occupational therapist in the screening and evaluation process along with the importance of and rationale for supervision and collaborative work between the occupational therapy assistant and occupational therapist in that process.

(Continued)

Standard Number	Accreditation Standards for a Doctoral-Degree-Level Educational Program for the Occupational Therapist	Accreditation Standards for a Master's-Degree-Level Educational Program for the Occupational Therapist	Accreditation Standards for an Associate-Degree-Level Educational Program for the Occupational Therapy Assistant
B.4.6.	Interpret criterion-referenced and norm-referenced standardized test scores on the basis of an understanding of sampling, normative data, standard and criterion scores, reliability, and validity.	Interpret criterion-referenced and norm-referenced standardized test scores on the basis of an understanding of sampling, normative data, standard and criterion scores, reliability, and validity.	*(No related Standard)*
B.4.7.	Consider factors that might bias assessment results, such as culture, disability status, and situational variables related to the individual and context.	Consider factors that might bias assessment results, such as culture, disability status, and situational variables related to the individual and context.	*(No related Standard)*
B.4.8.	Interpret the evaluation data in relation to accepted terminology of the profession, relevant theoretical frameworks, and interdisciplinary knowledge.	Interpret the evaluation data in relation to accepted terminology of the profession and relevant theoretical frameworks.	*(No related Standard)*
B.4.9.	Evaluate appropriateness and discuss mechanisms for referring clients for additional evaluation to specialists who are internal and external to the profession.	Evaluate appropriateness and discuss mechanisms for referring clients for additional evaluation to specialists who are internal and external to the profession.	Identify when to recommend to the occupational therapist the need for referring clients for additional evaluation.
B.4.10.	Document occupational therapy services to ensure accountability of service provision and to meet standards for reimbursement of services, adhering to the requirements of applicable facility, local, state, federal, and reimbursement agencies. Documentation must effectively communicate the need and rationale for occupational therapy services.	Document occupational therapy services to ensure accountability of service provision and to meet standards for reimbursement of services, adhering to the requirements of applicable facility, local, state, federal, and reimbursement agencies. Documentation must effectively communicate the need and rationale for occupational therapy services.	Document occupational therapy services to ensure accountability of service provision and to meet standards for reimbursement of services, adhering to the requirements of applicable facility, local, state, federal, and reimbursement agencies. Documentation must effectively communicate the need and rationale for occupational therapy services.

(Continued)

Standard Number	Accreditation Standards for a Doctoral-Degree-Level Educational Program for the Occupational Therapist	Accreditation Standards for a Master's-Degree-Level Educational Program for the Occupational Therapist	Accreditation Standards for an Associate-Degree-Level Educational Program for the Occupational Therapy Assistant
B.4.11.	Articulate screening and evaluation processes for all practice areas. Use evidence-based reasoning to analyze, synthesize, evaluate, and diagnose problems related to occupational performance and participation.	(No related Standard)	(No related Standard)
B.5.0.	INTERVENTION PLAN: FORMULATION AND IMPLEMENTATION The process of formulation and implementation of the therapeutic intervention plan to facilitate occupational performance and participation must be culturally relevant; reflective of current and emerging occupational therapy practice; based on available evidence; and based on theoretical perspectives, models of practice, and frames of reference. In addition, this process must consider the continuum of need from individual- to population-based interventions. The program must facilitate development of the performance criteria listed below. The student will be able to	INTERVENTION PLAN: FORMULATION AND IMPLEMENTATION The process of formulation and implementation of the therapeutic intervention plan to facilitate occupational performance and participation must be culturally relevant; reflective of current occupational therapy practice; based on available evidence; and based on theoretical perspectives, models of practice, and frames of reference. The program must facilitate development of the performance criteria listed below. The student will be able to	INTERVENTION AND IMPLEMENTATION The process of intervention to facilitate occupational performance and participation must be done under the supervision of and in cooperation with the occupational therapist and must be culturally relevant, reflective of current occupational therapy practice, and based on available evidence. The program must facilitate development of the performance criteria listed below. The student will be able to
B.5.1.	Use evaluation findings to diagnose occupational performance and participation based on appropriate theoretical approaches, models of practice, frames of reference, and interdisciplinary knowledge. Develop occupation-based intervention	Use evaluation findings based on appropriate theoretical approaches, models of practice, and frames of reference to develop occupation-based intervention plans and strategies (including goals and methods to achieve them) on the	Assist with the development of occupation-based intervention plans and strategies (including goals and methods to achieve them) on the basis of the stated needs of the client as well as data gathered during the evaluation

(Continued)

Standard Number	Accreditation Standards for a Doctoral-Degree-Level Educational Program for the Occupational Therapist	Accreditation Standards for a Master's-Degree-Level Educational Program for the Occupational Therapist	Accreditation Standards for an Associate-Degree-Level Educational Program for the Occupational Therapy Assistant
	plans and strategies (including goals and methods to achieve them) on the basis of the stated needs of the client as well as data gathered during the evaluation process in collaboration with the client and others. Intervention plans and strategies must be culturally relevant, reflective of current occupational therapy practice, and based on available evidence. Interventions address the following components: • The occupational profile, including participation in activities that are meaningful and necessary for the client to carry out roles in home, work, and community environments. • Client factors, including values, beliefs, spirituality, body functions (e.g., neuromuscular, sensory and pain, visual, perceptual, cognitive, mental) and body structures (e.g., cardiovascular, digestive, nervous, genitourinary, integumentary systems). • Performance patterns (e.g., habits, routines, rituals, roles). • Context (e.g., cultural, personal, temporal, virtual) and environment (e.g., physical, social). • Performance skills, including motor and praxis skills, sensory–perceptual skills, emotional regulation skills, cognitive skills, and communication and social skills.	basis of the stated needs of the client as well as data gathered during the evaluation process in collaboration with the client and others. Intervention plans and strategies must be culturally relevant, reflective of current occupational therapy practice, and based on available evidence. Interventions address the following components: • The occupational profile, including participation in activities that are meaningful and necessary for the client to carry out roles in home, work, and community environments. • Client factors, including values, beliefs, spirituality, body functions (e.g., neuromuscular, sensory and pain, visual, perceptual, cognitive, mental) and body structures (e.g., cardiovascular, digestive, nervous, genitourinary, integumentary systems). • Performance patterns (e.g., habits, routines, rituals, roles). • Context (e.g., cultural, personal, temporal, virtual) and environment (e.g., physical, social). • Performance skills, including motor and praxis skills, sensory–perceptual skills, emotional regulation skills, cognitive skills, and communication and social skills.	process in collaboration with the client and others. Intervention plans and strategies must be culturally relevant, reflective of current occupational therapy practice, and based on available evidence. Interventions address the following components: • The occupational profile, including participation in activities that are meaningful and necessary for the client to carry out roles in home, work, and community environments. • Client factors, including values, beliefs, spirituality, body functions (e.g., neuromuscular, sensory and pain, visual, perceptual, cognitive, mental) and body structures (e.g., cardiovascular, digestive, nervous, genitourinary, integumentary systems). • Performance patterns (e.g., habits, routines, rituals, roles). • Context (e.g., cultural, personal, temporal, virtual) and environment (e.g., physical, social). • Performance skills, including motor and praxis skills, sensory–perceptual skills, emotional regulation skills, cognitive skills, and communication and social skills.

(Continued)

Standard Number	Accreditation Standards for a Doctoral-Degree-Level Educational Program for the Occupational Therapist	Accreditation Standards for a Master's-Degree-Level Educational Program for the Occupational Therapist	Accreditation Standards for an Associate-Degree-Level Educational Program for the Occupational Therapy Assistant
B.5.2.	Select and provide direct occupational therapy interventions and procedures to enhance safety, health and wellness, and performance in ADLs, IADLs, education, work, play, rest, sleep, leisure, and social participation.	Select and provide direct occupational therapy interventions and procedures to enhance safety, health and wellness, and performance in ADLs, IADLs, education, work, play, rest, sleep, leisure, and social participation.	Select and provide direct occupational therapy interventions and procedures to enhance safety, health and wellness, and performance in ADLs, IADLs, education, work, play, rest, sleep, leisure, and social participation.
B.5.3.	Provide therapeutic use of occupation, exercises, and activities (e.g., occupation-based intervention, purposeful activity, preparatory methods).	Provide therapeutic use of occupation, exercises, and activities (e.g., occupation-based intervention, purposeful activity, preparatory methods).	Provide therapeutic use of occupation, exercises, and activities (e.g., occupation-based intervention, purposeful activity, preparatory methods).
B.5.4.	Design and implement group interventions based on principles of group development and group dynamics across the lifespan.	Design and implement group interventions based on principles of group development and group dynamics across the lifespan.	Implement group interventions based on principles of group development and group dynamics across the lifespan.
B.5.5.	Provide training in self-care, self-management, health management and maintenance, home management, and community and work integration.	Provide training in self-care, self-management, health management and maintenance, home management, and community and work integration.	Provide training in self-care, self-management, health management and maintenance, home management, and community and work integration.
B.5.6.	Provide development, remediation, and compensation for physical, mental, cognitive, perceptual, neuromuscular, behavioral skills, and sensory functions (e.g., vision, tactile, auditory, gustatory, olfactory, pain, temperature, pressure, vestibular, proprioception).	Provide development, remediation, and compensation for physical, mental, cognitive, perceptual, neuromuscular, behavioral skills, and sensory functions (e.g., vision, tactile, auditory, gustatory, olfactory, pain, temperature, pressure, vestibular, proprioception).	Provide development, remediation, and compensation for physical, mental, cognitive, perceptual, neuromuscular, behavioral skills, and sensory functions (e.g., vision, tactile, auditory, gustatory, olfactory, pain, temperature, pressure, vestibular, proprioception).

(Continued)

Standard Number	Accreditation Standards for a Doctoral-Degree-Level Educational Program for the Occupational Therapist	Accreditation Standards for a Master's-Degree-Level Educational Program for the Occupational Therapist	Accreditation Standards for an Associate-Degree-Level Educational Program for the Occupational Therapy Assistant
B.5.7.	Demonstrate therapeutic use of self, including one's personality, insights, perceptions, and judgments, as part of the therapeutic process in both individual and group interaction.	Demonstrate therapeutic use of self, including one's personality, insights, perceptions, and judgments, as part of the therapeutic process in both individual and group interaction.	Demonstrate therapeutic use of self, including one's personality, insights, perceptions, and judgments, as part of the therapeutic process in both individual and group interaction.
B.5.8.	Develop and implement intervention strategies to remediate and/or compensate for cognitive deficits that affect occupational performance.	Develop and implement intervention strategies to remediate and/or compensate for cognitive deficits that affect occupational performance.	Implement intervention strategies to remediate and/or compensate for cognitive deficits that affect occupational performance.
B.5.9.	Evaluate and adapt processes or environments (e.g., home, work, school, community) applying ergonomic principles and principles of environmental modification.	Evaluate and adapt processes or environments (e.g., home, work, school, community) applying ergonomic principles and principles of environmental modification.	Adapt environments (e.g., home, work, school, community) and processes, including the application of ergonomic principles.
B.5.10.	Articulate principles of and be able to design, fabricate, apply, fit, and train in assistive technologies and devices (e.g., electronic aids to daily living, seating and positioning systems) used to enhance occupational performance and foster participation and well-being.	Articulate principles of and be able to design, fabricate, apply, fit, and train in assistive technologies and devices (e.g., electronic aids to daily living, seating and positioning systems) used to enhance occupational performance and foster participation and well-being.	Articulate principles of and demonstrate strategies with assistive technologies and devices (e.g., electronic aids to daily living, seating and positioning systems) used to enhance occupational performance and foster participation and well-being.
B.5.11.	Provide design, fabrication, application, fitting, and training in orthotic devices used to enhance occupational performance and participation. Train in the use of prosthetic devices, based on scientific principles of kinesiology, biomechanics, and physics.	Provide design, fabrication, application, fitting, and training in orthotic devices used to enhance occupational performance and participation. Train in the use of prosthetic devices, based on scientific principles of kinesiology, biomechanics, and physics.	Provide fabrication, application, fitting, and training in orthotic devices used to enhance occupational performance and participation, and training in the use of prosthetic devices.

(Continued)

Standard Number	Accreditation Standards for a Doctoral-Degree-Level Educational Program for the Occupational Therapist	Accreditation Standards for a Master's-Degree-Level Educational Program for the Occupational Therapist	Accreditation Standards for an Associate-Degree-Level Educational Program for the Occupational Therapy Assistant
B.5.12.	Provide recommendations and training in techniques to enhance functional mobility, including physical transfers, wheelchair management, and mobility devices.	Provide recommendations and training in techniques to enhance functional mobility, including physical transfers, wheelchair management, and mobility devices.	Provide training in techniques to enhance functional mobility, including physical transfers, wheelchair management, and mobility devices.
B.5.13.	Provide recommendations and training in techniques to enhance community mobility, including public transportation, community access, and issues related to driver rehabilitation.	Provide recommendations and training in techniques to enhance community mobility, including public transportation, community access, and issues related to driver rehabilitation.	Provide training in techniques to enhance community mobility, including public transportation, community access, and issues related to driver rehabilitation.
B.5.14.	Provide management of feeding, eating, and swallowing to enable performance (including the process of bringing food or fluids from the plate or cup to the mouth, the ability to keep and manipulate food or fluid in the mouth, and swallowing assessment and management) and train others in precautions and techniques while considering client and contextual factors.	Provide management of feeding, eating, and swallowing to enable performance (including the process of bringing food or fluids from the plate or cup to the mouth, the ability to keep and manipulate food or fluid in the mouth, and swallowing assessment and management) and train others in precautions and techniques while considering client and contextual factors.	Enable feeding and eating performance (including the process of bringing food or fluids from the plate or cup to the mouth, the ability to keep and manipulate food or fluid in the mouth, and the initiation of swallowing) and train others in precautions and techniques while considering client and contextual factors.
B.5.15.	Demonstrate safe and effective application of superficial thermal and mechanical modalities as a preparatory measure to manage pain and improve occupational performance, including foundational knowledge, underlying principles, indications, contraindications, and precautions.	Demonstrate safe and effective application of superficial thermal and mechanical modalities as a preparatory measure to manage pain and improve occupational performance, including foundational knowledge, underlying principles, indications, contraindications, and precautions.	Recognize the use of superficial thermal and mechanical modalities as a preparatory measure to improve occupational performance. On the basis of the intervention plan, demonstrate safe and effective administration of superficial thermal and mechanical modalities to achieve established goals while adhering to contraindications and precautions.

(Continued)

(Continued)

Standard Number	Accreditation Standards for a Doctoral-Degree-Level Educational Program for the Occupational Therapist	Accreditation Standards for a Master's-Degree-Level Educational Program for the Occupational Therapist	Accreditation Standards for an Associate-Degree-Level Educational Program for the Occupational Therapy Assistant
B.5.16.	Explain the use of deep thermal and electrotherapeutic modalities as a preparatory measure to improve occupational performance, including indications, contraindications, and precautions.	Explain the use of deep thermal and electrotherapeutic modalities as a preparatory measure to improve occupational performance, including indications, contraindications, and precautions.	*(No related Standard)*
B.5.17.	Develop and promote the use of appropriate home and community programming to support performance in the client's natural environment and participation in all contexts relevant to the client.	Develop and promote the use of appropriate home and community programming to support performance in the client's natural environment and participation in all contexts relevant to the client.	Promote the use of appropriate home and community programming to support performance in the client's natural environment and participation in all contexts relevant to the client.
B.5.18.	Demonstrate an understanding of health literacy and the ability to educate and train the client, caregiver, family and significant others, and communities to facilitate skills in areas of occupation as well as prevention, health maintenance, health promotion, and safety.	Demonstrate an understanding of health literacy and the ability to educate and train the client, caregiver, family and significant others, and communities to facilitate skills in areas of occupation as well as prevention, health maintenance, health promotion, and safety.	Demonstrate an understanding of health literacy and the ability to educate and train the client, caregiver, and family and significant others to facilitate skills in areas of occupation as well as prevention, health maintenance, health promotion, and safety.
B.5.19.	Apply the principles of the teaching–learning process using educational methods to design experiences to address the needs of the client, family, significant others, communities, colleagues, other health providers, and the public.	Apply the principles of the teaching–learning process using educational methods to design experiences to address the needs of the client, family, significant others, colleagues, other health providers, and the public.	Use the teaching–learning process with the client, family, significant others, colleagues, other health providers, and the public. Collaborate with the occupational therapist and learner to identify appropriate educational methods.
B.5.20.	Effectively interact through written, oral, and nonverbal communication with the client, family, significant others, communities, colleagues, other health providers, and the public in a professionally acceptable manner.	Effectively interact through written, oral, and nonverbal communication with the client, family, significant others, colleagues, other health providers, and the public in a professionally acceptable manner.	Effectively interact through written, oral, and nonverbal communication with the client, family, significant others, colleagues, other health providers, and the public in a professionally acceptable manner.

Standard Number	Accreditation Standards for a Doctoral-Degree-Level Educational Program for the Occupational Therapist	Accreditation Standards for a Master's-Degree-Level Educational Program for the Occupational Therapist	Accreditation Standards for an Associate-Degree-Level Educational Program for the Occupational Therapy Assistant
B.5.21.	Effectively communicate, coordinate, and work interprofessionally with those who provide services to individuals, organizations, and/or populations in order to clarify each member's responsibility in executing components of an intervention plan.	Effectively communicate and work interprofessionally with those who provide services to individuals, organizations, and/or populations in order to clarify each member's responsibility in executing an intervention plan.	Effectively communicate and work interprofessionally with those who provide services to individuals and groups in order to clarify each member's responsibility in executing an intervention plan.
B.5.22.	Refer to specialists (both internal and external to the profession) for consultation and intervention.	Refer to specialists (both internal and external to the profession) for consultation and intervention.	Recognize and communicate the need to refer to specialists (both internal and external to the profession) for consultation and intervention.
B.5.23.	Grade and adapt the environment, tools, materials, occupations, and interventions to reflect the changing needs of the client, the sociocultural context, and technological advances.	Grade and adapt the environment, tools, materials, occupations, and interventions to reflect the changing needs of the client, the sociocultural context, and technological advances.	Grade and adapt the environment, tools, materials, occupations, and interventions to reflect the changing needs of the client and the sociocultural context.
B.5.24.	Select and teach compensatory strategies, such as use of technology and adaptations to the environment, that support performance, participation, and well-being.	Select and teach compensatory strategies, such as use of technology and adaptations to the environment, that support performance, participation, and well-being.	Teach compensatory strategies, such as use of technology and adaptations to the environment, that support performance, participation, and well-being.
B.5.25.	Identify and demonstrate techniques in skills of supervision and collaboration with occupational therapy assistants and other professionals on therapeutic interventions.	Identify and demonstrate techniques in skills of supervision and collaboration with occupational therapy assistants and other professionals on therapeutic interventions.	Demonstrate skills of collaboration with occupational therapists and other professionals on therapeutic interventions.

(Continued)

(Continued)

Standard Number	Accreditation Standards for a Doctoral-Degree-Level Educational Program for the Occupational Therapist	Accreditation Standards for a Master's-Degree-Level Educational Program for the Occupational Therapist	Accreditation Standards for an Associate-Degree-Level Educational Program for the Occupational Therapy Assistant
B.5.26.	Demonstrate use of the consultative process with groups, programs, organizations, or communities.	Understand when and how to use the consultative process with groups, programs, organizations, or communities.	Understand when and how to use the consultative process with specific consumers or consumer groups as directed by an occupational therapist.
B.5.27.	Demonstrate care coordination, case management, and transition services in traditional and emerging practice environments.	Describe the role of the occupational therapist in care coordination, case management, and transition services in traditional and emerging practice environments.	Describe the role of the occupational therapy assistant in care coordination, case management, and transition services in traditional and emerging practice environments.
B.5.28.	Monitor and reassess, in collaboration with the client, caregiver, family, and significant others, the effect of occupational therapy intervention and the need for continued or modified intervention.	Monitor and reassess, in collaboration with the client, caregiver, family, and significant others, the effect of occupational therapy intervention and the need for continued or modified intervention.	Monitor and reassess, in collaboration with the client, caregiver, family, and significant others, the effect of occupational therapy intervention and the need for continued or modified intervention, and communicate the identified needs to the occupational therapist.
B.5.29.	Plan for discharge, in collaboration with the client, by reviewing the needs of the client, caregiver, family, and significant others; available resources; and discharge environment. This process includes, but is not limited to, identification of client's current status within the continuum of care; identification of community, human, and fiscal resources; recommendations for environmental adaptations; and home programming to facilitate the client's progression along the continuum toward outcome goals.	Plan for discharge, in collaboration with the client, by reviewing the needs of the client, caregiver, family, and significant others; available resources; and discharge environment. This process includes, but is not limited to, identification of client's current status within the continuum of care; identification of community, human, and fiscal resources; recommendations for environmental adaptations; and home programming to facilitate the client's progression along the continuum toward outcome goals.	Facilitate discharge planning by reviewing the needs of the client, caregiver, family, and significant others; available resources; and discharge environment, and identify those needs to the occupational therapist, client, and others involved in discharge planning. This process includes, but is not limited to, identification of community, human, and fiscal resources; recommendations for environmental adaptations; and home programming.

Standard Number	Accreditation Standards for a Doctoral-Degree-Level Educational Program for the Occupational Therapist	Accreditation Standards for a Master's-Degree-Level Educational Program for the Occupational Therapist	Accreditation Standards for an Associate-Degree-Level Educational Program for the Occupational Therapy Assistant
B.5.30.	Organize, collect, and analyze data in a systematic manner for evaluation of practice outcomes. Report evaluation results and modify practice as needed to improve client outcomes.	Organize, collect, and analyze data in a systematic manner for evaluation of practice outcomes. Report evaluation results and modify practice as needed to improve client outcomes.	Under the direction of an administrator, manager, or occupational therapist, collect, organize, and report on data for evaluation of client outcomes.
B.5.31.	Terminate occupational therapy services when stated outcomes have been achieved or it has been determined that they cannot be achieved. This process includes developing a summary of occupational therapy outcomes, appropriate recommendations, and referrals and discussion of postdischarge needs with the client and with appropriate others.	Terminate occupational therapy services when stated outcomes have been achieved or it has been determined that they cannot be achieved. This process includes developing a summary of occupational therapy outcomes, appropriate recommendations, and referrals and discussion of postdischarge needs with the client and with appropriate others.	Recommend to the occupational therapist the need for termination of occupational therapy services when stated outcomes have been achieved or it has been determined that they cannot be achieved. Assist with developing a summary of occupational therapy outcomes, recommendations, and referrals.
B.5.32.	Document occupational therapy services to ensure accountability of service provision and to meet standards for reimbursement of services. Documentation must effectively communicate the need and rationale for occupational therapy services and must be appropriate to the context in which the service is delivered.	Document occupational therapy services to ensure accountability of service provision and to meet standards for reimbursement of services. Documentation must effectively communicate the need and rationale for occupational therapy services and must be appropriate to the context in which the service is delivered.	Document occupational therapy services to ensure accountability of service provision and to meet standards for reimbursement of services. Documentation must effectively communicate the need and rationale for occupational therapy services and must be appropriate to the context in which the service is delivered.
B.5.33.	Provide population-based occupational therapy intervention that addresses occupational needs as identified by a community.	*(No related Standard)*	*(No related Standard)*

(Continued)

B.6.0. CONTEXT OF SERVICE DELIVERY

Context of service delivery includes the knowledge and understanding of the various contexts, such as professional, social, cultural, political, economic, and ecological, in which occupational therapy services are provided. The program must facilitate development of the performance criteria listed below. The student will be able to

Standard Number	Accreditation Standards for a Doctoral-Degree-Level Educational Program for the Occupational Therapist	Accreditation Standards for a Master's-Degree-Level Educational Program for the Occupational Therapist	Accreditation Standards for an Associate-Degree-Level Educational Program for the Occupational Therapy Assistant
B.6.1.	Evaluate and address the various contexts of health care, education, community, political, and social systems as they relate to the practice of occupational therapy.	Evaluate and address the various contexts of health care, education, community, political, and social systems as they relate to the practice of occupational therapy.	Describe the contexts of health care, education, community, and social systems as they relate to the practice of occupational therapy.
B.6.2.	Analyze the current policy issues and the social, economic, political, geographic, and demographic factors that influence the various contexts for practice of occupational therapy.	Analyze the current policy issues and the social, economic, political, geographic, and demographic factors that influence the various contexts for practice of occupational therapy.	Identify the potential impact of current policy issues and the social, economic, political, geographic, or demographic factors on the practice of occupational therapy.
B.6.3.	Integrate current social, economic, political, geographic, and demographic factors to promote policy development and the provision of occupational therapy services.	Integrate current social, economic, political, geographic, and demographic factors to promote policy development and the provision of occupational therapy services.	(No related Standard)
B.6.4.	Advocate for changes in service delivery policies, effect changes in the system, and identify opportunities to address societal needs.	Articulate the role and responsibility of the practitioner to advocate for changes in service delivery policies, to effect changes in the system, and to identify opportunities in emerging practice areas.	Identify the role and responsibility of the practitioner to advocate for changes in service delivery policies, to effect changes in the system, and to recognize opportunities in emerging practice areas.

(Continued)

Standard Number	Accreditation Standards for a Doctoral-Degree-Level Educational Program for the Occupational Therapist	Accreditation Standards for a Master's-Degree-Level Educational Program for the Occupational Therapist	Accreditation Standards for an Associate-Degree-Level Educational Program for the Occupational Therapy Assistant
B.6.5.	Analyze the trends in models of service delivery, including, but not limited to, medical, educational, community, and social models, and their potential effect on the practice of occupational therapy.	Analyze the trends in models of service delivery, including, but not limited to, medical, educational, community, and social models, and their potential effect on the practice of occupational therapy.	(No related Standard)
B.6.6.	Integrate national and international resources in education, research, practice, and policy development.	Utilize national and international resources in making assessment or intervention choices and appreciate the influence of international occupational therapy contributions to education, research, and practice.	(No related Standard)
B.7.0.	LEADERSHIP AND MANAGEMENT Leadership and management skills include principles and applications of leadership and management theory. The program must facilitate development of the performance criteria listed below. The student will be able to	MANAGEMENT OF OCCUPATIONAL THERAPY SERVICES Management of occupational therapy services includes the application of principles of management and systems in the provision of occupational therapy services to individuals and organizations. The program must facilitate development of the performance criteria listed below. The student will be able to	ASSISTANCE WITH MANAGEMENT OF OCCUPATIONAL THERAPY SERVICES Assistance with management of occupational therapy services includes the application of principles of management and systems in the provision of occupational therapy services to individuals and organizations. The program must facilitate development of the performance criteria listed below. The student will be able to
B.7.1.	Identify and evaluate the impact of contextual factors on the management and delivery of occupational therapy services for individuals and populations.	Describe and discuss the impact of contextual factors on the management and delivery of occupational therapy services.	Identify the impact of contextual factors on the management and delivery of occupational therapy services.

(Continued)

Standard Number	Accreditation Standards for a Doctoral-Degree-Level Educational Program for the Occupational Therapist	Accreditation Standards for a Master's-Degree-Level Educational Program for the Occupational Therapist	Accreditation Standards for an Associate-Degree-Level Educational Program for the Occupational Therapy Assistant
B.7.2.	Identify and evaluate the systems and structures that create federal and state legislation and regulations and their implications and effects on practice and policy.	Describe the systems and structures that create federal and state legislation and regulations and their implications and effects on practice.	Identify the systems and structures that create federal and state legislation and regulations and their implications and effects on practice.
B.7.3.	Demonstrate knowledge of applicable national requirements for credentialing and requirements for licensure, certification, or registration under state laws.	Demonstrate knowledge of applicable national requirements for credentialing and requirements for licensure, certification, or registration under state laws.	Demonstrate knowledge of applicable national requirements for credentialing and requirements for licensure, certification, or registration under state laws.
B.7.4.	Demonstrate knowledge of various reimbursement systems (e.g., federal, state, third party, private payer), appeals mechanisms, and documentation requirements that affect society and the practice of occupational therapy.	Demonstrate knowledge of various reimbursement systems (e.g., federal, state, third party, private payer), appeals mechanisms, and documentation requirements that affect the practice of occupational therapy.	Demonstrate knowledge of various reimbursement systems (e.g., federal, state, third party, private payer) and documentation requirements that affect the practice of occupational therapy.
B.7.5.	Demonstrate leadership skills in the ability to plan, develop, organize, and market the delivery of services to include the determination of programmatic needs and service delivery options and formulation and management of staffing for effective service provision.	Demonstrate the ability to plan, develop, organize, and market the delivery of services to include the determination of programmatic needs and service delivery options and formulation and management of staffing for effective service provision.	Demonstrate the ability to participate in the development, marketing, and management of service delivery options.
B.7.6.	Demonstrate leadership skills in the ability to design ongoing processes for quality improvement (e.g., outcome studies analysis) and develop program changes as needed to ensure quality of services and to direct administrative changes.	Demonstrate the ability to design ongoing processes for quality improvement (e.g., outcome studies analysis) and develop program changes as needed to ensure quality of services and to direct administrative changes.	Participate in the documentation of ongoing processes for quality improvement and implement program changes as needed to ensure quality of services.

(Continued)

Standard Number	Accreditation Standards for a Doctoral-Degree-Level Educational Program for the Occupational Therapist	Accreditation Standards for a Master's-Degree-Level Educational Program for the Occupational Therapist	Accreditation Standards for an Associate-Degree-Level Educational Program for the Occupational Therapy Assistant
B.7.7.	Develop strategies for effective, competency-based legal and ethical supervision of occupational therapy and non–occupational therapy personnel.	Develop strategies for effective, competency-based legal and ethical supervision of occupational therapy and non–occupational therapy personnel.	Identify strategies for effective, competency-based legal and ethical supervision of nonprofessional personnel.
B.7.8.	Describe the ongoing professional responsibility for providing fieldwork education and the criteria for becoming a fieldwork educator.	Describe the ongoing professional responsibility for providing fieldwork education and the criteria for becoming a fieldwork educator.	Describe the ongoing professional responsibility for providing fieldwork education and the criteria for becoming a fieldwork educator.
B.7.9.	Demonstrate knowledge of and the ability to write program development plans for provision of occupational therapy services to individuals and populations.	*(No related Standard)*	*(No related Standard)*
B.7.10.	Identify and adapt existing models or develop new service provision models to respond to policy, regulatory agencies, and reimbursement and compliance standards.	*(No related Standard)*	*(No related Standard)*
B.7.11.	Identify and develop strategies to enable occupational therapy to respond to society's changing needs.	*(No related Standard)*	*(No related Standard)*
B.7.12.	Identify and implement strategies to promote staff development that are based on evaluation of the personal and professional abilities and competencies of supervised staff as they relate to job responsibilities.	*(No related Standard)*	*(No related Standard)*

(Continued)

Standard Number	Accreditation Standards for a Doctoral-Degree-Level Educational Program for the Occupational Therapist	Accreditation Standards for a Master's-Degree-Level Educational Program for the Occupational Therapist	Accreditation Standards for an Associate-Degree-Level Educational Program for the Occupational Therapy Assistant
B.8.0. SCHOLARSHIP **Promotion of scholarly endeavors will serve to describe and interpret the scope of the profession, establish new knowledge, and interpret and apply this knowledge to practice. The program must facilitate development of the performance criteria listed below. The student will be able to**			
B.8.1.	Articulate the importance of how scholarly activities contribute to the development of a body of knowledge relevant to the profession of occupational therapy.	Articulate the importance of how scholarly activities contribute to the development of a body of knowledge relevant to the profession of occupational therapy.	Articulate the importance of how scholarly activities and literature contribute to the development of the profession.
B.8.2.	Effectively locate, understand, critique, and evaluate information, including the quality of evidence.	Effectively locate, understand, critique, and evaluate information, including the quality of evidence.	Effectively locate and understand information, including the quality of the source of information.
B.8.3.	Use scholarly literature to make evidence-based decisions.	Use scholarly literature to make evidence-based decisions.	Use professional literature to make evidence-based practice decisions in collaboration with the occupational therapist.
B.8.4.	Select, apply, and interpret basic descriptive, correlational, and inferential quantitative statistics and code, analyze, and synthesize qualitative data.	Understand and use basic descriptive, correlational, and inferential quantitative statistics and code, analyze, and synthesize qualitative data.	*(No related Standard)*
B.8.5.	Understand and critique the validity of research studies, including their design (both quantitative and qualitative) and methodology.	Understand and critique the validity of research studies, including their design (both quantitative and qualitative) and methodology.	*(No related Standard)*

(Continued)

Standard Number	Accreditation Standards for a Doctoral-Degree-Level Educational Program for the Occupational Therapist	Accreditation Standards for a Master's-Degree-Level Educational Program for the Occupational Therapist	Accreditation Standards for an Associate-Degree-Level Educational Program for the Occupational Therapy Assistant
B.8.6.	Design a scholarly proposal that includes the research question, relevant literature, sample, design, measurement, and data analysis.	Demonstrate the skills necessary to design a scholarly proposal that includes the research question, relevant literature, sample, design, measurement, and data analysis.	*(No related Standard)*
B.8.7.	Implement a scholarly study that evaluates professional practice, service delivery, and/or professional issues (e.g., Scholarship of Integration, Scholarship of Application, Scholarship of Teaching and Learning).	Participate in scholarly activities that evaluate professional practice, service delivery, and/or professional issues (e.g., Scholarship of Integration, Scholarship of Application, Scholarship of Teaching and Learning).	Identify how scholarly activities can be used to evaluate professional practice, service delivery, and/or professional issues (e.g., Scholarship of Integration, Scholarship of Application, Scholarship of Teaching and Learning).
B.8.8.	Write scholarly reports appropriate for presentation or for publication in a peer-reviewed journal. Examples of scholarly reports would include position papers, white papers, and persuasive discussion papers.	Demonstrate skills necessary to write a scholarly report in a format for presentation or publication.	Demonstrate the skills to read and understand a scholarly report.
B.8.9.	Demonstrate an understanding of the process of locating and securing grants and how grants can serve as a fiscal resource for scholarly activities.	Demonstrate an understanding of the process of locating and securing grants and how grants can serve as a fiscal resource for scholarly activities.	*(No related Standard)*
B.8.10.	Complete a culminating project that relates theory to practice and demonstrates synthesis of advanced knowledge in a practice area.	*(No related Standard)*	*(No related Standard)*

(Continued)

Standard Number	Accreditation Standards for a Doctoral-Degree-Level Educational Program for the Occupational Therapist	Accreditation Standards for a Master's-Degree-Level Educational Program for the Occupational Therapist	Accreditation Standards for an Associate-Degree-Level Educational Program for the Occupational Therapy Assistant
B.9.0. PROFESSIONAL ETHICS, VALUES, AND RESPONSIBILITIES Professional ethics, values, and responsibilities include an understanding and appreciation of ethics and values of the profession of occupational therapy. The program must facilitate development of the performance criteria listed below. The student will be able to			
B.9.1.	Demonstrate knowledge and understanding of the American Occupational Therapy Association (AOTA) *Occupational Therapy Code of Ethics and Ethics Standards* and AOTA *Standards of Practice* and use them as a guide for ethical decision making in professional interactions, client interventions, and employment settings.	Demonstrate knowledge and understanding of the American Occupational Therapy Association (AOTA) *Occupational Therapy Code of Ethics and Ethics Standards* and AOTA *Standards of Practice* and use them as a guide for ethical decision making in professional interactions, client interventions, and employment settings.	Demonstrate knowledge and understanding of the American Occupational Therapy Association (AOTA) *Occupational Therapy Code of Ethics and Ethics Standards* and AOTA *Standards of Practice* and use them as a guide for ethical decision making in professional interactions, client interventions, and employment settings.
B.9.2.	Discuss and justify how the role of a professional is enhanced by knowledge of and involvement in international, national, state, and local occupational therapy associations and related professional associations.	Discuss and justify how the role of a professional is enhanced by knowledge of and involvement in international, national, state, and local occupational therapy associations and related professional associations.	Explain and give examples of how the role of a professional is enhanced by knowledge of and involvement in international, national, state, and local occupational therapy associations and related professional associations.
B.9.3.	Promote occupational therapy by educating other professionals, service providers, consumers, third-party payers, regulatory bodies, and the public.	Promote occupational therapy by educating other professionals, service providers, consumers, third-party payers, regulatory bodies, and the public.	Promote occupational therapy by educating other professionals, service providers, consumers, third-party payers, regulatory bodies, and the public.
B.9.4.	Identify and develop strategies for ongoing professional development to ensure that practice is consistent with current and accepted standards.	Discuss strategies for ongoing professional development to ensure that practice is consistent with current and accepted standards.	Discuss strategies for ongoing professional development to ensure that practice is consistent with current and accepted standards.

(Continued)

(Continued)

Standard Number	Accreditation Standards for a Doctoral-Degree-Level Educational Program for the Occupational Therapist	Accreditation Standards for a Master's-Degree-Level Educational Program for the Occupational Therapist	Accreditation Standards for an Associate-Degree-Level Educational Program for the Occupational Therapy Assistant
B.9.5.	Discuss professional responsibilities related to liability issues under current models of service provision.	Discuss professional responsibilities related to liability issues under current models of service provision.	Identify professional responsibilities related to liability issues under current models of service provision.
B.9.6.	Discuss and evaluate personal and professional abilities and competencies as they relate to job responsibilities.	Discuss and evaluate personal and professional abilities and competencies as they relate to job responsibilities.	Identify personal and professional abilities and competencies as they relate to job responsibilities.
B.9.7.	Discuss and justify the varied roles of the occupational therapist as a practitioner, educator, researcher, policy developer, program developer, advocate, administrator, consultant, and entrepreneur.	Discuss and justify the varied roles of the occupational therapist as a practitioner, educator, researcher, consultant, and entrepreneur.	Identify and appreciate the varied roles of the occupational therapy assistant as a practitioner, educator, and research assistant.
B.9.8.	Explain and justify the importance of supervisory roles, responsibilities, and collaborative professional relationships between the occupational therapist and the occupational therapy assistant.	Explain and justify the importance of supervisory roles, responsibilities, and collaborative professional relationships between the occupational therapist and the occupational therapy assistant.	Identify and explain the need for supervisory roles, responsibilities, and collaborative professional relationships between the occupational therapist and the occupational therapy assistant.
B.9.9.	Describe and discuss professional responsibilities and issues when providing service on a contractual basis.	Describe and discuss professional responsibilities and issues when providing service on a contractual basis.	Identify professional responsibilities and issues when providing service on a contractual basis.
B.9.10.	Demonstrate strategies for analyzing issues and making decisions to resolve personal and organizational ethical conflicts.	Demonstrate strategies for analyzing issues and making decisions to resolve personal and organizational ethical conflicts.	Identify strategies for analyzing issues and making decisions to resolve personal and organizational ethical conflicts.

Standard Number	Accreditation Standards for a Doctoral-Degree-Level Educational Program for the Occupational Therapist	Accreditation Standards for a Master's-Degree-Level Educational Program for the Occupational Therapist	Accreditation Standards for an Associate-Degree-Level Educational Program for the Occupational Therapy Assistant
B.9.11.	Demonstrate a variety of informal and formal strategies for resolving ethics disputes in varying practice areas.	Explain the variety of informal and formal systems for resolving ethics disputes that have jurisdiction over occupational therapy practice.	Identify the variety of informal and formal systems for resolving ethics disputes that have jurisdiction over occupational therapy practice.
B.9.12.	Describe and implement strategies to assist the consumer in gaining access to occupational therapy and other health and social services.	Describe and discuss strategies to assist the consumer in gaining access to occupational therapy services.	Identify strategies to assist the consumer in gaining access to occupational therapy services.
B.9.13.	Demonstrate advocacy by participating in and exploring leadership positions in organizations or agencies promoting the profession (e.g., AOTA, state occupational therapy associations, World Federation of Occupational Therapists, advocacy organizations), consumer access and services, and the welfare of the community.	Demonstrate professional advocacy by participating in organizations or agencies promoting the profession (e.g., AOTA, state occupational therapy associations, advocacy organizations).	Demonstrate professional advocacy by participating in organizations or agencies promoting the profession (e.g., AOTA, state occupational therapy associations, advocacy organizations).

SECTION C: FIELDWORK EDUCATION AND DOCTORAL EXPERIENTIAL COMPONENT

C.1.0. FIELDWORK EDUCATION

Fieldwork education is a crucial part of professional preparation and is best integrated as a component of the curriculum design. Fieldwork experiences should be implemented and evaluated for their effectiveness by the educational institution. The experience should provide the student with the opportunity to carry out professional responsibilities under supervision of a qualified occupational therapy practitioner serving as a role model. The academic fieldwork coordinator is responsible for the program's compliance with fieldwork education requirements. The academic fieldwork coordinator will

Standard Number	Doctoral	Master's	Associate
C.1.1.	Ensure that the fieldwork program reflects the sequence and scope of content in the curriculum design in collaboration with faculty so that	Ensure that the fieldwork program reflects the sequence and scope of content in the curriculum design in collaboration with faculty so that	Ensure that the fieldwork program reflects the sequence and scope of content in the curriculum design in collaboration with faculty so that

(Continued)

Standard Number	Accreditation Standards for a Doctoral-Degree-Level Educational Program for the Occupational Therapist	Accreditation Standards for a Master's-Degree-Level Educational Program for the Occupational Therapist	Accreditation Standards for an Associate-Degree-Level Educational Program for the Occupational Therapy Assistant
	fieldwork experiences strengthen the ties between didactic and fieldwork education.	fieldwork experiences strengthen the ties between didactic and fieldwork education.	fieldwork experiences strengthen the ties between didactic and fieldwork education.
C.1.2.	Document the criteria and process for selecting fieldwork sites, to include maintaining memoranda of understanding, complying with all site requirements, maintaining site objectives and site data, and communicating this information to students.	Document the criteria and process for selecting fieldwork sites, to include maintaining memoranda of understanding, complying with all site requirements, maintaining site objectives and site data, and communicating this information to students.	Document the criteria and process for selecting fieldwork sites, to include maintaining memoranda of understanding, complying with all site requirements, maintaining site objectives and site data, and communicating this information to students.
C.1.3.	Demonstrate that academic and fieldwork educators collaborate in establishing fieldwork objectives and communicate with the student and fieldwork educator about progress and performance during fieldwork.	Demonstrate that academic and fieldwork educators collaborate in establishing fieldwork objectives and communicate with the student and fieldwork educator about progress and performance during fieldwork.	Demonstrate that academic and fieldwork educators collaborate in establishing fieldwork objectives and communicate with the student and fieldwork educator about progress and performance during fieldwork.
C.1.4.	Ensure that the ratio of fieldwork educators to students enables proper supervision and the ability to provide frequent assessment of student progress in achieving stated fieldwork objectives.	Ensure that the ratio of fieldwork educators to students enables proper supervision and the ability to provide frequent assessment of student progress in achieving stated fieldwork objectives.	Ensure that the ratio of fieldwork educators to students enables proper supervision and the ability to provide frequent assessment of student progress in achieving stated fieldwork objectives.
C.1.5.	Ensure that fieldwork agreements are sufficient in scope and number to allow completion of graduation requirements in a timely manner in accordance with the policy adopted by the program as required by Standard A.4.14.	Ensure that fieldwork agreements are sufficient in scope and number to allow completion of graduation requirements in a timely manner in accordance with the policy adopted by the program as required by Standard A.4.14.	Ensure that fieldwork agreements are sufficient in scope and number to allow completion of graduation requirements in a timely manner in accordance with the policy adopted by the program as required by Standard A.4.14.

(Continued)

Standard Number	Accreditation Standards for a Doctoral-Degree-Level Educational Program for the Occupational Therapist	Accreditation Standards for a Master's-Degree-Level Educational Program for the Occupational Therapist	Accreditation Standards for an Associate-Degree-Level Educational Program for the Occupational Therapy Assistant
C.1.6.	The program must have evidence of valid memoranda of understanding in effect and signed by both parties at the time the student is completing the Level I or Level II fieldwork experience. (Electronic memoranda of understanding and signatures are acceptable.) Responsibilities of the sponsoring institution(s) and each fieldwork site must be clearly documented in the memorandum of understanding.	The program must have evidence of valid memoranda of understanding in effect and signed by both parties at the time the student is completing the Level I or Level II fieldwork experience. (Electronic memoranda of understanding and signatures are acceptable.) Responsibilities of the sponsoring institution(s) and each fieldwork site must be clearly documented in the memorandum of understanding.	The program must have evidence of valid memoranda of understanding in effect and signed by both parties at the time the student is completing the Level I or Level II fieldwork experience. (Electronic memoranda of understanding and signatures are acceptable.) Responsibilities of the sponsoring institution(s) and each fieldwork site must be clearly documented in the memorandum of understanding.
C.1.7.	Ensure that at least one fieldwork experience (either Level I or Level II) has as its focus psychological and social factors that influence engagement in occupation.	Ensure that at least one fieldwork experience (either Level I or Level II) has as its focus psychological and social factors that influence engagement in occupation.	Ensure that at least one fieldwork experience (either Level I or Level II) has as its focus psychological and social factors that influence engagement in occupation.
The goal of Level I fieldwork is to introduce students to the fieldwork experience, to apply knowledge to practice, and to develop understanding of the needs of clients. The program will			
C.1.8.	Ensure that Level I fieldwork is integral to the program's curriculum design and include experiences designed to enrich didactic coursework through directed observation and participation in selected aspects of the occupational therapy process.	Ensure that Level I fieldwork is integral to the program's curriculum design and include experiences designed to enrich didactic coursework through directed observation and participation in selected aspects of the occupational therapy process.	Ensure that Level I fieldwork is integral to the program's curriculum design and include experiences designed to enrich didactic coursework through directed observation and participation in selected aspects of the occupational therapy process.
C.1.9.	Ensure that qualified personnel supervise Level I fieldwork. Examples may include, but are not limited to, currently licensed or otherwise	Ensure that qualified personnel supervise Level I fieldwork. Examples may include, but are not limited to, currently licensed or otherwise	Ensure that qualified personnel supervise Level I fieldwork. Examples may include, but are not limited to, currently licensed or otherwise

(Continued)

Standard Number	Accreditation Standards for a Doctoral-Degree-Level Educational Program for the Occupational Therapist	Accreditation Standards for a Master's-Degree-Level Educational Program for the Occupational Therapist	Accreditation Standards for an Associate-Degree-Level Educational Program for the Occupational Therapy Assistant
	regulated occupational therapists and occupational therapy assistants, psychologists, physician assistants, teachers, social workers, nurses, and physical therapists.	regulated occupational therapists and occupational therapy assistants, psychologists, physician assistants, teachers, social workers, nurses, and physical therapists.	regulated occupational therapists and occupational therapy assistants, psychologists, physician assistants, teachers, social workers, nurses, and physical therapists.
C.1.10.	Document all Level I fieldwork experiences that are provided to students, including mechanisms for formal evaluation of student performance. Ensure that Level I fieldwork is not substituted for any part of Level II fieldwork.	Document all Level I fieldwork experiences that are provided to students, including mechanisms for formal evaluation of student performance. Ensure that Level I fieldwork is not substituted for any part of Level II fieldwork.	Document all Level I fieldwork experiences that are provided to students, including mechanisms for formal evaluation of student performance. Ensure that Level I fieldwork is not substituted for any part of Level II fieldwork.
	The goal of Level II fieldwork is to develop competent, entry-level, generalist occupational therapists. Level II fieldwork must be integral to the program's curriculum design and must include an in-depth experience in delivering occupational therapy services to clients, focusing on the application of purposeful and meaningful occupation and research, administration, and management of occupational therapy services. It is recommended that the student be exposed to a variety of clients across the lifespan and to a variety of settings. The program will	The goal of Level II fieldwork is to develop competent, entry-level, generalist occupational therapists. Level II fieldwork must be integral to the program's curriculum design and must include an in-depth experience in delivering occupational therapy services to clients, focusing on the application of purposeful and meaningful occupation and research, administration, and management of occupational therapy services. It is recommended that the student be exposed to a variety of clients across the lifespan and to a variety of settings. The program will	**The goal of Level II fieldwork is to develop competent, entry-level, generalist occupational therapy assistants. Level II fieldwork must be integral to the program's curriculum design and must include an in-depth experience in delivering occupational therapy services to clients, focusing on the application of purposeful and meaningful occupation. It is recommended that the student be exposed to a variety of clients across the lifespan and to a variety of settings. The program will**
C.1.11.	Ensure that the fieldwork experience is designed to promote clinical reasoning and reflective practice, to transmit the values and beliefs that enable	Ensure that the fieldwork experience is designed to promote clinical reasoning and reflective practice, to transmit the values and beliefs that enable	Ensure that the fieldwork experience is designed to promote clinical reasoning and reflective practice, appropriate to the occupational therapy assistant role,

(Continued)

Standard Number	Accreditation Standards for a Doctoral-Degree-Level Educational Program for the Occupational Therapist	Accreditation Standards for a Master's-Degree-Level Educational Program for the Occupational Therapist	Accreditation Standards for an Associate-Degree-Level Educational Program for the Occupational Therapy Assistant
	ethical practice, and to develop professionalism and competence in career responsibilities.	ethical practice, and to develop professionalism and competence in career responsibilities.	to transmit the values and beliefs that enable ethical practice, and to develop professionalism and competence in career responsibilities.
C.1.12.	Provide Level II fieldwork in traditional and/or emerging settings, consistent with the curriculum design. In all settings, psychosocial factors influencing engagement in occupation must be understood and integrated for the development of client-centered, meaningful, occupation-based outcomes. The student can complete Level II fieldwork in a minimum of one setting if it is reflective of more than one practice area, or in a maximum of four different settings.	Provide Level II fieldwork in traditional and/or emerging settings, consistent with the curriculum design. In all settings, psychosocial factors influencing engagement in occupation must be understood and integrated for the development of client-centered, meaningful, occupation-based outcomes. The student can complete Level II fieldwork in a minimum of one setting if it is reflective of more than one practice area, or in a maximum of four different settings.	Provide Level II fieldwork in traditional and/or emerging settings, consistent with the curriculum design. In all settings, psychosocial factors influencing engagement in occupation must be understood and integrated for the development of client-centered, meaningful, occupation-based outcomes. The student can complete Level II fieldwork in a minimum of one setting if it is reflective of more than one practice area, or in a maximum of three different settings.
C.1.13.	Require a minimum of 24 weeks' full-time Level II fieldwork. This may be completed on a part-time basis, as defined by the fieldwork placement in accordance with the fieldwork placement's usual and customary personnel policies, as long as it is at least 50% of an FTE at that site.	Require a minimum of 24 weeks' full-time Level II fieldwork. This may be completed on a part-time basis, as defined by the fieldwork placement in accordance with the fieldwork placement's usual and customary personnel policies, as long as it is at least 50% of an FTE at that site.	Require a minimum of 16 weeks' full-time Level II fieldwork. This may be completed on a part-time basis, as defined by the fieldwork placement in accordance with the fieldwork placement's usual and customary personnel policies, as long as it is at least 50% of an FTE at that site.
C.1.14.	Ensure that the student is supervised by a currently licensed or otherwise regulated occupational therapist who has a minimum of 1 year full-time (or its equivalent) of practice experience subsequent to initial certification and who is adequately prepared to serve as a fieldwork	Ensure that the student is supervised by a currently licensed or otherwise regulated occupational therapist who has a minimum of 1 year full-time (or its equivalent) of practice experience subsequent to initial certification and who is adequately prepared to serve as a fieldwork	Ensure that the student is supervised by a currently licensed or otherwise regulated occupational therapist or occupational therapy assistant (under the supervision of an occupational therapist) who has a minimum of 1 year full-time (or its equivalent) of practice experience subsequent

(Continued)

Standard Number	Accreditation Standards for a Doctoral-Degree-Level Educational Program for the Occupational Therapist	Accreditation Standards for a Master's-Degree-Level Educational Program for the Occupational Therapist	Accreditation Standards for an Associate-Degree-Level Educational Program for the Occupational Therapy Assistant
	educator. The supervising therapist may be engaged by the fieldwork site or by the educational program.	educator. The supervising therapist may be engaged by the fieldwork site or by the educational program.	to initial certification and who is adequately prepared to serve as a fieldwork educator. The supervising therapist may be engaged by the fieldwork site or by the educational program.
C.1.15.	Document a mechanism for evaluating the effectiveness of supervision (e.g., student evaluation of fieldwork) and for providing resources for enhancing supervision (e.g., materials on supervisory skills, continuing education opportunities, articles on theory and practice).	Document a mechanism for evaluating the effectiveness of supervision (e.g., student evaluation of fieldwork) and for providing resources for enhancing supervision (e.g., materials on supervisory skills, continuing education opportunities, articles on theory and practice).	Document a mechanism for evaluating the effectiveness of supervision (e.g., student evaluation of fieldwork) and for providing resources for enhancing supervision (e.g., materials on supervisory skills, continuing education opportunities, articles on theory and practice).
C.1.16.	Ensure that supervision provides protection of consumers and opportunities for appropriate role modeling of occupational therapy practice. Initially, supervision should be direct and then decrease to less direct supervision as appropriate for the setting, the severity of the client's condition, and the ability of the student.	Ensure that supervision provides protection of consumers and opportunities for appropriate role modeling of occupational therapy practice. Initially, supervision should be direct and then decrease to less direct supervision as appropriate for the setting, the severity of the client's condition, and the ability of the student.	Ensure that supervision provides protection of consumers and opportunities for appropriate role modeling of occupational therapy practice. Initially, supervision should be direct and then decrease to less direct supervision as appropriate for the setting, the severity of the client's condition, and the ability of the student.
C.1.17.	Ensure that supervision provided in a setting where no occupational therapy services exist includes a documented plan for provision of occupational therapy services and supervision by a currently licensed or otherwise regulated occupational therapist with at least 3 years' full-time or its equivalent of professional experience. Supervision must include a minimum of 8 hours	Ensure that supervision provided in a setting where no occupational therapy services exist includes a documented plan for provision of occupational therapy services and supervision by a currently licensed or otherwise regulated occupational therapist with at least 3 years' full-time or its equivalent of professional experience. Supervision must include a minimum of 8 hours	Ensure that supervision provided in a setting where no occupational therapy services exist includes a documented plan for provision of occupational therapy assistant services and supervision by a currently licensed or otherwise regulated occupational therapist or occupational therapy assistant (under the direction of an occupational therapist) with at least 3 years'

(Continued)

Standard Number	Accreditation Standards for a Doctoral-Degree-Level Educational Program for the Occupational Therapist	Accreditation Standards for a Master's-Degree-Level Educational Program for the Occupational Therapist	Accreditation Standards for an Associate-Degree-Level Educational Program for the Occupational Therapy Assistant
	of direct supervision each week of the fieldwork experience. An occupational therapy supervisor must be available, via a variety of contact measures, to the student during all working hours. An on-site supervisor designee of another profession must be assigned while the occupational therapy supervisor is off site.	of direct supervision each week of the fieldwork experience. An occupational therapy supervisor must be available, via a variety of contact measures, to the student during all working hours. An on-site supervisor designee of another profession must be assigned while the occupational therapy supervisor is off site.	full-time or its equivalent of professional experience. Supervision must include a minimum of 8 hours of direct supervision each week of the fieldwork experience. An occupational therapy supervisor must be available, via a variety of contact measures, to the student during all working hours. An on-site supervisor designee of another profession must be assigned while the occupational therapy supervisor is off site.
C.1.18.	Document mechanisms for requiring formal evaluation of student performance on Level II fieldwork (e.g., the AOTA *Fieldwork Performance Evaluation for the Occupational Therapy Student* or equivalent).	Document mechanisms for requiring formal evaluation of student performance on Level II fieldwork (e.g., the AOTA *Fieldwork Performance Evaluation for the Occupational Therapy Student* or equivalent).	Document mechanisms for requiring formal evaluation of student performance on Level II fieldwork (e.g., the AOTA *Fieldwork Performance Evaluation for the Occupational Therapy Assistant Student* or equivalent).
C.1.19.	Ensure that students attending Level II fieldwork outside the United States are supervised by an occupational therapist who graduated from a program approved by the World Federation of Occupational Therapists and has 1 year of experience in practice.	Ensure that students attending Level II fieldwork outside the United States are supervised by an occupational therapist who graduated from a program approved by the World Federation of Occupational Therapists and has 1 year of experience in practice.	Ensure that students attending Level II fieldwork outside the United States are supervised by an occupational therapist who graduated from a program approved by the World Federation of Occupational Therapists and has 1 year of experience in practice.
C.2.0. **DOCTORAL EXPERIENTIAL COMPONENT** **The goal of the doctoral experiential component is to develop occupational therapists with advanced skills (those that are beyond a generalist level). The doctoral experiential component shall be an integral part of the pro-**			

(Continued)

Standard Number	Accreditation Standards for a Doctoral-Degree-Level Educational Program for the Occupational Therapist	Accreditation Standards for a Master's-Degree-Level Educational Program for the Occupational Therapist	Accreditation Standards for an Associate-Degree-Level Educational Program for the Occupational Therapy Assistant
	gram's curriculum design and shall include an in-depth experience in one or more of the following: clinical practice skills, research skills, administration, leadership, program and policy development, advocacy, education, or theory development. The student must successfully complete all coursework and Level II fieldwork and pass a competency requirement prior to the commencement of the doctoral experiential component. The specific content and format of the competency requirement is determined by the program. Examples include a written comprehensive exam, oral exam, NBCOT certification exam readiness tool, and the NBCOT practice exams.		
C.2.1.	Ensure that the doctoral experiential component is designed and administered by faculty and provided in setting(s) consistent with the program's curriculum design, including individualized specific objectives and plans for supervision.	*(No related Standard)*	*(No related Standard)*
C.2.2.	Ensure that there is a memorandum of understanding that, at a minimum, includes individualized specific objectives, plans for supervision or mentoring, and responsibilities of all parties.	*(No related Standard)*	*(No related Standard)*
C.2.3.	Require that the length of this doctoral experiential component be a minimum of 16 weeks (640 hours). This may be completed on a part-	*(No related Standard)*	*(No related Standard)*

(Continued)

Standard Number	Accreditation Standards for a Doctoral-Degree-Level Educational Program for the Occupational Therapist	Accreditation Standards for a Master's-Degree-Level Educational Program for the Occupational Therapist	Accreditation Standards for an Associate-Degree-Level Educational Program for the Occupational Therapy Assistant
	time basis and must be consistent with the individualized specific objectives and culminating project. No more than 20% of the 640 hours can be completed outside of the mentored practice setting(s). Prior fieldwork or work experience may not be substituted for this experiential component.		
C.2.4.	Ensure that the student is mentored by an individual with expertise consistent with the student's area of focus. The mentor does not have to be an occupational therapist.	(No related Standard)	(No related Standard)
C.2.5.	Document a formal evaluation mechanism for objective assessment of the student's performance during and at the completion of the doctoral experiential component.	(No related Standard)	(No related Standard)

Glossary

Definitions given below are for the purposes of these documents.

ability to benefit—A phrase that refers to a student who does not have a high school diploma or its recognized equivalent but is eligible to receive funds under the Title IV Higher Education Act programs after taking an independently administered examination and achieving a score, specified by the Secretary of the U.S. Department of Education (USDE), indicating that the student has the ability to benefit from the education being offered.

academic calendar—The official institutional document that lists registration dates, semester/quarter stop and start dates, holidays, graduation dates, and other pertinent events. Generally, the academic year is divided into two major semesters, each approximately 14 to 16 weeks long. A smaller number of institutions have quarters rather than semesters. Quarters are approximately 10 weeks long; there are three major quarters and the summer session.

activity—A term that describes a class of human actions that are goal directed (AOTA, 2008b).

advanced—The stage of being beyond the elementary or introductory.

affiliate—An entity that formally cooperates with a sponsoring institution in implementing the occupational therapy educational program.

areas of occupation—Activities in which people engage: activities of daily living, instrumental activities of daily living, rest and sleep, education, work, play, leisure, and social participation.

assist—To aid, help, or hold an auxiliary position.

body functions—The physiological functions of body systems (including psychological functions).

body structures—Anatomical parts of the body, such as organs, limbs, and their components.

care coordination—The process that links clients with appropriate services and resources.

case management—A system to ensure that individuals receive appropriate health care services.

client—The term used to name the entity that receives occupational therapy services. Clients may include (1) individuals and other persons relevant to the client's life, including family, caregivers, teachers, employers, and others who may also help or be served indirectly; (2) organizations, such as businesses, industries, or agencies; and (3) populations within a community (AOTA, 2008b).

client-centered service delivery—An orientation that honors the desires and priorities of clients in designing and implementing interventions.

client factors—Factors that reside within the client and that may affect performance in areas of occupation. Client factors include body functions and body structures.

clinical reasoning—Complex multifaceted cognitive process used by practitioners to plan, direct, perform, and reflect on intervention.

collaborate—To work together with a mutual sharing of thoughts and ideas.

competent—To have the requisite abilities/qualities and capacity to function in a professional environment.

consumer—The direct and/or indirect recipient of educational and/or practitioner services offered.

context/contextual factors and environment:

> **context**—The variety of interrelated conditions within and surrounding the client that influence performance. Contexts include cultural, personal, temporal, and virtual aspects.

> **environment**—The external physical and social environment that surrounds the client and in which the client's daily life occupations occur.

context of service delivery—The knowledge and understanding of the various contexts in which occupational therapy services are provided.

criterion-referenced—Tests that compare the performance of an individual with that of another group, known as the *norm group.*

culminating project—A project that is completed by a doctoral student that demonstrates the student's ability to relate theory to practice and to synthesize advanced knowledge in a practice area.

curriculum design—An overarching set of assumptions that explains how the curriculum is planned, implemented, and evaluated. Typically, a curriculum design includes educational goals and curriculum threads and provides a clear rationale for the selection of content, the determination of scope of content, and the sequence of the content. A curriculum design is expected to be consistent with the mission and philosophy of the sponsoring institution and the program.

curriculum threads—Curriculum threads, or *themes,* are identified by the program as areas of study and development that follow a path through the curriculum and represent the unique qualities of the program, as demonstrated by the program's graduates. Curriculum threads are typically based on the profession's and program's vision, mission, and philosophy (e.g., occupational needs of society, critical thinking/professional reasoning, diversity/globalization; AOTA, 2008a).

diagnosis—The process of analyzing the cause or nature of a condition, situation, or problem. Diagnosis as stated in Standard B.4.0. refers to the occupational therapist's ability to analyze a problem associated with occupational performance and participation.

distance education—Education that uses one or more of the technologies listed below to deliver instruction to students who are separated from the instructor and to support regular and substantive interaction between the students and the instructor, either synchronously or asynchronously. The technologies may include

- The Internet;

- One-way and two-way transmissions through open broadcast, closed circuit, cable, microwave, broadband lines, fiber optics, satellite, or wireless communications devices;

- Audio conferencing; or

- Video cassettes, DVDs, and CD-ROMs, if the cassettes, DVDs, or CD-ROMs are used in a course.

driver rehabilitation—Specialized evaluation and training to develop mastery of specific skills and techniques to effectively drive a motor vehicle independently and in accordance with state department of motor vehicles regulations.

entry-level occupational therapist—The outcome of the occupational therapy educational and certification process; an individual prepared to begin generalist practice as an occupational therapist with less than 1 year of experience.

entry-level occupational therapy assistant—The outcome of the occupational therapy educational and certification process; an individual prepared to begin generalist practice as an occupational therapy assistant with less than 1 year of experience.

faculty:

> **faculty, core**—Persons who are resident faculty, including the program director, appointed to and employed primarily in the occupational therapy educational program.

> **faculty, full time**—Core faculty members who hold an appointment that is full time, as defined by the institution, and whose job responsibilities include teaching and/or contributing to the delivery of the designed curriculum regardless of the position title (e.g., full-time instructional staff and clinical instructors would be considered faculty).

> **faculty, part time**—Core faculty members who hold an appointment that is considered by that institution to constitute less than full-time service and whose job responsibilities include teaching and/or contributing to the delivery of the designed curriculum regardless of the position title.

> **faculty, adjunct**—Persons who are responsible for teaching at least 50% of a course and are part-time, nonsalaried, non-tenure-track faculty members who are paid for each class they teach.

fieldwork coordinator—Faculty member who is responsible for the development, implementation, management, and evaluation of fieldwork education.

frame of reference—A set of interrelated, internally consistent concepts, definitions, postulates, and principles that provide a systematic description of a practitioner's interaction with clients. A frame of reference is intended to link theory to practice.

full-time equivalent (FTE)—An equivalent position for a full-time faculty member (as defined by the institution). An FTE can be made up of no more than three individuals.

graduation rate—The total number of students who graduated from a program within 150% of the published length of the program, divided by the number of students on the roster who started in the program.

habits—"Automatic behavior that is integrated into more complex patterns that enable people to function on a day-to-day basis" (Neidstadt & Crepeau, 1998).

health literacy—Degree to which individuals have the capacity to obtain, process, and understand basic health information and services needed to make appropriate health decisions (National Network of Libraries of Medicine, 2011).

interprofessional collaborative practice—"Multiple health workers from different professional backgrounds working together with patients, families, careers, and communities to deliver the highest quality of care" (World Health Organization, 2010).

memorandum of understanding (MOU)—A document outlining the terms and details of an agreement between parties, including each party's requirements and responsibilities. A memorandum of understanding may be signed by any individual who is authorized by the institution to sign fieldwork memoranda of understanding on behalf of the institution.

mentoring—A relationship between two people in which one person (the mentor) is dedicated to the personal and professional growth of the other (the mentee). A mentor has more experience and knowledge than the mentee.

mission—A statement that explains the unique nature of a program or institution and how it helps fulfill or advance the goals of the sponsoring institution, including religious missions.

modalities—Application of a therapeutic agent, usually a physical agent modality.

deep thermal modalities—Modalities such as therapeutic ultrasound and phonophoresis.

electrotherapeutic modalities—Modalities such as biofeedback, neuromuscular electrical stimulation, functional electrical stimulation, transcutaneous electrical nerve stimulation, electrical stimulations for tissue repair, high-voltage galvanic stimulation, and iontophoresis.

mechanical modalities—Modalities such as vasopneumatic devices and continuous passive motion.

superficial thermal modalities—Modalities such as hydrotherapy, whirlpool, cryotherapy, fluidotherapy, hot packs, paraffin, water, and infrared.

model of practice—The set of theories and philosophies that defines the views, beliefs, assumptions, values, and domain of concern of a particular profession or discipline. Models of practice delimit the boundaries of a profession.

occupation—"Activities . . . of everyday life, named, organized and given value and meaning by individuals and a culture. Occupation is everything that people do to occupy themselves, including looking after themselves . . . enjoying life . . . and contributing to the social and economic fabric of their communities" (Law, Polatajko, Baptiste, & Townsend, 1997).

occupational profile—An analysis of a client's occupational history, routines, interests, values, and needs to engage in occupations and occupational roles.

occupational therapy—The art and science of applying occupation as a means to effect positive, measurable change in the health status and functional outcomes of a client by a qualified occupational therapist and/or occupational therapy assistant (as appropriate).

occupational therapy practitioner—An individual who is initially credentialed as an occupational therapist or an occupational therapy assistant.

participation—Active engagement in occupations.

performance patterns—Patterns of behavior related to daily life activities that are habitual or routine. Performance patterns include habits, routines, rituals, and roles.

performance skills—Features of what one does, not what one has, related to observable elements of action that have implicit functional purposes. Performance skills include motor and praxis, sensory–perceptual, emotional regulation, cognitive, and communication and social skills.

philosophy—The underlying belief and value structure for a program that is consistent with the sponsoring institution and which permeates the curriculum and the teaching learning process.

population-based interventions—Interventions focused on promoting the overall health status of the community by preventing disease, injury, disability, and premature death. A population-based health intervention can include assessment of the community's needs, health promotion and public education, disease and disability prevention, monitoring of services, and media interventions. Most interventions are tailored to reach a subset of a population, although some may be targeted toward the population at large. Populations and subsets may be defined by geography, culture, race and ethnicity, socioeconomic status, age, or other characteristics. Many of these characteristics relate to the health of the described population (Keller, Schaffer, Lia-Hoagberg, & Strohschein, 2002).

preparatory methods—Intervention techniques focused on client factors to help a client's function in specific activities.

program director (associate-degree-level occupational therapy assistant)—An initially certified occupational therapist or occupational therapy assistant who is licensed or credentialed according to regulations in the state or jurisdiction in which the program is located. The program director must hold a minimum of a master's degree.

program director (master's-degree-level occupational therapist)—An initially certified occupational therapist who is licensed or credentialed according to regulations in the state or jurisdiction in which the program is located. The program director must hold a doctoral degree.

program director (doctoral-degree-level occupational therapist)—An initially certified occupational therapist who is licensed or credentialed according to regulations in the state or jurisdiction in which the program is located. The program director must hold a doctoral degree.

program evaluation—A continuing system for routinely and systematically analyzing data to determine the extent to which the program is meeting its stated goals and objectives.

purposeful activity—"An activity used in treatment that is goal directed and that the [client] sees as meaningful or purposeful" (Low, 2002).

recognized regional or national accrediting authority—Regional and national accrediting agencies recognized by the USDE and/or the Council for Higher Education Accreditation (CHEA) to accredit postsecondary educational programs/institutions. The purpose of recognition is to ensure that the accrediting agencies are reliable authorities for evaluating quality education or training programs in the institutions they accredit.

Regional accrediting bodies recognized by USDE:

- Accrediting Commission for Community and Junior Colleges, Western Association of Schools and Colleges (ACCJC/WASC)

- Accrediting Commission for Senior Colleges and Universities, Western Association of Schools and Colleges (ACSCU/WASC)

- Commission on Colleges, Southern Association of Colleges and Schools (SACS)

- Commission on Institutions of Higher Education, New England Association of Schools and Colleges (CIHE/NEASC)

- Higher Learning Commission, North Central Association of Colleges and Schools (HLC)

- Middle States Commission on Higher Education, Middle States Association of Colleges and Schools (MSCHE)

- Northwest Commission on Colleges and Universities (NWCCU).

National accrediting bodies recognized by USDE:

- Accrediting Bureau of Health Education Schools (ABHES)

- Accrediting Commission of Career Schools and Colleges (ACCSC)

- Accrediting Council for Continuing Education and Training (ACCET)

- Accrediting Council for Independent Colleges and Schools (ACICS)

- Council on Occupational Education (COE)

- Distance Education and Training Council Accrediting Commission (DETC).

reflective practice—Thoughtful consideration of one's experiences and knowledge when applying such knowledge to practice. Reflective practice includes being coached by professionals.

release time—Period when a person is freed from regular duties, especially teaching, to allow time for other tasks or activities.

retention rate—A measure of the rate at which students persist in their educational program, calculated as the percentage of students on the roster, after the add period, from the beginning of the previous academic year who are again enrolled in the beginning of the subsequent academic year.

scholarship—"A systematic investigation . . . designed to develop or to contribute to generalizable knowledge" (45 CFR § 46). Scholarship is made public, subject to review, and part of the discipline or professional knowledge base (Glassick, Huber, & Maeroff, 1997). It allows others to build on it and further advance the field (AOTA, 2009).

> **scholarship of discovery:** Engagement in activity that leads to the development of "knowledge for its own sake." The Scholarship of Discovery encompasses original research that contributes to expanding the knowledge base of a discipline (Boyer, 1990).

> **scholarship of integration:** Investigations making creative connections both within and across disciplines to integrate, synthesize, interpret, and create new perspectives and theories (Boyer, 1990).

> **scholarship of application:** Practitioners apply the knowledge generated by scholarship of discovery or integration to address real problems at all levels of society (Boyer, 1990). In occupational therapy, an example would be the application of theoretical knowledge to practice interventions or to teaching in the classroom.

> **scholarship of teaching and learning:** "Involves the systematic study of teaching and/or learning and the public sharing and review of such work through presentations, publications, and performances" (McKinney, 2007, p. 10).

skill—The ability to use one's knowledge effectively and readily in execution or performance.

sponsoring institution—The identified legal entity that assumes total responsibility for meeting the minimal standards for ACOTE accreditation.

strategic plan—A comprehensive plan that articulates the program's future vision and guides the program development (e.g., faculty recruitment and professional growth, changes in the curriculum design, priorities in academic resources, procurement of fieldwork sites). A program's strategic plan must include, but need not be limited to,

- Evidence that the plan is based on program evaluation and an analysis of external and internal environments,

- Long-term goals that address the vision and mission of both the institution and program as well as specific needs of the program,

- Specific measurable action steps with expected timelines by which the program will reach its long-term goals,

- Person(s) responsible for action steps, and

- Evidence of periodic updating of action steps and long-term goals as they are met or as circumstances change.

supervise—To direct and inspect the performance of workers or work.

supervision, direct—Supervision that occurs in real time and offers both audio and visual capabilities to ensure opportunities for timely feedback.

supervisor—One who ensures that tasks assigned to others are performed correctly and efficiently.

theory—A set of interrelated concepts used to describe, explain, or predict phenomena.

transfer of credit—A term used in higher education to award a student credit for courses earned in another institution prior to admission to the occupational therapy or occupational therapy assistant program.

References

American Occupational Therapy Association. (2008a). *Occupational therapy model curriculum.* Bethesda, MD: Author. Retrieved from www.aota.org/Educate/EdRes/COE/Other-Education-Documents/OT-Model-Curriculum.aspx

American Occupational Therapy Association. (2008b). Occupational therapy practice framework: Domain and process (2nd ed.). *American Journal of Occupational Therapy, 62,* 625–683. http://dx.doi.org/10.5014/ajot.62.6.625

American Occupational Therapy Association. (2009). Scholarship in occupational therapy. *American Journal of Occupational Therapy, 63,* 790–796. http://dx.doi.org/10.5014/ajot.63.6.790

Boyer, E. L. (1990). *Scholarship reconsidered: Priorities of the professoriate.* San Francisco: Jossey-Bass.

Crepeau, E. B., Cohn, E., & Schell, B. (Eds.). (2008). *Willard and Spackman's occupational therapy* (11th ed.). Philadelphia: Lippincott Williams & Wilkins.

Glassick, C. E., Huber, M. T., & Maeroff, G. I. (1997). *Scholarship assessed: Evaluation of the professoriate.* San Francisco: Jossey-Bass.

Interprofessional Education Collaborative Expert Panel. (2011). *Core competencies for interprofessional collaborative practice: Report of an expert panel.* Washington, DC: Interprofessional Education Collaborative.

Keller, L., Schaffer, M., Lia-Hoagberg, B., & Strohschein S. (2002). Assessment, program planning and evaluation in population-based public health practice. *Journal of Public Health Management and Practice, 8*(5), 30–44.

Law, M., Polatajko, H., Baptiste, W., & Townsend, E. (1997). Core concepts of occupational therapy. In E. Townsend (Ed.), *Enabling occupation: An occupational therapy perspective* (pp. 29–56). Ottawa, ON: Canadian Association of Occupational Therapists.

Low, J. (2002). Historical and social foundations for practice. In C. A. Trombly & M. V. Radomski (Eds.), *Occupational therapy for physical dysfunction* (5th ed., pp. 17–30). Philadelphia: Lippincott Williams & Wilkins.

McKinney, K. (2007). *Enhancing learning through the scholarship of teaching and learning.* San Francisco: Jossey-Bass.

National Network of Libraries of Medicine. (2011). *Health literacy.* Retrieved February 3, 2012, from http://nnlm.gov/outreach/consumer/hlthlit.html

Schon, D. A. (1987). *Educating the reflective practitioner.* San Francisco: Jossey-Bass.

Part 5.

THE PATH TO BECOMING A FIELDWORK EDUCATOR

OVERVIEW OF PART 5

Donna Costa, DHS, OTR/L, FAOTA

The path to becoming a fieldwork educator includes becoming familiar with numerous documents, policies, forms, and role development. In this section, you will find two important official documents. Chapter 26 contains the "Specialized Knowledge and Skills of Occupational Therapy Educators of the Future," which replaced the role competency documents many of us were familiar with. The document emphasizes a progression in the development of competencies, from novice through intermediate and on to advanced roles. You will find competencies in this document for fieldwork educators, academic fieldwork coordinators, faculty members, and program directors.

The other important document for fieldwork educators is the "The American Occupational Therapy Association Self-Assessment Tool for Fieldwork Educator Competency," which you will find in Chapter 27. This document is designed to facilitate the identification of competencies and areas for professional development in the fieldwork educator. The Fieldwork Educator Certificate Program Workshop, offered by AOTA (see Chapter 69, "AOTA Fieldwork Educators Certificate Program Workshop") follows the outline of this document and addresses the competencies that fieldwork educators need in the areas of clinical practice, administration, education, supervision, and evaluation.

The remaining chapters in this section are articles that have appeared in *OT Practice* or the *AOTA Special Interest Section Quarterlies.* The first of these in Chapter 23 is "Supervision Competencies for Fieldwork Educators," and, as the title suggests, focuses on the supervisory aspect of the fieldwork educator's role. The second is Chapter 24, "Becoming a Fieldwork Educator: Enhancing Your Teaching Skills," which addresses the teaching aspect of being a fieldwork educator. Chapter 25 contains "Creating Congruence Between Identities as a Fieldwork Educator and a Practitioner," which focuses on the added role we take when we become fieldwork educators. The roles of practitioner and fieldwork educator partially overlap and are complementary rather than opposing. The last chapter in this section, Chapter 28, "Collaborative Intraprofessional Education With Occupational Therapy and Occupational Therapy Assistant Students," focuses on ways that fieldwork educators can and should be taking occupational therapy and occupational therapy assistant students together. If we expect these individuals to work together in clinical practice, what better way is there than educating them together? The collaborative learning model is particularly well-suited for educating groups of students at the same time.

Chapter 23.

SUPERVISION COMPETENCIES FOR FIELDWORK EDUCATORS

Caryn Johnson, MS, OTR/L, FAOTA
Academic Fieldwork Coordinator and Assistant Professor
Thomas Jefferson University, Philadelphia, PA

Cynthia Haynes, MEd, MBA, OTR/L
Academic Fieldwork Coordinator and Assistant Professor
Philadelphia University, Philadelphia, PA

Joanne Oppermann Ames, MS, OT/L
Formerly Academic Fieldwork Coordinator
University of the Sciences, Philadelphia, PA

Abstract

The Level II fieldwork experience is arguably the most influential piece of a student's preparation for practice. The role that the supervisor plays in this process and the type of relationship that develops between the supervisor and the student are critical aspects of a successful fieldwork experience. According to the Self-Assessment Tool for Fieldwork Educator Competency (American Occupational Therapy Association [AOTA], 1997; Chapter 27), supervisors must develop competence in the areas of practice, supervision, education, evaluation, and administration as they relate to student supervision. This article focuses specifically on those competencies associated with supervision. The fieldwork supervisor is able to influence the student's experience significantly by using strategies that facilitate a collaborative relationship with the student and foster a student-centered approach that emphasizes the student's independent thinking and problem solving. The development of supervision competency is enhanced when the style of supervision selected balances the student's needs and the clinical environment. This article explores the styles outlined in the Situational Leadership model (Costa, 2007b) and discusses how they can be applied to fieldwork supervision. Finally, to use any of these supervision strategies and styles, the supervisor must learn how to give and receive feedback effectively, yet being able to do both skillfully is one of the most difficult professional behaviors to develop. Thus, the last portion of this article explores methods for developing this critical skill.

Learning Objectives

After reading this article, you should be able to:

1. Identify supervision skills required for competent student supervision.
2. Identify strategies to promote student-centered supervision.
3. Understand the Situational Leadership model of supervision and the four supervisor interactive styles delineated.
4. Identify effective methods for providing feedback.

A note on terminology: Much of the study of supervision in clinical education has been performed by scholars outside of occupational therapy. For purposes of this article, the terms *clinical education* and *fieldwork education* are used interchangeably, as are the terms *supervisor* and *fieldwork educator.*

Introduction

A number of recent developments are having an impact on the future of fieldwork education. The newest standards for occupational therapy education require academic programs to educate students about the "professional responsibility for providing fieldwork education and the criteria for becoming a fieldwork educator" (Accreditation Council for Occupational Therapy Education, 2007, p. 36). Unlike the existing "catch as catch can" approach to fieldwork educator training, this standard essentially mandates that all occupational therapy practitioners begin developing some supervisory competencies and a commitment to fieldwork education early in their careers. Further, in response to a report from the Commission on Education, the 2007 AOTA Representative Assembly initiated a process to develop a voluntary credentialing program for fieldwork educators. Such a program would both recognize individuals who have achieved a level of competence in fieldwork education and provide highly desirable resources and structure for those who are interested in developing those competencies. Finally, leaders in the profession have called on fieldwork educators to help achieve the profession's *Centennial Vision* (AOTA, 2006) by influencing students during their fieldwork experiences. In a recent article, Crist (2006) called on fieldwork educators to not only educate for today, but also "accept the charge to address 'what can be'" (p. 9) by engaging in evidence- and occupation-based practice, encouraging cultural competence, and empowering students to advocate for the profession. Costa's (2007b) "vision of fieldwork excellence" envisions "fieldwork education as

the primary driver in transforming practice" (p. 9) and calls for the development of a set of fieldwork educator competencies, training resources, and research on supervision and fieldwork education.

The impact supervision has on the fieldwork experience has long been recognized in the literature. In a survey of 122 occupational therapists more than 2 decades ago (Christie, Joyce, & Moeller, 1985a), 75 respondents identified fieldwork as the most influential aspect of their professional development compared with preprofessional and academic experiences. The most frequently mentioned contributing factors were the supervisor's attitude, interpersonal skills, organization, and creative problem solving. Recent studies have shown similar themes, such as having a positive attitude, regularly engaging in self-assessment and reflection, taking a proactive approach, giving constructive and timely feedback, being consistent with expectations, taking a collaborative approach, and embracing the importance of the gatekeeper role (Banks, Bell, & Smits, 2000; Dimeo, Malta, & Bruns, 2004; Farber & Koenig, 2008; McCarron & Crist, 2000; Scheerer, 2003).

AOTA's (1997) Self-Assessment Tool for Fieldwork Educator Competency (Chapter 27) provides a useful structure for identifying the competencies a fieldwork educator should have. This tool organizes the skills required of fieldwork educators into five areas:

1. *Professional practice:* Competencies related to knowledge, skills, and judgment in occupational therapy practice
2. *Education:* Competencies related to teaching and learning

3. *Supervision:* Competencies related to communication, guidance, and the supervisory relationship
4. *Evaluation:* Competencies related to evaluating student performance
5. *Administration:* Competencies related to developing and implementing a fieldwork program with attention to legal, professional, environmental, and cultural issues.

Exhibit 23.1 lists the 12 supervision competencies identified in the Self-Assessment Tool for Fieldwork Educator Competency (AOTA, 1997). The majority of these competencies pertain to communication

---

Exhibit 23.1. *Supervision Competencies From the Self-Assessment Tool for Fieldwork Educator Competency (AOTA, 1997)*

1. Presents clear performance expectations initially and throughout the experience appropriate to occupational therapy practice (e.g., student occupational therapist/occupational therapy assistant role delineation, Level I or II fieldwork, practice environment).
2. Collaborates with the student in setting learning goals, objectives, and expectations, and makes modifications accordingly.
3. Anticipates and prepares student for challenging situations.
4. Provides activities to challenge student's optimal performance.
5. Provides the student with prompt, direct, specific, and constructive feedback throughout the fieldwork experience.
6. Makes specific suggestions to the student for improvement in performance.
7. Uses verbal, nonverbal, and written communication effectively.
8. Initiates interaction to resolve conflict and to raise issues of concern.
9. Uses a variety of supervisory approaches to facilitate student performance (e.g., written, support/confrontation, multiple supervisors).
10. Elicits and responds to student's feedback and concerns.
11. Collaborates with the student and academic fieldwork coordinator to identify and modify learning situations when the student experiences difficulty.
12. Acts as a role model of professional behavior (e.g., separates personal vs. professional issues with students and staff, addresses diversity issues, uses humor appropriately).

---

and the supervisory process as well as to the application of models of supervision that guide students' progression toward entry-level competence. *(Note: To learn about competencies in the remaining areas, such as role modeling and handling particularly difficult situations, readers will need to pursue additional study.)*

Contemporary Approaches to Student Supervision

Student-Centered Supervision

A *student-centered* approach to fieldwork supervision recognizes the student as the driver of the experience and the supervisor as the navigator who provides the resources, guidance, and support to provide the student with what is needed for a challenging, yet successful journey. Ultimately, the student must choose to use these provisions to reach the destination; hence, his or her attitudes and actions are equally important to the success of the fieldwork experience (Banks et al., 2000; Christie, Joyce, & Moeller, 1985b; Farber & Koenig, 1999; Sladyk & Sheckley, 1999) and should not be overlooked. Studies have found that students have a positive experience when they take the initiative to ask questions regarding clinical reasoning, value the process of learning, appreciate the use of theoretical constructs (Banks et al., 2000), engage in self-reflection (Sladyk & Sheckley, 1999), and initiate problem solving (Farber & Koenig, 1999; Schkade, 1999). Although the student plays an integral role in the supervisory relationship, the scope of this article focuses on the *supervisor's* role.

Strategies for Promoting Student-Centered Supervision

This section explores specific strategies that supervisors can use to create a positive supervisory experience for both the students and themselves and to provide an environment where optimal learning and professional skill development in the areas of initiative taking, problem solving, decision making, and self-reflection can occur. In keeping with the competencies identified in the Self-Assessment Tool for Fieldwork Educator Competency (AOTA, 1997), these strategies support the concept of a student-centered approach to supervision that promotes collaborative problem solving and independent thinking. A review of the literature yields three broad types of strategies for promoting student success: organizational, collaborative, and adaptive.

Organizational Strategies

These strategies involve planning the learning process (Banks et al., 2000) and taking a proactive approach to structure the fieldwork experience before the student even arrives (Farber & Koenig, 1999). The following are examples of organizational strategies:

- *Provide written descriptions of student expectations:* These can be in the form of professional behavior, weekly clinical expectations (e.g., caseload requirements, assessment and treatment expectations), special projects, and assignments with due dates. Providing these expectations in writing not only will give the student an understanding of what the affiliation will be like, but also puts the onus on the student to organize time effectively and take the initiative to meet the expectations. Accordingly, one of the professional behavior expectations may be that the student is responsible for staying on track with the scheduled outline. A written record can promote consistency and direct communication for a student having difficulty.
- *Provide the student with the department's site-specific objectives that correlate with the Fieldwork Performance Evaluation (AOTA, 2002a):* This document enhances the student's understanding of the expectations of an entry-level therapist at this specific clinical setting, as well as provides an objective tool with which both the supervisor and the student can evaluate the student's performance.
- *Conduct formal feedback sessions weekly at a designated time mutually agreed on by the supervisor and student:* The day and time may be established during the first week of the affiliation.
- *Create special projects and assignments that require the student to demonstrate initiative:* Examples for this strategy include conducting an evidence-based literature search using a variety of scholarly resources that are not present in the department; building independent thinking by writing a case study review of a client the student has worked with that includes input from practitioners from other disciplines involved in the client's care; and

developing other professional skills, such as public speaking, writing, and presenting a formal poster.

Collaborative Strategies

These strategies embrace a spirit of mutual responsibility between the supervisor and student (Farber & Koenig, 1999; McCarron & Crist, 2000) and recognize that learning is a process that requires the supervisor's nurturing and guidance (Banks et al., 2000; Sladyk & Sheckley, 1999). Supervisors who are collaborative demonstrate flexible problem solving and engage in mutual activities for self-assessment and reflection (Banks et al., 2000; Farber & Koenig, 1999, 2008; McCarron & Crist, 2000). Examples of collaborative strategies include the following:

- *Acknowledge that professional learning is an ongoing process:* The supervisor discusses and demonstrates methods for learning new information for the purpose of providing best practice in the treatment setting.
- *Engage in reflective dialogue activities regularly with students* (Sladyk & Sheckley, 1999): For example, during the first week of the affiliation, the supervisor reflects on the thought process during client sessions and the reasoning for using or modifying specific evaluation or treatment methods. When students begin working with clients, they discuss their own clinical reasoning process. Students have indicated that this back-and-forth dialogue is a powerful tool in teaching them how to think like occupational therapists (Sladyk & Sheckley, 1999).
- *Give the student responsibility to identify two or three possible ways to improve a challenging situation:* The student and supervisor then discuss these possibilities. This strategy takes the onus off the supervisor to have all the answers and forces more independent thinking on the part of the student (Farber & Koenig, 1999).
- *Expect the student to engage in a reflective activity before the weekly feedback sessions by identifying that week's achievements and challenges and then establishing new learning goals:* The student also can be expected to provide formal written feedback to the supervisor, thus further emphasizing the concept of a *mutual* learning process. For more structured reflective activities, the Fieldwork Experience Assessment Tool (FEAT, Chapter 13;

AOTA, 2001) provides an excellent opportunity for both the supervisor and the student to participate in mutual reflection.

Adaptive Strategies

One of the keys to successful supervision is the ability to be flexible—to try different approaches to guiding the student throughout the learning process, and to address difficulties that emerge during the affiliation (Farber & Koenig, 1999; McCarron & Crist, 2000). Helpful to both the supervisor and the student is maintaining an attitude of willingness to see problems as challenges and to seek alternate solutions. Strategies that facilitate more flexible thinking include the following:

- *Expect the student, not the supervisor, to generate ideas for addressing challenging issues:* This strategy will give the supervisor new options to consider.
- *Provide the student with regular, structured opportunities to give feedback to the supervisor:* This strategy provides the supervisor with suggestions and opportunities to modify certain supervisory skills.
- *Discuss supervisory situations with colleagues for their input and support* (Farber & Koenig, 1999).
- *Engage in continuing education for fieldwork supervision:* Congratulations! You are already engaging in this one.

These strategies can be a useful start to implementing a student-centered approach to supervision. However, as with all intervention techniques, they can be ineffective if not used as part of a theoretical framework. The next section describes a model that can be used to promote effective supervision using student-centered concepts.

The Situational Leadership Model

Occupational therapy practitioners may supervise students with the best of intentions, using supervision styles they encountered during their own work experiences or when they were students. However, according to Competencies 3, 4, and 9 of the Self-Assessment Tool for Fieldwork Educator Competency (AOTA, 1997), a fieldwork educator should demonstrate the ability to use a variety of supervisory models that will challenge the student and facilitate growth and development. Fieldwork educator competencies also include a positive attitude toward practice, supervision, and mentoring students

(Dickerson, 2006). Costa (2007a) described several models of supervision appropriate to fieldwork education, particularly the Situational Leadership model, which is a student-centered approach.

The Situational Leadership model of supervision has been adapted from Hershey's work in the area of leadership (Costa, 2007a; Hershey, Blanchard, & Johnson, 1996; Meyer, 2002) because of its relevance to clinical student supervision. It focuses on the match among the supervisor's styles, the demands of the task, and the student's readiness in the areas of competence and confidence. This model describes how a supervisor progressively facilitates a student's development of professional competencies across several domains: assessment and intervention skills, interpersonal assessment, treatment planning, adherence to ethical standards, integration of theoretical frameworks, and an understanding of clients and cultural differences (Costa, 2007a).

In selecting supervisory styles, the supervisor must address the student's readiness and learning needs. The match among supervisory styles, the student's needs, and the demands of the environment starts with understanding the student's competence and confidence. Each factor varies during the student's fieldwork experience, and the supervisor must be willing to assess the student's progress and alter the supervisory style with changes in the student (Blanchard, 2007; Costa, 2007a).

Students show confidence through motivation, commitment, interest, and enthusiasm as they progress through the fieldwork placement (Meyer, 2002). Student competence is demonstrated by progress toward achieving site-specific learning objectives and weekly learning targets and objectives that match items on the Fieldwork Performance Evaluation (AOTA, 2002a; Chapters 58 and 59). Competence is achieved through a variety of instructional methods and can be measured by changes in the student's demonstrated behaviors and a gradual progression in supervision strategies from directive to coaching, supportive, and ultimately, delegation. The supervisor can have a positive impact on competence and confidence by clearly communicating the importance of each task, skill, or duty the student is responsible for (Crist, 2006).

The Situational Leadership model delineates four supervisor interaction styles, which are developmental in nature. The supervisor selects one of the following styles based on the task or activity and on the student's motivation, confidence, and competence (Costa, 2007a).

Directive

A directive style is applied when a student presents with a low level of competence or confidence (readiness), needing direction and guidance to complete most tasks (Meyer, 2002). The supervisor must orient the student, closely observe performance, provide feedback, and lead discussions. Additionally, the supervisor should maintain clear expectations, establish weekly goals, and provide additional reading materials. Many of the *organizational* strategies previously discussed are examples of a directive approach. Some activities appropriate for a student at this level may include having the student explain how to follow the facility's policies for standard precautions, complete a chart review and make a list of a client's strengths and needs, and read an occupational therapy evaluation and explain the focus of intervention.

Coaching

A coaching style is used with the student who demonstrates a higher level of readiness. The supervisor facilitates clinical reasoning through two-way communication and encourages the student to generate intervention ideas. The supervisor provides feedback and positive reinforcement and carefully allows increased independence with demonstrated competence through increasingly complex clinical situations (Meyer, 2002). Many of the *collaborative* and *adaptive* strategies previously discussed lend themselves well to the coaching approach. A student at this level could be asked to observe an intervention session and clearly document observations, explain why a specific intervention was appropriate to the client's occupational roles, and select several assessments based on a chart review and client interview.

Supportive

As student competence and confidence levels improve, the supervisor can move on to a supportive style of supervision. At this point, the student is treating an entry-level caseload, seeking input, demonstrating self-directed learning, and showing an ability to work independently. The supervisor acts primarily as a consultant, monitor, or overseer. Many of the *collaborative* and *adaptive* strategies discussed previously are appropriate to the supervisory process at this point. Additional student activities could include grading interventions appropriate to the client's needs and conducting an

assessment and interpreting it based on the client's occupational roles and desired outcomes.

Delegation

When the student demonstrates sufficient competence and confidence throughout the scope of practice, the supervisor may apply a delegation style. The supervisor acts as a consultant, allowing the student to function more or less autonomously, and provides input for more complex, unfamiliar situations. Supervision at this level should encourage students to articulate their clinical reasoning process so the supervisor can ask probing questions and facilitate critical thinking. Students become increasingly confident in their skills and their roles as occupational therapy professionals. They have reached a level of autonomy and can identify their unique strengths and weaknesses as entry-level practitioners (Costa, 2007a). Higher-level *organizational, collaborative,* and *adaptive* strategies can be applied at this level. Examples of activities that may be delegated include scheduling and carrying a full caseload, completing all documentation accurately and on time, and explaining clinical reasoning to substantiate intervention plans (Costa, 2007a; McCarron & Crist, 2000).

Students are not uniform in their progression across domains. It is not unusual for students to take detours, wavering between confidence and confusion, dependence and independence, inexperience and competence. These normal behaviors will require adaptations in supervision style to progress the student toward increasing independence (Meyer, 2002). Matching supervision styles to the student's needs is a dynamic, challenging process; however, the effective match can ultimately enhance the student's learning experience, enthusiasm, and commitment to the profession as well as provide the supervisor with the satisfaction of facilitating entry-level practice competencies in a new member of the profession.

Feedback, Communication, and the Supervision Process

If effective supervision is the most crucial component of the successful fieldwork experience, then communication and feedback are undisputedly among the most important components of supervision. In fact, in the Self-Assessment Tool for Fieldwork Educator Competency (AOTA, 1997), half of the supervision competencies (i.e., 1–2, 5–7, 10) involve communication and feedback.

Students must be able to ask for, accept, and apply feedback. Supervisors must be able to provide feedback effectively. Evidence regarding the importance of effective communication and feedback in clinical education is abundant (Bruns, Dimeo, & Malta, 2003; Cross, 1995; Falender & Shafranske, 2004; Heine & Bennett, 2003). This section provides strategies to develop feedback skills.

In a study of 207 fieldwork educators, Farber (1998) reported that feedback was a primary strategy to address problematic behaviors in students. Hughes, Mangold, Thuss, Buckley, and Lennon (1999) found that students "believed that the supervisor's ability as well as their own to communicate their needs effectively was essential to their success" (p. 16). Christie et al. (1985b) reported that the critical components of a good fieldwork experience most frequently mentioned by students and supervisors included an individualized approach, an organized and well-structured program, effective feedback, and open communication. In addition, both student and supervisor respondents "perceived the supervisory process as the most critical element in distinguishing the good versus poor fieldwork experience" (p. 681). For many of us, the ability to give effective feedback does not come naturally. The good news is that providing feedback uses a variety of skills that can be learned.

Feedback often is used to heighten awareness of strengths and weaknesses, develop solutions to facilitate and manage change, empower students to develop new strategies, and clarify expectations and objectives. Even after reading weekly expectations and site-specific objectives, many students still do not really understand what the desired behavior should actually look like.

Feedback and Timing

Timing is an essential component of feedback. Feedback should be provided as soon as possible and often. Waiting too long to provide feedback may lead the student to see it as invalid, irrelevant, or unimportant, lessening the effect.

Formative feedback is provided to inform students about their performance. It may be formal or informal and is provided throughout the fieldwork experience, allowing change and development to occur (Moore, Hilton, Morris, Caladine, & Bristow, 1997). *Summative* feedback, on the other hand, occurs at the end of the fieldwork experience. Because it summarizes the student's overall performance, potential for further growth and change is limited (Moore et al., 1997). The Fieldwork Performance Evaluation (AOTA, 2002a), for example, provides formative feedback at midterm and summative feedback at the completion of the Level II experience. When formative feedback is provided effectively, there are no surprises at the final evaluation.

The FEAT (AOTA, 2001) and weekly supervision forms are two additional methods for providing formative feedback. The FEAT usually is used at midterm or earlier and provides a structured way to elicit feedback from both the student and fieldwork educator. It helps to facilitate dialogue by examining how the student, supervisor, and environment are functioning and interacting, and it examines how these interactions are affecting the student's learning and performance. The information obtained can be used to enhance the fieldwork program for stronger students or to help weaker students verbalize their needs and identify strategies.

Many fieldwork sites have developed their own version of a weekly supervision form to review the previous week's goals, address what went well that week and which areas need improvement, and identify goals for the following week. This tool helps to ensure a balance of positive and constructive feedback and provides documentation of the student's progress, strengths, and areas of concern over time.

Types of Feedback

A number of different types of feedback exist, and each has its role. *Constructive* feedback, also known as *critical* feedback, commonly is used to provide students with information about areas of their performance that need improvement. Providing effective constructive feedback consists of two parts: (a) identify the problem and the consequences that may result, and (b) identify possible solutions and strategies. An example of the need for constructive feedback is when a student consistently arrives 10 to 15 minutes late to fieldwork. The supervisor would explain that arriving on time is an expectation in the area of professional behavior, and that being late makes the student appear rushed and disorganized; does not allow time to set up the treatment area; and causes client intervention to be behind schedule, possibly compromising the client's confidence and trust in the student. Consistent lateness disrupts the rest of the department, affects the quality of care the student is providing, and affects the student's midterm evaluation score. The supervisor would follow up on this feedback by collaborating with the student to develop solutions and strategies.

Positive feedback is just as essential. It increases morale and, more importantly, reinforces performance. In the absence of positive feedback, the student may not recognize when the desired behavior has been achieved or when goals have been accomplished. The student may become frustrated or confused, or revert to previous, less successful behaviors.

Destructive, or *negative,* feedback often is the result of constructive feedback gone awry. Statements like, "You never remember to lock the brakes," or "That activity will never work," provide the student with no useful information and have no educational benefit. Negative feedback decreases student commitment and confidence, and results in conflict.

Instructive feedback is a process that allows the student to react to feedback, enables self-assessment, and helps the student to develop strategies for improvement (Holmboe, Yepes, Williams, & Huot, 2004).

The Challenge of Giving Feedback

One might ask, "Why is it so difficult to give feedback?" For those who are conflict adverse, it simply is easier *not* to. Many supervisors are concerned about how a student may respond, anticipating an emotional reaction or being fearful of damaging the relationship or challenging a student's individuality. Less experienced supervisors may lack confidence in their own judgment or abilities. Still others may have a "gut" feeling but no facts to back up their concerns.

The logical next question would be, "Why do people have trouble receiving feedback?" Feedback often can elicit emotional reactions. Some individuals only hear the good parts of feedback, whereas others only hear the bad. Still others just sit there, hearing nothing and waiting for it to be over. Some recipients regard feedback as invalid because they do not respect or trust the provider. Others are overwhelmed by too much information being provided at one time.

Effective Feedback

Skilled delivery of feedback is essential to a positive outcome. The method of delivery may vary from a formal appointment to informal discussions as the supervisor and student travel from one location to another. Feedback can be provided verbally or in written form. Nonverbal communication, such as a nod, a frown, or clenched teeth, also conveys information. To ensure that feedback is effective, provide it in a prompt and timely manner; be specific and direct, with clear behavioral objectives; balance the positive and constructive by "sandwiching" a critical statement between two positive statements; remain nonjudgmental, focusing on the behavior, not the person; give constructive feedback privately; use "I" statements to lessen the chances of a defensive response; and deliver feedback that is appropriate for the student's stage of development.

The supervisor must confirm the message by having the student reflect or restate what he or she heard. Then the student and supervisor collaborate to develop strategies to address areas of need. Some students benefit from written feedback that they can reflect on later.

Conclusion

Building competency as a fieldwork educator is a gradual process. The Self-Assessment Tool for Fieldwork Educator Competency (AOTA, 1997) can help both experienced and inexperienced fieldwork educators to identify areas of competency as well areas requiring further development. When students begin to examine prospective Level II fieldwork options, many focus on the sites with the "best" reputations. The evidence presented in this article, however, indicates that it is not necessarily the site, but the supervisor that truly makes the fieldwork experience a successful one.

References

Accreditation Council for Occupational Therapy Education. (2007). *Accreditation Council for Occupational Therapy Education (ACOTE) standards and interpretive guidelines.* Retrieved October 1, 2007, from http://www.aota.org/educate/accred it/standardsReview/40601.aspx

American Occupational Therapy Association. (1997). *Self-assessment tool for fieldwork educator competency.* Retrieved October 21, 2007, from http://www.aota.org/Educate/ EdRes/Fieldwork/Supervisors/Forms/38251.aspx

American Occupational Therapy Association. (2001). *The Fieldwork Experience Assessment Tool.* Bethesda, MD: Author.

American Occupational Therapy Association. (2002a). *Field-work performance evaluation for the occupational therapy or occupational therapy assistant student.* Bethesda, MD: Author.

American Occupational Therapy Association. (2002b). Occupational therapy practice framework: Domain and process. *American Journal of Occupational Therapy, 56,* 609–639. http://dx.doi.org/10.5014/ajot.56.6.609

American Occupational Therapy Association. (2006). *Centennial vision.* Retrieved October 26, 2007, from http://www.aota.org/News/Centennial.aspx

Banks, S., Bell, E., & Smits, E. (2000). Integration tutorials and seminars: Examining the integration of academic and fieldwork learning by student occupational therapists. *Canadian Journal of Occupational Therapy, 67,* 93–100.

Blanchard, K. (2007). *Manage and develop people to do their best: Ignite! newsletter.* Retrieved October 11, 2007, from http://www.kenblanchard.com/ignite/april_2007/april2007_main/Default.asp?

Bruns, C., Dimeo, S. B., & Malta, S. (2003). Journey into supervision. *OT Practice, 8*(6), 19–22.

Christie, B. A., Joyce, P. C., & Moeller, P. L. (1985a). Fieldwork experience, part I: Impact on practice preference. *American Journal of Occupational Therapy, 39,* 671–674. http://dx.doi.org/10.5014/ajot.39.10.671

Christie, B. A., Joyce, P. C., & Moeller, P. L. (1985b). Fieldwork experience, part II: The supervisor's dilemma. *American Journal of Occupational Therapy, 39,* 675–681. http://dx.doi.org/10.5014/ajot.39.10.675

Costa, D. M. (2006). Fieldwork Issues: A vision of fieldwork excellence. *OT Practice, 11*(8), 9–10.

Costa, D. M. (2007). *Clinical supervision in occupational therapy: A guide for fieldwork and practice.* Bethesda, MD: AOTA Press.

Crist, P. A. (2006, May 15). Start now, if you want to educate for 2017. *Advance for Occupational Therapy Practitioners,* p. 9.

Cross, V. (1995). Perceptions of the ideal clinical educator in physiotherapy education. *Physiotherapy, 81,* 506–513.

Dickerson, A. (2006). Role competencies for a fieldwork educator. *American Journal of Occupational Therapy, 60,* 650–651. http://dx.doi.org/10.5014/ajot.60.6.650

Dimeo, S. B., Malta, S. L., & Bruns, C. J. (2004). The supervisory journey. In D. M. Costa (Ed.), *The essential guide to occupational therapy fieldwork education: Resources for today's educators and practitioners* (pp. 69–77). Bethesda, MD: AOTA Press.

Falender, C. A., & Shafranske, E. P. (2004). *The practice of clinical supervision: A competency-based approach.* Washington, DC: American Psychological Association.

Farber, R. S. (1998, March). Supervisory relationships: Snags, stress, and solutions. *Education Special Interest Section Quarterly, 8*(1), 2–3.

Farber, R. S., & Koenig, K. P. (1999). Examination of fieldwork educators' responses to challenging situations. In P. Crist (Ed.), *Innovations in occupational therapy education, 1999* (pp. 89–101). Bethesda, MD: American Occupational Therapy Association.

Farber, R. S., & Koenig, K. P. (2008). Facilitating clinical reasoning in fieldwork: The relational context of the supervisor and student. In B. A. B. Schell & J. W. Schell (Eds.), *Clinical and professional reasoning in occupational therapy* (pp. 335–368). Baltimore: Lippincott Williams & Wilkins.

Heine, D., & Bennett, N. (2003). Student perceptions of Level I fieldwork supervision. *Occupational Therapy in Health Care, 17*(2), 89–97.

Hershey, P., Blanchard, K., & Johnson, D. (1996). *Management of organizational behavior: Utilizing human resources* (7th ed.). Upper Saddle River, NJ: Prentice Hall.

Holmboe, E. S., Yepes, M., Williams, F., & Huot, S. J. (2004). Feedback and the mini clinical evaluation exercise. *Journal of General Internal Medicine, 19*(5 Pt. 2), 558–561.

Hughes, K. A., Mangold, S. M., Thuss, S. L., Buckley, S. M., & Lennon, J. K. (1999). Success of Level II fieldwork: The student's perspective. In P. A. Crist (Ed.), *Innovations in occupational therapy education 1999* (pp. 7–19). Bethesda, MD: American Occupational Therapy Association.

McCarron, K., & Crist, P. A. (2000). Supervision and mentoring, lesson 5. In S. C. Merrill & P. A. Crist (Eds.), *Meeting the fieldwork challenge* (pp. 1–27). Bethesda, MD: American Occupational Therapy Association.

Meyer, L. P. (2002). Athletic training clinical instructors as situational leaders. *Journal of Athletic Training, 37*(4), 261S–265S.

Moore, A. P., Hilton, R. W., Morris, D. J., Caladine, L. K., & Bristow, H. R. (1997). *The clinical educator: Role development.* New York: Churchill Livingstone.

Scheerer, C. R. (2003). Perceptions of effective professional behavior feedback: Occupational therapy student voices. *American Journal of Occupational Therapy, 57,* 205–214. http://dx.doi.org/10.5014/ajot.57.2.205

Schkade, J. K. (1999). Student practitioner: The adaptive transition. In P. A. Crist (Ed.), *Innovations in occupational therapy education 1999* (pp. 147–156). Bethesda, MD: American Occupational Therapy Association.

Sladyk, K., & Scheckley, B. G. (1999). Differences between clinical reasoning gainers and decliners during fieldwork. In P. A. Crist (Ed.), *Innovations in occupational therapy education 1999* (pp. 157–176). Bethesda, MD: American Occupational Therapy Association.

Chapter 24.

BECOMING A FIELDWORK "EDUCATOR": ENHANCING YOUR TEACHING SKILLS

Ingrid Provident, EdD, OTR/L
Assistant Professor and Academic Fieldwork Coordinator
Duquesne University, Pittsburgh, PA

Mary Lou Leibold, MS, OTR/L
Assistant Professor and Academic Fieldwork Coordinator
University of Pittsburgh, Pittsburgh, PA

Cathy Dolhi, OTD, OTR/L, FAOTA
Associate Professor and Academic Fieldwork Coordinator
Chatham University, Pittsburgh, PA

Joanne Jeffcoat, MEd, OTR/L
Professor and Academic Fieldwork Coordinator
Community College of Allegheny County, Monroeville, PA

This article was developed in collaboration with AOTA's **Education Special Interest Section.**

Abstract

Level II fieldwork education can be one of the most influential elements of a student's preparation for practice. The 2007 American Occupational Therapy Association's (AOTA's) Ad Hoc Committee to Explore and Develop Resources for Occupational Therapy Fieldwork Educators stated that "fieldwork education is a primary driver in transforming our current practice into meeting the 2017 *Centennial Vision*" (AOTA, 2007a, p. 14). Often, fieldwork educators taking their first student have only their own Level II fieldwork experiences to guide their teaching. Few occupational therapy practitioners have formal training in education. The purpose of this article is to provide the fieldwork educator with teaching tools and strategies that can be incorporated to enhance efficiency and effectiveness as a fieldwork educator and to maximize the student's learning during the fieldwork experience. Being aware of teaching–learning styles will also aid in setting realistic expectations for the fieldwork experience. Although this continuing education article provides an overview of these topics, it should be noted that a more thorough presentation of this material is available through AOTA's Fieldwork Educators Certificate Program (AOTA, 2009a), which is being offered nationwide by regional trainers.

Learning Objectives

After reading this article, you should be able to:

1. Identify the importance of customizing the fieldwork experience by incorporating the student's strengths, liabilities, academic preparation, and curriculum design into the experience.
2. Identify students' learning styles.
3. Identify teaching styles to facilitate student learning.
4. Recognize the value of developing student-specific learning objectives for fieldwork experiences.
5. Identify tools available through AOTA to maximize the fieldwork experience for the fieldwork educator and student.

Introduction

Although not often recognized as a primary job responsibility, most occupational therapy practitioners routinely incorporate "teaching" into practice. From showing a client how to use a piece of adaptive equipment to instructing a caregiver on how to prevent injury by using appropriate body mechanics, occupational therapy practitioners teach on a daily basis. Most practitioners were not, however, formally trained as teachers. This lack of training in education techniques can result in unnecessary problems during fieldwork. The fieldwork educator who uses proper teaching tools can effectively influence the student's experience by using strategies that facilitate learning. By understanding the student's learning style and unique characteristics, the fieldwork educator can use the teaching style that will best facilitate the student's thinking and problem solving. As the fieldwork educator becomes more cognizant of his or her role as teacher and more skilled at using appropriate teaching strategies, learning experiences can be sequenced to grade the student's progression toward entry-level practice in an efficient and effective manner.

AOTA's Self-Assessment Tool for Fieldwork Educator Competency (2009b; Chapter 27) provides a useful structure for identifying the competencies a fieldwork educator should have. This tool organizes the skills required of fieldwork educators into five areas: professional practice, education, supervision, evaluation, and administration.

The majority of these competencies pertain to understanding the student's learning needs and designing the fieldwork experience to adapt the teaching style to guide student performance. The complete Self-Assessment Tool for Fieldwork Educator Competency listing all 14 education competencies is available on the AOTA website. The reader is encouraged to access this document in its original format and use it as a tool for self-assessment related to the skills necessary for being a fieldwork educator.

Teaching Skills

Think about the interactions that occupational therapy practitioners have with clients on a daily basis. In the early stages of the practitioner–client relationship, practitioners talk with the client (or family and significant others) to gather basic information. During the initial interview and evaluation, occupational therapy practitioners gain information about the client's strengths and problem areas; the contexts that have an impact on the client's performance; and the client's personal needs, wants, and expectations. Practitioners then collaborate with the client to establish goals based on that information.

As a fieldwork educator, it is reasonable to use a similar process with students. In doing so, the fieldwork educator can design a teaching–learning plan that will guide the experience and best meet the student's needs. Some basic tools and strategies can be used for soliciting student perceptions and input throughout the occupational therapy fieldwork experience.

Fieldwork Personal Data Sheet

The Personal Data Sheet for Student Fieldwork Experience (AOTA, 1999) was developed by AOTA as a method of student introduction to the Level II fieldwork site. The form is provided to the fieldwork educator by the academic institution prior to the student's arrival at the fieldwork site to provide background information and the student's self-appraisal of strengths and areas for growth. After reviewing the Personal Data Sheet with the student, the fieldwork educator can consider asking questions such as: "I see that you have identified _____ as a strength. Why do you consider that to be a strength? Can you give me an example of when or how you were able to use that characteristic effectively?" or "I see that you have identified _____ as an area for growth. Tell me what you know about _____ and give me some specifics that you would like to learn."

These types of questions encourage introspection by the student and enable the fieldwork educator to gain a deeper understanding of the student's perspectives. In addition, the Personal Data Sheet asks the student to identify preferred learning and supervision styles. Insight into these preferences is useful as the fieldwork educator plans feedback strategies with the student, as will be presented later in this article.

Observe, Question, and Listen

Observing and listening to the student will provide the fieldwork educator with additional information about strengths and areas for growth that can be incorporated into the fieldwork experience. As noted above, asking the student to reflect and elaborate on the self-assessment of strengths and areas for growth is an appropriate strategy. To have a thorough understanding of the student's background and its potential impact on the fieldwork experience, it is important for the fieldwork educator to become familiar with the student's work, volunteer, and Level I fieldwork experiences and the curriculum design of the student's academic

program, all of which are included on the Personal Data Sheet. As required by the Accreditation Council for Occupational Therapy Education (ACOTE®, 2007a, 2007b), academic programs should make this information available to the fieldwork educator prior to the student's arrival. As the student's experience is reviewed, the fieldwork educator should consider asking questions such as, "Can you tell me about the occupational performance deficits experienced by the clients in your Level I fieldwork experience?" "What occupational therapy evaluations were used in that setting and which ones did you administer?" or "What types of occupational therapy interventions did you implement with the clients at that setting?" Asking the student to provide a thorough description of his or her experiences will enhance the fieldwork educator's perspective on the student's background with clients in various settings. Also, asking what the student needs, wants, and expects out of the fieldwork experience can be a useful way to gather information at the beginning of fieldwork.

Writing Learning Objectives

The concept of learning objectives is familiar to fieldwork students because they are routinely exposed to them in the academic setting. Each course they take has objectives to give them a "roadmap" of where they should be upon successful completion of the course. Similarly, having specific learning objectives during fieldwork facilitates the student's understanding of the expected outcomes of the experience.

The student's self-identified areas for growth are a good starting point for developing learning objectives to be addressed during fieldwork. In addition, the fieldwork educator will likely have ideas about what the student may need to be successful in the fieldwork setting. These ideas will be based on the fieldwork educator's understanding and knowledge of the intricacies of the facility and its clients, experience with previous students, and an understanding of the curriculum design of the student's academic institution. As fieldwork educators begin to identify learning objectives for a particular student, collaboration with the student to generate a list of learning priorities is essential so the student begins to take responsibility for his or her own education.

Practitioners develop occupational therapy goals with clients so that both parties have a common understanding of where the intervention is headed as well as the expected outcomes, so there is a mutual understanding of when the intervention has been successful. Using the same approach during fieldwork will help ensure that the student and the fieldwork educator are operating under the same expectations. Generating specific learning objectives enables the fieldwork educator to make certain that the student has a clear understanding of what is expected during the fieldwork experience and provides parameters that measure successful achievement.

The fieldwork educator's ability to turn a learning need into a learning objective is one teaching tool that can help clarify expectations and maximize the student's learning experience. The practice of writing learning objectives specific to individual students helps ensure that the teaching and learning are targeted to the individual student's ability to meet the site-specific behavioral objectives. In addition, using learning objectives is a strategy for increasing the student's responsibility for learning. It is imperative to use learning objectives because they (1) increase the student's responsibility for learning, (2) require student input into the evaluation methods, and (3) enhance the student's sense of competence and accountability in the learning environment (Bossers et al., 2007).

When To Use Learning Objectives

The question of when to use student-specific learning objectives can be complex. Objectives are commonly developed when a student shows signs of difficulty during the fieldwork experience that, in turn, require remediation. In light of the described benefits of learning objectives, they could be valuable for all students when a learning need is identified. There is no reason why these types of learning objectives could not be used for all students, but because they are student-specific, they do take time to generate and to monitor. Like client goals related to occupational therapy intervention, student learning objectives need to be specific and measurable with regard to the outcome and should have a time frame associated with them. Early identification of potential problems, along with specific and measurable learning objectives, may circumvent problems by redirecting the student onto a successful pathway early in the fieldwork.

Several models are available to assist the fieldwork educator in writing student learning objectives.

The major components identified in most models include (1) outcomes (what the student will be able to do); (2) measurement method (how the student's performance will be evaluated); (3) time frame (when the objective will be accomplished); and (4) resources (the methods, processes, procedures, and/or strategies that the student will use to facilitate success). Clear behavioral learning objectives reduce the opportunity for miscommunication and increase potential for success.

Incorporating Bloom's Taxonomy

Learning objectives can also be used when the student is able to perform a particular skill at a basic level but is not performing consistently or is not progressing to a more advanced, professional level of performance. This is a common concern and frequent challenge for the fieldwork educator to express, as well as for the student to understand how to improve performance. One tool that can be helpful for both the fieldwork educator and student in this and other situations is Bloom's Taxonomy (Bloom, Englehart, Furst, Hill, & Krathwohl, 1956). Widely used in education, this classification system was developed as a method of categorizing intellectual behavior that is important for learning. Bloom's work includes six hierarchically oriented levels of cognitive thinking. The levels progress from the lowest level (knowledge), which includes basic recall and recognition, to the highest level of learning (evaluation), which includes skills such as judging, defending, and justifying. In the late 1990s, a group of cognitive psychologists updated Bloom's original taxonomy to reflect work being done in education in the 21st century (Anderson et al., 2001). Of significance was the change from Bloom's use of nouns to illustrate the levels to the use of verbs. This change in and of itself is indicative of "doing" by the learner. This hierarchy helps the fieldwork educator understand and anticipate the trajectory of the student's learning. In other words, the student must first remember the information before progressing to understanding it. In turn, the student applies information, followed by analyzing and evaluating information. Finally, the student can create new information. Table 24.1 provides a synopsis of the major categories of the two taxonomies, with examples of skills associated with each level.

Table 24.1. Cognitive Process Dimension of Bloom's Taxonomy and Revisions by Anderson

Bloom et al., 1956	Anderson et al., 2001
Knowledge: define, recall, list, repeat, recognize	**Remember:** recognize, recall
Comprehension: describe, explain, discuss, demonstrate	**Understand:** interpret, classify, summarize, explain
Application: interpret, illustrate, solve, use	**Apply:** execute, implement
Analysis: organize, choose, compare, contrast	**Analyze:** differentiate, organize, attribute
Synthesis: devise, create, support, design	**Evaluate:** check, critique
Evaluation: choose, judge, defend, justify	**Create:** generate, plan, produce

If a student is having difficulty with a procedure or fieldwork item, the fieldwork educator should consider developing a learning objective that reflects a lower level of achievement as a building block. For example, if a student is having trouble demonstrating the facility's safety procedures, that objective could be broken down in the following way:

REMEMBER: The student is able to (1) list fire safety procedures and (2) identify sequential steps for activating the emergency system.

UNDERSTAND: The student is able to (1) offer examples of potentially hazardous situations related to fire safety and (2) predict the consequences of specific client emergency situations.

The verbiage available in the taxonomy provides a way to "grade" student learning objectives. Sequencing learning experiences for a student is similar to grading the activities of a client's occupational therapy intervention plan. Clearly, students are not expected to demonstrate all of the skills and knowledge of a practitioner on the first day of fieldwork. The goal is for the student to demonstrate the skills similar to those of an entry-level practitioner by the end of the fieldwork experience. By being engaged in a sequenced, graded approach using his or her preferred learning style, each student can become effectively integrated into the practitioner role. Although there is no "one right way," this

sequencing and graded approach doesn't just happen. Rather, it requires thought and planning on the part of the fieldwork educator.

Grading Learning Experiences

AOTA's Fieldwork Experience Assessment Tool (FEAT, Chapter 13) was designed to promote discussions between students and fieldwork educators to facilitate reflection and problem solving (AOTA, 2001). Providing graded learning experiences is identified in the FEAT as a teaching strategy for the fieldwork educator. One of the first suggested activities focuses on clinical practice through observation and modeling. By providing an opportunity for students to observe therapeutic interactions between a client and practitioner before requiring involvement in an evaluation or intervention session, students gain an appreciation for "how it's done" without anxiety associated with having to "perform." Fieldwork educators model appropriate behaviors to demonstrate acceptable and expected performance for the student to emulate. Some students will benefit, initially, from a more guided observation where the fieldwork educator outlines specific areas of observation and subsequent discussion. Guided observations could be built by the fieldwork educator using the *Occupational Therapy Practice Framework: Domain and Process* (2nd ed.; AOTA, 2008) as an infrastructure. For example, in the first session, the student could be directed to observe and describe the client's performance in self-feeding and eating. In a subsequent session, the student could be further challenged to identify the client factors and performance skills that are contributing to the client's occupational performance deficits in self-feeding and eating.

After the student's comfort and confidence levels stabilize, he or she will benefit from being challenged. Fieldwork educators can facilitate this process by asking probing questions to develop clinical reasoning skills (i.e., "Why do you think that will work?" "What might you try instead?" "How could you get that information?" "What is the evidence that this approach might be effective?"). As the student progresses, the fieldwork educator gradually reduces the amount of direction provided. This sequence can effectively help the student transition from the role of passive observer to active student-practitioner. Furthermore, the student should be guided to independently seek out additional resources to facilitate new learning and, once researched, initiate discussions with the fieldwork educator for application to clients in the fieldwork setting. These strategies can help students develop a repertoire of skills for use in future practice and contribute to their development as life-long learners.

Reflection

Reflection is another teaching tool fieldwork educators can use with students to critically evaluate their professional reasoning skills and, hence, promote further learning. Dewey (1933) was the first to define reflective thinking as "the active, persistent, and careful consideration of any belief or supposed form of knowledge in the light of the grounds that support it and the further conclusion to which it tends" (p. 7).

Andersen and Moyers (2002) go on to claim that reflection involves thinking both retrospectively and prospectively. Retrospective reflection facilitates processing what has already occurred and requires careful consideration and dissection of what happened and one's response to it. Questions such as, "What was the client's response to that intervention?" "How could that intervention have been more effective?" and "What did I learn about the client from that session?" will promote ongoing insight and growth on the part of the student.

Prospective reflection, on the other hand, promotes the student's consideration for future planning (Andersen & Moyers, 2002). Questions may include, "What did I learn from this treatment session that can be beneficial in future sessions with clients?" "What skills do I need to develop to improve my effectiveness?" and "What characteristics of effective practitioners have I observed others using that were positive that I would like to develop in myself?"

To get the student started, fieldwork educators can generate an initial list of "Reflection Questions." As the students progress, they can be encouraged to expand into questions and topics of their choice.

Teaching and Learning Styles

The concept of teaching and learning styles is based on the premise that fieldwork education is a shared responsibility between the fieldwork educator and the student, where the educator has a wealth of information to share and the student has a deep desire to learn. It is important to keep in mind that most students have recently left the "traditional" learning environment (of classrooms and laboratories) and moved to a new "clinical or professional" setting that has very different expectations. Students may find this change to be an exciting, yet daunting, leap into the "real world." Learning for the fieldwork student may not come as easily as it did even a few weeks or months ago due to multiple new circumstances. It is important that fieldwork educators help bridge this gap for students by customizing the fieldwork experience to meet their individual learning needs.

Literature in the education research suggests that students learn better when there is congruency between the teacher's learning and teaching styles and the student's learning style (Canfield & Canfield, 1988; Stitt-Gohdes, Crews, & McCannon, 1999). When students are able to learn in the way that is most natural for them, more can be retained and achieved. How, then, can fieldwork educators assist students in achieving their highest potential? The use of a learning style inventory can be an important first step in making the fieldwork experience a win-win situation for both the student and fieldwork educator.

Using a Learning Style Inventory

There are numerous learning style inventories that can be completed in 30 minutes, either online or as a "paper-and-pencil" activity. The fieldwork educator should select one and complete it before introducing it to the student. By doing so, the fieldwork educator will be familiar with the content and be prepared to answer questions that the student may have. Most learning style inventories categorize learners into one of four distinct categories: (1) visual/verbal, (2) visual/nonverbal, (3) tactile/kinesthetic, or (4) auditory/verbal.

The **visual/verbal learner** will benefit from assignments or key information supplied in handouts and other written formats, videos, or DVDs. Encourage the student to take brief notes for review at a later time. For example, it might be suggested that the student review a range-of-motion video before working with a client's upper extremity. Additionally, treatment protocols may be written as a flow chart or with diagrams for this learner. Approximately 40% of college students are visual learners (Clarke, Flaherty, & Yankey 2006).

The **auditory/verbal learner** will benefit from any instructions or explanations given orally. This student may wish to tape conferences or supervisory meetings for use or review at a later time. He or she will gain skills by discussions, and by talking through a new situation or circumstance. The fieldwork educator should encourage well thought out spoken questions. The tone or pitch of one's voice or the speed with which one speaks may have an impact on this student. Fast talkers should ask the student to remind them to slow down.

The **visual/nonverbal learner** benefits from visual presentations. The use of flash cards, highlighters to color-code information, and diagrams or pictures assist this type of learner to grasp concepts. Introducing small amounts of information at a time is beneficial. This learner works well in learning groups where responsibilities are specific or assigned to the group members and information is verbally reinforced. This tactic may be beneficial when there are multiple fieldwork students at the fieldwork site simultaneously. Visual input is key to effective learning for this group, as is step-by-step sequencing of an activity.

The **tactile/kinesthetic learner** is the hands-on learner. Touching, holding, moving, or manipulating objects or materials is beneficial to this learner. Tactile learners need to actively explore the world around them. They may have difficulty sitting still for extended periods. This type of learner might be given the opportunity to practice with assistive equipment, for example, prior to introducing the device to a client. Similarly, permitting the student to actively participate in making or adjusting a client's splint when appropriate will promote active learning.

Teaching Style

Teaching a student to be an effective occupational therapy practitioner is one of the motives for becoming a fieldwork educator. Fieldwork students typically place a great deal of faith and trust in the fieldwork educator who will guide their occupational therapy future in this new learning environment. Many occupational therapy practitioners gladly accept the opportunity to supervise or mentor a fieldwork student. As a fieldwork educator, it is important to acknowledge one's teaching style, or the identifiable sets of behaviors that are consistent even though the content being taught may change (Conti & Welborn, 1986).

Consider these questions:

1. Were my own fieldwork experiences good examples of fieldwork education? Did I do the best I could in those settings?
2. What skills does a fieldwork educator need to guide a student through the transition from student to practitioner?
3. What is my teaching style?

Similar to learning styles, there are a number of teaching styles as well as surveys used to identify these styles, available online or via paper. Although the formal surveys are geared toward teaching in the classroom, they appear applicable to fieldwork education as well. The Grasha-Reichmann Teaching Style Inventory (Grasha & Reichmann-Hruska, 1996) is one such example. It consists of 40 questions that result in five possible teaching styles: (1) expert, (2) formal authority, (3) personal model, (4) facilitator, and (5) delegator. Exhibit 24.1 includes a description of each style. Effective teachers do not simply have one style of teaching for use in every situation. Rather, a blend of teaching styles is used depending on individual circumstances, whether one is working with clients in practice or with students during fieldwork. For fieldwork students, one's teaching style may vary as the following questions are considered: (1) Is this fieldwork experience the first or second assignment for this student? (2) Is this fieldwork environment familiar to the student? (3) How many weeks has the student completed in the fieldwork thus far, and how has he or she responded?

Conclusion

Effective fieldwork education requires understanding and implementing multiple teaching strategies to meet the student's learning needs. The following suggestions are offered for consideration before, during, and after the student fieldwork experience.

Before the fieldwork experience, the fieldwork educator should:

1. Complete the Self-Assessment Tool for Fieldwork Educator Competency.
2. Understand the range of teaching styles and indications for their use.

Exhibit 24.1. *Teaching Styles*

- **Expert:** Possesses knowledge and expertise that students need; strives to maintain status as an expert among students by displaying detailed knowledge and by challenging students to enhance their competence. Concerned with transmitting information and ensuring that students are well prepared.
- **Formal Authority:** Possesses status among students because of knowledge and role as a faculty member. Concerned with providing positive and negative feedback, and establishing learning goals, expectations, and rules of conduct for students. Concerned with correct, acceptable, and standard ways to do things and with providing students with the structure they need to learn.
- **Personal Model:** Believes in "teaching by personal example" and establishes a prototype for how to think and behave. Oversees, guides, and directs by showing how to do things, and encouraging students to observe and then to emulate the instructor's approach.
- **Facilitator:** Emphasizes the personal nature of the teacher–student interactions. Guides and directs students by asking questions, exploring options, suggesting alternatives, and encouraging them to develop criteria to make informed choices.
- **Delegator:** Concerned with developing students' capacity to function in an autonomous fashion. Students work independently on projects as part of autonomous teams.

Adapted from "The Teacher as Expert, Formal Authority, Personal Model, Facilitator, and Delegator," by A. F. Grasha, 1994, *College Teaching, 42,* p. 143. Copyright © 1994 by Taylor & Francis. Adapted with permission.

3. Select a learning style inventory for completion by the fieldwork student.
4. Review the student's Personal Data Sheet.

During the fieldwork experience, the fieldwork educator should:

1. Ask the student to complete the selected learning style inventory.
2. Customize student learning objectives for remediation and growth.
3. Determine the student's current performance and provide graded learning opportunities to challenge and promote clinical competence.
4. Be cognizant of and modify one's teaching style for efficacy in various student learning situations.

After the fieldwork experience, the fieldwork educator should:

1. Evaluate the student's feedback regarding the fieldwork experience for use with future students.
2. Use the Self-Assessment Tool for Fieldwork Educator Competency to reassess competencies.
3. Design and implement a personal learning plan for mastery in the fieldwork educator role.

References

Accreditation Council for Occupational Therapy Education. (2007a). Accreditation standards for a master's-degree-level educational program for the occupational therapist. *American Journal of Occupational Therapy, 61,* 652–661. http://dx.doi .org/10.5014/ajot.61.6.652

Accreditation Council for Occupational Therapy Education. (2007b). Accreditation standards for an educational program for the occupational therapy assistant. *American Journal of Occupational Therapy, 61,* 662–671. http://dx.doi .org/10.5014/ajot.61.6.662

American Occupational Therapy Association. (1999). *Personal data sheet for student fieldwork experience.* Retrieved August 24, 2009, from http://www.aota.org/Educate/EdRes/Field work/Supervisor.aspx

American Occupational Therapy Association. (2001). *Fieldwork experience assessment tool.* Retrieved August 23, 2009, from http:// www.aota.org/Students/Current/Fieldwork/Tools/38220.aspx

American Occupational Therapy Association. (2007). *Ad hoc committee to explore and develop resources for OT fieldwork educators* [Unpublished report to the Commission on Education, Chairperson, Pat Crist].

American Occupational Therapy Association. (2008). Occupational therapy practice framework: Domain and process (2nd ed.). *American Journal of Occupational Therapy, 62,* 625–683. http:// dx.doi.org/10.5014/ajot.62.6.625

American Occupational Therapy Association. (2009a). *Fieldwork educators certificate workshop.* Retrieved August 23, 2009, from http://www.aota.org/Educate/EdRes/Fieldwork/Workshop.aspx

American Occupational Therapy Association. (2009b). *Self-assessment tool for fieldwork educator competency.* Retrieved August 17, 2009, from http://www. aota.org/Educate/ EdRes/Fieldwork/Supervisor/Forms/38251.aspx

Andersen, L. T., & Moyers, P. (2002). Reflection and continuing competence. *OT Practice, 7*(22), 11–12.

Anderson, L. W., Krathwohl, D. R., Airasian, P. W., Cruikshank, K. A., Mayer, R. E., Pintrich, P. R., et al. (Eds.). (2001). *A taxonomy for learning, teaching, and assessing: A revision of Bloom's taxonomy of educational objectives* (abridged edition). New York: Addison Wesley Longman.

Bloom, B. S., Englehart, M. D., Furst, E. J., Hill, W. H., & Krathwohl, D. R. (1956). *Taxonomy of educational objectives: Handbook I: Cognitive domain.* New York: David McKay.

Bossers, A., Bezzina, M. B., Hobson, S., Kinsella, A., MacPhail, A., Schurr, S., et al. (2007). *Preceptor education program for health professionals and students.* Retrieved November 25, 2008, from http://www.preceptor.ca/

Canfield, A., & Canfield, J. (1988). *Canfield instructional styles inventory manual.* Los Angeles: Western Psychological Services.

Clarke, I., Flaherty, T. B., & Yankey, M. (2006). Teaching the visual learner: The use of visual summaries in marketing education. *Journal of Marketing Education, 28*(3), 218–226.

Conti, G., & Welborn, R. (1986). Teaching learning styles and the adult learner. *Lifelong Learning, 9*(8), 20–24.

Dewey, J. (1933). *How we think: A restatement of the relation of reflective thinking to the educative process.* Boston: D. C. Heath.

Grasha, A. F., (1994). The teacher as expert, formal authority, personal model, facilitator, and delegator. *College Teaching, 42,* 142–149.

Stitt-Gohdes, W. L., Crews, T. B., & McCannon, M. (1999, Spring). Business teachers' learning and instructional styles. *The Delta Pi Epsilon Journal, 41,* 1–9.

Chapter 25.

CREATING CONGRUENCE BETWEEN IDENTITIES AS A FIELDWORK EDUCATOR AND A PRACTITIONER

Patricia Stutz-Tanenbaum, MS, OTR, and Barbara Hooper, PhD, OTR, FAOTA

When we, the authors, first became fieldwork educators, we identified ourselves primarily as occupational therapy practitioners who, secondarily, "took" Level I and Level II fieldwork students. Identifying ourselves primarily as practitioners rather than educators shaped what we imagined we were supposed to do when we "took" students. We were supposed to share our expertise in our particular practice area; demonstrate how to perform certain procedures; and observe, assess, and give feedback as students applied the knowledge they received from their academic education. But the more students we took, the more we came to see that being practitioners did not fully prepare us for being educators. We found that we increasingly wanted to become as knowledgeable about how to design good learning experiences as we were about occupational therapy; thus, new professional identities as educators began to emerge. Assuming stronger identities as educators reshaped what we imagined we were supposed to do with students. We weren't necessarily supposed to make students competent in *our* skills, but rather create learning experiences that nurtured *their* skills, knowledge, and expertise.

Similar to our experience, Abreu (2006) described a portion of her career development as "a tale of two loves—clinician and educator" (p. 598). She created congruence between her two loves and discovered how each informed and changed how she performed the other. Peloquin (2006) also created congruence between her identities as an occupational therapy educator and a practitioner, stating "the best of my teaching has been like occupational therapy. And the best of occupational therapy [with clients] has felt like collaborative learning" (p. 239).

Most fieldwork educators wear at least two hats—the hat of a practitioner and the hat of a fieldwork educator. Sometimes, however, a fieldwork educator may naturally identify himself or herself more strongly as a practitioner than as an educator. Consequently, neither students nor fieldwork educators benefit as fully as they might from the student–educator relationship in the practice environment.

In this article, we propose that assuming a stronger identity as an educator can help fieldwork educators integrate multiple dimensions of the role and more fully engage students in deep personal and professional learning.

"Supervising" the Fieldwork Student: How and Who

Fieldwork education has been described as "supervising students." *Supervising* is defined as "a critical watching and directing" (Merriam-Webster Online, n.d.). In occupational therapy, supervising students has involved directing them through increasingly more responsibility for clients over time. Fieldwork supervisors observe, assess, and give feedback based on the student's competence with clients and related duties, such as documentation, time management, and professional communication (Crist, 1986). Supervisors are also expected to understand and implement well-designed teaching and learning experiences (American Occupational Therapy Association [AOTA], 1997; American Occupational Therapy Foundation, 2001; Costa, 2004, 2007). Yet the role of "supervisor" typically is not associated with applying instructional design principles to create powerful learning experiences. Thus, framing the role as "supervisor" can occlude from view the important dimension of intentional, systematic learning design.

In addition, the key questions we ask about the role can occlude from view the importance of instructional design principles in planning the fieldwork experience. The question most commonly asked in becoming a fieldwork educator is, "How?" (Palmer, 1998). How do we effectively supervise students? What methods, techniques, and skills are considered effective in clinical supervision (e.g., AOTA, 1997; Christie, Joyce, & Moeller, 1985; Costa, 2007; Herkt, 2005; Ilott, 1995; Johnson, Haynes, & Oppermann, 2007; Kautzmann, 1990; Quilligan, 2007)? Of course, how to effectively supervise students is a very important question. But if "how" is presented as the primary question, it can overshadow the equally important, "Who?" Who is the self that supervises students? If one's practitioner-self is the sole supervisor, then his or her knowledge and expertise in a particular practice area will be the central guiding force in the learning experience. If the educator-self and the practitioner-self are equally robust, then knowledge and expertise in instructional design will gain prominence.

Asking the "who" question (i.e., Who is the self that supervises students?) could help to address the disconnect that some supervisors experience between being a practitioner and being a fieldwork educator. Practitioners sometimes experience a disassociation between the roles, not because they lack skills in *how*

to be a supervisor, but because they have not formed a sense of self as an educator who is fully integrated with a sense of self as a practitioner (Costa, 2007; Higgs & McAllister, 2005). Consequently, they may not have integrated strong instructional design into their role as much as they have integrated strong supervision skills.

Identity and Instructional Design in Fieldwork Education

According to Fink (2003), instructional design involves a dynamic interaction among four elements: (a) knowledge of the subject matter, (b) interaction with students, (c) management and administration skills, and (d) skills in designing learning experiences (see Figure 25.1). The degree to which all four elements are done well determines the quality of the student's learning experience. However, the degree to which all four elements are done well can hinge on how a practitioner sees himself or herself—as practitioner, as educator, or as both (Fink, 2003). For example, therapists whose primary identity rests in being a practitioner may not have in view the element of designing intentional learning experiences. They may have in view knowledge of the subject matter (e.g., passing on knowledge and expertise, assessing student performance in light of that knowledge and expertise), interaction with students (e.g., communicating clearly, giving feedback, observing, supporting), and management/administration skills (e.g., completing the fieldwork performance evaluation). From this view, which

Figure 25.1 Four elements of quality learning experiences.

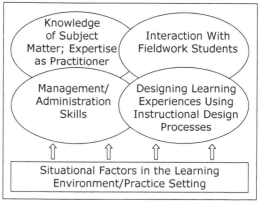

Modified from *Creating Significant Learning Experiences: An Integrated Approach to Designing College Courses* by D. Fink, 2003, San Francisco: Jossey-Bass.

is focused on three of Fink's four elements, a learning experience is considered positive if the practitioner has a high degree of competence and has been able to communicate that competence well to the student (Fink, 2003). In such a scenario, a focused identity as a practitioner can keep the supervisor from seeing and attending carefully to the fourth element of quality learning: designing learning experiences.

When an identity as educator emerges, it provides "an important central figure in a self-narrative or life story that provides coherence and meaning for everyday events" (Christiansen, 1999, p. 550). In addition to being a practitioner, an educator begins to see more clearly and adopts more consciously the previously underregarded element of designing learning experiences.

Applying Instructional Design Principles to Fieldwork Education

As an identity as educator emerges, the supervisor may reinterpret the fieldwork placement as a "course" taught in the context of the practice setting and apply course design principles when anticipating a student. The steps of good course design include many components typically found in a fieldwork experience; however, one key difference is the upfront, intentional deliberation and design of the learning goals, the learning activities to meet the learning goals, and the plan for assessment and feedback.

Student learning goals go beyond the goals received from the academic program. The learning goals are site specific, building on the fieldwork educator's dreams for where this particular student will be at the end of this particular placement, given all the opportunities the setting offers, and the student's own dreams and learning styles. Table 25.1 presents six areas of learning from which goals can be crafted. Deeper learning occurs when all six areas are covered (Fink, 2003). For example, a goal reflecting the human dimension in Table 25.1 might be as follows: "Student will demonstrate effective interview skills in order to establish the client's and family's occupational interests and priorities." A goal reflecting the integration dimension in Table 25.1 might be as follows: "Student will demonstrate narrative, procedural, and pragmatic reasoning while performing assessment and interventions and concurrently interacting with clients and families."

Table 25.1. Taxonomy of Goal Areas to Promote Significant Learning

Term	Definition
Application	Clinical reasoning, assessment, intervention, communication, use of self, and management skills that need to be applied.
Caring	Developing new feelings, interests, and values that support client-centered, evidence-based, and occupation-centered practice.
Foundational knowledge	Information and ideas that need to be remembered and understood.
Human dimension	Learning about self and others that enable the student to be more effective (abilities, limits, potentials, assumptions, feelings, responses, etc.)
Integration	Ideas, perspectives, people, resources, and skills that need to be combined to do a task well.

Note. Modified from *Creating Significant Learning Experiences: An Integrated Approach to Designing College Courses* by D. Fink, 2003, San Francisco: Jossey-Bass.

The next step of selecting learning activities may seem redundant. Aren't the learning activities built into the everyday activities of the setting and based on the role of occupational therapy at the site? Yes, the setting provides opportunities for direct observation and real doing in an authentic practice context. A practitioner identity may lead one to focus on the current caseload and to assign clients to the student that are believed to produce optimum learning. However, an educator identity expands that perspective somewhat. Educators intentionally will augment students' experiences with clients by asking them:

1. What information and data will you need to prepare for, or to process what happened in, experience X? The student decides and obtains the information through readings, talking to people, searching the Internet, and reviewing course materials.
2. What indirect experiences will help you to prepare for the real experience of X? The student decides what combination of indirect experiences, such as role plays, simulations, case studies, and observations, might help to prepare for a direct experience.

3. What do you anticipate will happen, or what do you think happened, during experience X? The student may verbally process anticipations or what happened. He or she also may write a 1-minute response on his or her anticipation or perception of the experience.

4. As a follow-up, what did you learn from experience X? How did having the experience change what the student knows, how the student feels, what the student cares about, and the student's self-perception as an emerging occupational therapy practitioner?

The selected learning activities should be sequenced carefully and plugged into a weekly schedule (Fink, 2003). With time, the plan is individualized to the student's needs.

Fieldwork assessment strategies often include observing the student's performance, having the student complete a weekly self-assessment on his or her progress, and conducting a weekly review of learning goals. The educator assesses learning by how the depth and breadth of the student's approach to clients grows with time. The educator's criteria for critical appraisal are based on how closely the student's performance resembles client-centered, evidence-based, and occupation-centered practice rooted in current discourse in the profession.

Strengthening an Educator Identity

Identity is not a fixed state. Rather, individuals possess multiple identities that change over time through experiences and by how we ascribe meaning to those experiences. Identities can be developed through social engagement, emotional awareness, and a process of "selfing" to actively tie together the roles of practitioner and educator (Christiansen, 1999; McAdams, 1996; Peloquin, 2006).

Get Involved With a Supportive Group

According to Christiansen (1999), "identity is an overarching concept that shapes and is shaped by our relationship with others" (p. 548). Thus, we gain an identity through identification with others in a social group. However, Abreu (2006) noted that there are at least two modes by which our social engagements can shape our identities. One mode is through those whom we consider to be mentors, and the second is

through those whom we consider to be our "symbolic others" (p. 596). Mentors are those groups and individuals who reflect to us who we hope to become. We all remember the exceptional educator to whom we listened with captivated attention to every word and followed every therapeutic footstep, awe-inspired by his or her magical way and eloquence. Symbolic others are groups or individuals with whom we do not identify (Abreu, 2006). They teach us through negative example how we do not want to be. We remember acutely the fieldwork educator intent on intimidation over collaboration. Mentors and symbolic others for fieldwork educators can be found among students, other fieldwork educators, past teachers, clients, and authors who write about fieldwork education and learning. Higgs and McAllister (2005) suggested that clinical educators regularly come together to share educational stories, including stories of mentors and symbolic others. Sharing educational stories and peer support can help to strengthen one's identity as educator.

Attend to Emotional Responses

Emerging identities also can be detected by paying careful attention to our internal responses as we go through experiences with students and clients. Whyte (2001) proposed that "paying close attention to an astonishing world and the way each of us is made differently and uniquely for that world" results in self-knowledge that can create coherence between one's self and one's work (as cited in Peloquin, 2006, p. 236). We learn from our flashes of joy, anger, exasperation, and elation—all of which will be part of the fabric of feeling rightly related to educating students. Journals, meditation, and mindfulness can be tools to help with attending to emotional responses.

Tie the Roles Together

"Selfing" is a process by which we unify, integrate, and synthesize the various strands of our lives, such as the strand of educator and the strand of practitioner (Peloquin, 2006). Peloquin recommended tracing each strand backward in time, exploring how it emerged, became expressed over time, and continues today. Selfing is similar to what Higgs and McAlister (2005) described as the process of creating "dynamic self-congruence" (p. 164) or living out who we are through what we do. Self-congruence, or a sense of self as educator, can be created by shared discussions, role playing, journaling, and videotaping experiences with students.

Opportunities to Develop a Stronger Identity as Educator

Academic programs, fieldwork education consortia, and fieldwork sites where there is a cluster of fieldwork educators can support the building of social networks. Also, for the first time in the history of occupational therapy, there is a voluntary, nationwide training program promoting the role of fieldwork educators. Regional trainers for the Fieldwork Educators Credentialing Program will offer workshops across the country and provide opportunities for educator communities to network and share their wisdom and experience. Watch for details about upcoming workshops in *OT Practice*. The new OT Connections website (www.otconnections.org) is another resource for networking.

Summary

This article explored how an identity as educator can help fieldwork educators integrate multiple dimensions of their role and more fully engage students in deep personal and professional learning. Overall, an identity as educator expands the clinical supervisor role to include designing learning experiences through which the student learns to care deeply about clients, be more aware of self, use evidence, stay tightly honed on the occupational needs of clients, engage in lifelong learning, and become an active member of the larger professional society.

The 2007 AOTA Ad Hoc Committee to Explore and Develop Resources for OT Fieldwork Educators concluded that "fieldwork education is a primary driver in transforming our current practice into meeting the 2017 *Centennial Vision*" (Commission on Education, 2007, p. 14). The committee named 2007 to 2017 as the "Decade of Fieldwork." We will shape identities as fieldwork educators through the meaning we ascribe to nurturing future occupational therapy practitioners.

References

Abreu, B. C. (2006). A firm persuasion in our work: Professional identity and workplace integration. *American Journal of Occupational Therapy, 60*, 596–599. http://dx.doi.org/10.5014/ajot.60.5.596

American Occupational Therapy Association. (1997). *Self-assessment tool for fieldwork educator competency*. Retrieved January 8, 2009, from http://www.aota.org/Educate/EdRes/Fieldwork/Supervisor/Forms/38251.aspx

American Occupational Therapy Foundation. (2001). *Fieldwork Experience Assessment Tool*. Retrieved January 8, 2009, from http://www.aota.org/Educate/EdRes/Fieldwork/StuSuprvsn/38220.aspx

Christiansen, C. (1999). Defining lives: Occupation as identity: An essay on competence, coherence, and the creation of meaning (Eleanor Clarke Slagle Lecture). *American Journal of Occupational Therapy, 53*, 547–558. http://dx.doi.org/10.5014/ajot.53.6.547

Christie, B., Joyce, P. C., & Moeller, P. (1985). Fieldwork experience, part II: The supervisor's dilemma. *American Journal of Occupational Therapy, 39*, 675–681. http://dx.doi.org/10.5014/ajot.39.10.675

Commission on Education. (2007). *Ad hoc committee to explore and develop resources for OT fieldwork educators* [Unpublished report to the Commission on Education, Chairperson, Pat Crist].

Costa, D. (2004). *The essential guide to fieldwork education: Resources for today's educators and practitioners*. Bethesda, MD: AOTA Press.

Costa, D. (2007). *Clinical supervision in occupational therapy: A guide for fieldwork and practice*. Bethesda, MD: AOTA Press.

Crist, P. (1986). *Contemporary issues in clinical education* [Current practice series in occupational therapy]. Thorofare, NJ: Slack.

Fink, D. (2003). *Creating significant learning experiences: An integrated approach to designing college courses*. San Francisco: Jossey-Bass.

Herkt, A. (2005). *Exploring the supervision of occupational therapists in New Zealand*. Unpublished master's thesis, Auckland University of Technology, New Zealand.

Higgs, J., & McAllister, L. (2005). The lived experiences of clinical educators with implications for their preparation, support, and professional development. *Learning in Health and Social Care, 4*(3), 156–171.

Ilott, I. (1995). To fail or not to fail? A course for fieldwork educators. *American Journal of Occupational Therapy, 49*, 250–255. http://dx.doi.org/10.5014/ajot.49.3.250

Johnson, C., Haynes, C., & Oppermann, J. (2007). Supervision competencies for fieldwork educators. *OT Practice, 12*(22), CE-1–CE-8.

Kautzmann, L. (1990). Clinical teaching: Fieldwork supervisors' attitudes and values. *American Journal of Occupational Therapy, 44*, 835–838. http://dx.doi.org/10.5014/ajot.44.9.835

McAdams, D. P. (1996). Personality, modernity, and the storied self: A contemporary framework for studying persons. *Psychological Inquiry, 7*, 295–321.

Merriam-Webster Online. (n.d.). [Definition of supervision]. Retrieved January 8, 2009, from http://www.merriam-webster.com/dictionary/supervision

Palmer, P. (1998). *The courage to teach: Exploring the inner landscape of a teacher's life.* San Francisco: Jossey-Bass.

Peloquin, S. M. (2006). A firm persuasion in our work: Occupations strands of coherence in a life. *American Journal of Occupational Therapy, 60,* 236–239. http://dx.doi.org/10.5014/ajot.60.2.236

Quilligan, S. (2007). Communication skills teaching: The challenge of giving effective feedback. *Clinical Teacher, 4*(2), 100–105.

Stutz-Tanenbaum, P., & Hooper, B. (2009, June). Creating congruence between identities as a fieldwork educator and a practitioner. *Education Special Interest Section Quarterly, 19*(2), 1–4.

Patricia Stutz-Tanenbaum, MS, OTR, is Assistant Professor and Academic Fieldwork Coordinator, Department of Occupational Therapy, Colorado State University, 217 Gibbons, Fort Collins, CO 80523-1501; Tanenbaum@cahs.colostate.edu.

Barbara Hooper, PhD, OTR, FAOTA, is Assistant Professor, Department of Occupational Therapy, Colorado State University, Fort Collins, CO.

Chapter 26.

SPECIALIZED KNOWLEDGE AND SKILLS OF OCCUPATIONAL THERAPY EDUCATORS OF THE FUTURE

American Occupational Therapy Association

Introduction

In 2006, the American Occupational Therapy Association (AOTA) articulated a *Centennial Vision* statement for the profession as it nears its 100th anniversary. This statement affirms that

> We envision that occupational therapy is a powerful, widely recognized, science-driven, and evidence-based profession with a globally connected and diverse workforce meeting society's occupational needs. (AOTA, 2007, p. 613)

This vision reflects the longstanding commitment of the profession to serve society in ways that are relevant and forward-thinking. As social concerns evolve, occupational therapy practitioners must understand the occupational implications of broad contextual issues that affect health and well-being directly and indirectly. Global efforts to deal with climate change, for example, are causing downward economic pressures on middle-class living standards, thus altering daily routines, limiting occupational opportunities, increasing chronic health conditions, and reducing access to health care (Kawachi &

Wamala, 2006). Occupational therapy practitioners need not only know how to respond to evolving social needs; they need to do so quickly, creatively, and proactively.

Occupational therapy education is critical to the achievement of this vision in 2017 and beyond. The constellation of skills and attitudes that occupational therapy practitioners must possess are the result of their inherent abilities and motivations refined into longstanding dispositions through a deliberate educational process. Indeed, occupational therapy education embodies the aspirations for the kind of society we wish to see. To talk about the purpose of the profession is also to talk about the purpose of occupational therapy education, as it is here, where these aspirations are nurtured and shaped.

Use of This Document

Occupational therapy is essentially an educative profession. Occupational therapy practitioners are skilled at analyzing limitations that may result in diminished occupational participation and designing therapeutic programs through which people learn new skills or re-learn skills lost to illness, injury, or contextual constraints. While to some degree all occupational therapy practitioners are educators, this document focuses on recognized roles related to education in the profession (Academic Program Director, Academic Faculty, Academic Fieldwork Coordinator, and Fieldwork Educator). The purpose is to articulate the attributes practitioners should possess in such roles in order to have an enduring legacy in the fulfillment of the *Centennial Vision* and beyond. These attributes are described in the language of possibility, including the characteristics of innovator/visionary, scholar/explorer, leader, integrator, and mentor. Because the embodiment of these attributes is developmental, they are described in a continuum of experience from novice, intermediate, and advanced practitioner.

The context surrounding the educator will determine which attributes are most needed and/or appropriate. While all professionals will demonstrate some aspects of the attributes, not everyone is expected to achieve the advanced level in all the attributes. Indeed, because of experience, available opportunities, and personal curiosities and strengths, an educator may demonstrate some attributes at the novice level while demonstrating others at the intermediate and advanced levels. Therefore, the purpose of this document is not to identify rigid standards of performance but rather to serve as a guide of desired attributes toward which an educator may aspire in order to contribute to the fulfillment of the *Centennial Vision* and beyond.

It is recommended that this document be used as an aid in the articulation of the professional development plans of faculty. Such plans are essential in their growth and are required by the Accreditation Council for Occupational Therapy Education (ACOTE®) for all program directors and faculty who teach two or more courses (ACOTE, 2006, Standard A.5.2).

Desired attributes include the following:

- *Innovator/Visionary:* Someone who embraces new directions, is forward-thinking, projecting into the future. This person thinks outside of the traditional confines of the profession to predict and propose how to meet future societal needs. A visionary can see past traditional boundaries to new possibilities at all levels of personal and societal life.
- *Scholar/Explorer:* A scholar/explorer is someone who seeks, uses, and produces knowledge and

effectively disseminates new findings to internal and external audiences. These individuals use a critical, theoretically grounded, and systematic approach in their scholarly endeavors to produce outcomes that inform and address societal needs.
- *Leader:* Someone who analyzes past, present, and future trends and develops solutions to problems or strategies for taking advantage of opportunities by collaborating, inspiring, and influencing people to create a desired future.
- *Integrator:* Someone who seeks and finds divergent information, perceives meaningful relationships, and makes connections through analysis to create a new, more coherent understanding.
- *Mentor:* A trusted role model who inspires, encourages, influences, challenges, and facilitates the growth and development of others' goals and aspirations. This involves a collaborative process that may be among peers, colleagues, experienced and inexperienced individuals, practitioners and academicians, and others. The mentor may function in various roles such as educator, tutor, coach, counselor, encourager, consultant, etc.

As stated earlier, the embodiment of these attributes is developmental, and not all attributes are likely to be developed at the same time nor needed equally. An educator can demonstrate an attribute at a novice level while demonstrating another at an advanced level. In this document, *novice* performance is understood as beginning expertise, as when a person has had limited experience in an area and therefore has limited familiarity with the associated knowledge or its application. *Intermediate* performance is understood as consistent demonstration of an attribute in specific situations as a result of prior experience in those situations. Finally, *advanced* performance is understood as the ability to demonstrate an attribute in multiple situations, including some in which a person has no prior experience. Advanced performance denotes a high level of expertise.

In Tables 26.1–26.5, each attribute is represented, summarizing how it might be demonstrated in each educator role. It is assumed that the incumbent in a role has met or exceeded occupational therapy practitioner competencies described in the *Standards for Continuing Competence* (AOTA, 2005). The attributes are general statements and specific characteristics may not apply to all situations.

Table 26.1. Innovator/Visionary

Experience	Academic Program Director	OT/OTA Faculty Member	Academic Fieldwork Coordinator	Fieldwork Educator
Novice	1. Analyzes the current curriculum to reflect the future needs of the program, profession, and society. 2. Analyzes institutional needs in order to identify new ways that the program can fulfill the institution's mission. 3. Develops curriculum that challenges and prepares students to identify and fulfill innovative practice roles.	1. Demonstrates the ability to prepare ethical and competent practitioners for both traditional and emerging practice settings. 2. Develops plan to maintain self abreast of the breadth and depth of knowledge of the profession in order to incorporate such knowledge in student learning. 3. Assists with the development of new learning processes that can enhance learning opportunities for students in the program. 4. Develops a plan of continued proficiency in emerging pedagogy through investigation, and formal and informal education.	1. Embraces new approaches for fieldwork, including in non-OT practice settings, international fieldwork, diverse settings. 2. Projects an exemplary curricular model representing the OT/OTA academic program.	1. Embraces new approaches for fieldwork in traditional or emerging practice settings. 2. Implements a model fieldwork program that reflects the curricular design of the academic program. 3. Uses innovation within own fieldwork setting to enhance student learning experience during fieldwork.
Intermediate	1. Projects future trends and societal needs of the profession and appropriately adapts the curriculum, including both the academic and fieldwork components. 2. Establishes a management plan that guides student development in the OT program and facilitates faculty development within the OT unit and the college/university community.	1. Proposes and implements nontraditional learning environments that facilitate development of competent and ethical professionals. 2. Participates in college-/university-wide committees and assists in propelling the institution forward in the future in order to meet projected societal needs. 3. Embraces the use and development of course materials and experiences that are innovative and nontraditional. 4. Assesses and predicts the effectiveness of new learning processes to enhance learning opportunities for students in the program.	1. Proposes strategies that facilitate linkages between academic program curriculum and fieldwork practice opportunities. 2. Proposes strategies to support client-centered, meaningful, occupation-based, and evidence-based outcomes of the OT process during fieldwork experiences.	1. Proposes strategies that facilitate collaborative partnerships between academic program curricula and fieldwork practice opportunities. 2. Proposes strategies to support client-centered, meaningful, occupation-based, and evidence-based outcomes of the OT process during fieldwork experiences. 3. Promotes innovation among fieldwork educators in OT as well as other disciplines in own and other related settings to enhance student learning experiences and interdisciplinary collaboration.

(Continued)

Table 26.1. Innovator/Visionary *(Cont.)*

Experience	Academic Program Director	OT/OTA Faculty Member	Academic Fieldwork Coordinator	Fieldwork Educator
Advanced	1. Anticipates future directions of the profession in meeting societal needs by exploring new possibilities for strategic planning and identifying factors related to funding, resources, etc. 2. Identifies opportunities to engage with the community to promote OT as a profession in order to serve society's evolving needs. 3. Identifies new ways of applying the use of occupation that will lead to societal growth, prosperity and social justice.	1. Proposes innovative solutions and designs innovative strategies to address predicted future trends in education, practice, and research. 2. Proposes, builds, and sustains novel integrative collaborations across disciplines.	1. Predicts future directions for fieldwork environments in emerging practice areas and proposes fieldwork opportunities for students. 2. Innovates strategies for providing fieldwork in emerging practice areas. 3. Anticipates and prepares for the direction of legal and health care policy that influences fieldwork and designs strategies for compliance.	1. Predicts future directions of practice and fieldwork in emerging environments and develops fieldwork opportunities for students. 2. Consults with other fieldwork educators and sites to develop creative learning experiences for students. 3. Innovates strategies for providing fieldwork in emerging practice areas. 4. Anticipates and prepares for the direction of legal and health care policy that influences fieldwork and designs strategies for compliance.

Note: OT = occupational therapy; OTA = occupational therapy assistant.

Table 26.2. Scholar/Explorer

Experience	Academic Program Director	OT/OTA Faculty Member	Academic Fieldwork Coordinator	Fieldwork Educator
Novice	1. Possesses requisite knowledge and skills to design and conduct independent research relevant to OT practice and education and to disseminate results. 2. Recognizes the importance of scholarship within the academic community in general and within own educational institution in particular. 3. Designs a curriculum that meets accreditation	1. Effectively critiques and uses new research literature and educational materials that will promote critical thinking, evidence-based practice, and lifelong learning in preparing future practitioners. 2. Critically integrates theory and research evidence into practice and facilitates that process in learners.	1. Effectively critiques and utilizes new research literature and educational materials that will promote critical thinking, evidence-based practice, and lifelong learning in preparing future practitioners. 2. Facilitates fieldwork educators' ability to effectively critique and use new research literature and educational materials that will promote	1. Critically evaluates current research to reflect best practice in teaching and practice. 2. Engages in systematic literature reviews to support and enhance practice. 3. Recognizes scholarly role in client service provision and program evaluation. 4. Models engagement in evidence-based practice specific to setting and populations served.

(Continued)

Table 26.2. Scholar/Explorer *(Cont.)*

Experience	Academic Program Director	OT/OTA Faculty Member	Academic Fieldwork Coordinator	Fieldwork Educator
	standards relating to the scholarly role and skills of entry-level practitioners. 4. Actively engages in scholarly activities within area of expertise. 5. Creates a scholarly environment in which faculty and students have substantive resources and infrastructure necessary for productive scholarship.	3. Models behaviors that demonstrate the importance of scholarship to learners and practitioners. 4. Initiates research inquiry within contextually determined expectations, either independently or with a mentor.* 5. Initiates the processes to develop a line of inquiry for research.* *May not always be possible for faculty in an OTA program.*	critical thinking, evidence-based practice, and lifelong learning in preparing future practitioners. 3. Critically integrates theory and research evidence into practice and facilitates that process in fieldwork educators. 4. Facilitates integration and agreement of the academic philosophy and curriculum design within the fieldwork site. 5. Identifies questions about the fieldwork learning experiences for future research. 6. Facilitates best practices in using scholarship of teaching and learning in practice settings.	5. Seeks current evidence and information regarding effective fieldwork education and educational methodologies. 6. Translates practice knowledge into learning modes appropriate for fieldwork students. 7. Identifies questions about the fieldwork learning experiences for future research. 8. Monitors and interprets fieldwork student learning outcomes and effectiveness of student fieldwork program. 9. Coordinates with the academic fieldwork coordinator to monitor and interpret student fieldwork learning outcomes.
Intermediate	1. Coordinates active research agenda within the occupational therapy program. 2. Facilitates interdisciplinary collaboration and cooperation in research.	1. Contributes to the production of new findings and educational materials that add to the knowledge base of the profession. 2. Actively cultivates knowledge, skills, and interests in students by incorporating evidence from research into practice. 3. Conducts scholarship independently and begins to identify	1. Synthesizes new research literature and educational materials that will promote critical thinking, evidence-based practice, and lifelong learning in preparing future practitioners. 2. Conducts workshops and training programs to facilitate fieldwork educators' ability to use evidence in fieldwork education. 3. Plans and engages in the	1. Designs evidence-based practice learning opportunities for fieldwork students to enhance understanding of the OT process. 2. Contributes to the breadth and body of knowledge through collaborative research projects. 3. Generates a clinical research agenda in collaboration with clinical and academic colleagues. 4. Collaborates with academic fieldwork coordinator and

(Continued)

Table 26.2. Scholar/Explorer *(Cont.)*

Experience	Academic Program Director	OT/OTA Faculty Member	Academic Fieldwork Coordinator	Fieldwork Educator
		a coherent line(s) of inquiry.* 4. Successfully advises and guides students and practitioners in research.* 5. Disseminates findings in a public format such as presentations and publications. 6. Seeks opportunities to serve as a reviewer, editor, or publisher of scholarly work to internal and external audiences. *May not always be possible for faculty in an OTA program.*	scholarship of teaching and learning regarding fieldwork education. 4. Collaborates with fieldwork educators and faculty to conduct research regarding fieldwork.	faculty to conduct research regarding fieldwork.
Advanced	1. Provides national leadership in the development of and/or implementation of scholarship that further establishes foundational knowledge and efficacy of occupational therapy interventions. 2. Contributes to and/or leads national dialogue concerning the advancement of OT theory and practice through research and scholarship.	1. Develops collaborative opportunities in research and scholarly work with other faculty. 2. Effectively produces and disseminates new findings within and outside of the profession. 3. Establishes a well-defined scholarly agenda or lines of inquiry. 4. Provides leadership in advancing the profession's knowledge base. 5. Uses innovative methodologies to identify, analyze, and effectively address the changing needs of society at the local, national, or global levels. 6. Establishes a national or international reputation or recognition as an expert in his or her area of inquiry.	1. Creates and disseminates new resources for fieldwork educators and academic fieldwork coordinators to incorporate best practices in fieldwork education through student–fieldwork educator collaboration. 2. Conducts research with other academic fieldwork coordinator and fieldwork educators. 3. Conducts research with other academic fieldwork coordinator and fieldwork educators. 4. Uses research evidence to inform professional educational policy.	1. Models for students the importance of practitioner scholarship by engaging in independent and/or collaborative research projects and program evaluation. 2. Engages in multisite research.

Note: OT = occupational therapy; OTA = occupational therapy assistant.

Table 26.3. Leader

Experience	Academic Program Director	OT/OTA Faculty Member	Academic Fieldwork Coordinator	Fieldwork Educator
Novice	1. Uses management and leadership skills related to finance, planning, policy, marketing, public relations, and legal issues in order to meet accreditation standards and fulfill the program and institutional missions within an increasingly challenging educational environment. 2. Uses excellent interpersonal skills and demonstrates the ability to relate to diverse groups, constituencies, and organizations. 3. Takes responsibility for the assessment process for specific and overall program evaluation to enable the individual faculty to assess, diagnose, and apply interventions necessary to ensure quality.	1. Facilitates student development toward leadership roles. 2. Models ethical and professional behavior to facilitate the transition from student to clinician, advocate, and future fieldwork educator. 3. Assesses course materials, objectives, and educational experiences to promote optimal learning for students. 4. Develops plan of continued competency in leadership skills as related to role of teaching. 5. Participates with faculty in identifying trends that may influence future student learning and preparation.	1. Takes responsibility to develop systems to manage data for recordkeeping, fieldwork contract agreements, confidential student health records, and so on, to ensure compliance with standards and legal requirements of local, state, and federal jurisdictions. 2. Develops a working relationship between the institution and fieldwork sites to facilitate ongoing collaborative partnerships to support education and practice. 3. Assists and monitors students in the development of their successful transition from the academic to the fieldwork portion of the educational program. 4. Evaluates the ongoing effectiveness of the fieldwork program, including student performance and fieldwork site integration of academic curricular design.	1. Critically reviews site-specific fieldwork program to ensure that quality learning experiences reflect best practice. 2. Advocates for department-wide participation in fieldwork education. 3. Facilitates student's transition into practice.
Intermediate	1. Forms strategic alliances with critical constituent groups within and outside the program's organization that can assist and promote the program's goals. 2. Builds and maintains systems that ensure that the program operates in concert with the mission of the institution and the mission of the academic unit in which the program is housed. 3. Seeks and accepts institutional leadership roles.	1. Seeks and obtains leadership role as representative from OTA/OT/OS department on institution-wide committees and organizations where collaboration occurs between various disciplines of study. 2. Analyzes past, present, and future trends to integrate practice, theory, literature, and research for instruction in evidence-based practice. 3. Collaborates with other faculty members on	1. Analyzes current and future trends in OT practice to develop fieldwork settings to reflect emerging practice. 2. Develops or explores innovative strategies of supervision for students in emerging practice areas. 3. Collaborates with other clinical coordinators within the institution to streamline policies and procedures with regard to student placements in fieldwork.	1. Modifies site-specific fieldwork objectives to ensure that high-quality learning experiences reflect best practice. 2. Educates colleagues and develops networks and programs to ensure fieldwork excellence. 3. Participates in knowledge generation by contributing to local, regional, and/or national fieldwork discussion/dialogues.

(Continued)

Table 26.3. Leader *(Cont.)*

Experience	Academic Program Director	OT/OTA Faculty Member	Academic Fieldwork Coordinator	Fieldwork Educator
		scholarship research activities related to the advancement of occupational therapy, occupational science, teaching, and outcomes assessment.		4. Participates in national initiatives that are collaborative efforts between educational institutions and fieldwork sites (e.g., backpack awareness month).
Advanced	1. Applies the processes of advancement (philanthropy), including identifying, cultivating, and securing gifts through the matching of potential donors with well-articulated needs. 2. Seeks and accepts leadership roles within the community as well as within state, national, and international associations.	1. Proposes innovative solutions and designs innovative strategies to address predicted future trends in education, practice, and research. 2. Proposes, builds, and sustains novel integrative collaborations across disciplines.	1. Develops national and international fieldwork student exchanges, placements, and programs. 2. Provides national and global leadership in the development of fieldwork education. 3. Develops and evaluates the ongoing effectiveness and quality of national and international fieldwork education. 4. Seeks and fully embraces the leadership role in the education of regional fieldwork consortiums.	1. Develops national models for fieldwork education in collaboration with other fieldwork educators and academic fieldwork coordinators across disciplines. 2. Shares innovative models of fieldwork supervision on a state, national, and international levels. 3. Seeks leadership roles in regional, national, and international fieldwork education.

Note: OS = occupational science; OT = occupational therapy; OTA = occupational therapy assistant.

Table 26.4. Integrator

Experience	Academic Program Director	OT/OTA Faculty Member	Academic Fieldwork Coordinator	Fieldwork Educator
Novice	1. Forms strategic alliances with critical constituent groups within and outside the program's organization that can assist and promote the program's goals.	1. Develops a plan to continue proficiency in teaching through investigation, continuing education, and self-investigation. 2. Meets diverse learning needs of students and faculty. 3. Creates learning environments that facilitate the	1. Seeks close collaboration with fieldwork educators to facilitate student fieldwork learning and align clinical fieldwork program with curriculum design/ outcomes. 2. Facilitates partnerships between program faculty and fieldwork educators. 3. Supports communication,	1. Seeks close collaboration with academic programs to facilitate student fieldwork learning and align clinical fieldwork program with curriculum design/outcome. 2. Develops and/or modifies clinical fieldwork manual/ objectives to

(Continued)

Table 26.4. Integrator *(Cont.)*

Experience	Academic Program Director	OT/OTA Faculty Member	Academic Fieldwork Coordinator	Fieldwork Educator
		development of culturally sensitive, competent, and ethical professionals. 4. Independently seeks, selectively chooses relevant resources from OT and other disciplines, and disseminates information to promote advanced understanding in a variety of areas. 5. Develops a strategic plan for professional development that combines teaching, scholarship, and service.	collaboration, and connections between students and fieldwork educators to support the selection, matching, and scheduling of appropriate fieldwork experiences. 4. Designs culturally sensitive fieldwork programs and fieldwork objectives. Advocates for interdisciplinary fieldwork learning opportunities. 5. Collaborates with fieldwork educators and faculty to facilitate congruence of curriculum design and best practice.	reflect national standards and academic fieldwork objectives. 3. Collaborates with academic fieldwork coordinator to ensure integration of curriculum design into the practice setting. 4. Designs culturally sensitive fieldwork programs and fieldwork objectives. 5. Facilitates collaborative learning among fieldwork students within the profession and across disciplines.
Intermediate	1. Integrates increasingly diverse sources of information in order to define problems, explore solutions, and formulate appropriate decisions that result in effective management of the academic unit to meet its mission.	1. Develops a framework from which to practice using divergent resources. 2. Demonstrates progress of professional development plan that combines teaching, scholarship, and service.	1. Analyzes current trends to create new fieldwork opportunities. 2. Facilitates development of academic fieldwork advisory panels that integrate diverse perspectives from the community. 3. Forms strategic alliances across disciplines to advance the profession.	1. Serves on academic fieldwork advisory panels. 2. Actively facilitates interdisciplinary fieldwork learning opportunities. 3. Develops and/or modifies fieldwork student manual/objectives to reflect national standards and academic fieldwork objectives. 4. Functions as a practice resource for academic fieldwork coordinators to enhance fieldwork collaboration and academic outcomes. 5. Models cultural sensitivity when designing fieldwork programs and fieldwork objectives.

(Continued)

Table 26.4. Integrator *(Cont.)*

Experience	Academic Program Director	OT/OTA Faculty Member	Academic Fieldwork Coordinator	Fieldwork Educator
Advanced	1. Fosters ongoing relationships among educators, researchers, and practitioners that address the needs of both the profession and society. 2. Creatively collaborates with consumers, interdisciplinary educators, and researchers to meet the increasingly complex needs of national and global communities. 3. Effectively utilizes various venues, such as regulatory bodies, non-governmental organizations, legislatures, and other bodies such as the World Health Organization or the Centers for Disease Control and Prevention in order to promote the health and well-being of people through occupation.	1. Collaborates with diverse disciplines for information synthesis and dissemination. 2. Articulates and represents the role of OT in emerging areas of practice at the local, national, and international levels. 3. Creatively collaborates with consumers, interdisciplinary educators, and researchers to meet the increasingly complex needs of national and global communities. 4. Effectively uses various venues, such as regulatory bodies, nongovernmental organizations, legislatures, and other internationally recognized agencies in order to promote the health and well-being through occupation.	1. Bridges the gap between OT/OTA practitioner needs (evidence-based practice) and resources available through OT/OTA academic program and student fieldwork experiences. 2. Enhances relationships with regional/national/international fieldwork committees. 3. Creatively contributes to a national/international understanding of the importance of fieldwork education by facilitating meaningful relationships and networking among practitioners, students, and educators.	1. Contributes to a more coherent understanding of health care service provision and a national fieldwork student network. 2. Develops/contributes to interdisciplinary experimental learning modules. 3. Serves on regional/national/international fieldwork committees. 4. Creatively contributes to a national and international understanding of the importance of fieldwork education by facilitating meaningful relationships and networking among practitioners, students, and educators.

Note: OT = occupational therapy; OTA = occupational therapy assistant.

Table 26.5. Mentor

Experience	Academic Program Director	OT/OTA Faculty Member	Academic Fieldwork Coordinator	Fieldwork Educator
Novice	1. Serves as a model to mentor diverse faculty, students, alumni, and occupational therapy practitioners in their area of expertise. 2. Facilitates mentoring	1. Demonstrates a competent and positive attitude that results in the mentoring of students in professional development in scholarship, research, and/or service. 2. Develops and fosters trusting relationships	1. Coaches and guides students to engage in appropriate professional and fieldwork education activities. 2. Creates a collaborative process between academic faculty and fieldwork educators. 3. Serves as a model and consultant for	1. Mentors students prior to and during fieldwork by functioning as a model. 2. Serves as a model to mentor diverse individuals and occupational therapy

(Continued)

Table 26.5. Mentor *(Cont.)*

Experience	Academic Program Director	OT/OTA Faculty Member	Academic Fieldwork Coordinator	Fieldwork Educator
	relationships within the academic institution. 3. Models professional and ethical behavior within the academic setting. Instills in students the professional responsibility of seeking and offering mentoring relationships. 4. Analyzes personal and professional goals and acquires resources necessary to attain professional growth.	with practitioners interested in transitioning from practice into academia. 3. Identifies a variety of tangible and intangible resources that can enhance the professional growth of self and others. 4. Analyzes personal and professional goals and acquires resources necessary to attain professional growth. 5. Encourages potential students to develop relationships with OT/OTA practitioners, alumni, students, and faculty prior to entering the profession. 6. Facilitates the inclusion of a diverse community of faculty and students through the mentoring process.	fieldwork educators to facilitate development of quality fieldwork programs. 4. Facilitates the growth of practitioners and fieldwork educators for implementing best practice principles during fieldwork education. 5. Analyzes personal and professional goals and acquires resources necessary to attain professional growth. 6. Encourages potential students to develop relationships with occupational therapy practitioners, students, alumni, and faculty prior to entering the profession. 7. Facilitates the inclusion of a diverse community of faculty and students through the mentoring process. 8. Serves as a model representative of the academic program locally and regionally.	practitioners in their area of expertise. 3. Encourages potential students to develop relationships with occupational therapy practitioners, students, and faculty prior to entering the profession. 4. Analyzes personal and professional goals and acquires resources necessary to attain professional growth.
Intermediate	1. Develops innovative strategies for negotiating creative, constructive, and ethical solutions to address interpersonal and academic issues within a complex environment. 2. Develops resources, policies, and procedures/ guidelines for faculty that can be used to facilitate progressively higher levels of responsibility at the department, university, community,	1. Identifies individuals or groups in need of mentoring who would otherwise not seek mentorship and encourages them to develop mentoring relationships to maximize their potential. 2. Participates in mentoring or coaching of junior faculty through constructive feedback and role modeling of work with students, practitioners, and peers. 3. Effectively mentors and functions as faculty advisor for student organizations. 4. Inspires others to serve as mentor to students, alumni, practitioners, and faculty.	1. Collaborates with fieldwork educators to promote effective and innovative learning opportunities for students. 2. Tutors and coaches non-OT fieldwork educators in their development as supervisors and their implementation of fieldwork experiences reflecting OT practice. 3. Models and facilitates development of innovative strategies to obtain excellence within the constraints of the fieldwork practice environment. 4. Coaches students, fieldwork educators, and academic fieldwork coordinators to negotiate and problem solve challenging fieldwork dilemmas.	1. Identifies a variety of tangible and intangible resources that can be used to enhance the professional growth of self and others. 2. Recruits and guides inexperienced OT/OTA staff to develop in the role as a fieldwork educator. 3. Models excellence as a fieldwork educator and fieldwork site coordinator. 4. Models excellence and commitment to the tenets of the profession using occupation-based and evidence-based

(Continued)

Table 26.5. Mentor *(Cont.)*

Experience	Academic Program Director	OT/OTA Faculty Member	Academic Fieldwork Coordinator	Fieldwork Educator
	and professional levels. 3. Uses a variety of methods and technology to expand mentoring relationships beyond the academic institution and the community it serves.	5. Actively contributes to the accomplishment of long-term expectations and outcomes of mentor relationships necessary for own personal and professional growth. 6. Uses a variety of methods and technology to expand mentoring relationships beyond the academic institution and the community it serves.	5. Creates effective resources reflecting current trends and emerging practice areas to sustain excellence in fieldwork education. 6. Influences the development of innovative programs to bridge the gap between fieldwork and didactic content into a cohesive curriculum design. 7. Uses a variety of methods and technology to expand mentoring relationships beyond existing fieldwork education network.	practice during the OT process. 5. Develops mentorship programs within the facility that reflect and promote interdisciplinary and intradisciplinary fieldwork excellence. 6. Uses a variety of methods and technology to expand mentoring relationships beyond the fieldwork site. 7. Develops innovative strategies for negotiating creative, constructive, and ethical solutions to address interpersonal and practice issues within a complex environment. 8. Serves as role model for other fieldwork educators.
Advanced	1. Anticipates and facilitates the development of future mentoring relationships within and outside the educational program to meet the needs of the profession and society. 2. Facilitates intra- and interdisciplinary mentoring relationships for faculty, students, alumni, and practitioners. 3. Models advocacy and acts as a change agent to fulfill the	1. Creates and shares networks, resources, and opportunities for growth of mentees at the national and international levels. 2. Develops and sustains programs across disciplines and geographical regions to foster mentees' successful performance in scholarship, teaching, and practice. 3. Models advocacy and acts as a change agent to fulfill the occupational and social justice vision of the profession both nationally and globally. 4. Develops innovative strategies for facilitating connections among students, educators, alumni,	1. Models the creation of innovative fieldwork training programs globally to anticipate and meet the needs of the profession in the future. 2. Facilitates national and international networks among academic fieldwork coordinators to collectively and systematically address fieldwork issues. 3. Develops innovative strategies for negotiating creative, constructive, and ethical solutions that address interpersonal and academic issues within a complex environment. 4. Develops and sustains programs across disciplines and geographical	1. Consults on the development of new fieldwork programs, supporting at other fieldwork sites, settings, and practice areas. 2. Develops national and international programs of mentorship excellence that connect students, practitioners, fieldwork educators, and academic fieldwork coordinators. 3. Anticipates and develops mentoring opportunities and programs designed to address disparities in health care,

(Continued)

Table 26.5. Mentor *(Cont.)*

Experience	Academic Program Director	OT/OTA Faculty Member	Academic Fieldwork Coordinator	Fieldwork Educator
	occupational and social justice vision of the profession both nationally and globally. 4. Identifies and addresses professional and societal trends that may present new ethical challenges for the profession and society. 5. Inspires others to develop new strategies and paradigms in response to societal issues.	practitioners, and other colleagues for unusual, challenging, and/or complex mentee needs or situations. 5. Anticipates and develops mentoring opportunities and programs designed to address disparities in health care, social injustices, issues within the profession, and society. 6. Develops innovative strategies for negotiating creative, constructive, and ethical solutions to address interpersonal and academic issues within a complex environment.	regions to foster mentees' successful performance in scholarship, teaching, and practice. 5. Anticipates and develops mentoring opportunities and programs designed to address disparities in health care, social injustices, issues within the profession, and society. 6. Models advocacy and acts as a change agent to fulfill the occupational and social justice vision of the profession both nationally and globally.	social injustices, issues within the profession, and society. 4. Models advocacy and acts as a change agent to fulfill the occupational and social justice vision of the profession both nationally and globally.

Note: OT = occupational therapy; OTA = occupational therapy assistant.

References

Accreditation Council for Occupational Therapy Education. (2006). *Standards and interpretive guidelines.* Available at http://www.aota.org/Educate/Accredit/StandardsReview/guide/42369.aspx

American Occupational Therapy Association. (2005). Standards for continuing competence. *American Journal of Occupational Therapy, 59,* 661–662. http://dx.doi.org/10.5014/ajot.59.6.661

American Occupational Therapy Association. (2007). AOTA's *Centennial Vision* and executive summary. *American Journal of Occupational Therapy, 61,* 613–614. http://dx.doi.org/10.5014/ajot.61.6.413

Kawachi, I., & Wamala, S. (2006). *Globalization and health.* New York: Oxford University Press.

by

Commission on Education:

René Padilla, PhD, OTR/L, FAOTA, *Chairperson*
Andrea Bilics, PhD, OTR/L
Judith C. Blum, MS, OTR/L
Paula C. Bohr, PhD, OTR/L, FAOTA
Jennifer C. Coyne, COTA/L
Jyothi Gupta, PhD, OTR/L
Linda Musselman, PhD, OTR, FAOTA

Linda Orr, MPA, OTR/L
Abbey Sipp, *ASD Liaison*
Patricia Stutz-Tanenbaum, MS, OTR
Neil Harvison, PhD, OTR/L, *AOTA Staff Liaison*

Adopted by the Representative Assembly 2009FebCS112

Note: This document replaces the following documents: *Role Competencies for a Professional-Level Program Director in an Academic Setting, 2003M167; Role Competencies for a Program Director in an Occupational Therapy Assistant Academic Setting, 2005C239; Role Competencies for a Professional-Level Occupational Therapist Faculty Member in an Academic Setting, 2003M168; Role Competencies for a Faculty Member in an Occupational Therapy Assistant Academic Setting, 2005C240; Role Competencies for an Academic Fieldwork Coordinator, 2003M169;* and *Role Competencies for a Fieldwork Educator, 2005M284.*

Chapter 27.

THE AMERICAN OCCUPATIONAL THERAPY ASSOCIATION SELF-ASSESSMENT TOOL FOR FIELDWORK EDUCATOR COMPETENCY

American Occupational Therapy Association Commission on Education

Fieldwork education is a vital component in preparing students for entry-level occupational therapy practice. This voluntary self-assessment tool supports the development of skills necessary to be an effective fieldwork educator (FWE) whose role is to facilitate the progression from student to entry-level practitioner. This tool was designed to provide a structure for FWEs to assess their own level of competence and to identify areas for further development and improvement of their skills. Competency as a FWE promotes the practitioner's pursuit of excellence in working with students and ensures the advancement of the profession.

Purpose

Both novice and experienced OTA and OT FWEs can use this tool as a guide for self-reflection to target areas for professional growth. Proficiency as a FWE is an ongoing process of assessment, education, and practice. It is essential for FWEs to continually work toward improving their proficiency in all competency areas as they supervise OTA/OT students. Use of this assessment tool is intended to be the foundation from which each FWE will create a professional growth plan with specific improvement strategies and measurable outcomes to advance development in this area of practice.

Content

The self-assessment tool includes the following features:

1. Addresses FWE competencies in the areas of professional practice, education, supervision, evaluation, and administration.
2. Uses a numerical rating (Likert) scale from 1 (*Low Proficiency*) to 5 (*High Proficiency*) to aid in self-assessment.

3. Includes a "Comment Section" intended to be used by the FWE in identifying aspects of competency for self improvement.
4. Results in a "Fieldwork Educator Professional Development Plan." FWEs can use the suggested format for recording a professional development plan of action. The suggested format or chart may be copied for additional space. Such a plan helps FWEs meet the standards established for FWEs as stated in the Accreditation Council for Occupational Therapy Education (ACOTE®) Standards and Interpretive Guidelines (2006).
5. Explains terminology, which is based on the *Occupational Therapy Practice Framework: Domain and Process* (2nd ed.), AOTA, 2008.

Who Should Use the Tool

This self-assessment tool is designed to be used by OTA and OT FWEs at all levels of expertise in supervising students. While the tool is primarily oriented toward OTA/OT practitioners who directly supervise OTA and/or OT Level II fieldwork, it can easily be applied to Level I fieldwork and to non-OT supervisors.

Directions

FWEs should determine the relevance of each competency to the role of the OTA/OT in their setting. Some competency statements may not be applicable in their setting and/or in their state (refer to the appropriate OTA/OT role delineation documents). In addition, the "Self-Assessment Tool for Fieldwork Educator Competency" is to be used for professional development only. It is not intended to be used as a performance appraisal. However, the FWE may certainly include goals articulated in the "Fieldwork Educator Professional Development Plan" in their annual professional goals.

Self-Assessment Tool

Circle the number that correlates with your level of competence for each item. The "Comments" section can be used to highlight strengths, areas that need improvement, and so on.

Development Plan

It is helpful to prioritize the competency areas that need improvement and to select only a few areas that can realistically be accomplished. Write goals for each of the selected areas and identify strategies to meet the goals and establish a deadline for meeting the goals.

OT practitioners are adept in assessing, planning, and implementing practical and meaningful continuous quality improvement plans. It is this attribute, plus a desire to support the growth of future practitioners, that motivates OTAs and OTs to seek methods for gaining and maintaining their competence as FWEs. We hope this tool is helpful in guiding FWEs on a journey of self-appraisal and professional development. It meets the immediate need of defining basic competencies of fieldwork educators. It is in this spirit that the "Self-Assessment Tool" was drafted and offered as a means for better serving the needs of individuals and the future of occupational therapy.

Originally developed in 1997 by the COE Fieldwork Issues Committee.

Revised in 2009 by the Commission on Education:

René Padilla, PhD, OTR/L, FAOTA, *Chairperson*
Andrea Billics, PhD, OTR/L
Judith Blum, MS, OTR/L
Paula Bohr, PhD, OTR/L, FAOTA
Jennifer Coyne, COTA/L
Jyothi Gupta, PhD, OTR/L
Linda Musselman, PhD, OTR, FAOTA
Linda Orr, MPA, OTR/L
Abbey Sipp, OTS
Patricia Stutz-Tanenbaum, MS, OTR
Neil Harvison, PhD, OTR/L *(AOTA Liaison)*

SELF-ASSESSMENT TOOL FOR FIELDWORK EDUCATOR COMPETENCY

A. PROFESSIONAL PRACTICE COMPETENCIES

KEY DEFINITION STATEMENT: *The fieldwork educator demonstrates competencies in professional knowledge, skills, and judgment in occupational therapy practice that supports the client's engagement in meaningful occupation*

The fieldwork educator:	CIRCLE ONE					COMMENTS
	Low Proficient			High Proficient		
1. Uses a systematic approach to evaluation and intervention that is science-driven and focused on clients' occupational performance needs.	1	2	3	4	5	
2. Skillfully collects and analyzes clients' occupational profile and performance in order to develop and implement OT services.	1	2	3	4	5	
3. Considers context, activity demands, and client factors when determining feasibility and appropriateness of interventions.	1	2	3	4	5	
4. Understands clients' concerns, occupational performance issues, and safety factors for participation in intervention.	1	2	3	4	5	
5. Articulates the rationale and theoretical model, frame of reference, and/or therapeutic approach for OT services.	1	2	3	4	5	
6. Incorporates evidence-based research into occupational therapy practice.	1	2	3	4	5	
7. Collaborates with the OT/OTA to provide evaluation, interpretation of data, intervention planning, intervention, discharge planning, and documentation.	1	2	3	4	5	
8. Collaborates with individuals, colleagues, family/support system, and other staff or professionals with respect, sensitivity, and professional judgment.	1	2	3	4	5	
9. Works to establish a collaborative relationship that values the client perspective, including diversity, values, beliefs, health, and well-being as defined by the client.	1	2	3	4	5	
10. Addresses psychosocial factors across the OT practice setting as a reflection of a client-centered approach.	1	2	3	4	5	
11. Effectively manages and prioritizes client-centered services (e.g., intervention, documentation, team meetings) that support occupation-based outcomes.	1	2	3	4	5	
12. Incorporates legal, ethical, and professional issues that influence practice (e.g., reimbursement, confidentiality, role delineation).	1	2	3	4	5	
13. Articulates and implements OTA/OT role delineations as relevant to the practice setting.	1	2	3	4	5	
14. Adheres to professional standards of practice and Code of Ethics as identified by AOTA and state regulatory boards.	1	2	3	4	5	
15. Assumes responsibility for and pursues professional development to expand knowledge and skills (e.g., understands own strengths and limitations).	1	2	3	4	5	
16. Is knowledgeable regarding entry-level practice skills for the OT and OTA.	1	2	3	4	5	

KEY DEFINITION STATEMENT: *The fieldwork educator facilitates the student's development of professional clinical reasoning and its application to entry-level practice. The fieldwork educator assumes responsibility for ensuring her or his own competence as a fieldwork educator.*

B. EDUCATION COMPETENCIES

The fieldwork educator:	CIRCLE ONE					COMMENTS
	Low Proficient			High Proficient		
1. Provides ongoing assessment of a student's individual learning needs based on review of academic curriculum design, OTA and OT roles, prior experiences, and current performance level.	1	2	3	4	5	
2. Collaboratively develops student and fieldwork learning contracts to support occupation-based fieldwork experience (develop outcome-based measurable learning objectives).	1	2	3	4	5	
3. Sequences learning experiences to grade progression toward entry-level practice.	1	2	3	4	5	
4. Facilitates student-directed learning within the parameters of the fieldwork environment.	1	2	3	4	5	
5. Maximizes opportunities for learning by using planned and unplanned experiences within the fieldwork environment.	1	2	3	4	5	
6. Uses a variety of instructional strategies to facilitate the learning process (e.g., role modeling, co-intervention, videotaping).	1	2	3	4	5	
7. Adapts approach to work effectively with all students, including those who have physical and/ or psychosocial impairment(s).	1	2	3	4	5	
8. Demonstrates sensitivity to student learning style to adapt teaching approach for diverse student populations.	1	2	3	4	5	
9. Guides student integration of therapeutic concepts and skills (e.g., facilitates discussions to elicit clinical/professional reasoning, convert practice situations into learning experiences, and/ or to process personal feelings/values that interface with practice).	1	2	3	4	5	
10. Reflects upon educator role as complementary to OT practitioner role.	1	2	3	4	5	
11. Self-identifies and implements a Fieldwork Educator Professional Development Plan.	1	2	3	4	5	
12. Identifies resources to promote student and fieldwork educator professional development (e.g., academic program, student and supervisor mentors, AOTA, Commission on Education, Education Special Interest Section, workshops, in-services, etc.).	1	2	3	4	5	
13. Provides reference materials to promote student and fieldwork educator professional development and use of evidence-based practice (e.g., publications, texts, videos, Internet, etc.).	1	2	3	4	5	
14. Uses evidence-based research to guide student performance and learning for effective teaching strategies.	1	2	3	4	5	

C. SUPERVISION COMPETENCIES

KEY DEFINITION STATEMENT: *The fieldwork educator facilitates student achievement of entry-level practice through a student-centered approach.*

The fieldwork educator:	CIRCLE ONE					COMMENTS
	Low Proficient			High Proficient		
1. Uses current supervision models and theories to facilitation student performance and professional behavior	1	2	3	4	5	
2. Presents clear expectations of performance throughout the fieldwork experience, appropriate to entry level OT practice (e.g., student OTA/OT role delineation, Level I/II fieldwork, practice environment).	1	2	3	4	5	
3. Anticipates and prepares student for challenging situations.	1	2	3	4	5	
4. Provides activities to challenge student's optimal performance.	1	2	3	4	5	
5. Provides the student with prompt, direct, specific, and constructive feedback throughout the fieldwork experience.	1	2	3	4	5	
6. Uses a progression of supervisory approaches throughout the student learning cycle (adapts the amount and type of supervision, changes approach to support student learning, challenges student at current level of performance) to facilitate student performance.	1	2	3	4	5	
7. Uses a variety of strategies to provide communication and feedback to promote student professional development (verbal, nonverbal, group, direct, indirect).	1	2	3	4	5	
8. Is aware of his or her own personal style of supervision and is able to adapt the approach in response to student performance.	1	2	3	4	5	
9. Initiates interaction to resolve conflict and to raise issues of concern.	1	2	3	4	5	
10. Elicits and responds to student's feedback and concerns.	1	2	3	4	5	
11. Collaborates with the student and academic fieldwork coordinator to identify and modify learning environments when student experiences difficulty.	1	2	3	4	5	
12. Models appropriate professional behaviors when interacting with students, clients, and peers.	1	2	3	4	5	
13. Consults with other fieldwork educators and sites to develop creative learning experiences for the student.	1	2	3	4	5	
14. Uses innovation within own fieldwork setting to enhance the student learning experience during fieldwork.	1	2	3	4	5	

D. EVALUATION COMPETENCIES

KEY DEFINITION STATEMENT: *The fieldwork educator evaluates student performance to achieve entry-level practice in the fieldwork setting.*

The fieldwork educator:	Low Proficient			High Proficient		COMMENTS
	1	2	3	4	5	
1. Reviews the evaluation tool and expected entry-level expectations (e.g., behavioral objectives, weekly objectives) with student prior to midterm and final.	1	2	3	4	5	
2. Assesses student according to performance standards based on objective information (e.g., direct observation, discussion with student, review of student's documentation, observation by others, etc.).	1	2	3	4	5	
3. Assesses student's performance based on appropriate OTA/OT entry-level roles of the fieldwork practice setting.	1	2	3	4	5	
4. Facilitates student self-reflection and self-assessment throughout the fieldwork and evaluation process.	1	2	3	4	5	
5. Uses an evaluation process to advise and guide the student regarding strengths and opportunities for growth based on site-specific objectives.	1	2	3	4	5	
6. Uses fieldwork evaluation tools to accurately measure student performance and provide feedback.	1	2	3	4	5	
7. Completes and distributes in a timely manner all evaluations regarding student performance, including but not limited to the midterm and final evaluation (e.g., AOTA Fieldwork Performance Evaluation, Fieldwork Experience Assessment Tool [FEAT]).	1	2	3	4	5	
8. Guides the student in the use of the Fieldwork Performance Evaluation as a method of promoting continued professional growth and development.	1	2	3	4	5	
9. Documents student's fieldwork performance recognizing ethical and legal rights (e.g., due process, confidentiality, Americans with Disabilities Act, integrity).	1	2	3	4	5	

ADMINISTRATION COMPETENCIES

KEY DEFINITION STATEMENT: *The fieldwork educator develops and/or implements an organized fieldwork program in keeping with legal and professional standards and environmental factors (physical, social, and cultural).*

The fieldwork educator:	Low Proficient			High Proficient		COMMENTS
1. Communicates and collaborates with academic programs to integrate the academic curriculum design during fieldwork.	1	2	3	4	5	
2. Implements a model FW program that supports the curriculum of the academic program.	1	2	3	4	5	
3. Seeks support from fieldwork site administration and staff to develop and implement the student fieldwork program.	1	2	3	4	5	
4. Designs and implements the fieldwork program in collaboration with the academic programs served and in accordance to ACOTE® standards for Level I and Level II fieldwork (2008; e.g., academic and fieldwork setting requirements, Standards of Practice, Code of Ethics).	1	2	3	4	5	
5. Ensures that the fieldwork program is sensitive to diversity and multicultural issues.	1	2	3	4	5	
6. Documents an organized, systematic fieldwork program (e.g., fieldwork manual, student expectations, weekly sequence of expectations).	1	2	3	4	5	
7. Schedules formal and informal meetings with the student to guide the fieldwork experience.	1	2	3	4	5	
8. Collaborates with the student to develop student learning objectives.						
9. Documents behavioral objectives to achieve fieldwork objectives and learning experiences appropriate for entry-level practice.	1	2	3	4	5	
10. Is knowledgeable in legal and health care policies that directly influence fieldwork.	1	2	3	4	5	
11. Defines essential functions and roles of a fieldwork student, in compliance with legal and accreditation standards (e.g., ADA, Family Education Rights and Privacy Act, Joint Commission, fieldwork agreement, reimbursement mechanism, state regulations).	1	2	3	4	5	
12. Provides student work areas appropriate to fieldwork site (e.g., student safety, accessibility, supplies).	1	2	3	4	5	
13. Provides a complete orientation for student to fieldwork site (e.g., policies, procedures, student expectations, and responsibilities).	1	2	3	4	5	
14. Requires student compliance with the fieldwork site policies and procedures (HIPAA, OSHA regulations), mission, goals, philosophy, and safety standards.	1	2	3	4	5	
15. Submits required fieldwork documents to academic program in a timely manner to ensure current data is available (e.g., fieldwork evaluation, fieldwork agreements, fieldwork data form).	1	2	3	4	5	
16. Conducts ongoing fieldwork program evaluations and monitors changes in the program with student and staff input (e.g., Student Evaluation of Fieldwork Experience, Self-Assessment Tool for Fieldwork Competencies).	1	2	3	4	5	

FIELDWORK EDUCATOR PROFESSIONAL DEVELOPMENT PLAN

NAME: _____

DATE: _____

Strengths:

Areas to Develop:

Competency Areas to Address	Goals	Independent Study	Academic Coursework	Workshops/Continuing Education	Student Feedback	Consult With Academic Fieldwork Coordinator	Presentations	Publications	Research Activities	Mentorship	Peer Review	Shared Supervision of Student	Target Date	Completed Date

AMERICAN OCCUPATIONAL THERAPY ASSOCIATION RESOURCE LIST

Atler, K. (2003). *Using the fieldwork performance forms: The complete guide.* Bethesda, MD: American Occupational Therapy Association.

Atler, K. & Wimmer, R. (2003). *Online course—Using the Fieldwork Performance Evaluation forms: An interactive approach.* Bethesda, MD: American Occupational Therapy Association.

Accreditation Council for Occupational Therapy Education. (2009). *Standards and interpretive guidelines.* Downloaded June 8, 2009 from http://www.aota.org/Educate/Accredit/StandardsReview/guide/42369.aspx

American Occupational Therapy Association. (2005). *Occupational therapy code of ethics.* Bethesda, MD: Author.

American Occupational Therapy Association. (2008). *Occupational therapy practice framework: Domain and process* (2nd ed.). *American Journal of Occupational Therapy, 62,* 625–683. http://dx.doi.org/10.5014/ajot.62.6.625

American Occupational Therapy Association. (2008). *Recommendations for occupational therapy fieldwork experiences.* Bethesda, MD: Author.

American Occupational Therapy Association. (2009). Guidelines for supervision, roles, and responsibilities during the delivery of occupational therapy services. *American Journal of Occupational Therapy, 63,* 797–803. http://dx.doi.org/10.5014/ajot.63.6.797

American Occupational Therapy Association. (2009). Occupational therapy fieldwork education: Value and purpose. *American Journal of Occupational Therapy, 63,* 821–822. http://dx.doi.org/10.5014/ajot.63.6.821

American Occupational Therapy Association. (2009). Specialized knowledge and skills of occupational therapy educators of the future. *American Journal of Occupational Therapy, 63,* 804–818. http://dx.doi.org/10.5014/ajot.63.6.804

Costa, D. (2004). *Essential guide to occupational therapy fieldwork education: Resources for today's educators and practitioners.* Bethesda, MD: American Occupational Therapy Association.

Costa, D. (2007). *Clinical supervision in occupational therapy: A guide for fieldwork and practice.* Bethesda, MD: American Occupational Therapy Association.

Moyers, P. A. (2007). *The guide to occupational therapy practice.* Bethesda, MD: American Occupational Therapy Association.

Chapter 28.

COLLABORATIVE INTRAPROFESSIONAL EDUCATION WITH OCCUPATIONAL THERAPY AND OCCUPATIONAL THERAPY ASSISTANT STUDENTS

Donna Costa, DHS, OTR/L, FAOTA
University of Utah, Salt Lake City, UT

Rivka Molinsky, OTR/L
Touro College, New York, NY

Camille Sauerwald, EdM, OTR/L
The Richard Stockton College of New Jersey, Galloway, NJ

This CE Article was developed in collaboration with AOTA's Education Special Interest Section.

ABSTRACT

Graduates of occupational therapy and occupational therapy assistant programs are expected to work collaboratively as practitioners. Preparing competent practitioners is the goal and outcome of all professional programs. Developing opportunities for students to work together during their fieldwork experience enhances their skills for that collaboration in their future as practitioners. Academic and fieldwork (clinical) educators are encouraged to create opportunities for occupational therapy and occupational therapy assistant students to learn together, both in the classroom and during fieldwork experiences.

Learning Objectives

1. Recognize the main components of the collaborative learning model.
2. Identify a supervision strategy with multiple fieldwork students from different levels and schools.
3. Identify learning experiences for occupational therapy and occupational therapy assistant students that lead to increased collaboration.

Introduction

It is important to start with some common definitions currently used in academic and fieldwork education. A term that needs definition is *intraprofessional education*, which is defined as "an educational activity that occurs between two or more professionals within the same discipline, with a focus on the participants to work together, act jointly, and cooperate" (Jung, Solomon, & Martin, 2010, p. 235). This concept has received considerable attention in the fields of nursing, physical therapy, and occupational therapy, in which there is more than one professional level. In nursing, there is the licensed practical nurse and registered nurse; in physical therapy, there is the physical therapist (PT) and physical therapy assistant (PTA); and in occupational therapy, there is the occupational therapist (OT) and occupational therapy assistant (OTA). In intraprofessional education, students and practitioners within the same profession are engaged in learning together and subsequently collaborating in the workplace.

The second concept that warrants defining is the *collaborative learning model*, a method used in both interprofessional and intraprofessional education. "Collaborative learning refers to pairs or small groups engaging in reciprocal learning experiences whereby knowledge and ideas are exchanged" (Rozsa & Lincoln, 2005, p. 229).

The collaborative learning model is based on work by Russian educational psychologist Lev Vygotsky (Costa, 2007). He theorized that learning has a social component and that people learn best through interaction. The collaborative learning model, which is an expansion of constructivist learning theory, is the opposite of the traditional 1:1 model, in which the fieldwork educator is the expert. Instead, students help each other learn, and the educator guides the learning process (Table 28.1).

Collaborative learning is based on four principles:

1. Knowledge is constructed, discovered, transformed, and extended by the students. The educator creates a setting where students, when given a subject, can explore, question, research, interpret, and solidify the knowledge they feel is important.
2. Students actively construct their own knowledge. Students guided by the instructor actively seek out knowledge.

Table 28.1. Traditional vs. Collaborative Learning Model

Traditional or 1:1 Model	Collaborative Model
Competitive	**Cooperative**
Passive learning	Active learning
Students work on own	Interaction required
Fieldwork educator is the expert	Fieldwork educator is co-learner
Fieldwork educator controls time, content, and structure	Control is within group for time, content, and structure
Fieldwork educator is autonomous	Interdependence
Learning objectives established in advance	Learning objectives set by group
Traditional assignments	Multidimensional assignments

From "Collaboration in Clinical Education" by M. Rozsa & M. Lincoln, in *Transforming Practice Through Clinical Education, Professional Supervision, and Mentoring* (p. 231), by M. Rose and D. Best (Eds.), 2005, Philadelphia: Elsevier. Used with permission.

3. Education is a personal transaction among students and between educators as they work together.
4. All of the above can only take place within a cooperative context. There is no competition among students to strive to be better than the other. Students take responsibility for each other's learning. (Calm, Dooley, & Simmons, 2001, p. 71)

Background Literature

Thomas Dillon (2001), in interviewing OT/OTA teams in Pennsylvania, Ohio, and West Virginia, found that "both OTRs and COTAs expressed that effective intraprofessional relationships enhance the quality of OT services provided, and strengthen their desire to practice in the field" (Dillon, 2001, p. 1). Dillon said that the essence of the relationship between OTs and OTAs cannot be learned by reading articles on professional role delineation and supervisory guidelines. Supervision of an OTA by an OT is an ongoing process that should mutually enhance the professional growth of each individual; both parties have their own set of responsibilities. Themes that emerged in this study included the necessity of effective two-way communication, the need for mutual respect, and the importance of professionalism.

Carol Scheerer (2001) described a partnering model used in Ohio between an OT and OTA program in the classroom. "Partnering between the OT/OTA team needs to become a habit so that future practitioners can use it as part of their daily occupation. To develop this partnership, practice needs to be embedded in the educational curriculum of future occupational therapy practitioners" (p. 204). Scheerer paired students from OT and OTA programs in a series of classroom learning activities. The first sessions involved learning about each other's curriculum and role delineation, and then the pairs applied the American Occupational Therapy Association's (AOTA's) *Standards of Practice for Occupational Therapy* (AOTA, 2010c) to a hypothetical case. The second set of sessions focused on working on cases in OT/OTA pairs, then using a Scattergories game format to identify one-word descriptors of an "ideal" OT/OTA relationship. In the third and final set of sessions, OT and OTA students were assigned to work as teams to complete joint assignments related to a group process course. Later, they worked as collaborative research teams, with the OTA students serving as research assistants to the OT students. All students reported benefitting from the hands-on learning. "Practicing interaction, teamwork, and collaboration as students should provide a lifetime habit of partnering as practitioners" (Scheerer, 2001, p. 204).

Jung, Salvatori, and Martin (2008) described a fieldwork study in which seven pairs of OT and OTA students in Canada were jointly assigned to fieldwork placements. "Student participants all agreed that working together in a clinical setting not only enhanced their understanding of each other's roles, including similarities and differences, but also fostered the development of competence and confidence in one's own skills and abilities as well as one's partner" (Jung et al., 2008, p. 48). They further wrote, "pairing OT and OTA students in collaborative fieldwork placements … has not been common practice. Nevertheless, there is increasing evidence that such collaborative learning experiences can generate positive learning outcomes that include learning about the roles of OTs and OTAs, emulating real world practice by pairing student OTs and student OTAs to provide client care, and expanding opportunities for collaboration and teamwork" (Jung et al., 2008, p. 43). The students in this study reported that they

learned the importance of developing a working relationship through shared learning, effective communication, and mutual trust and respect. "Through understanding each other's roles and effective communication, there emerged a sense of teamwork and genuine interest in collaborating on a comprehensive client plan that ultimately complemented the delivery of occupational therapy services" (Jung et al., 2008, p. 46).

Another study from Canada by Jung, Sainsbury, Grum, Wilkins, and Tryssenar (2002) reported on a joint clinical learning experience between OT and OTA students. "The strength of this collaborative model included allowing students to learn about the roles of OTs and OTAs, emulating real world practice by pairing the student OTs and student OTAs to work together to provide client care" (Jung et al., 2002, p. 96). "The importance of collaborative learning, which included ideas about partnership and teamwork, was evident. Learning together led to feelings of respect and trust about the different knowledge and skills each brought to the client as well as the different responsibilities each had in the care of the client" (Jung et al., 2002, p. 99).

Higgins (1998) described her experience with supervising OT and OTA students in Massachusetts. "Although collaboration among practitioners is an everyday occurrence, collaboration among students is not. The OT/OTA collaborative model of student education provides opportunities that parallel those in the working environment while promoting positive fieldwork experiences, enhanced clinical reasoning development, and continued personal and professional educational opportunities" (Higgins, 1998, p. 41).

The physical therapy literature yields articles focusing on intraprofessional education between PT and PTA students. Matthews, Smith, Hussey, and Plack (2010) reported on a 4-week joint placement between PTs and PTAs in North Carolina and South Carolina that employed a 2:1 supervision model. The placements were designed to provide an authentic experience that enhanced the students' knowledge of, skills for, and attitudes about working together. Students kept reflective journals, and 14 jurors reviewed these for themes. The researchers noted ongoing "misperceptions regarding the roles among both PTs and PTAs that may have impeded a preferred PT–PTA relationship" (p. 50). The authors concluded with recommendations: Establish clear expectations of collaboration, not competition;

provide structured feedback; develop clear learning contracts; clarify individual student roles; establish ground rules to facilitate collaborative learning; and pair students in the later phases of their educational preparation so that PT students will feel better prepared to delegate patient care to the PTA.

In the same article, the authors cited Robinson, McCall, and DePalma (1995), who reported that more than 50% of PTs surveyed in 1992 said they received no information during their professional education on the role of the PTA. Subsequently, other studies done in the 1990s indicated that both PTs and PTAs had erroneous perceptions of their respective roles (Robinson et al., 1994, 1995). PTs were noted to be either overly restrictive or permissive in working with PTAs. Similarly, PTAs also varied between being overly restrictive or permissive when interpreting their job roles and responsibilities. "To facilitate effective teamwork of PT and PTA practitioners, it may be helpful to not only educate students about the legal and education requirements of each role, but also to provide them with the skills, attitudes, and abilities needed to effectively communicate and interact with each other in clinical practice. Designing an educational experience that pairs PT and PTA students in clinical studies in the clinical setting may provide the authentic experience needed to enhance their knowledge, skills, and attitudes" (Matthews et al., 2010, p. 51).

Jelley, Larocque, and Patterson (2010) reported on a pilot study in Canada that paired PT and PTA students on a 5-week placement:

> Unfortunately, PT and PTA students get little or no experience in working together as a team during their education, despite the fact that in the workforce, PTs and PTAs are expected to practice collaboratively. It should also be noted that a lack of familiarity with scope of practice significantly reduces the ability to work collaboratively....An unexpected benefit reported by participants was the value of learning through the interview process and by writing in journals. This finding is consistent with those of past research, since the reflective journals kept by participants were deemed useful both by participants and researchers in understanding the shared placement experience.... A teacher cannot do the learning for a student but can only support and encourage a learner. (p. 76)

The Commission on Accreditation in Physical Therapy Education (CAPTE) reviewed 10 self-study reports from physical therapy programs and found that not all of them were providing learning opportunities to adequately address direction and supervision of PTAs or the role of the PTA in clinical care. Similarly, 10 self-study reports from PTA programs found that there were instances in which learning experiences went beyond the accepted role of the PTA, exceeding the foundation upon which PTA education is based. CAPTE developed a revised position paper in response to these findings—*The Evaluative Criteria That Address the Relationship Between Physical Therapists and Physical Therapist Assistants.* This document states that:

> PT education programs will be cited for conditional or noncompliance when there are not didactic and clinical learning experiences that lead to the ability to (1) direct and supervise the PTA in the application of appropriate interventions, or (2) recognize those elements of the clinical care process that may not be directed to the PTA. PTA education programs will be cited for conditional or noncompliance when didactic or clinical experiences or assessments go beyond the application of appropriate interventions under the direction and supervision of a PT. (CAPTE, 2005, p. 13)

The Mayo Clinic in Rochester, Minnesota, extensively uses the collaborative model of clinical education, which it has named the Mayo Collaborative Model of Clinical Education; this model has been used by OTs and PTs since 1930. Rindflesch et al. (2009) reported that:

> The collaborative model does not merely mean that there is more than one student supervised by each clinical instructor. In this model, students collaborate with each other, share learning experiences, adopt the role of teacher in addition to the student role, and take on some of the responsibility for their legal and ethical supervision. (p. 133)

Students at the Mayo Clinic are asked to teach their peers about patients and conditions they have encountered and must use evidence-based practice. When students graduate from their respective programs, they will not likely have a 1:1 mentor. "The collaborative model encourages students to develop helpful habits that emulate what it will be like for them when they become licensed" (Rindflesch et al., p. 136).

Academic Curricula

There are many sources of information within the profession of occupational therapy that contribute to our understanding of the intended relationship between OTs and OTAs. Higgins (1998) cited the need for students to have knowledge of the official documents of the professional association for a collaborative model of fieldwork to be successful. These documents must be included within any curriculum for occupational therapy practitioners. Current official documents of AOTA include, among others, the Scope of Practice for OTs and OTAs (AOTA, 2010b). This official document provides definitions of supervision and descriptions of the cooperative nature of the OT/OTA relationship, the outcome of which is to benefit the client by providing effective services. The Accreditation Council for Occupational Therapy Education (ACOTE®) sets standards for the education of all OT and OTA students, and those standards further describe the relationship between those sets of practitioners (ACOTE, 2007a, b, c). In addition to the guidance provided by AOTA and ACOTE, individual states may have regulations in their licensing statute documents that further mandate the supervisory relationship between OTs and OTAs.

ACOTE standards due to take effect in July 2013 state in the preamble that occupational therapy practitioners "be prepared to effectively communicate and work interprofessionally with those who provide care for individuals and/or populations in order to clarify each member's responsibility in executing components of an intervention plan" and to "understand the distinct roles and responsibilities of the occupational therapist and occupational therapy assistant in the supervisory process" (ACOTE, 2012). All students who aspire to be occupational therapy practitioners are also schooled in professional ethics, values, and responsibilities, which apply not only to client care but also to interactions among occupational therapy practitioners and other professionals (ACOTE, 2007a, b, c). The "commitment [to act ethically] extends beyond service recipients to include professional colleagues, students, educators, businesses, and

the community" (AOTA, 2010a, p. S17) and therefore compels us to work intraprofessionally in a way that upholds those ethical standards.

Arguably, the most informative document for understanding the delineation of duties between OTs and OTAs is the *Guidelines for Supervision, Roles, and Responsibilities During the Delivery of Occupational Therapy Services* (AOTA, 2009). This document provides statements on supervision and outlines general principles involved in the supervisory relationship both inside and outside of the provision of occupational therapy services. In addition, the document contains statements about the roles and responsibilities of OTs and OTAs during the process of occupational therapy. For both sets of students, and for practitioners who are in settings where occupational therapy clinicians include both OTs and OTAs, this document can assist in understanding role delineation.

An important concept contained in all documents is that of the supervisory relationship. In *Guidelines for Supervision, Roles, and Responsibilities During the Delivery of Occupational Therapy Services,* supervision is defined as "a cooperative process... based on mutual understanding" that "promotes effective utilization of resources" and that is "aimed at the safe and effective delivery of occupational therapy services" (AOTA, 2009, p. 797). It is also defined as "a joint effort" that must include "mutual understanding between the supervisor and the supervisee about each other's competence, experience, education, and credentials" and that encompasses "professional competence and development" (AOTA, 2009, p. 797). The Scope of Practice further emphasizes the cooperative nature of the OT/OTA relationship in its inclusive use of the term *occupational therapy practitioner* (AOTA, 2010b) for both OTs and OTAs. ACOTE Standard B.4.4 for OTA education states that in addition to being able to "articulate the role of the occupational therapy assistant and occupational therapist in the screening and evaluation process," the OTA student must understand "the rationale for supervision and collaborative work between the occupational therapy assistant and occupational therapist in that process"(ACOTE 2007c, p. 667). Doctoral and master's level OT students must learn to "explain and justify the importance of supervisory roles, responsibilities, and collaborative professional relationships between the occupational therapist and the occupational therapy assistant" (ACOTE 2007a, p. 649; 2007b, p. 660). All students in the states in which they will practice must learn the regulations that govern the supervisory relationship between them.

These documents are often provided as part of coursework in professional issues or health administration services and professional development, or a course with similar content, and may in fact be explored in more than one course within the curriculum. Because OTA education is most often found at the community college level and OT education is most often found at the university level, most programs would need to plan intraprofessional activities between institutions, or between OT and OTA programs in the same institution, to allow students to practice skills related to the supervisory relationship during their academic coursework. It is common for academic programs to offer lectures regarding role delineation and supervision, or to plan guest speakers and panels to address the topic.

In an already crammed curriculum with different class schedules, programs may find it difficult to realize plans to connect OT and OTA students, and often the first intraprofessional or interprofessional interaction students have is during fieldwork. When there is an opportunity for students to interact in a classroom, it is often for 1 day, and learning activities may include case-based assignments that include opportunities to practice roles.

Fieldwork Education

In the field of occupational therapy, most of the literature on the collaborative model has focused on its application to fieldwork education. In fieldwork education, collaboration can occur:

- Between pairs or groups of students (peers)
- Between two or more fieldwork educators (same profession)
- Between clinical educators and/or students from different disciplines
- Between all stakeholders in the clinical education process.

In the collaborative fieldwork model, the student relies less on the fieldwork educator's expert knowledge to learn skills, with a trend to move away from *received* or *passive* knowledge to more *process-oriented* or *active* knowledge creation. As an added benefit, the latter process prepares future practitioners for lifelong learning. Responsibility is shifted to the learners to solve the problems they encounter in clinical practice. "Collaborative learning calls on levels of ingenuity and inventiveness that many students never knew they had. And it teaches interdependence in an increasingly collaborative world that requires greater flexibility and adaptability to change than ever before" (Bruffee, cited in Cohn et al., 2001, p. 74).

Research has shown that if educators carefully structure collaborative learning, students will achieve at a higher level, apply clinical reasoning more frequently, and be more intrinsically motivated (Johnson & Johnson, cited in Cohn et al., 2001, p. 74).

An understanding of standards for occupational therapy fieldwork education and supervision is necessary for students and fieldwork educators alike. Current ACOTE standards for supervising OT and OTA students are identical. Standard B.10.12 states that Level I OT and OTA students may receive supervision from currently licensed or credentialed OTs and OTAs. For Level II fieldwork, supervision requirements differ. OTs may receive supervision from a qualified OT, and OTAs can be supervised by a qualified OT or OTA. Certainly, different states may have more strict regulations that supersede those guidelines. The Fieldwork Performance Evaluation for OT and OTA students in Level II placements contains items describing the competencies needed for each to demonstrate a satisfactory performance in understanding the supervisory relationship.

In many fieldwork settings, OT students do not have opportunities to observe or work with OTAs and must imagine that interaction through academic exercises such as writing a sample state regulation governing that relationship, or composing an essay explaining the legal and interpersonal aspects of OT/OTA relationships. Anecdotal information suggests that many OT fieldwork educators have not had the experience of working with OTAs themselves and may have difficulty helping fieldwork students understand the professional, interpersonal, and legal requirements of the OT/OTA relationship. Often they do not have a practical understanding of role delineation and may need assistance from academic programs to review and understand how OTAs may contribute to client care. It is incumbent on OTA academic programs, in that case, to interact with fieldwork sites so that OTA students can receive appropriate supervision and practice the interactions necessary to benefit clients.

The Philadelphia Region Fieldwork Consortium (PRFC) is currently managing challenges related to density of academic programs within a relatively small geographic area. In the Philadelphia and southern New Jersey region, there are six entry-level OT programs. There are two newer OTA programs, with another in development. There are two OTD programs and a new entry-level OTD program, with another in development. In addition, there are established programs within 2 hours of Philadelphia in every direction that seek fieldwork sites in and around the Philadelphia region, and demand for placements is intense. Academic fieldwork coordinators for the OTA programs have been challenged to develop traditional and nontraditional sites that will accept students, which requires educating fieldwork educators on basic requirements for OTA students for fieldwork, on role delineation, and on state regulations that have a bearing on supervision. This information has been provided in one-on-one meetings, through electronic communication, and through formalized meetings. In addition, because increased numbers of OT students in the region demand increased numbers of placements, the PRFC has already provided an introduction to an intraprofessional collaborative supervision model to fieldwork educators who attended the organization's annual Clinical Council Day in March 2012 in an effort to introduce fieldwork educators to this model (Costa, 2012).

A proposal to coordinate placements so that OT and OTA students might be assigned deliberately to specific and willing sites across programs encountered barriers that included nonuniform fieldwork dates and insufficient preparation of sites for a collaborative intraprofessional fieldwork experience. Therefore, the PRFC is exploring more limited options between programs in the same institution or between programs that may have similar fieldwork dates. The PRFC appears to be positioned ideally to explore the use of a collaborative model of intraprofessional fieldwork.

An analysis by Rodger et al. (2008) of the changing environment of health care provision identified some key themes of change that may affect fieldwork education, including fiscal restraints, new models of care, reduced staffing, and increased productivity expectations. In addition, they found that clinical educators report having decreased time for direct patient care due to increased documentation requirements and ongoing staffing challenges. These may be some of the factors that decrease the availability of fieldwork placements.

Curtin University in Perth, Australia, established a program of partnership with stakeholders that included a complete overhaul of their fieldwork sequence to meet the demands of placing their students (Rosenwax, Gribble, & Margalia, 2010). In addition, Touro College's occupational therapy program developed student clinic placement with faculty on release time as a supervisor for both OT and OTA students. Although these may seem extremely ambitious, every accredited program can understand the pressures for student placement that would lead to such a drastic response.

Intraprofessional fieldwork options require managing logistics and continually evaluating the current team of students' clinical skills, knowledge set, and interpersonal skills—in addition to providing traditional supervision of each student's developing competence as an entry-level clinician. The prospect might be somewhat daunting; however, the pressure to find and secure quality sites in which to place students is sufficiently overwhelming to justify the effort. Preparing students for collaborative learning on fieldwork involves recognizing that students have been socialized in the classroom to compete more than cooperate, and moving away from the model where professors are the authority in the classroom. To understand how the expectations are different in this model, students can read articles and participate in meetings and seminars. The fieldwork educator will have to take a step back and facilitate more than teach.

Strategies that can be used to prepare students can include planning start and end dates to accommodate for differences in length of fieldwork placements, with OTA students starting later; assigning reading about the collaborative model; holding group supervision sessions at least weekly; setting clear expectations for all that will be required on fieldwork, including job delineation; holding joint treatment/co-treatment sessions; assigning cases jointly, with expectations for mutual problem solving; structuring entire fieldwork placements in advance, so that educators don't "wing it"; and assigning group projects and final projects to teams.

There are a number of examples of intraprofessional clinical education currently in practice. An in-depth interview by the authors with two skilled clinicians currently running intraprofessional fieldwork supervision models indicated that the challenges are manageable. The one thing both clinicians share is a passion for what motivates them.

Sean Getty, MS, OTR/L, rehab director at Roads to Recovery and assistant clinical professor at Stony Brook University, is passionate about supervision being a critical competency requirement for occupational therapy practitioners (personal communication, July 13, 2012). He feels that without modeling the process and practice during fieldwork, few occupational therapy clinicians develop quality supervision skills to meet the learning needs of students. In addition, occupational therapy assistants need to develop the ability to participate in the supervisory experience in a way that enhances clinical competence, Getty says. Again, without actively learning this skill on a fieldwork placement, it is difficult to really use supervision effectively.

Melanie Austin, MPA, OTR/L, clinician at Henry Street Settlement Community Consultation Center and assistant professor at New York Institute of Technology (NYIT), is passionate about mental health practice (personal communication, July 11, 2012). According to Austin, occupational therapy practitioners at every level of practice need to be clear what they are offering clients, to "grasp hold of the core of OT" so that the value of occupation-based treatment is clear to themselves, their clients, and the clinics that offer mental health care. There are other professionals addressing a range of client needs, so without passion for who we are as a profession and what each offers as a practitioner, the value of occupational therapy to day treatment centers such as Henry Street is unclear. Austin's passion for her area of practice has led her to develop a system of intraprofessional supervision to increase in the number of occupational therapy clinicians who are passionate about evidence-based quality care in the mental health practice arena.

Austin requires two students to co-run groups at Henry Street. This may be two OT students, or one OT and one OTA student. Austin takes OT students from NYIT and Touro College, and OTA students from Touro College. There is some challenge related to the different requirements—whereas the OT students complete 12-week rotations, the OTA students generally complete 9 weeks at the site.

In contrast, Getty takes students from many schools. With a constant flow of incoming and outgoing students, he reports that the challenge is balancing the education students receive from different programs. Programs emphasize different theories and focus on different aspects of the profession's domain, impacting clinical style and readiness. In addition, students at Roads to Recovery are working with and receiving supervision from a multidisciplinary team in addition to the two levels of occupational therapy practice.

Whenever a diverse group works together, there are inevitably conflicts. Resolving them professionally in a way that meets client needs is a vital clinical skill, Getty and Austin note. They both feel that the interprofessional and multiprofessional interactions required at their site offer students unique opportunities to learn how to interact appropriately, professionally, and effectively with clients and coworkers. *All* practitioners, whatever their level of practice, work with others. Getting along in a way that is professional and effective for client care is best developed on fieldwork so that it becomes an integral part of the students' developing professional persona.

Both Getty and Austin report that the difference between OT and OTA levels of practice is clear in the clinic. Getty has a clearly defined process of mentoring OT students to develop supervisory skills and for OTA students to become active participants in the process. Austin generally provides group and individual supervision to the students at her site. Austin reports that the OTA students are weaker in evidence-based practice in comparison with OT students, but are strongest in their eagerness to engage. Getty reports that the OT students are best at understanding concepts and theory, whereas the OTA students tend to be effectively creative in their treatment application. Both Getty and Austin are working at sites that are committed to enabling community integration. The groups run at both sites are core to occupational therapy values, history, and philosophy. These include a range of activities of daily living, from grooming to banking. They both believe that by taking students at both levels of practice, they are enhancing the profession as a whole and within every area of practice.

Both Getty and Austin understand the importance of role delineation between practice levels, and both are clear about the strengths each level offers to the clinic. It is likely this value of both levels of practice that enables their respective programs to be effective. Each manages the process distinctly differently, with different clinic management styles and different student management methods. However, they both have passion for enhancing the profession, which was evident throughout the interviews.

Conclusion

Creating learning opportunities that enhance lifelong learning and clinical competency is a vital component of every professional program. Within occupational therapy, the multiple levels of entry-level practice provide a unique opportunity to promote access to quality care with a focus on occupation and living life to its fullest. The support for collaborate fieldwork education is found in the literature, in the success of intraprofessional student supervision models, and in the pragmatics of fieldwork placements for educational programs. It is necessary to recognize the components of a collaborative learning model in order to implement supervision strategies that encourage intraprofessional collaboration and communication skills. Learning experiences for OT and OTA students while at a clinical placements will lead to increased collaboration in practice.

References

Accreditation Council for Occupational Therapy Education. (2007a). Accreditation standards for doctoral-degree-level educational program for the occupational therapist. *American Journal of Occupational Therapy, 61,* 641–651. http://dx.doi.org/10.5014/ajot.61.6.641

Accreditation Council for Occupational Therapy Education. (2007b). Accreditation standards for a master's-degree-level educational program for the occupational therapist. *American Journal of Occupational Therapy, 61,* 652–661. http://dx.doi.org/10.5014/ajot.61.6.652

Accreditation Council for Occupational Therapy Education. (2007c). Accreditation standards for an educational program for the occupational therapy assistant. *American Journal of Occupational Therapy, 61,* 662–671. http://dx.doi.org/10.5014/ajot.61.6.662

Accreditation Council for Occupational Therapy Education. (2012). *2011 Accreditation Council for Occupational Therapy Education (ACOTE®) standards and interpretive guide.* Retrieved from http://www.aota.org/Educate/Accredit/DraftStandards/50146.aspx?IT=.pdf

American Occupational Therapy Association. (2009). Guidelines for supervision, roles, and responsibilities during the delivery of occupational therapy services. *American Journal of Occupational Therapy, 63,* 797–803. http://dx.doi.org/10.5014/ajot.63.6.797

American Occupational Therapy Association. (2010a). Occupational therapy code of ethics and ethics standards. *American Journal of Occupational Therapy, 64,* S17–S26. http://dx.doi.org/10.5014/ajot.2010.64S17

American Occupational Therapy Association. (2010b). Scope of practice. *American Journal of Occupational Therapy, 64,* S70–S77. http://dx.doi.org/10.5014/ajot.2010.64S70

American Occupational Therapy Association. (2010c). Standards of practice for occupational therapy. *American Journal of Occupational Therapy, 64,* S106–S111. http://dx.doi.org/10.5014/ajot.2010.64S106

Commission on Accreditation in Physical Therapy Education. (2005). Revised position paper: The evaluative criteria that address the relationship between physical therapists and physical therapist assistants. *CAPTE Accreditation Update, 10*(2), 13–14

Cohn, E., Dooley, N., & Simmons, L. (2001). Collaborative learning applied to fieldwork education. *Occupational Therapy in Health Care, 15*(112), 69–83.

Costa, D. (2007). *Clinical supervision in occupational therapy: A guide for fieldwork practice.* Bethesda, MD: AOTA Press.

Costa, D. (2012, March). *Using a collaborative/concurrent model of supervision for OT and OTA students.* Presentation at the Philadelphia Region Fieldwork Consortium Annual Clinical Council Day, Philadelphia.

Dillon, T. (2001). Practitioner perspectives: Effective intraprofessional relationships in occupational therapy. *Occupational Therapy in Health Care, 14*(3/4), 1–15.

Higgins, S. (1998). The OT/OTA collaborative model of fieldwork education. *OT Practice, 3*(9), 41–44.

Jelley, W., Larocque, N., & Patterson, S. (2010). Intradisciplinary clinical education for physiotherapists and physiotherapist assistants: A pilot study. *Physiotherapy Canada, 62,* 75–80.

Jung, B., Sainsbury, S., Grum, R., Wilkins, S., & Tryssenar, J. (2002). Collaborative fieldwork education with student occupational therapists and student occupational therapist assistants. *Canadian Journal of Occupational Therapy, 69,* 95–103.

Jung, B., Salvatori, P., & Martin, A. (2008). Intraprofessional fieldwork education: Occupational therapy and occupational therapist assistant students learning together. *Canadian Journal of Occupational Therapy, 75,* 42–50.

Jung, B., Solomon, P., & Martin, A. (2010). Collaborative fieldwork education: Exploring the intraprofessional and interprofessional context. In L. McAllister, M. Paterson, J. Higgs, & C. Bithell (Eds.), *Innovations in allied health fieldwork education: A critical appraisal* (pp. 235–246). Rotterdam, Netherlands: Sense Publishers.

Matthews, H., Smith, S., Hussey, J., & Plack, M. (2010). Investigation of the preferred PT–PTA relationship in a 2:1 clinical education model. *Journal of Physical Therapy Education, 24*(3), 50–61.

Rindflesch, A., Dunfee, H., Cieslak, K., Trenary, T., Calley, D., & Heinle, D. (2009). Collaborative model of clinical education in physical and occupational therapy at the Mayo Clinic. *Journal of Allied Health, 38*(3), 132–142.

Robinson, A., McCall, M., & DePalma, M. (1995). Physical therapist assistants' perceptions of the documented roles of the physical therapist assistant. *Physical Therapy, 75,* 1054–1064.

Robinson, A., McCall, M., DePalma, M., Clayton-Krasinski, D., Tingley, S., Simoncelli, S., & Harnish, L. (1994). Physical therapists' perceptions of the roles of the physical therapist assistant. *Physical Therapy, 74,* 571–582.

Rodger, S., Webb, G., Devitt, L., Gilbert, J., Wrightson, P., & McMeeken, J. (2008). Clinical education and practice placements in the allied health professions: An international perspective. *Journal of Allied Health, 37*(1), 53–62.

Rosenwax, L., Gribble, N., & Margaria, H. (2010). GRACE: An innovative program of clinical education in allied health. *Journal of Allied Health, 39*(1), e11–e16.

Rozsa, M., & Lincoln, M. (2005). Collaboration in clinical education. In M. Rose & D. Best (Eds.), *Transforming practice through clinical education, professional supervision, and mentoring* (pp. 229–248). Philadelphia: Elsevier.

Scheerer, C. (2001). The partnering model: Occupational therapy assistant and occupational therapy students working together. *Occupational Therapy in Health Care, 15*(112), 193–208.

Part 6.

FIELDWORK RESOURCES FOR STUDENTS

OVERVIEW OF PART 6

Donna Costa, DHS, OTR/L, FAOTA

Part 6 provides resources that may be helpful to students beginning their fieldwork experiences. Students across the country tend to ask the same kinds of questions, some of which are asked of American Occupational Therapy Association (AOTA) staff, so Chapter 29 is a reprint of an article from the AOTA website, "Answers to Your Fieldwork Questions," which contains the most frequently asked questions.

At the end of a Level II fieldwork experience, occupational therapy and occupational therapy assistant students are asked to complete the "Student Evaluation of Fieldwork Experience," reproduced in Chapter 30. Academic programs often use the results from this form for program evaluation purposes, and the form often is expanded to include additional information. Some programs keep these forms on file for future students to read to gain more information on a particular fieldwork site. Fieldwork educators should keep copies of this form and also use it as a way to evaluate the effectiveness of their fieldwork programs and provide feedback to fieldwork educators about the supervision they provided.

International fieldwork is a popular topic among students, who often ask their academic programs if they can complete fieldwork in another country. This book has several resources on international fieldwork, including Chapter 31, "Student Guide to Planning International Fieldwork."

Chapter 32, "Top 9 Things You Should Know Before Transitioning From the Classroom to Level II Fieldwork," Chapter 33, "Top 6 Tips for Navigating Relationships With Fieldwork Educators," and Chapter 34, "Framework for Fieldwork: Making the Most of Student–Educator Collaboration" contain reprints of articles from *OT Practice* or the AOTA website and contain helpful advice for students about to begin their fieldwork. Lastly, Chapter 35, "Fieldwork Opportunities at AOTA," contains information for students interested in doing fieldwork at the AOTA headquarters in Bethesda, MD. This is an experience that is particularly suited to students who want to focus on learning more about advocacy and organizational effectiveness.

Chapter 29.

ANSWERS TO YOUR FIELDWORK QUESTIONS

American Occupational Therapy Association

This information provides answers to students about fieldwork requirements, supervision, grading, difficulties with supervisors, failing, unfair treatment, accommodations for a disability, and international fieldwork.

Who Sets Fieldwork Requirements?

The Accreditation Council for Occupatioal Therapy Education (ACOTE®) Standards (ACOTE, 2012) are the official document that govern the length and types of fieldwork required for all students.

How Many Hours Are Required for Level I and Level II Fieldwork?

For Level I fieldwork, the American Occupational Therapy Association (AOTA) does not require a minimum number of hours. Each program sets the time requirements for students on Level I fieldwork. For Level II fieldwork, the Standards require a minimum of 24 weeks full-time for occupational therapy students and 16 weeks full-time for occupational therapy assistant students. This may be completed on a full-time or part-time basis, but may not be less than half-time, as defined by the fieldwork site. Your academic program determines the required time needed to complete both Level I and II fieldwork in your program. All students must complete the fieldwork required by their academic programs.

Are There Mandatory Types of Level II Fieldwork Required for All Students?

The Standards recommend that the student be exposed to a variety of clients across the lifespan and to a variety of settings. While AOTA does not mandate specific types of fieldwork, such as pediatrics or physical disabilities, individual academic programs do have the right to require specific types of fieldwork placement for their students.

How Many Days Off Are Allowed?

Time off during fieldwork is decided by the fieldwork site **and** the academic program. You should direct any questions about taking time off to your academic fieldwork coordinator and your fieldwork educator.

How Many Times May a Student Repeat Level II Fieldwork?

Because fieldwork is considered a part of your academic program, your school sets the policy on repeating Level II fieldwork. Check your college catalog or student handbook for a statement of your program's policy. Also, discuss this issue with your academic fieldwork coordinator to be sure that you understand the policy at your institution.

How Much Time Do You Have to Finish Level II Fieldwork?

The Standards do not specify time requirements for completion of Level II fieldwork. It should be completed in a reasonable amount of time. You should consult with your academic program if there are unusual circumstances that might make it difficult for you to complete fieldwork within their required time period.

Who Is Permitted to Supervise Students?

For Level I fieldwork, a student can be supervised by qualified personnel including, but not limited to, occupational therapy practitioners with initial national certification, psychologists, physician assistants, teachers, social workers, nurses, and physical therapists.

For Level II fieldwork, an occupational therapist can supervise an occupational therapy student as long as the therapist meets state regulations and has a minimum of 1 year of practice experience subsequent to the requisite initial certification. An occupational therapist or occupational therapy assistant who meets state regulations and has 1 year of practice experience subsequent to the requisite initial certification can supervise an occupational therapy assistant student.

What Is a Passing Grade for Level II Fieldwork?

Each academic program is responsible for determining its grading criteria. The academic program has the responsibility to assign a letter grade or pass/fail grade, and to determine the number of credit hours to be awarded for fieldwork.

What Should You Do If Your Fieldwork Grade Is Lower Than You Believe You Deserve?

Because fieldwork is considered part of your academic program, you will need to follow whatever grade appeal process your program or college requires. The steps involved in that process should be outlined in your college catalog or student handbook. Your academic program makes the final decision on your fieldwork grade.

What Should You Do If You Are Asked to Perform Above or Outside Your Level of Practice?

First, discuss this with your fieldwork educator. You may wish to check with the licensure board in the state where you are doing fieldwork for information defining the scope of practice. If you are unable to resolve this issue with the fieldwork site, contact your academic fieldwork coordinator.

What Should You Do If You Are Experiencing Difficulty During Level II Fieldwork?

The first step is to talk with your fieldwork educator. Before your meeting, try to write down what you perceive as the problems and develop a list of possible solutions. If you are still experiencing difficulty after meeting with your fieldwork educator, contact the academic fieldwork coordinator at your school for a different perspective and advice on other possible solutions. It is very important that the academic fieldwork coordinator hear from you if you are experiencing difficulty.

What Happens If You Fail Fieldwork and You Believe You Should Pass?

First, discuss the situation with your academic fieldwork coordinator. Should you wish to appeal your grade, you must follow the procedures required by your academic program or college. Check your student handbook or college catalog, or contact the Student Affairs office to learn about your school's procedure. Also, find out what your program's policy is on repeating a failed fieldwork. If repeating is a possibility, you should request another fieldwork placement to make up for the prior failure.

Can Your School Drop You From the Program for Failing Fieldwork? What Options Would You Have to Get a Degree?

Each academic program determines its own criteria for dropping a student from the program. You need to find out your school's policy. You may wish to appeal the decision according to the procedure for your school or program. Some possible options for students who have been dropped from occupational therapy education programs include transfer to another major that may have similar course requirements; career counseling; or application to another occupational therapy program. Should you decide to apply to another occupational therapy education program, be aware that the prospective school decides on whether or not your course credits will be accepted.

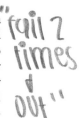

Are You Required to Tell the Fieldwork Site That You Have a Disability?

Under the Americans with Disability Act, occupational and occupational therapy assistant students with disabilities have the right to decide if and when they disclose their disability to the fieldwork site. Students with disabilities have the right to be seen as qualified capable students first, and second as students who have a disability. Discuss your decision to disclose with your academic fieldwork coordinator. Determine if you will need accommodations to fulfill the essential job functions for a student in your fieldwork setting. After a student is accepted for the fieldwork placement, the student, academic fieldwork coordinator, and fieldwork educator should determine the appropriate and most effective accommodations.

How Can You Find a Fieldwork Site Outside of Your State or Region?

First, you should talk with your academic fieldwork coordinator for suggestions. Generally speaking, it is not appropriate for students to contact fieldwork sites independently unless they are told to do so by their school. Another source of information is the state occupational therapy association in the state where you wish to find a fieldwork site. View a list of state occupational therapy associations contacts at http://www.aota.org/Advocacy-Policy/State-Policy.aspx. AOTA does not maintain a listing of current fieldwork sites.

Can You Do a Level II Fieldwork Outside of the United States?

Yes, depending on the policies of your academic program, you can do fieldwork outside the U.S., as long as the criteria listed in the Standards are followed. This is the criterion that must be met: "Ensure that the student completing Level II fieldwork outside the U.S. is supervised by an occupational therapist who has graduated from a program approved by the World Federation of Occupational Therapists (WFOT) and has 1 year of experience in practice. Such fieldwork shall not exceed 12 weeks."

How Do You Go About Filing a Formal Complaint If You Feel That You Have Been Treated Unfairly?

If you have not been able to resolve an unsatisfactory fieldwork situation with your academic program, you may wish to pursue a formal grievance procedure at your school. To do so, you must follow the steps outlined in the written information on your school or program's grievance process. See your program director for details.

What If You Believe That the Occupational Therapy Program at Your School Is Not in Compliance With the Standards?

You may initiate a formal complaint in letter form to ACOTE. ACOTE requires the complainant to demonstrate that reasonable efforts have been made to resolve the complaint, or to demonstrate that such efforts would be unsuccessful. ACOTE will not intervene on behalf of individuals or act as a court of appeal for students in matters of admission or dismissal. ACOTE will intervene only when it believes practices or conditions indicate the program may not be in substantial compliance with accreditation standards or established policies. For more information on the complaint procedure, see Accreditation Administrative Procedures (at http://www.aota.org/Education-Careers/Accreditation/Policies.aspx).

What If You Believe That Your Legal Rights Have Been Violated?

In this case, you may wish to consider seeking legal counsel. You should be aware that the courts have a history of upholding the judgment of professional educators on questions of student performance, but may rule in favor of the student when due process or civil rights have been violated.

Reference

Accreditation Council for Occupational Therapy Education. (2012). 2011 Accreditation Council for Occupational Therapy Education (ACOTE) Standards. *American Journal of Occupational Therapy, 66* (Suppl.), 56–74. http://dx.doi .org/10.5014/ajot.2012/6656

Reprinted from http://www.aota.org/Education-Careers/Fieldwork/Answers.aspx

Chapter 30.

STUDENT EVALUATION OF THE FIELDWORK EXPERIENCE (SEFWE)

American Occupational Therapy Association SEFWE Task Force

Purpose

This evaluation serves as a tool for fieldwork sites, academic programs, and students. The main objectives of this evaluation are to:

- Enable the Level II fieldwork student who is completing a placement at the site to evaluate and provide feedback to the supervisor and fieldwork setting;
- Enable academic programs, fieldwork sites, and fieldwork educators to benefit from student feedback in order to develop and refine their Level II fieldwork programs;
- Ensure that all aspects of the fieldwork program reflect the sequence, depth, focus, and scope of content of the curriculum design;

- Provide objective information to students who are selecting sites for future Level II fieldwork; and
- Provide a means of evaluation to ensure that fieldwork is performed in settings that provide educational experiences applicable to the academic program.

This form is designed to offer each program the opportunity to gather meaningful and useful information. Sections outlined with thick black double borders are designed to be customized by your program as needed. Pages involving evaluation of individual fieldwork educators have been positioned at the end of the form to allow academic programs to easily remove these pages before making them available for student review, if they choose to do so.

STUDENT EVALUATION OF THE FIELDWORK EXPERIENCE (SEFWE)

Instructions to the Student:
Complete this STUDENT EVALUATION OF THE FIELDWORK EXPERIENCE (SEFWE) form before your final meeting with your fieldwork supervisor(s). It is imperative that you review the form with your supervisor and that both parties sign on page 1. Copy the form so that a copy remains at the site and a copy is forwarded to your academic fieldwork coordinator at your educational program. This information may be reviewed by future students as well. The evaluation of the student Fieldwork Performance Evaluation (FWPE) should be reviewed first, followed by the Student Evaluation of the Fieldwork Experience (SEFWE), allowing the student to be honest and constructive.

Fieldwork Site _____ Site Code _____

Address _____

Placement Dates: from _____ to _____

Order of Placement: [ ] First   [ ] Second   [ ] Third   [ ] Fourth

Living accommodations: *(include type, cost, location, condition)*

Public transportation in the area:

Please write your email address here if you don't mind future students contacting you to ask you about your experience at this site: _____

We have mutually shared and clarified this Student Evaluation of the Fieldwork Experience report.

_____   _____
Student's Signature   FW Educator's Signature

_____   _____
Student's Name *(Please Print)*   FW Educator's Name and Credentials *(Please Print)*

FW Educator's years of experience _____

ORIENTATION

Indicate your view of the orientation by *checking* "Satisfactory" (S) or "Needs Improvement" (I) regarding the three factors of adequacy, organization, and timeliness.

TOPIC	Adequate		Organized		Timely		NA
	S	I	S	I	S	I	
1. Site-specific fieldwork objectives							
2. Student supervision process							
3. Requirements and assignments for students							
4. Student schedule (daily, weekly, monthly)							
5. Staff introductions							
6. Overview of physical facilities							
7. Agency or department mission							
8. Overview of organizational structure							
9. Services provided by the agency							
10. Agency or department policies and procedures							
11. Role of other team members							
12. Documentation procedures							
13. Safety and emergency procedures							
14. Confidentiality, HIPAA							
15. OSHA—Standard precautions							
16. Community resources for service recipients							
17. Department model of practice							
18. Role of occupational therapy services							
19. Methods for evaluating occupational therapy services							
20. Other							

Comments or suggestions regarding your orientation to this fieldwork placement:

_____

_____

_____

CASELOAD

List approximate number of each age category in your caseload.

Age	Number
0–3 years old	
3–5 years old	
6–12 years old	
13–21 years old	
22–65 years old	
>65 years old	

List approximate number of each primary condition, problem, or diagnosis in your caseload

Condition or Problem	Number

OCCUPATIONAL THERAPY PROCESS

Indicate the approximate number of screenings or evaluations you did; also indicate their value to your learning experience by *circling* the appropriate number, with #1 being *least valuable* and #5 being the *most valuable*.

	REQUIRED		HOW MANY	EDUCATIONAL VALUE
	Yes	No		
1. Client or patient screening				1 2 3 4 5
2. Client or patient evaluations *(Use specific names of evaluations)*				
				1 2 3 4 5
				1 2 3 4 5
				1 2 3 4 5
				1 2 3 4 5
				1 2 3 4 5
				1 2 3 4 5
				1 2 3 4 5
				1 2 3 4 5
				1 2 3 4 5
3. Written treatment or care plans				1 2 3 4 5
4. Discharge summary				1 2 3 4 5

List major therapeutic interventions frequently used and indicate whether it was provided individually, in group, co-treatment, or consultation. List other professionals involved.

Therapeutic Interventions	Individual	Group	Co-Tx	Consultation
Occupation-based activity, such as play, shopping, ADL, IADL, work, school activities (within client's own context with his or her goals)				
1.				
2.				
3.				
4.				
Purposeful activity (therapeutic context leading to occupation)				
1.				
2.				
3.				
4.				
Preparatory methods, such as sensory, PAMs, splinting, exercise (preparation for occupation-based activity)				
1.				
2.				
3.				
4.				

THEORY, FRAMES OF REFERENCE, MODELS OF PRACTICE

Indicate frequency of theory or frames of reference used.

	Never	Rarely	Occasionally	Frequently
Model of Human Occupation				
Occupational Adaptation				
Ecology of Human Performance				
Person–Environment–Occupation Model				
Biomechanical Frame of Reference				
Rehabilitation Frame of Reference				
Neurodevelopmental Theory				
Sensory Integration				
Behaviorism				
Cognitive Theory				
Cognitive Disability Frame of Reference				
Motor Learning Frame of Reference				
Other (list)				

FIELDWORK ASSIGNMENTS

List the types of assignments required of you at this placement (check all that apply), and indicate their educational value (1 = *not valuable*, 5 = *very valuable*).

	Case study applying the *Practice Framework*	1 2 3 4 5 N/A
	Evidence-based practice presentation: Topic:	1 2 3 4 5 N/A
	Revision of site-specific fieldwork objectives	1 2 3 4 5 N/A
	Program development Topic:	1 2 3 4 5 N/A
	In-service or presentation Topic:	1 2 3 4 5 N/A
	Research Topic:	1 2 3 4 5 N/A
	Other (list)	1 2 3 4 5

	1 = *Rarely* 2 = *Occasionally* 3 = *Frequently* 4 = *Consistently*			
ASPECTS OF THE ENVIRONMENT	1	2	3	4
Staff and administration demonstrated cultural sensitivity				
The *Practice Framework* was integrated into practice				
Student work area, supplies, and equipment were adequate				
Opportunities to collaborate with or supervise OTs, OTAs, or aides				
Opportunities to network with other professionals				
Opportunities to interact with other OT students				
Opportunities to interact with students from other disciplines				
Staff used a team approach to care				
Opportunities to observe role modeling of therapeutic relationships				
Opportunities to expand knowledge of community resources				
Opportunities to participate in research				
Additional educational opportunities (*specify*):				
How would you describe the pace of this setting? (circle one)	Slow	Med	Fast	
Types of documentation used in this setting:				
Ending student caseload expectation: _____ # of clients per week or day				
Ending student productivity expectation: _____ % per day (direct care)				

SUPERVISION

What was the primary model of supervision used? (check one)
- ☐ One supervisor : one student
- ☐ One supervisor : group of students
- ☐ Two supervisors : one student
- ☐ One supervisor : two students
- ☐ Distant supervision (primarily off-site)
- ☐ Three or more supervisors : one student (count person as supervisor if supervision occurred at least weekly)

List fieldwork educators who participated in your learning experience.

	Name	Credentials	Frequency	Individual	Group
1.					
2.					
3.					
4.					
5.					

ACADEMIC PREPARATION

Rate the relevance and adequacy of your academic coursework relative to the needs of **THIS** fieldwork placement, *circling* the appropriate number. (Note: may attach own course number.)

	Adequacy for Placement					Relevance for Placement				
	Low				High	Low				High
Anatomy and Kinesiology	1	2	3	4	5	1	2	3	4	5
Neurodevelopment	1	2	3	4	5	1	2	3	4	5
Human development	1	2	3	4	5	1	2	3	4	5
Evaluation	1	2	3	4	5	1	2	3	4	5
Intervention planning	1	2	3	4	5	1	2	3	4	5
Interventions (individual, group, activities, methods)	1	2	3	4	5	1	2	3	4	5
Theory	1	2	3	4	5	1	2	3	4	5
Documentation skills	1	2	3	4	5	1	2	3	4	5
Leadership	1	2	3	4	5	1	2	3	4	5
Professional behavior and communication	1	2	3	4	5	1	2	3	4	5
Therapeutic use of self	1	2	3	4	5	1	2	3	4	5
Level I fieldwork	1	2	3	4	5	1	2	3	4	5
Program development	1	2	3	4	5	1	2	3	4	5

What were the strongest aspects of your academic program relevant to preparing you for **THIS** Level II fieldwork experience? Indicate your top 5.

☐ Informatics	☐ Occ. as Life Org	☐ A & K	☐ Foundations	☐ Level I FW
☐ Pathology	☐ Neuro	☐ Administration	☐ Theory	☐ Peds electives
☐ Env. Competence	☐ Research courses	☐ Prog. design/eval	☐ Consult/collab.	☐ Older adult elect.
☐ Interventions	☐ Evaluations	☐ Adapting Env.	☐ Human comp.	☐ Community elect.
☐ Social Roles	☐ History	☐ Occupational Sci.	☐ Other:	

What changes would you recommend in your academic program relative to the needs of **THIS** Level II fieldwork experience?

_____

_____

_____

SUMMARY	1 = *Strongly disagree* 2 = *Disagree* 3 = *No opinion* 4 = *Agree* 5 = *Strongly agree*				
	1	2	3	4	5
Expectations of fieldwork experience were clearly defined					
Expectations were challenging but not overwhelming					
Experiences supported student's professional development					
Experiences matched student's expectations					

What particular qualities or personal performance skills do you feel that a student should have to function successfully on this fieldwork placement?

_____

_____

_____

What advice do you have for future students who wish to prepare for this placement?

• Study the following evaluations:

_____

_____

_____

• Study the following intervention methods:

_____

_____

_____

• Read up on the following in advance:

_____

_____

_____

Overall, what changes would you recommend in this Level II fieldwork experience?

_____

_____

_____

_____

Please feel free to add any further comments, descriptions, or information concerning your fieldwork at this site.

_____

_____

_____

_____

_____

Indicate the number that seems descriptive of each fieldwork educator. Please make a copy of this page for each individual.

	1 = *Strongly disagree* 2 = *Disagree* 3 = *No opinion* 4 = *Agree* 5 = *Strongly agree*

FIELDWORK EDUCATOR NAME: _____

FIELDWORK EDUCATOR YEARS OF EXPERIENCE: _____

	1	2	3	4	5
Provided ongoing positive feedback in a timely manner					
Provided ongoing constructive feedback in a timely manner					
Reviewed written work in a timely manner					
Made specific suggestions to student to improve performance					
Provided clear performance expectations					
Sequenced learning experiences to grade progression					
Used a variety of instructional strategies					
Taught knowledge and skills to facilitate learning and challenge student					
Identified resources to promote student development					
Presented clear explanations					
Facilitated student's clinical reasoning					
Used a variety of supervisory approaches to facilitate student performance					
Elicited and responded to student feedback and concerns					
Adjusted responsibilities to facilitate student's growth					
Supervision changed as fieldwork progressed					
Provided a positive role model of professional behavior in practice					
Modeled and encouraged occupation-based practice					
Modeled and encouraged client-centered practice					
Modeled and encouraged evidence-based practice					

Frequency and types of meetings with supervisor (value and frequency):

_____

_____

_____

_____

General comments on supervision:

_____

_____

_____

_____

AOTA SEFWE Task Force, June 2006

Chapter 31.

STUDENT GUIDE TO PLANNING INTERNATIONAL FIELDWORK

American Occupational Therapy Association Commission on Education

Purpose

1. Provide information and resources to support U.S. and non-U.S. student efforts in preparing to do fieldwork placements in countries other than where they received their academic preparation.
2. Facilitate the process of preparing for an international fieldwork by introducing issues to consider.
3. Ensure students are prepared for and able to meet expectations of an international fieldwork experience.
4. Promote questions to consider about international fieldwork.

Introduction

Preparing for fieldwork can be a daunting task, especially when doing so for a placement outside of the country where one's academic preparation took place. This document is intended to be an introduction to topics and issues that should be addressed prior to embarking on an international fieldwork. Addressing the issues raised in this document is only one aspect of preparation for successful international fieldwork. It is recommended that the accompanying documents and guides be reviewed as well.

Items to Consider

For occupational therapy (OT) students prepared in the U.S. and doing fieldwork in another country:

- Meet the Accreditation Council for Occupational Therapy Education's (ACOTE®) Standard for international fieldwork educator: Identify methods of documentation to address ACOTE B.10.22 that ensure that students attending Level II fieldwork outside the United States are supervised by an occupational therapist who graduated from a program approved by the World Federation of Occupational Therapists and has 1 year of experience in practice. Such fieldwork must not exceed 12 weeks for occupational therapy students and 8 weeks for occupational therapy assistant students (ACOTE, 2007a, b, & c).
- Identify the national model (if any) for OT fieldwork implementation that may influence the fieldwork experience (e.g., in Japan, fieldwork can be separated into different areas of focus, such as evaluation and intervention).

- Increase student familiarity with the service system in the receiving country, potentially including the following: national health care policies, community practice norms, reimbursement policies, documentation expectations, and attitudes toward disability.
- Identify the fieldwork site's requirements for student professional liability insurance, workers' compensation insurance, immunizations, criminal background checks, health requirements (e.g., bloodwork, medical exam, drug screening), and so forth.
- Determine the fieldwork administration process, including student fieldwork objectives, student evaluation, student evaluation of fieldwork experience, system for communicating with and providing feedback to the student, and strategies to prevent problems.
- Identify cultural and unique aspects of language (terminology, idioms) to become familiar with prior to fieldwork (e.g., in the UK, *learning disability* is a broad term that includes developmental disability).
- Understand OT entry-level practice expectations and adequate preparation for taking the National Board for Certification in Occupational Therapy (NBCOT) certification exam. Consider whether the fieldwork experience at this potential fieldwork site will provide an applicable/generalizable background in OT practice that supports knowledge, clinical reasoning, and judgment to be successful in taking the NBCOT certification exam.

Items to Consider

For OT students prepared in another country and doing fieldwork in the U.S.:
- Become familiar with common practice models and legislation reflecting the OT practice setting (e.g., IDEA public school laws related to provision of OT, Medicare guidelines for OT reimbursement).
- Understand U.S. OT service reimbursement models (Medicare, Medicaid, workers' compensation).
- Explore potential fieldwork site's requirements for student professional liability insurance, workers' compensation insurance, immunizations, criminal background checks, health requirements (e.g., bloodwork, medical exam, drug screening), and so forth.

- Understand OT entry-level practice expectations and adequate preparation for meeting home country expectations for OT practice. Ensure that the fieldwork experience in the U.S. will provide an applicable/generalizable background in OT practice that supports knowledge, clinical reasoning, and judgment to be successful as an OT in home country.
- Explore cultural and unique aspects of language (terminology, idioms) to become familiar with prior to fieldwork (e.g., in the UK, *learning disability* is a broad term that includes developmental disability while in the U.S. it does not).
- Provide support for the student's transition back to the home country, culture, and OT practice.

Student-Centered Issues

- Explore characteristics of the potential OT practice setting to ensure there is a good match for student, fieldwork site, supervisory style, and student learning needs.
- Ensure there is a support system that fully endorses the placement academically, professionally, and personally.
- Ensure the student is aware of cultural diversity issues that may have an impact on OT practice and personal life while abroad.
- Ensure there is an emotional/social support system for the student.
- Ensure student has the financial wherewithal to afford day-to-day expenses to live, eat, and shelter.
- Ensure the student has an appropriate passport and/or visa to enter and remain in the receiving country.
- Ensure the student has the means for health insurance coverage in the receiving country and access to medical health services if needed.
- Ensure the student has the necessary vaccinations and medications for the receiving country.
- Ensure the student has access to emergency evacuation resources (e.g., International Student Travel Card).
- Prepare an emergency plan, including contact information and contingency plan for emergencies.
  - Specify contingency plan for emergencies.
  - Register time abroad with the U.S. Department of State if the student is a U.S. citizen.
  - Identify if the student's country of origin requires registration with the country's embassy in the U.S.

- Obtain emergency contact information for the student and the academic OT/OTA program.
- Obtain home country embassy contact information.
- Obtain State Department travel advisory information, which can be received via email from the U.S. Department of State.
- Prepare a terrorist attack contingency plan.
- Obtain waiver of liability for academic OT/OTA program.

Student responsibilities to ensure shared/realistic expectations of international fieldwork:

- Be responsible for clarifying the learning opportunities and ensuring quality OT practice should be shared between the academic fieldwork coordinator (AFWC), student, and fieldwork educator.
- Communicate with the AFWC about and advocate for their corresponding academic OT/OTA preparation and curriculum model (e.g., Is student adequately prepared to meet expectations for OT practice in this setting?).
- Explore cultural differences (e.g., tea breaks in some cultures allow networking with team) and unique aspects of language (e.g., idioms) to become familiar with prior to fieldwork.
- Identify whether the student possesses sufficient verbal and written fluency with potential clients' language.
- Become familiar with customary etiquette in another country (cultural and social norms are often taken for granted until broken).

Considering international OT practice:

- Explore certification and licensure procedures for practice within the receiving country in order to determine the required academic and fieldwork standards and requirements that must be complied with prior to completion of the academic OT/OTA program.

Resources

1. U.S. Department of State, regarding international travel: http://travel.state.gov/content/passports/english.html
2. Centers for Disease Control and Prevention, regarding international travel: http://wwwnc.cdc.gov/travel/
3. International Student Identity Card: http://www.isic.org
4. STA Travel: http://www.statravel.com/
5. AOTA website with content related to fieldwork: http://www.aota.org/Educate/EdRes/Fieldwork.aspx
6. WFOT Accredited OT programs: http://www.wfot.org/schoolLinks.asp
7. WFOT country profiles: http://www.wfot.org/countries.asp
8. NBCOT: http://www.nbcot.org/
9. OT Connections: http://otconnections.aota.org/; a few groups currently exist about international OT, including "Global Initiatives" and "OTs in Developing Countries"
10. Embassies and Consulates Around the World: http://www.embassy.goabroad.com

References

Accreditation Council for Occupational Therapy Education. (2007a). Accreditation standards for a doctoral-degree-level educational program for the occupational therapist. *American Journal of Occupational Therapy, 61,* 641–651. http://dx.doi.org/10.5014/ajot.61.6.641

Accreditation Council for Occupational Therapy Education. (2007b). Accreditation standards for a master's-degree-level educational program for the occupational therapist. *American Journal of Occupational Therapy, 61,* 652–661. http://dx.doi.org/10.5014/ajot.61.6.652

Accreditation Council for Occupational Therapy Education. (2007c). Accreditation standards for an educational program for the occupational therapy assistant. *American Journal of Occupational Therapy, 61,* 662–671. http://dx.doi.org/10.5014/ajot.61.6.662

Prepared by

International Fieldwork Ad Hoc Committee for the Commission on Education (1/26/09).

Patricia Crist, PhD, OTR/L, FAOTA *(Chair)— Duquesne University, PA*
Naomi Greenberg, MPH, PhD, OTR—*LaGuardia Community College, NY*

Susan K. Meyers, EdD, OTR—*Private Foundation, IN*

Susan Mullholland MSc (rehab), BScOT, OT(c)—*University of Alberta*

Patty Stutz-Tanenbaum, MS, OTR—*Colorado State University, CO*

Pamela Richardson, PhD, OTR/L, FAOTA—*San Jose University, CA*

Debra Tupe, MS, OTR—*Columbia University, NY*

Neil Harvison, PhD, OTR/L—*AOTA Staff*

Emerging Leaders Development Program Participant:
Juleen Rodakowski, OTD, OTR/L

Reprinted from http://www.aota.org/-/media/Corporate/Files/EducationCareers/Educators/International/Student%20Guide%20to%20Planning%20International%20FWfinalnh.pdf

Chapter 32.

TOP 9 THINGS YOU SHOULD KNOW BEFORE TRANSITIONING FROM THE CLASSROOM TO LEVEL II FIELDWORK

Scott Ingraham, OTR/L
Assembly of Student Delegates Advocacy and Communications Chairperson
The University of Findlay, Findlay, OH

As soon-to-be occupational therapy (OT) practitioners, we know how important transitions can be for our clients. But what are we doing ourselves to prepare for the transition from the classroom to fieldwork? Here are some tips to help ease you into fieldwork:

1. **Read up on prior students' experiences.** It is likely that your academic program keeps files from past students that you can review. Use this information when choosing a fieldwork placement and when preparing for your fieldwork site after it has been confirmed. These files can provide valuable information on what subject material to review, populations you may work with, services that you may provide, and other helpful details.

2. **Prior to your fieldwork, contact your fieldwork educator (FWE) through a formal letter or email to introduce yourself.** Consider asking about the following:
   - Subject material that you should review (e.g., theories or frames of reference, screens, assessments, evaluations, typical diagnoses)
   - Any paperwork, training, medical examinations, or testing you must complete
   - Dress code
   - Directions, parking, where and when to meet on the first day
   - If your FWE would like to talk further over the phone or arrange a site visit prior to your fieldwork.

3. **If you need to take time off, plan it ASAP!** If you know you will need to miss days or need to come in late or leave early, speak with your FWE as soon as you can so that plans can be made for caseload coverage and makeup time.

4. **Ask the fieldwork coordinator (FWC) at your school for support and assistance when you need it.** Make sure you are open and clear with your FWC about your interests and needs so that he or she can find a site that is a good fit for you. If you have concerns about your fieldwork site and don't feel comfortable addressing your FWE directly, your FWC is there to help you work out your issues.

5. **Rest assured that your education has prepared you for fieldwork.** You are where you need to be—you attended an accredited school and you passed your classes to this point. The most important knowledge you have yet to gain will come from hands-on clinical experience. If you are feeling lost and overwhelmed, remind yourself that you are just beginning in the field, almost every student and entry-level practitioner can sympathize, and you will feel more competent with time.

6. **You won't always be placed at your ideal fieldwork and that is okay.** While your program makes every attempt to place you in a setting and location that you choose, sometimes fate intervenes and you end up in places and settings you never imagined. Approach this as an opportunity with a positive attitude and learn as much as you can. This will help you develop into a well-rounded practitioner and you might end up loving it! Whether your experience is positive or negative, realize that you will learn a lot. When you are feeling stressed or overworked, keep in mind the skills you are gaining. If your environment isn't as supportive as you had hoped, you will learn what not to do when you are a practitioner and how to face challenging situations. Keeping that in mind, don't hesitate to speak with your FWC at your school if your concerns are related to ethical, safety, or more serious issues.

7. **Staying professional at all times also means keeping your fieldwork life and your personal social media life separate.** Do not consider adding staff members to your social media accounts until after you have completed your fieldwork. Never share pictures, information about clients or coworkers, or mention your fieldwork setting in social media. Likewise, monitor your posts and pictures to make sure you aren't sharing anything that you wouldn't want your FWE or clients to see. Keep in mind that no matter how much you protect your accounts, information can become public.

8. **Meet with your FWE regularly.** During a busy day, it can be hard to find an appropriate time to address your questions and concerns. Schedule time to meet with your FWE regularly to ask questions and gather feedback on your performance. Ask about what you are doing well and what you need to focus on next. Consider filling out a weekly student review form.

9. **Make time for yourself outside of fieldwork to do something that makes you feel at ease and competent.** Fieldwork can be stressful in a different way than school and can leave you questioning your abilities as a future OT practitioner. Whether it is yoga, counseling, reading, time with friends and family, or pursing other interests, you need time to step away, decompress, and feel good about yourself. With the right balance of work and personal time, you will likely find yourself feeling more refreshed and confident on fieldwork.

Good luck!

Special acknowledgment and thanks to Heather Meredith, OTR/L, Fieldwork Coordinator at the University of Findlay for her support during my fieldwork transition.

Reprinted from http://www.aota.org/Education-Careers/Students/Pulse/Archive/fieldwork/Transition-to-Fieldwork.aspx

Chapter 33.

TOP 6 TIPS FOR NAVIGATING RELATIONSHIPS WITH FIELDWORK EDUCATORS

Melissa S. Reed
Springfield College, Springfield, MA

Heidi Carpenter
Creighton University, Omaha, NE

When you are a student, the prospect of leaving the safety and comfort of the classroom; campus resources; and familiar professors, staff, and friends for Level II fieldwork can be unsettling. Fieldwork placements vary tremendously, and each site holds unique challenges. When transitioning to your fieldwork site, it is important to remember that as a student, you are there to learn, first and foremost.

Most fieldwork educators (FWEs) recognize that students will make mistakes, ask a plethora of questions, come from diverse backgrounds, and have different experiences and comfort levels with the setting. Your supervisor is likely to be understanding and helpful through this experience, but as a student you may find it stressful to be observed and critiqued on a regular basis and to navigate a relationship with someone who is likely to be different from you in some aspects, whether it be communication style, personality, routines, organization, or learning and teaching approaches.

Building a relationship with your FWE requires skills that are similar to building a relationship with your clients. A candid relationship between fieldwork student and educator can facilitate successful application of classroom knowledge into clinical practice and prepare students to confidently enter into the profession. To gain the most out of your fieldwork experience, consider using the following tips for developing a strong relationship with your FWE.

1. **Communicate often** with your FWE. Schedule regular meetings to discuss your caseload, ask questions, discuss concerns, and set goals for your remaining time during fieldwork. Consider filling out a weekly review form. Setting this time aside should make it easier to approach your FWE and ensures that important issues are discussed in a timely way, and not put to the side.

2. **Be professional** at all times. Remember, this is a professional job (even though a paycheck is not involved). The impressions you make during fieldwork matter and can make or break the ability to use your FWE as a reference for a future job. We all get frustrated and need to vent, but save this for your mother, friend, or cat. Your FWE does not need to hear about it. If you are feeling overwhelmed during fieldwork, find a way to vent in a healthy manner, such as taking a short walk or stepping outside to practice some deep breathing. Avoid addressing difficult issues with your FWE when your emotions are high. If there are serious concerns you feel need to be addressed with your FWE, find a way to do it calmly and professionally. Sometimes writing down the concerns and reading them helps and takes some pressure off. Consider refining professional behavior as important as demonstrating competency with clinical skills.

3. **Be open** to suggestions for improvement and feedback from your FWE. Unless you're one of that rare breed who agrees with everything everyone says, you are going to disagree with your FWE, and that is okay—in fact it is good, because it means you are able to think for yourself. Keep in mind that your FWE has a different perspective and experience level than you and offers critiques not to make you feel bad, but to help you learn. Encourage your FWE to express feedback to you and let yourself be open and listen to what he or she has to say.

4. **Share** what you learned in school. Most FWEs value not only teaching students, but learning from them as well. If you find your supervisor using techniques that are outdated or conflict with current evidence-based practice, take the time to understand why your FWE uses those techniques and ask if he or she would be open to a possible adjustment. When trying new approaches at your fieldwork site, you must be able to point to the evidence and be able to have a well-versed conversation to justify your approach.

5. **Be the best you can be** in every moment, every day of your fieldwork. You don't have to give 110% all of the time, and you will not know all the answers, but your FWE does not expect that. However, your FWE does expect you to be fully engaged, and by trying your best with every client encounter, every note, and every interaction, you will increase the likelihood of retaining and learning more than you thought possible. Even when you make mistakes, which will be inevitable, your FWE will appreciate your hard work and good intentions to make the most out of your experience.

6. **Be proactive** when it comes to identifying the needs of your patients and the site. Review clinical conditions, assessments, and evidence-based practice techniques; always be prepared for your sessions; and try to anticipate what your FWE might need you to do. Most FWEs appreciate not having to delegate tasks at every moment and will value your proactivity, as long as you have demonstrated your competence and you do not overstep supervision policies and guidelines.

Reprinted from http://www.aota.org/Education-Careers/Students/Pulse/Archive/fieldwork/RelationshipsonFieldwork.aspx

Chapter 34.

FRAMEWORK FOR FIELDWORK: MAKING THE MOST OF STUDENT–EDUCATOR COLLABORATION

Ideas from the Cleveland Clinic Children's Hospital for Rehabilitation for successfully organizing the occupational therapy fieldwork experience

Danielle R. Petrozelle MS, OTR/L, and Rebecca Iscrupe, MS

As university programs swell with occupational therapy students, a new challenge emerges: The need for fieldwork educators (FWE) is at an all-time high (Kirke, Layton, & Sim, 2007). At Cleveland Clinic Children's Hospital for Rehabilitation (CCCHR), Level II fieldwork students frequent the facility during summer and fall months. Hosting fieldwork students has been beneficial for all involved parties: Students gain clinical skills in a challenging pediatric environment, fieldwork educators earn continuing education units (CEUs) necessary for licensure, and the student contributes fresh ideas to the facility. This article, written in collaboration between a Level II fieldwork student and her fieldwork educator, outlines the teaching approach used at CCCHR, with the aim of providing fieldwork educators with ideas for successfully organizing the fieldwork experience.

A quality student placement is one in which learning is optimal and individualized to meet students' needs (Kirke et al., 2007). A recent study completed in Australia identified a welcoming atmosphere, detailed orientation, clear expectations, graded learning experiences, and quality modeling as key factors in a successful fieldwork experience (Rodger, Fitzgerland, Davila, Millar, & Allison, 2011). At CCCHR, these factors are addressed with pre-fieldwork recommendations for preparation, a 12-week student schedule with graded learning opportunities, structured journaling, and project/in-service completion that is research-based and provides opportunity to reflect on what is learned during the fieldwork experience.

Pre-Fieldwork Preparation

Research shows that students who considered pre-fieldwork preparation to be beneficial tended to have a higher degree of satisfaction with their fieldwork experience (Chiang, Pang, Li, Shin, & Su, 2012).

Fieldwork educators indicate that they have limited time to re-teach basic skills due to the demands of clinical practice, and therefore greatly appreciate a student who reviews these concepts prior to beginning the fieldwork experience. Students, in consultation with their academic advisors, should review basic skills, including manual muscle testing; range of motion; subjective, objective, assessment, and plan (SOAP) notes; and medical terminology. They should also have a general understanding of occupation and activities of daily living (Knecht-Sabres, Kovic, St. Amand, & Wallingford, 2012). This prior level of knowledge is important because it is necessary in order for new skills to be learned, implemented, and refined (Holmes et al., 2010).

In addition, the fieldwork educator can facilitate student preparedness with pre-fieldwork communication. At CCCHR, the student receives a letter at least 1 month prior to arrival indicating more advanced materials for review. These include a list of frequently treated conditions, recommended readings specific to the areas of practice to be covered during the experience, and a list of assessment tools used at the facility. Recommended readings and review items serve as a beginning point for conversations between the fieldwork educator and student.

At some point prior to beginning the fieldwork, it is also important that the student and fieldwork educator exchange general knowledge of one another in preparation for future interactions. Important details that a fieldwork educator should gather about the student include settings of previous fieldwork experiences, preferred learning and communication styles, and long-term clinical interests. The student will be interested in knowing the fieldwork educator's number of years in practice and areas of expertise. AOTA offers a Fieldwork Data Form and Personal Data Sheet that can be helpful in gathering and exchanging this information between the student and fieldwork educator (www.aota.org).

Elements of the 12-Week Schedule

Developing and implementing a 12-week schedule is another opportunity to outline clear expectations for the student. Of course, the original plan can be altered to meet the individual needs of the fieldwork educator and the student as time passes. The CCCHR Level II fieldwork schedule incorporates several important principles:

a checklist for orientation, a list of clinical practices and modalities (e.g., casting, splinting, taping) that the student should be exposed to during the experience, graded exposure and expectations for documentation, and recommendations for a workload that increases in both number of clients and level of difficulty over time.

Checklist for orientation. Orientation should be thorough, and for larger facilities may take 1 to 2 days to complete. The fieldwork educator should introduce the student to clinical staff, including other occupational therapists, occupational therapy assistants, students, physical therapists, speech therapists, managers, and rehab assistants/techs. Special attention should be given to the individuals with whom the student will be in contact most often. The fieldwork educator should provide a tour of the facility, detailing locations for treatment materials, evaluation materials, and available treatment spaces. Easily overlooked, but perhaps most important, the fieldwork educator should show the student the locations of restrooms and staff lounges, point out spaces for storing materials and personal belongings, and explain the lunch procedure. Chiang, Pang, Li, Shih, and Su (2012) found that 49.3% of fieldwork students surveyed were not sure of or not satisfied with the personal space provided at fieldwork sites, with the greatest percentage of these students completing fieldwork in the hospital setting. To improve the level of satisfaction and student perceptions of the therapy department, all students should be granted some space, regardless of how small, that they can call their own during the 12-week experience. Students who receive personal space in an office shared by other occupational therapy practitioners will also benefit from informal learning opportunities. Community office space enables collaboration and interactions with practitioners that further promotes clinical growth.

Clinical practices and modalities. The fieldwork educator is responsible for exposing the student to the intervention process, including evaluating, treating, and discharging the clients. At CCCHR, daily exposure to sensory integrative approaches, self-care development, bilateral upper extremity strengthening, and neurodevelopmental techniques is typical. Treatment strategies—including casting, splinting, constraint-induced therapy, and Kinesio taping—occur at varying rates, depending on the needs of current clients. Although the student's workload may not warrant these less common modalities, it is expected that the fieldwork educator expose the student to these forms of practice. This can be done through hands-on demonstration with the student, or by permitting the student to spend time observing other therapists when they are using these techniques. A checklist of these and similar items is placed at the beginning of the 12-week schedule. Although the student will not gain independence performing these somewhat advanced techniques, the ability to observe them promotes a better understanding of total practice and the necessity for ongoing continuing education.

Graded exposure to documentation. The 12-week schedule at CCCHR begins with SOAP notes, which promote organized note taking for the student, leaving less room for errors and omissions. Students begin documentation during their first or second day of fieldwork, learning to document the intervention strategies and client response for sessions modeled by the fieldwork educator. The fieldwork educator encourages the student to write notes detailing the level of assistance provided by the treating fieldwork educator, the client's physical and emotional response to treatment, adaptive responses, and client position during targeted occupations. Initial review of student documentation allows the fieldwork educator to evaluate the student's clinical reasoning skills and level of knowledge retained from previous course work. In 2010, Holmes et al. indicated that students who completed 1,000 hours of fieldwork (the standard established by the World Federation of Occupational Therapists) frequently still fell below competence in practice knowledge, clinical reasoning, and facilitating change, as measured by the Competency Based Fieldwork Evaluation Scale. Therefore, it is important to introduce, model, and review these skills early in the fieldwork experience.

During the first week, focus is placed solely on daily intervention notes. Once the student becomes efficient with SOAP note documentation, the transition to narrative documentation is made if desired. The skills developed during the SOAP note process allow for greater clarity and thoroughness in narrative documentation. During the second and consecutive weeks, the student is introduced to progress summaries, written home exercise programs, evaluations, and discharge summaries. Sufficient time is allowed for skill mastery in each category prior to introducing a new documentation domain.

Workload recommendations. The 12-week schedule provides graded expectations for developing workloads. The schedule provides ample time for observation and hands-on learning. Depending on the treatment setting and complexity of the client population, the student begins planning and leading treatment sessions in the first or second weeks of placement. The workload can further be graded by building the student's workload, with the least complicated clients initially and more complicated clients later in the fieldwork experience. Students also benefit from sustained workloads, which can be defined as maintaining the same clients over time, with occasional gaps in workload growth. Students completing their outpatient fieldworks at CCCHR maintain a workload, without adding new clients, in weeks 6, 8, and 10 to 12. This provides the student with additional time to focus on current clients, equipment requests, and documentation for those clients. A sustained workload is most beneficial in settings requiring long-term care—skilled nursing facilities, outpatient facilities, and inpatient rehabilitation hospitals. This is not a practical approach to be used in acute care settings, where clients are quickly discharged.

Structured Journaling

Journaling is a critical aspect of a successful fieldwork at CCCHR. A template is used for a structured one-page journal entry that the student completes each week. Each journal entry consists of a clinical observation reflecting a specific client or treatment session. Specific skills, such as formulating a detailed description of a client's body mechanics, analyzing a task, and creating a relevant treatment note, can be addressed in this section of the journal template.

Other sections of the journal include things the student did well, things the student would like to improve, and methods to improve these skills. The journal template at CCCHR also includes a space to record the number of clients on the student's workload, a 1 to 5 scale (very easy to very difficult) for how the student regards the current workload, and a similar scale for how the student is generally feeling (bored to overwhelmed). The journal is mainly completed by the student, but each entry does reserve a section for fieldwork educator comments. In a study done in 2011, Rodger, Fitzgerald, Davila, Miller, and Allison stated that the single most important part of students' learning during their placement was the timely feedback given by their fieldwork educator.

During the journaling process, both constructive criticism and strengths are shared with the student. This is also a place for the fieldwork educator to establish goals for the student in upcoming weeks that the 12-week fieldwork schedule may not illustrate (such as improving caregiver interactions).

The structured journaling process is used to document both strengths and weaknesses. This gives the student opportunity to track progression throughout the 12 weeks, and also to review previous weeks and self-reflect when necessary. Successful Level II fieldwork placements are focused on an overall flourishing learning experience. Self-reflection allows a student to self-identify strengths and weaknesses and to focus on specific skill acquisition throughout the learning process (Hanson, Larsen, & Nielsen, 2011). Positive self-reflection promotes an overall feeling of accomplishment and personal growth.

Student In-Service and Project

Students at CCCHR complete an in-service presentation and project prior to completing fieldwork. The in-service presentation allows the student to reflect on what he or she learned during the fieldwork experience. The student can choose a topic that occupational therapists and occupational therapy assistants within the department want to learn more about or simply one that the student finds interesting. In-service topics may include client case studies, recent medical developments, emerging treatment techniques, or demonstrations of treatment equipment. Most important, because evidence-based practice is what provides meaning to our work as practitioners, the in-service should reference research and include an accurate bibliography.

Project completion is an excellent approach to developing student creativity. The student should choose a project that will fulfill a facility need. Ideas for projects that have benefitted our facility include fabricating low-tech equipment (e.g., buttoning boards, fine motor games), implementing facility blogs or websites, and developing family resource handouts. The possibilities are endless.

These assignments allow the student and facility to grow. The therapy department gains new knowledge, while the student becomes an overall contributor to the therapy team.

Other Ways to Make Fieldwork Successful

There are many other approaches to developing successful fieldwork education programs. A fieldwork educator can implement all or some of the following strategies to make the fieldwork experience unique. The fieldwork educator may also want to review the options on this list with the student to determine what is attainable, as a collaborative approach to planning the 12-week experience.

Attend a continuing education course. Practitioners are required to constantly learn new techniques and keep up-to-date with emerging practice areas, and therefore they should model advanced learning for their students. Fieldwork educators and fieldwork sites should require students to attend conferences or continuing education courses if offered by the facility during the student's 12-week placement. Attendance at a course provides the student with an opportunity to learn more in-depth material about a specific area of practice, and a better understanding of requirements to retain licensure and registration.

Promote interactions with other students. Interaction among fieldwork students in occupational therapy and other disciplines is an important contributor to a successful fieldwork experience. It establishes a peer outlet in which successes and failures can be shared. Students are likely to feel equal to their peers, as compared with inferior to licensed practitioners, and therefore may be more inclined to exchange ideas and collaborate to solve problems.

Promote interactions with other occupational therapists and occupational therapy assistants. The fieldwork educator should encourage the student to spend time observing other staff practitioners. This exposes the student to a variety of personalities and intervention approaches. When treating, the student will develop autonomy by imitating the skills acquired from several role models and develop a unique treatment style.

Determine learning styles. A study by Jensen and Daniel (2010) found that a student's learning and communication styles are two very important factors affecting the fieldwork experience. Knowledge of these factors permits the fieldwork educator to present material in a way that best accommodates the student, based on whether the student is a visual or hands-on learner, and to know how the student may react to and prefer to receive feedback. Preferred learning and communication styles can be determined through informal conversation, or by using a structured learning inventory.

Involve a third party. Third-party involvement can benefit both the student and the fieldwork educator. At CCCHR, a fieldwork coordinator assigns and supervises fieldwork educators and students. During the 12-week placement, this coordinator serves as third-party support, monitoring the fieldwork experience by meeting regularly with both parties. If a serious problem were to arise, the fieldwork educator and/or student would be able to report the concern to the coordinator and the coordinator would then mediate as necessary. The third-party participant should emphasize an "open-door" policy for the student. This person should also have previous experience as an educator in order to provide guidance, when necessary, to the fieldwork educator.

Complete the AOTA Fieldwork Educator Certificate Program. Prior to hosting a Level II student, attend the AOTA-sponsored Fieldwork Educator Certificate Program (www.aota.org). Course attendees receive a certificate and 15 contact hours toward licensure renewal. Course objectives include: obtain a deeper understanding for the fieldwork educator role, integrate learning theories and supervisory models, and increase skills to provide high-quality educational opportunities.

Maintain communication. Communication between the student's university and the fieldwork placement site throughout the entire fieldwork process is crucial for program success. In 2011, Hanson recommended beginning consistent communication with the academic program within the second week of placement and maintaining open communication throughout the fieldwork experience. Open communication further enhances the experience for the academic program and the fieldwork site. The academic program becomes increasingly familiar with the demands of the fieldwork site, as well as the strengths and weaknesses exhibited by their own students. The fieldwork site grows increasingly knowledgeable about academic standards and university expectations. The student

significantly benefits from this interaction as well. Academic advisors from the student's university can assist the fieldwork educator in handling problematic student situations. The student will likely feel more comfortable discussing problems with a familiar advisor from the university.

Conclusion

Academic programs continue to grow, requiring an increased number of students to complete Level I and Level II placements. There are many ways to build and structure the fieldwork as an educator. The strategies outlined in this article, used together or separately, can help provide a foundation for successful fieldwork experiences.

References

Chiang, H., Pang, C., Li, W., Shih, Y., & Su, C. (2012). An investigation of the satisfaction and perception of fieldwork experiences among occupational therapy students. *Hong Kong Journal of Occupational Therapy, 22*(1), 9–16. http://dx.doi.org/10.1016/j.hkjot.20112.04.001

Hanson, D. (2011). The perspectives of fieldwork educators regarding Level II fieldwork students. *Occupational Therapy in Health Care, 25*, 164–177. http://dx.doi.org/10.3109/0738 0577.2011.561420

Hanson, D., Larsen, J. K., & Nielsen, S. (2011). Reflective writing in Level II fieldwork: A tool to promote clinical reasoning. *OT Practice, 16*(7), 11–14.

Holmes, J., Bossers, A., Polatajko, H., Drynan, D., Gallagher, M., O'Sullivan, C., & Denney, J. (2010). 1000 fieldwork hours: Analysis of multi-site evidence. *Canadian Journal of Occupational Therapy, 77*, 135–143. http://dx.doi.org/10.2182/cjot.2010.77.3.2

Jensen, L., & Daniel, C. (2010). A descriptive study on Level II fieldwork supervision in hospital settings. *Occupational Therapy in Health Care, 24*(4), 341.

Kirke, P., Layton, N., & Sim, J. (2007). Informing fieldwork design: Key elements to quality in fieldwork education for undergraduate occupational therapy students. *Australian Occupational Therapy Journal, 44*, 147–157. http://dx.doi.org/10.1111/j.1440-1630.2007.00696.x

Knecht-Sabres, L., Kovic, M., St. Amand, L., & Wallingford, M. (2012, April/May). OT students: Meeting the current demands of

OT practice. *The Communique, 2,* 6–8. Retrieved from http://www.ilota.org/assets/documents/communique/ilota_may2012.pdf

Rodger, S., Fitzgerald, C., Davila, W., Millar, F., & Allison, H. (2011). What makes a quality occupational therapy practice placement? Students' and practice educators' perspectives. *Australian Occupational Therapy Journal, 58,* 195–202. http://dx.doi.org/10.1111/j.1440-1630.2010.00903.x

Danielle Petrozelle, MS, OTR/L, is a pediatric occupational therapist at Cleveland Clinic Children's Hospital for Rehabilitation and Cleveland Clinic Center for Autism. She graduated from Gannon University with a master's in occupational therapy in 2007. She completed a collaborative learning fieldwork at the Mayo Clinic in 2006. Petrozelle attended AOTA's Fieldwork Educator Certificate Workshop.

Rebecca Iscrupe, MS, completed her Level II occupational therapy fieldwork at Cleveland Clinic Children's Hospital for Rehabilitation. She earned her bachelor's degree in health science in 2012 and graduated with her master's in occupational therapy in May 2013 from Gannon University. Iscrupe's future includes seeking a career in pediatric occupational therapy.

See more at: http://www.aota.org/Publications-News/otp/Archive/2013/7-22-13/Framework.aspx#sthash.ZQYVC1Sl.dpuf

Chapter 35.

FIELDWORK OPPORTUNITIES AT AOTA

American Occupational Therapy Association

Fieldwork experience at the American Occupational Therapy Association's (AOTA's) headquarters is available to occupational therapy student members who will have completed their academic coursework prior to an AOTA fieldwork experience. (Special exceptions may be made on a case-by-case basis.) Occupational therapy assistant (OTA) students may apply for an OTA fieldwork opportunity as an optional third fieldwork.

Fieldwork at AOTA headquarters offers students the opportunity to gain and strengthen their analytical, organizational, communications, and advocacy skills while increasing their knowledge of AOTA. In addition, students will have the opportunity to meet national volunteer leaders. Finally, students may be involved in national projects and activities in the following areas:

- Practice (e.g., pediatrics, driving, ethics)
- Evidence-based practice (e.g., help create and communicate EBP resources)
- Research dissemination and advocacy (e.g., assist with creating resources, writing comments to National Institutes of Health)

- Annual Conference & Expo planning
- Professional development (continuing education)
- Federal affairs* (assist with monitoring legislation, advocacy, AOTPAC)
- Reimbursement and regulatory policy*
- State policy.*

How to Apply

Interested candidates should contact AOTA's Academic Affairs for an application packet via email at slin@aota.org. A fieldwork agreement will need to be established between the student's academic program and AOTA before the student starts fieldwork.

1. The candidate completes the application, selecting a first and second preference for placement among the selections and indicating the desired time frame for the placement. *[Note that AOTA cannot guarantee that the student will be placed in the preferred selections.]* Two reference letters from academic or clinical instructors are to be included with the application.

Requires 12 weeks minimum.

2. The student writes and submits an essay describing his or her interests; a description of prior (or anticipated) fieldwork experiences; information about related projects or activities; and the rationale for requesting an AOTA fieldwork experience, as well as expectations and objectives for the experience.

3. The potential supervisors will review the application and essay. A telephone interview will be scheduled.

4. A letter of acceptance or denial will be sent to the student and his or her academic fieldwork coordinator. If the student is accepted, the notification will include confirmation of dates, information about AOTA work policies, and instructions for the first day. On receipt of this packet, the student should contact his or her designated contact person to discuss objectives and expectations.

Students are responsible for arranging their own housing. AOTA headquarters is accessible to Metro, which is the subway system of metropolitan Washington, DC.

Reprinted from http://www.aota.org/Education-Careers/Fieldwork/AOTA-Fieldwork.aspx

Part 7.

ESTABLISHING NEW FIELDWORK PROGRAMS

OVERVIEW OF PART 7

Donna Costa, DHS, OTR/L, FAOTA

Given the numbers of students in all of the educational programs in the United States, we all need to be looking for ways to expand fieldwork options for students. Academic fieldwork coordinators need to be constantly recruiting new fieldwork sites and new fieldwork educators. Some universities and colleges are developing more community-based programs and using faculty to provide program development and student supervision. Some people say we have a critical shortage of fieldwork placements, and this may be the case in parts of the country where there has been an increase in the number of academic programs. The shortage is compounded by recent changes in Medicare regulations that preclude students from providing hands-on reimbursable services to patients under Medicare Part B.

Starting a new fieldwork program can seem like a daunting task, but there are resources to help. Perhaps you have developed a new program with a health care facility that you think would be a great setting for students to learn clinical practice skills. Or maybe you have been employed by a new health care facility and setting up a new fieldwork program seems like a natural progression. Students are learning about program development in the classroom; being involved in the development of a new fieldwork program can be a tremendous learning opportunity.

Chapter 36, "Strategies for Creative Fieldwork Opportunities," contains information such as a list of community sites that might be great community partners for academic programs to consider when thinking about developing fieldwork programs. Chapter 37, "Steps to Starting a New Fieldwork Program," focuses on the steps a fieldwork educator needs to take in setting up a new fieldwork program. And Chapter 38, "AOTA-Recommended Content for a Student Fieldwork Manual," contains a suggested outline that the American Occupational Therapy Association has put together to help fieldwork educators write a fieldwork manual. As mentioned in a later chapter, putting together a student fieldwork manual can be a great learning activity/assignment for a student.

Also of interest is the flash drive included with this book. The flash drive contains a few of the book's chapters as well as its appendixes. The appendixes consist of examples of fieldwork manuals from Washington University, Colorado State University, Penn State–Mont Alto, and Barnes Jewish Hospital for multiple levels of students, from first year students to students participating in Level II fieldwork, and include additional review forms and suggestions for a successful fieldwork experience. The flash drive also includes Chapters 9 ("Sample Level I Fieldwork Assignments"), 10 ("Sample Level I Fieldwork Evaluation Forms"), 13 ("Fieldwork Experience Assessment Tool [FEAT]"), 14 ("Suggestions for Level II Fieldwork Assignments"), 15 ("Sample 12-Week Assignment Outlines for Level II Fieldwork"), 16 ("Sample Weekly Supervisor–Student Feedback Forms"), 27 (AOTA's "Self-Assessment Tool for Fieldwork Educator Competency"), and 30 ("Student Evaluation of Fieldwork Experience").

Chapter 36.

STRATEGIES FOR CREATIVE FIELDWORK OPPORTUNITIES

American Occupational Therapy Association

There have been many recent discussions among American Occupattional Therapy Association (AOTA) members regarding the shortage of traditional fieldwork sites. This general decrease in available sites was exacerbated by the recent Medicare regulation that precludes students from providing hands-on reimbursable services to patients under Medicare Part B.

In an ongoing effort to assist our members, the National Office staff have compiled the following suggestions.

Considerations for Clinical Fieldwork Coordinators at Fieldwork Sites With a Medicare Part B Population

Occupational therapy students in fieldwork internships can engage in many activities in addition to hands-on patient care that provide rich learning opportunities and that meet the Accreditation Council for Occupational Therapy Education Standards. One of the first rules of thumb for fieldwork site coordinators is to think creatively about the experiences and opportunities available at your site before agreeing to take a student.

Specific suggestions include:

- Identify appropriate screening and assessment tools for specific patients.
- Review evaluations performed by the therapists, and make recommendations for initial treatment interventions and changes in treatment goals and activities as a patient's status changes.
- Develop patient or client intervention plans for review by, and discussion with, the clinical supervisor.
- Make recommendations for discharge summary.
- Practice clinical interviewing skills.
- Accompany therapists on home assessment visits, make recommendations, and write up reports for review by therapists.
- Select and use correct billing procedures and codes (e.g., helping therapists research CCI edits, other payer requirements).
- Provide discharge-planning assistance to the therapists to include
  - providing family education,
  - researching and determining available community resources,
  - determining accessibility issues and problems and developing solutions, and
  - recommending possible adaptive devices and advantages and disadvantages of prescribing a specific device.

- Use videotapes of treatment sessions as a means of developing clinical reasoning skills and critical observation skills.
- Design a beginning clinical research project involving direct interaction with patients. Students would be
  - gathering data,
  - assessing results of study,
  - writing results, and
  - presenting results to staff.
- Prepare presentations for staff (including other non–occupational therapy staff when appropriate). In case study presentations, progress from simple to complex cases and analyze applicability of case results to develop practice parameters or protocols.
  - Use role-playing with other students and with the clinical supervisor to improve clinical decision making and appropriate therapeutic interpersonal skills.
  - Evaluate the department's operations using a systems analysis and prepare recommendations that address
    ○ operational improvements,
    ○ operational effectiveness,
    ○ work flow,
    ○ productivity,
    ○ billing accuracy,
    ○ time management, and
    ○ documentation timelines.
- Develop quality assurance activities and measures in implementing a client-care program.
- Provide opportunities for the student to meet with local support groups:
  - Evaluate his or her needs and develop a plan of action (use knowledge of groups, condition-specific information, and observations and interactions from the meeting).
  - Develop patient education materials for support groups and families of group members.
- Provide opportunities for the student to explore community groups, city planners, agencies (e.g., Office on Aging) for a broad perspective of the occupational therapy "fit" and needs that may exist.
- Provide extra supervised hands-on treatment time for Medicare Part B patients, if appropriate and amenable to the facility and management staff.
- Provide the student with opportunities to assist in the treatment of Medicare Part B patients, as long as the supervisor provides the hands-on treatment at all times.

- Rotate students between inpatient and outpatient units whenever possible in facilities with both types of programs because the inpatient and outpatient payment rules differ.
- Consider how to enrich the clinical learning experience by including observation of clinicians performing components of the patient management model at varied levels of clinical experience and expertise.
- Develop critical skills that students usually associate with nonpatient care, such as peer review, quality assurance, administrative management, billing procedures, education, and documentation.
- Provide opportunities for students to strengthen their clinical reasoning abilities by seeking evidence to justify care delivered (compare observational learning experience of similar patient diagnoses) and developing a systematic approach to patient examination, including histories and assessments.
- Provide opportunities for students to make initial or follow-up calls to physicians' offices to clarify orders, obtain records, report progress, and obtain information (e.g., *ICD–10* codes).
- Assign students to develop a resource center of community contacts (e.g., volunteer organizations, sample equipment, pro bono support services for families).

Considerations for Fieldwork Coordinators at Universities and Colleges

- Look for sites that have a diverse case mix, including some Medicare Part B but not exclusively Medicare Part B patients.
- Look for sites providing more traditional occupational therapy services that do not rely on Medicare Part B reimbursement, such as workers' compensation and community programs with non-insurance funding.
- Consider community-based practice areas that do not rely on Medicare or other health insurance for funding, such as
  - senior centers,
  - congregate meals,
  - assisted living centers,

- clubhouses and community mental health centers,
- supported employment,
- homeless shelters,
- wellness centers,
- continence clinics,
- public service screenings,
- prisons and correctional facilities,
- area agencies on aging,
- Building Together With Christmas in April,
- Head Start and other early intervention programs,
- school-based programs,
- Lifestyle Redesign programs,
- home builders,
- the Salvation Army,
- life coaching programs,
- adult day care centers,
- the YMCA or YWCA,
- safe houses for abused women, and
- health promotion programs.
- Consider alternative funding to subsidize students and supervisors in areas of practice where occupational therapy services are appropriate but are not provided.
  - Consider having faculty members supervise students if the fieldwork site requires supervision.
  - Contract with adjunct faculty to serve as fieldwork educators and supervise students at several sites.
  - Provide opportunities for independent thinking, decision making, and critical reasoning.

General Comments

- To be considered viable as a fieldwork option, facilities that treat a high volume of patients covered by Medicare Part B must
  - be part of a larger system that allows for rotation through the non–Medicare Part B parts of the system that do not rely on Part B reimbursement, **or**
  - be willing to design a creative fieldwork experience for students.
- In fieldwork sites where there is no occupational therapist and the question of students writing progress notes arises, be cognizant of the following:
  - All student documentation must be cosigned by a qualified occupational therapist.
  - Discussions should be pursued between the program and the site to see whether a statement could be included in the memorandum of understanding (Educational Standard, A.1.4) allowing the off-site qualified occupational therapy supervisor to cosign documentation (in effect "credentialing" the off-site supervisor).

We would love to hear about other innovative ways you are solving the fieldwork dilemma. Please send your own tried-and-true solutions to mpeterson@ aota.org.

Reprinted from http://www.aota.org/Education-Careers/Fieldwork/NewPrograms/Strategies.aspx

Chapter 37.

STEPS TO STARTING A NEW FIELDWORK PROGRAM

Donna Costa, DHS, OTR/L, FAOTA

Imagine that you have taken a job at a new health care facility and the administrator would like you to develop a fieldwork program for students from the local community college and large university nearby. Where do you begin?

Learn About Fieldwork

You might start learning about fieldwork from a fieldwork educator's perspective:

- Take the American Occupational Therapy Association (AOTA) 2-day course, Fieldwork Educator Certificate Program Workshop (see Chapter 69).
- Browse the AOTA website and become familiar with all of its fieldwork resources.
- Consider reading articles in occupational therapy journals about fieldwork or books about fieldwork education.
- Attend a session focused on fieldwork education at an AOTA conference.

Conduct an Analysis of Your Facility

Conduct an analysis of your facility. Does your facility's mission and philosophy support the training of future occupational therapy practitioners? Discuss the formation of a student program with facility practitioners to determine how receptive they are to participating in a fieldwork program. Review your occupational therapy program: Can it provide a student with the number of appropriate clients and learning opportunities needed to develop entry-level skills?

Gaining support of your facility's management staff is vital for a successful fieldwork program. Arrange a time to meet with your administrator with the sole purpose of discussing the student program. Come prepared with a plan for the fieldwork program and a list of the benefits that a student program can bring to your facility. Take the time to understand the issues that management faces, and work together on addressing any areas of concern. As part of your analysis, you might consider doing a SWOT analysis (consisting of four steps: *s*trengths, *w*eaknesses, *o*pportunities, and *t*hreats), a widely used planning method in business and health care.

In the *strengths* step of the analysis, look at the pluses of your facility. In this case, a plus is that the facility is located near a community college that has an occupational therapy assistant program and is close to a large university that has an occupational therapy program. Academic programs are always looking for new clinical sites to collaborate with and provide quality fieldwork experiences for their students. Another plus in this scenario is that the administrator wants you to develop a fieldwork program.

In the *weaknesses* step of the analysis, look at all of the negatives associated with developing a program. They might include not feeling ready yet because you were just hired, having never developed such a program before, being only one person and this program adding to all of your other work demands, and having never trained a fieldwork student.

In the *opportunities* step of the analysis, think outside of the box. What could be the benefits of starting a fieldwork program, both to the facility and to you (personally and professionally)? It is a tremendous opportunity to build something from the bottom up. It is a way of giving back to the profession by providing quality fieldwork experiences. It's a way of putting this health care facility on the map as a community resource. It will get you known in the local community. It will look great on your résumé if you've always envisioned yourself in a teaching role someday. It will help with future hiring of occupational therapy practitioners at your facility.

The *threats* step focuses on elements in the environment that might become problematic. Practitioners almost always cite a lack of space for students. However, students do not need a dedicated office; a drawer or locker for their belongings will suffice. In addition, other health care facilities in the area may be competing for the same fieldwork students. However, in my experience, there is almost always a shortage rather than a surplus of fieldwork slots. Academic programs are increasing class size in response to increased demand for occupational therapy.

Develop a Fieldwork Program Action Plan

Next, start an action plan to develop the fieldwork program; the steps to starting a fieldwork program are outlined below. Do not think that you need to have an elaborate program in place before you accept your first student. Start with the basics, and add as you learn from the students and staff who participate in the fieldwork program.

Collaborate With an Academic Program

In the preliminary stages of developing a fieldwork program, it is helpful to contact at least one academic program. Each occupational therapist or occupational therapy assistant program has an academic fieldwork coordinator (AFWC) who can provide you with guidance and resource material needed to start a student program.

The academic programs with which you contract will provide specific information on their program. This information may include the program's fieldwork objectives, course syllabi, program curricula, and other related information. Note that active, ongoing collaboration between the fieldwork educator and the AFWC is an essential component of a positive fieldwork experience.

Create a Fieldwork Contract or Letter of Agreement

Next, develop a contract or letter of agreement (sometimes called a *memorandum of understanding,* or *MOU*) that serves as a legal document between the fieldwork site and the academic program. The contract should state the rights, fieldwork requirements, and obligations of the academic program, fieldwork site, and students. A written agreement is required for all fieldwork Level I and II placements. The academic program will have a standard contract that you can use. Be sure to have your facility's legal counsel review the document before it is signed. Begin this step early because the contract may require several revisions between both legal counsels. It can sometimes be executed in a month, but can take up to a year or longer if contractual issues arise.

Develop Student Resources

Now you can start establishing the foundation of your fieldwork program by developing and implementing the following student resources.

Create a Fieldwork Data Form

This form describes your fieldwork program to the AFWC and the student. The completed form should be sent to each academic program with which you have a contract (see http://thyurl.com/FWContract).

Develop Fieldwork Objectives

Fieldwork objectives are those that a student must achieve to successfully complete the fieldwork placement. Level I fieldwork objectives are usually provided by the academic program. Level II fieldwork objectives—specific behavioral objectives reflecting the entry-level competencies that the student is required to achieve by the end of the affiliation—are developed by the fieldwork site. These objectives serve to guide the student through sequential learning activities that lead to entry-level competency.

Some fieldwork programs correlate their objectives with AOTA's fieldwork evaluations. Other programs write weekly objectives that culminate in entry-level skills. Writing the learning objectives is invaluable to both students and fieldwork educators. Obtain examples of objectives from an AFWC or your regional fieldwork consultant. The AOTA website also has sample objectives for a variety of practice settings (see http://www.aota.org/education-careers/fieldwork/supervisor.aspx).

Produce a Fieldwork Student Manual

A fieldwork manual will serve as a valuable resource for students and fieldwork educators. Some fieldwork sites have had the first few fieldwork students help them create a student manual. Some of the content in the manual might come from other departments within your health care facility such as Human Resources or Infection Control. See Chapter 38, "AOTA-Recommended Content for a Student Fieldwork Manual," or http://www.aota.org/Education-Careers/Fieldwork/NewPrograms/Content.aspx for suggested content.

Establish a Schedule of Weekly Activities

Develop a list of learning activities and assignments that will guide a student developmentally toward the acquisition of entry-level skills. Some fieldwork programs have a week-by-week outline with increasing responsibilities, learning activities, and assignments that students must successfully complete. Your partner academic program may have sample learning activities and may even take the lead in

mandating that certain assignments be done while on fieldwork, especially in the case of Level I fieldwork.

Prepare an Orientation

A thorough orientation provides students with the knowledge and understanding needed for a successful fieldwork experience. Topics can include an overview of the fieldwork site and its fieldwork program, safety procedures, specific evaluation or treatment interventions used by the facility, documentation, and equipment use. Try to make the sessions as participatory as possible, with presentations made by different staff members or experienced students.

Decide on an Interview Format

Most fieldwork sites have some kind of interview so that the student and fieldwork educator can become acquainted. In some situations, the interview is competitive, meaning that multiple students are applying for the same fieldwork slot. Other interviews are more informative in nature, providing an opportunity for the student to see the fieldwork site, ask questions, and learn what they have to do in advance to prepare.

Create a Fieldwork Calendar

In this scenario, there are two schools in the area, both of which potentially could send students to you. Eventually, word will get out and you will be contacted by other schools outside the immediate area who have students to send to you. Decide how many students you and your staff can take at once, and then create a rotation schedule on the calendar.

For the occupational therapy assistant student, the length of the Level II experience is 8 weeks, and for the occupational therapist student, it is 12 weeks. There is no reason to take only one student at a time. Students are used to learning in groups and do well with a collaborative model. Consider taking occupational therapist and occupational therapy assistant students at the same time so they have an opportunity while still in school to learn how to best work in a collaborative manner with each other. In this instance, you may want to schedule the occupational therapist student 2 to 4 weeks before the start of the occupational therapy assistant student so that the occupational therapist student has a chance to get organized before beginning to take on some responsibility with the occupational therapy assistant student.

Create a Filing System

Create a filing system to store all the paperwork that comes from each school. Paperwork should be kept a locked drawer to protect students' confidentiality.

Create a Program Evaluation System

Create a program evaluation system whereby you review the outcomes of the fieldwork experiences you provide to students. This system should include copies of students' Fieldwork Performance Evaluations (see http://tinyurl.com/pwrjfle) and Student

Evaluation of Fieldwork Experience (see http://tinyurl.com/StudentEvaluation). This information will be invaluable in your end-of-year report to your administrator.

Summary

Do not spend excess time reinventing the wheel. Contact your AFWC or regional fieldwork consultant for program and resource examples and assistance.

Note: This chapter expands on the information found in steps to starting a Fieldwork Program, by the American Occupational Therapy Association, 1998, available at http://www.aota.org/Education-Careers/Fieldwork/NewPrograms/Steps.aspx

Chapter 38.

AOTA-RECOMMENDED CONTENT FOR A STUDENT FIELDWORK MANUAL

American Occupational Therapy Association

1. Orientation outline
2. Assignments
3. Safety procedures and codes
4. Behavioral objectives
5. Week-by-week schedule of responsibilities
6. Patient confidentiality information (patient rights)
7. Guidelines for documentation:
   - Completed samples of all forms
   - Acceptable medical abbreviations
   - Discharge plan
   - Billing
   - Dictation directions, if applicable.
8. *Occupational Therapy Practice Framework: Domain and Process*, 3rd Edition

Additional Information That Can Gradually Be Added to the Student Manual

1. Organizational chart of the fieldwork setting
2. History of the fieldwork setting
3. Department information
   - Policy and procedures
   - Mission statement
   - Organizational chart
   - Essential job functions
   - Dress code.
4. Regularly scheduled meetings
   a. Dates and times
   b. Purpose of meeting.
5. Special client-related groups and programs
   a. Purpose
   b. Referral system
   c. Operation
   d. Transport.
6. Guidelines for documentation
7. Responsibilities of
   a. Fieldwork educator
   b. Student
   c. Fieldwork coordinator (if position exists).
8. Performance evaluation
   a. Procedure and guidelines used in the evaluation of
      i. Student
      ii. Fieldwork educator
      iii. Fieldwork experience.

Material for your student manual can be gathered from other sources within your facility (e.g., employee handbooks, human resources department). Feel free to call the academic programs that you have contracts with to get the names of nearby facilities that are similar to your site. Call those facilities and see if they are willing to share their student manual with you.

Don't feel that you need to have a separate manual for students and fieldwork educators. The manuals can be the same.
October 2, 2000

Reprinted from http://www.aota.org/Education-Careers/Fieldwork/NewPrograms/Content.aspx#sthash.qPnIi8ES.dpuf

Part 8.

EXPANDING FIELDWORK OPPORTUNITIES

OVERVIEW OF PART 8

Donna Costa, DHS, OTR/L, FAOTA

Part 8 examines expanding fieldwork opportunities. The American Occupational Therapy Association (AOTA) has developed a list of recommendations for expanding fieldwork, found in Chapter 39, "Recommendations for Expanding Fieldwork." Many academic programs are developing innovative programs in the community in an attempt to create more fieldwork sites for students and to meet underserved populations in the community. The term *role-emerging* is used to refer to sites that do not currently have occupational therapy services or employ occupational therapy practitioners. More often than not, this practice leads to the facility hiring an occupational therapy practitioner. New to this edition of this book is a chapter on setting up role-emerging fieldwork placements, Chapter 40, "Introduction to Role-Emerging Fieldwork."

Many students ask to be placed outside the United States for their fieldwork assignments. This requires many additional considerations that academic programs will have to address, such as the establishment of contracts, requirements for additional liability insurance coverage, and student supervision requirements. Chapter 41, "General Guide for Planning International Fieldwork," and Chapter 42, "Ethical Considerations Related to International Fieldwork," cover the general guidelines for international fieldwork as well as the ethical considerations surrounding these placements.

Chapter 43, "Excellence in Fieldwork: Criteria for Fieldwork Educator Excellence and Criteria for Fieldwork Site Excellence," contains the criteria for recognizing excellence in fieldwork education, both for the individual fieldwork educator as well as for the fieldwork site. Sometimes fieldwork consortia and/or academic programs want to recognize individuals or facilities for their contributions to fieldwork education, and this list of criteria for excellence will come in handy. You will note that AOTA membership as well as state association membership is listed. Student membership in AOTA is either strongly encouraged or mandated in most academic programs as a professional responsibility, and so students are learning early the value of membership in national and state associations. Students often report being surprised when they get out to fieldwork and find out that their fieldwork educators are not AOTA members. That is why it is listed as one of the criteria for excellence as a fieldwork educator. Remember, you are a role model for students!

The final chapter in this section, "The Multiple Mentoring Model of Student Supervision: A Fit for Contemporary Practice," describes a model of supervision that is particularly useful in role-emerging fieldwork in community practice settings. The multiple mentoring model involves more than one fieldwork educator supervising a student; this is particularly useful when therapists work part-time, when therapists work in a highly specialized program, or when there is a person new to the role of fieldwork educator.

Chapter 39.

RECOMMENDATIONS FOR EXPANDING FIELDWORK

American Occupational Therapy Association

Rationale

Traditionally, fieldwork has been an experience in which a student spends 6 weeks to 3 months at one facility with a single supervisor, often at a hospital or primary health care setting. Many factors influence the way occupational therapy (OT) practice and clinical education are provided. These factors include an increasing demand for OT services in expanding practice arenas, manpower shortages, increasing numbers of students needing fieldwork placements, students with special needs, and a shrinking number of fieldwork placements.

Occupational therapy's growth into broader practice arenas provides us with an opportunity to expand and improve the fieldwork education component to reflect current practice. This is an essential consideration in preparing students for entry-level practice.

Examples

Alternative fieldwork options that reflect current practice might include:

- Part-time scheduling (e.g., half-days for 6 months)

- Flexible fieldwork schedule (e.g., longer than 3 months at one setting)
- Part-time OT supervisor (e.g., placement with consulting OT)
- Rotating through several programs at one setting
- Multiple sites, with similar or different caseloads or focus, and with one or more supervisors
- Combined experiences (e.g., psychiatric and physical dysfunction, adult and pediatrics)
- One supervisor supervising more than one student simultaneously
- Newer practice or setting areas such as:
  - Chronic pain program
  - Private practice
  - Alzheimer program
  - Forensic mental health unit
  - Head trauma program
  - Adaptive living skills program
  - Head Start center
  - Prevocational or vocational
  - Senior citizen center
  - Cognitive retraining
  - Special education center
  - Health education center
  - Work hardening/industrial
  - Administration or supervision
  - Injury center

- Hospice programs
- Rural home health
- Adaptive sports
- Geropsychiatry
- Family crisis centers
- Wellness program
- AIDS clinics and programs
- Department of corrections
- Camps
- Substance abuse centers
- Homeless shelters
- Soup kitchens
- School affirmative action programs
- Community-based programs, retirement homes.

Criteria

Fieldwork is a collaborative effort among students, clinicians, and educators. Ideas for placement may originate with an academic program or with a practitioner. The following criteria may help indicate whether your practice would be appropriate as a fieldwork placement.

- Your practice provides opportunities for a student to:
  - Learn OT skills and concepts, either general or specialized
  - Apply OT skills and concepts learned in the academic setting

- Experience success as a result of their OT intervention
- Communicate with other individuals in a professional manner.
- You are interested in supervising students.
- You are willing to collaborate with an academic fieldwork coordinator to plan and implement a student placement.

Resources

Any of the following resources will be able to offer further assistance:

- Education Department, AOTA
  4720 Montgomery Lane
  PO Box 31220
  Bethesda, MD 20824-1220
  301-652-2682, ext. 2932
- Academic fieldwork coordinators (at all occupational therapy or occupational therapy assistant educational programs)

Revised September 2000

Reprinted from http://www.aota.org/Education-Careers/Fieldwork/Supervisor/Expanding.aspx

Chapter 40.

INTRODUCTION TO ROLE-EMERGING FIELDWORK

Debra J. Hanson, PhD, OTR/L, FAOTA, and Sarah K. Nielsen, PhD, OTR/L

Role-emerging fieldwork placements are described in the literature as occurring in settings that do not traditionally offer occupational therapy services (Mulholland & Derdall, 2005; Wood, 2005). The intention of such placements is that students engage in promoting and increasing awareness of the profession and create a demand for occupational therapy services, which may or may not result in the emergence of an occupational therapy role in that setting (Mulholland & Derdall, 2005; Prigg & Mackenzie, 2002). This chapter explores the terms, definitions, and associated characteristics of role-emerging fieldwork and presents processes for academic program readiness, recruitment of sites, implementation of the fieldwork experience, and evaluation procedures to improve the quality of the role-emerging fieldwork experience.

Why Should Alternative Fieldwork Structures Be Considered?

Traditional placement structures, also known as *clinical* or *role-established placements,* are characterized by a one-to-one ratio of students to occupational therapy practitioners, following an apprenticeship model of supervision. Fieldwork occurs within a setting in which the occupational therapy role is well-established. The focus of student learning is to practice skills and perform tasks following the pattern of an established occupational therapy position. This model, although widely used, has been criticized for reinforcing dependency on fieldwork educators and limiting opportunities for the development of student initiative and problem-solving and critical-thinking skills (Martin, Morris, Moore, Sadlo, & Crouch, 2004; Thomas, Penman, & Williamson, 2005). Specifically, Bonello (2001) observed that fieldwork educators primarily rely on demonstration and imitation for teaching direct practice skills rather than promoting problem-solving skills and creative and independent thinking. This approach is in contrast to the opportunities available during role-emerging fieldwork for students to assume responsibility for their own learning as they gain the confidence needed to practice in innovative settings (Clarke, Martin, Sadlo, & de-visser, 2014).

Changes in health care have created a need for students to acquire skills and confidence for interaction in multidisciplinary and community-based environments so they can successfully work in emerging areas of practice (Fisher & Savin-Baden, 2002; Holmes & Scaffa, 2009; Prigg & Mackenzie,

2002; Thomas et al., 2005). From the perspective of higher education, current accreditation standards place increasing emphasis on skills in interprofessional learning and population-focused interventions that can be effectively addressed through the use of alternative fieldwork education models (Accreditation Council for Occupational Therapy Education [ACOTE®], 2012; Fortune & McKinstry, 2012; Overton, Clark, & Thomas, 2009).

Nontraditional placement structures, such as role-emerging fieldwork models, have been identified as a vehicle for broadening the student learning experience. Students gain confidence as they use education, advocacy, and consultancy skills while articulating the role of occupational therapy in a nontraditional setting. In addition, students are better able to both appreciate and use occupational therapy theory in the process (Dancza et al., 2013; Fortune & McKinstry, 2012).

Role-Emerging Fieldwork Options

Because many differing characteristics and variables describe the role-emerging model in the literature, it is important that readers have an appreciation for the unique options associated with this model to effectively develop a structure best suited to his or her academic program. Some elements to consider are

- Traditional versus role-emerging practice settings
- Placement goals
- Supervisory structures
- Collaborative approach to supervision
- Time frames for the placement
- Degree of fieldwork learning structure and student initiative
- Teaching and learning approaches.

Traditional vs. Emerging Practice Settings

Traditional practice settings have been associated with medical facilities such as acute, inpatient, and outpatient care and nursing homes, whereas nontraditional practice settings have been associated with community and nonprofit contexts such as low vision clinics, welfare-to-work programs, homeless shelters, and college campuses (Molineux & Baptiste, 2011; Smith, Cornella, & Williams, 2014). In a nontraditional setting, services might focus on prevention, wellness, or population health and require that occupational therapy practitioners be prepared for the varied roles of educator, consultant, administrator, entrepreneur, and leader that are needed to be successful in a new practice area (Holmes & Scaffa, 2009; Prigg & Mackenzie, 2002). However, defining the term *nontraditional* is problematic because placements once considered nontraditional might now be routinely used for fieldwork, such as school system placement (Mulholland & Derdall, 2005). Emerging practice areas might include service delivery at sites that once provided occupational therapy services but now do not (e.g., mental health centers) or sites that have only recently offered occupational therapy services, such as specialty areas of medical practice (e.g., primary health care, lymphedema clinics; Gregory, Quelch, & Watanabe, 2011; Rodger et al., 2009; Smith et al., 2014).

It is important to remember that what is considered an emerging practice setting is highly variable. The usual assumption that role-emerging fieldwork placement can occur solely in a community-based nonprofit setting is limiting. The academic program considering the development of a role-emerging fieldwork program needs to judiciously choose practice settings that best reflect the skills desired rather than rely on standard definitions of such settings.

Placement Goals

Implementing an occupational therapy fieldwork placement in settings without an established occupational therapy role often requires a change in fieldwork structure, depending on the placement goals. These goals may emphasize student skills for direct practice, the development of program planning and project management skills, or both.

When the focus is on developing student skills for direct practice, the supervising occupational therapy practitioner helps the student identify an occupational therapy perspective and role during the placement (Mulholland & Derdall, 2005; Smith et al., 2014). Students learn to differentiate the occupational therapy role from that of others and apply their academic knowledge to the delivery of services to the client. When the focus is on program planning or project management, the student considers the needs of the setting from an occupational therapy perspective and establishes an occupational therapy role through program development, implementation, and evaluation or carries out a project that demonstrates an occupational perspective that will benefit the practice setting (Edwards & Thew, 2011). When the focus is on developing skills for direct practice and program development or project management, students may provide direct services to clients as they test the effectiveness of the program or project developed.

Fieldhouse and Fedden (2009) identified a framework and sequence for building skills for direct practice in a setting without occupational therapy services. They identified dimensions of students' learning as they gained a greater awareness of the therapeutic use of self and understanding of oneself as an occupational being, developed skills in occupational therapy assessment and observation, and enabled occupation through the use of activity analysis and adaptation. Students completing this type of placement recognized the importance of person-centered goal setting and learned to differentiate occupational therapy services from services already provided by the site through the use of a guiding theory or practice framework.

Although students in this type of placement work under limited supervision of the occupational therapist as in all role-emerging placements, the development of client programming is not the focus of their learning; instead, their learning focus is directed to building skills for direct service delivery. Often, the framework or boundaries for the occupational therapy services to be provided have already been set in place by the supervising therapist, though it is up to students to determine the specific interventions needed for each client or client group. In one example of this type of placement, students delivered life skills programming, designed by their supervising therapist, to people with refugee backgrounds to increase occupational participation and independence (Smith et al., 2014). Students worked in client homes and the community and gained valuable skills as they helped clients increase their participation and independence in daily and meaningful occupations within the home and community. In another example, an occupational therapist employed part-time as a consultant in an acute psychiatric inpatient unit of a general hospital had already established the basic framework for

occupational therapy programming, but because she was only on-site for 8 hours a week, the students actually carried out the programming she had developed (Costa, 2007).

As described by Edwards and Thew (2011), the project placement experience emphasizes skills in program development and project management. Preparation for this type of placement includes discussion of the needs of the setting and potential student roles and projects before the placement. All stakeholders are aware that students will be evaluating how an occupational therapy role might complement existing services provided in the setting. The fieldwork educator and on-site supervisor help students orient to the facility and facilitate student completion of processes such as a needs assessment and program planning. In addition to learning to meet the needs of the people with whom they work, students develop project management skills as they initiate, plan, execute, and evaluate a project that will benefit the facility (Thew, Hargreaves, & Cronin-Davis, 2008). They strengthen their professional identity as they use occupational therapy theoretical models or frames of reference to structure their project- and program-planning efforts (Clarke et al., 2014). Stages of student learning and experience correspond to behaviors and emotions encountered when first initiating the project, planning and managing the project, collecting outcomes, and ensuring that the outcomes are communicated as the project comes to an end (Thomas & Rodger, 2011).

Role-emerging project-based placements have been implemented in settings such as a domestic violence shelter, a city library, a refuge detention center, and a community cardiac rehabilitation center (Edwards & Thew, 2011). Examples of projects undertaken by students include a program to increase social interactions for mothers and children affected by domestic violence, a sensory play project for a public kindergarten classroom, a stress and lifestyle management program for university employees, and a program for people learning to drive after a head injury (Edwards & Thew, 2011; Hunt, 2006).

The role-emerging placement may also include a mix of direct service components and program or project development. Note that although occupational therapy and occupational therapy assistant students might augment or complement the existing services provided at the site, they should not simply be put in the role of carrying out these preexisting services, regardless of the unique features of the setting. The expectation of role-emerging placement is that irrespective of a site's current programming or services, the placement will introduce or extend the unique perspective of occupational therapy, leading to programming that enhances the client experience.

Supervisory Structures

During role-emerging placements, students generally receive on-site supervision from a facility employee, such as a social worker, psychologist, or nurse, but are provided with overall supervision and support by an occupational therapy practitioner serving as fieldwork educator for a specific amount of time during the week (Mulholland & Derdall, 2005). ACOTE (2012) standards require an established plan for supervision and at least 8 hours of on-site fieldwork educator supervision per week.

Many occupational therapist and occupational therapy assistant programs that implement role-emerging fieldwork placements provide supervision by an occupational therapy educator; some involve fieldwork educators employed at other facilities within the community (Bossers, Cook, Polatajko, & Laine, 1997). For example, supervision may be provided by a placement coordinator who has been hired by the academic program specifically to supervise students in emerging practice settings (Mulholland & Derdall, 2005) or by program faculty members who oversee student learning or project management (Prigg & Mackenzie, 2002). Thomas et al. (2005) proposed an interagency model of supervision, where students divide their time between an occupational therapy practitioner in an established role and another agency in the community where project or program development is needed. The student might develop programming in practice settings affiliated with the fieldwork educator's practice or independent settings in the community. Following this model, role-emerging fieldwork might occur within a practice area that is situated in a traditional setting. For example, the student might complete mental health fieldwork on the behavioral health unit of a hospital, with the fieldwork educator being an occupational therapy practitioner who is working in the area of physical rehabilitation in the same hospital.

Collaborative Approach to Supervision

Although an apprenticeship model is commonly used for traditional fieldwork placements, the literature is widely supportive of using a collaborative approach to supervision for role-emerging placements (Dancza et al., 2013; Rodger et al., 2009). Collaborative learning can occur whenever two or more individuals learn together by capitalizing on the resources and skills of each other. The fieldwork educator might be an expert on some topics, but the student might have more experience or information for others. There is reciprocity evident in the learning process that propels the learners toward positive interdependence (Hanson & DeIuliis, 2015). Collaborative learning can occur between one student and one fieldwork educator, or might be employed when two or more students are supervised by one or more fieldwork educators. The key is not in the number of students or number of fieldwork educators, but in the learning approach employed.

There are some advantages to two or more students completing a role-emerging fieldwork placement at one time, in that they have a source of support to build each other's confidence and can plan and strategize together as they engage in the learning experience (Martin et al., 2004). Students find the opportunity to have immediate feedback on their performance from peers particularly helpful if they have limited occupational therapy practitioner on-site supervision (Dancza et al., 2013). Fieldwork educators supervising more than one student at a time find the collaborative supervision approach helpful because peer-learning activities can be introduced to foster student clinical reasoning (Bartholomai & Fitzgerald, 2007).

The collaborative model might be used to promote self-directed learning, sharing of work responsibilities, team building, and communication skills. Fieldwork educators using this approach create opportunities for giving and receiving feedback and sharing the teaching and learning roles between students if there is more than one, and between the student and the fieldwork educator if there is only one student. The approach is most effective when a balance exists between working together and individual ownership of learning (Thomas & Rodger, 2011). When used in a setting where no occupational therapy is provided, this model can foster peer learning that focuses on direct care to clients and also teamwork and collaboration in project or program planning (Fortune & McKinstry, 2012).

Time Frames for the Placement

Role-emerging placements vary in purpose and structure depending on where the student is in the academic cycle, the length of the placement, and whether the placement is required or an elective. Role-emerging placements can range in length from 3 to 12 weeks and are most commonly identified as a second, third, or fourth rather than a first Level II fieldwork experience (Fortune & McKinstry, 2012; Mulholland & Derdall, 2005). Earlier in the education cycle, students may have limited knowledge of the occupational therapy role and have difficulty recognizing or promoting the role in a new environment (Fisher & Savin-Baden, 2002; Thomas et al., 2005). Prigg and McKenzie (2002) compared the perceptions of second- and third-year students completing project placements and found that second-year students expressed a need for more hands-on supervision and were less able to value and transfer the skills acquired during a placement to other client-related activities. The researchers concluded that specific guidance and increased structure were required from supervisors to help students identify the value of the generic skills they were learning and their relevance for practice.

Degree of Fieldwork Learning Structure and Student Initiative

The academic fieldwork coordinator, placement site, and fieldwork educator collaborate to develop learning objectives in advance of the placement. However, a hallmark of the role-emerging fieldwork experience is that students are expected to identify personal learning goals consistent with the established learning objectives as they explore aspects of the occupational therapy role in a new setting. When the focus for learning is on direct practice, student-identified learning goals may lead to revision of or additions to identified site learning activities. When the focus is on

program development, the fieldwork site and the academic program might have identified focus areas for program development prior to student arrival or the student might have a great deal of input on program development focus. The degree of learning structure provided by the fieldwork and site educator, coupled with the degree of student initiative taken to accomplish personal learning goals, will ultimately shape the student learning process during a role-emerging fieldwork placement.

Teaching and Learning Approaches

Fieldwork educators supervising students during a role-emerging placement must balance providing direct supervision and promoting autonomy on the part of the student. Teaching and learning approaches that promote reflection and help students find the answers to their questions rather than providing answers are most successful (Thomas & Rodger, 2011). The supervision approaches of adult learning principles, problem-based learning, and experiential and peer learning have been identified as helpful to the development of student autonomy and reflection (Boniface, Seymour, Polglase, Lawrie, & Clarke, 2012; Bossers et al., 1997; Fieldhouse & Fedden, 2009; Thew et al., 2008).

Laying the Groundwork for Role-Emerging Fieldwork

Historically, academic programs have implemented role-emerging fieldwork placements for a plethora of reasons, including as a response to increased enrollments requiring additional fieldwork placements (Mulholland & Derdall, 2005; Prigg & Mackenzie, 2002) and global pressures to prepare students to work in community placements or increase the workforce in a particular practice area (Cooper & Raine, 2009; Fortune, Farnworth, & McKinstry, 2006; Overton et al., 2009; Rodger et al., 2009). Regardless of these pressures, the planning process is critical to launching role-emerging fieldwork in an organized and pragmatic fashion (Cooper & Raine, 2009; Mulholland & Derdall, 2005; Prigg & Mackenzie, 2002; Thew et al., 2008). Much of the literature on role-emerging fieldwork discusses the importance of planning learning objectives and communicating with facilities, but little discussion is given to an academic program preparing its own definitions of *role-emerging fieldwork, desired outcomes,* and *internal procedures.* In addition, this has raised concern about the sustainability of role-emerging fieldwork placements because of the demand on academic staff and students for individualized planning and supervision (Clark, 2004; Cooper & Raine, 2009). Lack of advanced planning could lead to ill-prepared students and a chaotic approach to developing role-emerging placements, which contribute greatly to the workload of the academic fieldwork coordinator (AFWC).

Level I and II fieldwork experiences must be reflective of and integral to the academic curriculum (Amini & Gupta, 2012), whether they are traditional or role-emerging. Academic programs just beginning to participate in role-emerging fieldwork should engage in a readiness process that includes the following three steps:

1. Defining *role-emerging fieldwork* and setting desired broad learning outcomes
2. Reviewing the curriculum to ensure students are adequately prepared
3. Developing policies and procedures to determine student eligibility requirements and the application process for successful role-emerging placements.

As discussed previously in this chapter, many factors may influence the structure of the role-emerging fieldwork placement. Consideration of these variables is essential to establishing what criteria the academic program will use to form its definition of role-emerging fieldwork. Concurrently, the academic program should review its mission and vision to confirm that the chosen definition reflects the program's beliefs and values. In addition, programs should set desired broad learning outcomes of role-emerging fieldwork placements. For example, the program might establish that the role-emerging fieldwork must result in the student being able to develop programming. The definition and learning outcomes will serve as a benchmark in evaluating potential placement sites.

Exhibit 40.1. *Student Fieldwork Eligibility Requirements and Application Procedures*

1. Student reviews description of role-emerging fieldwork and describes how he or she would accomplish the goals of this experience.
2. Student provides evidence of previous independent learning.
3. Student self-assesses domains of competency for placement.
4. Student interviews a student who has completed a role-emerging placement.
5. Student meets with academic fieldwork coordinator.
6. Student seeks faculty approval.

The next step in academic program readiness is to evaluate the curriculum to determine whether students are being adequately prepared to meet the desired learning outcomes of role-emerging fieldwork. Although this step should be guided by the desired broad learning outcomes, additional resources to understand specific competencies are necessary. Holmes and Scaffa (2009) set forth 104 potential competencies that practitioners need for emerging practice areas. This resource is particularly useful in developing a tool to evaluate whether the curriculum provides the content and learning activities related to desired outcomes. A positive outcome of this step is an understanding by all faculty of the nature and complexity of role-emerging fieldwork and the connection of the curriculum content to the role-emerging placement.

Finally, the academic program must establish policies and procedures to determine student eligibility requirements and the application process for successful role-emerging placements. For example, the University of North Dakota occupational therapy program developed six steps for students to follow for placement (Exhibit 40.1), including student self-assessment of five domains of competency. These domains of competency were based on the work of Holmes and Scaffa (2009) and include ethics, critical thinking, interpersonal abilities, knowledge, and performance. Exhibit 40.2 provides an example of the rating scale for the competency domain of interpersonal abilities to be used by students and faculty.

Exhibit 40.2. Rating Scale for Competency of Interpersonal Abilities

Interpersonal Ability	Student Rating	Faculty Rating
Can communicate occupational therapy concepts effectively to a variety of audiences		
Has the potential to engage in an interactive collaborative learning process		
Consistently demonstrates initiation, time management, and organizational skills without direct supervision		
Is able to reasonably self-assess strengths and needs independently		

Note. Rating scale: 2 = *acceptable,* 1 = *some concern,* 0 = *unacceptable.*

Site Recruitment

The academic programs' definitions and desired outcomes for the role-emerging placement should be considered when pursuing site recruitment. Although the referral sources for identifying potential sites might vary, the identification of specific sites will always be based on the program's criteria for role-emerging placements. The first stage of recruitment is identification of potential sites and the second is the process of securing the site. (See Appendix 40.A for a case example describing the two stages of site recruitment.)

Identification of Potential Sites

Exploring potential sites may occur in many ways. Faculty involvement, awareness of community initiatives, or membership in community organizations or governing boards provide opportunities for learning partnerships. Students may identify learning interests based on personal or work experiences, or organizations may contact the university requesting resources (Edwards & Thew, 2011). A conversation between the AFWC or another faculty member with an organization may lead to further exploration of learning possibilities. For example, the AFWC, when conducting fieldwork visits or otherwise in communication with local agencies, organizations, or facilities, may listen for key elements that have been identified as central to the role-emerging fieldwork placement, including

- Facility structure that is organized to support or enable occupational performance
- Organization structures or key personnel that are open and supportive of change
- A desire on the part of the organization to invest resources to further learning and change potentials.

If further questioning demonstrates that a good fit does not exist, the potential for a successful learning partnership may be limited. However, if all three elements are present, steps should be taken to earnestly pursue the possibility of developing a learning partnership.

In initial conversations, care must be taken to understand the purpose, values, and organizational structure of the potential placement setting to create a win–win situation, that is, meet organizational needs and provide a learning opportunity for students. A site visit is helpful to view the potential practice setting and meet relevant agency stakeholders; if it is not possible to visit in person, use of technology for a virtual visit may be helpful. An understanding of the organization and attending social structures will also make it easier when it is time to pursue the development of a memorandum of understanding with the site, which requires making explicit the expectations of both parties.

While the academic program is trying to understand the agency, the agency is evaluating the fit of the content, structure, and processes of the curriculum and academic program in relation to agency needs. It is important that the academic representative articulate the following elements of fieldwork placement:

- Skills and content the student will bring to the site from his or her academic experience
- Central purpose established by the academic program for the role-emerging placement
- Basic supervisory structures required for the placement.

Both parties should be alert for the match between these three elements and the purpose, values, and organizational structure of the potential placement.

When working with an agency that does not employ an occupational therapy practitioner, it is essential to discuss the supervision requirements. The academic program should know in advance what supervision options they will provide and be prepared to request on-site supervision provision from the agency. There will need to be some negotiation about reimbursement for supervision and whether the student will be asked to share in those costs.

It is important to consider whether a conflict of interest will arise in helping the agency either meet the direct needs of the client or establish new programs that will affect clients. Consider whether any occupational therapy practitioners in the community provide the same type of services and what the costs are. Role-emerging placements should demonstrate to an agency that hiring an occupational therapy practitioner is in their best interests; if they end up relying on students for this service, their motivation to hire an occupational therapy practitioner will decrease.

The academic program should provide the agency with a short summary about the curriculum or a link to the program website and the basic elements of the role-emerging fieldwork model, including the supervision structure. Table 40.1 is a sample handout comparing the supervisory

Table 40.1. Traditional and Role-Emerging Fieldwork Model Handout

	Traditional Fieldwork Model	**Role-Emerging Fieldwork Model**
Role of Fieldwork Educator	• The occupational therapy supervisor must have at least 1 year of experience after initial certification. • The occupational therapy supervisor is the expert and model; the student mirrors the activities of the supervisor. • The occupational therapy supervisor uses one-to-one direct supervision with the student. • The occupational therapy supervisor decides what skills the student will learn. • The student observes and practices skills and performs tasks within an established occupational therapy role. • The emphasis is on the student's development of skills needed for delivery of direct occupational therapy intervention.	• The occupational therapy supervisor must have a minimum of 3 years of experience after initial certification. • The occupational therapy supervisor is off-site and a non–occupational therapy on-site supervisor directs daily tasks. • The occupational therapy supervisor provides a minimum of 8 hours of supervision per week following a consultancy model. • The focus is on creating or expanding the role of occupational therapy at the site to complement existing services. • The emphasis is on the student's development of skills needed for program development of occupational therapy services.
Learning Objectives and Activities	• The student participates in site orientation provided by the occupational therapy supervisor. • Site-specific learning objectives focus on direct practice. • The student may possibly generate learning objectives. • The student practices skills identified by the supervisor. • A common learning activity involves the student observing the supervisor doing a procedure and then completing parts of the procedure under direct supervision.	• The student participates in site orientation provided by the non–occupational therapy on-site supervisor. • Site-specific learning objectives may focus on both direct service and program development or exclusively on program development. • The student generates learning objectives. • The student provides direct services (e.g., interprofessional therapy services, one-to-one or group delivery of nonbillable occupational therapy services directly supervised by the non–occupational therapy on-site supervisor) to cultivate skills and learn about the site.

(Continued)

Table 40.1. Traditional and Role-Emerging Fieldwork Model Handout *(Cont.)*

	Traditional Fieldwork Model	Role-Emerging Fieldwork Model
	• Supervision is withdrawn as the student demonstrates increased competency in patient care. • The supervisor identifies learning opportunities for the student within the facility setting. • The fieldwork educator supports development of the student's clinical reasoning skills through modeling, reflecting actions out loud, asking questions, or making assignments such as journaling. • The weekly review of student progress focuses on skills in direct practice. • The student needs to achieve the learning objectives as established by the site. • The student practices and learns specific skills and asks questions or seeks clarification as needed. • The student reflects on his or her practice and emerging clinical reasoning skills and develops increasing abilities in clinical reasoning. • The student demonstrates increasing levels of competency in his or her direct work with clients. • The student responds to direct feedback provided by the occupational therapy supervisor. • The student gradually learns to seek information from other sources and ultimately share ideas with the fieldwork educator.	• The student completes a needs assessment and proposes viable programming options for occupational therapy to fit the site's needs. • The student initiates and carries out assessment, treatment implementation, and outcomes collection for one new program, providing formative and summative assessment data to inform the site of progress made. • Ongoing supervision is provided to the student by the occupational therapy supervisor through telephone and electronic contacts, journaling, work samples, and reading assignments. • The weekly review of student progress by both supervisors may direct attention to both direct practice and program development skills. • The student may participate in the development of site-specific learning objectives for both direct practice and program development. • The student identifies learning opportunities within the site and negotiates a plan to accomplish learning objectives with the on-site and occupational therapy supervisor. • The student must seek out feedback from multiple sources and have a self-directed approach to learning, making the best use of the consultancy provided. • The student must work cooperatively with others. • The student must articulate potential linkages between occupational therapy philosophy, occupational behavior models, and practice opportunities at the setting. • The student develops project management skills and engages in a continuous process of reflection.
Benefits	• The apprenticeship approach is widely familiar and popular and presumed effective to foster direct practice skills. • One-to-one supervision supports an individualized student evaluation process. • One-to-one supervision provides the opportunity for direct role modeling of practice skills. • The strength of the student learning experience is directly related to the skills of the supervisor.	• Students are independent and autonomous, resulting in increased professional growth. • Students develop and refine lifelong learning and clinical reasoning skills. • Students apply research evidence and their knowledge of occupational behavior models to practice. • Students gain skills in program development and skills in education, advocacy, and consultation roles. • The potential exists for the expansion of an occupational therapy role at the fieldwork site.
Drawbacks	• The program may not foster innovation, critical thinking, or reflective practice. • The program may foster dependency. • The program is difficult to implement with part-time staff. • Negative role modeling may occur.	• No one is available to model specific application of occupational therapy skills. • Placement is challenging for students with limited confidence or knowledge of the occupational therapy role. • Therapy models used at the site may not align with an occupational therapy perspective. • The set-up and monitoring process can be challenging.

structure and expectations of a traditional and a role-emerging placement. A sample of learning objectives and weekly schedules of learning activities developed for other similar sites in the community may help the agency staff better understand how their agency needs might be met. The agency should also be aware of the resources it is expected to provide to make the experience successful, such as on-site supervision and space or materials for developing programs.

Securing the Site

After the academic program and the agency agree on a plan, they negotiate a formal memorandum of understanding (MOU). Negotiating an MOU can be time-consuming; therefore, the process should start early. The MOU must list the various components agreed upon for the placement such as the purpose and nature of the agreement, the purpose of the fieldwork, the nuances of a role-emerging placement, the provision of occupational therapy fieldwork educator supervision and on-site supervision, reasons for termination of student placement, and financial considerations. Financial considerations should include detailed information, for example, the hourly rate for service, the approximate hours to be invoiced, the expected dates of payment, and the specific activities or outcomes expected for payment received.

Once the MOU has been finalized, comprehensive planning for the fieldwork placement begins, starting with the establishment of site-specific learning objectives. To facilitate this process, the academic program may provide a learning-objectives template (see Exhibit 40.A.1 in Appendix 40.A), keeping in mind the site's purpose, values, and organizational structures. Because the site-specific objectives spell out the expectations for student performance in a particular setting, it is not acceptable to use objectives from another program.

The overall design of the learning activities for the placement should be built on the learning objectives. For example, if the role-emerging placement emphasizes skills in both direct service and program development, both of these components should be evident in the learning objectives and should be evaluated at midterm and at the conclusion of the placement. Direct services learning objectives involve delivery of direct care to clients and might include working collaboratively with other disciplines and working directly with residents in new development programming. Program development learning objectives are directed toward assessment of existing programs and creation of new programs and might include needs assessment, program planning, program implementation, and formative and summative evaluation.

Specific and sequential learning activities are needed to accomplish the learning objectives. Learning activities should be mapped out over the expected duration of the placement. To be flexible and responsive to student and agency needs, it may be more effective to plan learning activities over a select block of time rather than week by week. Because three stakeholders are involved in the learning process—the student, the on-site supervisor, and the occupational therapy fieldwork educator—care should be taken to spell out the responsibilities of each to minimize confusion and maximize accountability. See Exhibit 40.A.2 in Appendix 40.A for a sample of direct service and program development learning objectives and the responsibilities of all stakeholders.

Implementation

Laying the groundwork for fieldwork that includes development of learning outcomes, objectives, and learning activities prepares the site, university, and student for implementation of a successful fieldwork experience. Specifically, critical attention should be given to role delineation and facilitation of the learning experience. Exhibit 40.A.2 illustrates these concepts.

Role Delineation

Key players to be considered include the student, supervisors (occupational therapy fieldwork educator and non–occupational therapy on-site supervisor), and the AFWC. The plan for supervision should specifically and clearly delineate and describe the role of each participant and how the learning experience will be structured. Determining each participant's role in the experience will depend on the defined purpose of the placement as expressed in the learning objectives.

Students must be able to identify their learning needs and actively communicate with their fieldwork educator and others within the practice environment. When two or more students are paired together, they must effectively communicate while working with one another. Many of the students' learning activities are then shared among the student cohort, and students have an opportunity to be responsible for a particular aspect or component of learning and therefore can undertake a teaching role with peers. When the collaborative supervision model is used, all students are accountable to their supervisors, and to one another, and must be open to both giving and receiving feedback from one another during the learning process (Cohn, Dooley, & Simmons, 2002; Flood, Haslam, & Hocking, 2010).

Although the AFWC is not mentioned in the responsibilities sections of Exhibit 40.A.2 in Appendix 40.A, he or she is instrumental in planning weekly objectives and schedules before the placement begins. In some ways, the role of the AFWC in role-emerging fieldwork does not differ from a typical fieldwork placement because he or she supports the site by providing resources and problem solving as necessary. However, roles of the AFWC may vary depending on the supervisors and their experience with role-emerging placements. For example, if the supervisor has a good understanding of facilitating autonomous learning and application of occupation-based theoretical models, the AFWC may be less formally involved; however, if the supervisor does not have sufficient experience, consistent and more formal meetings and mentoring may be needed. Either way, it is likely that the AFWC will communicate with all parties more frequently during role-emerging than traditional fieldwork placements.

Facilitation of Learning

Facilitation of student learning is central to the learning process. Several resources in this chapter and in Appendix 40.A can be used to help guide the learning process. It is important for each program to ensure that students learn and use occupational therapy models to develop professional identity and that appropriate learning approaches that are consistent with the program's curriculum design and desired outcomes for the role-emerging fieldwork experience are implemented. It is also important to develop appropriate learning activities and assignments that meet fieldwork objectives. In addition, reflective journaling and weekly student feedback are essential components in facilitating student learning.

Participation in a role-emerging fieldwork placement has been associated with the development of autonomy, skills for independent practice, and strong professional identity (Cooper & Raine, 2009; Fieldhouse & Fedden, 2009; Overton et al., 2008; Rodger et al., 2009; Wood, 2005). Positive outcomes are more likely when fieldwork educators focus learning efforts on the development or refinement of clinical reasoning, take on a role of guiding instead of teaching, and

facilitate an understanding of professional identity (Mulholland & Derdall, 2005; Overton et al., 2008). Although development of a strong professional identity has been determined to be a positive outcome of role-emerging fieldwork (Fieldhouse & Fedden, 2009; Mulholland & Derdall, 2005), some research has found that students struggle to navigate their own profession's models within interagency models and remain focused on occupational therapy (Dancza et al., 2013; Rodger et al., 2009). In fact, practitioners have raised concern over whether or not a student can learn occupational therapy philosophy in a setting that does not already have an established occupational therapy presence (Fisher & Savin-Baden, 2002). Therefore, an important element of the fieldwork experience is critical attention to navigating the development of professional occupational therapy identity.

Each occupation-based theoretical model provides a unique way of organizing and describing the theoretical assumptions of occupational therapy for the purpose of guiding practice and distinguishing occupational therapy from other disciplines. It is essential that fieldwork educators be able to comfortably use these theoretical models to help students demonstrate the unique contributions of occupational therapy and guide students' learning throughout the fieldwork experience (Edwards & Thew, 2011). Moreover, because students are likely to have knowledge of theoretical models from classwork, they might join with the AFWC and other faculty to teach or provide resources to update the knowledge of the fieldwork educator if needed in this area (Thomas & Rodger, 2011).

Expertise in learning approaches is essential when collaborating with the facility to form weekly objectives and learning activities. Although discussion of adult learning principles is beyond the scope of this chapter, it is critical that AFWCs instruct fieldwork educators on learning approaches to facilitate desired outcomes. Typically, these learning approaches would be consistent with the academic program's curriculum design and be familiar to students. Additionally, the development of site-specific fieldwork objectives provides an orienting structure for a weekly road map for the fieldwork experience, as well as an objective measure for evaluating students' skills. Key players can review site-specific learning objectives and responsibilities each week to keep learning focused on desired outcomes.

Learning activities and assignments play a key role in meeting fieldwork objectives. Although potential assignments should be described in advance, AFWCs, occupational therapy fieldwork educators, on-site supervisors, and students should collaborate throughout the experience to develop and refine the learning activities and assignments. AFWCs may often be called upon for resources to supplement or refine these learning experiences. In the case example in Appendix 40.A, to meet the learning objective of interprofessional collaboration and dialogue with other disciplines, the AFWC and fieldwork educator collaborated to develop questions to guide the student's efforts (Exhibit 40.3).

Reflective journaling is recommended as a means to assist students in processing the learning experience and to assist occupational therapy supervisors in understanding students' strengths and weaknesses to better facilitate future learning. It can be especially beneficial for students working at an agency without an occupational therapy practitioner so that they are ready to raise discussion points and make best use of meeting times when the occupational therapy supervisor is present. A weekly formal meeting between the student or students and supervisors ensures that the student receives formative feedback throughout the experience and that learning objectives are accomplished in a timely fashion. Use of a weekly meeting guide (Exhibit 40.A.3 in Appendix 40.A) during the meeting to note student strengths and challenges and to identify goals for the coming week provides a record of student accomplishments. This guide can be referred to when completing the midterm and final evaluations and can provide a record of student performance in situations in which remediation was needed. In addition, when the form is completed by both the fieldwork educator and the student in advance of the weekly meeting, they can clarify perceptions and expectations to ensure that the learning objectives can be accomplished.

Evaluation

In this section, processes of evaluation are described relating to assessment of student learning and assessment of the fieldwork program from the perspective of the student, the fieldwork educator, the fieldwork site, and the academic program.

Assessment of Student Learning

Assessment of student learning should occur from both a formative and summative perspective. Providing student feedback throughout the fieldwork is essential to forming skills, attitudes, and behaviors that result in better client services and developing student professionalism. This feedback may occur during weekly meetings, as discussed previously, or at key transition points in the fieldwork. Transition points might include student completion of an important fieldwork task, such as a program evaluation or trial run with a difficult population. Feedback may also occur at preset time frames (e.g., 3-week intervals) throughout the fieldwork. The format for student assessment can be as simple as a summary of strengths and weaknesses in relation to key learning objectives. The American Occupational Therapy Association (AOTA) Fieldwork Performance Evaluation (FWPE; Chapters 58 and 59 in this book) form, if used for the final assessment, provides useful categories for the weekly meeting guide (Exhibit 40.A.3 in Appendix 40.A).

The AOTA Fieldwork Experience Assessment Tool (FEAT; AOTA, 2001; Chapter 13 in this book)

Exhibit 40.3. *Questions for the Interprofessional Collaboration Meeting*

- What is your educational background in (counseling vs. social work)?
- What frames of reference or models do you use to guide your practice?
- Can you tell me more about your approach to therapy? How does this guide your practice?
- What is your goal for the residents during process groups?
- What types of skills groups do you lead?
- What are some of the common ways you engage the residents during individual therapy sessions?
- During the individual therapy sessions, do you primarily utilize talk therapy or do you incorporate activities? If so, what types of activities?

is another formative assessment tool to assess the just-right fit between the student and the fieldwork experience. When a group collaborative model of supervision is used, it is important that the evaluation occur both individually and as a group to measure individual skills and abilities and the group's ability to work collaboratively. As with any fieldwork experience, it is necessary that the fieldwork educator notify the AFWC at the first sign of any difficulties or problems in student performance.

Fieldwork educators are responsible for evaluation of the clinical and professional performance of fieldwork students. The FWPE form might be used as a formative assessment at the midterm mark and as a summative measure at the completion. The fieldwork educator should refer back to the learning objectives to determine the student's level of performance in relation to desired outcomes. When both direct practice and program development are identified as learning outcomes, the fieldwork educator needs to translate the language of the FWPE form to address program development goals. For example, the "Assessment" category of the FWPE form is written to evaluate student assessment of a client, and the fieldwork educator will have to translate the items to assess the student's ability to complete a program needs assessment.

Assessment of the Fieldwork Program

Thorough assessment of the fieldwork program requires the perspective of all stakeholders—student, fieldwork educator, fieldwork facility, and academic program. The AFWC, representing the academic program, should evaluate the learning opportunities offered by the facility in view of curricular goals and accreditation standards. The assessment tool should mirror the definitions and learning outcomes established by the academic program in relation to the role-emerging placement. In addition, data may be gathered regarding the quality of the procedures and processes used to achieve the stated outcomes, such as student knowledge or experience in the area of program development. If gathering data from the student, the Student Evaluation of the Fieldwork Experience (SEFWE; Chapter 30 of this book) form could be revised to include factors that are identified as salient by the academic program. A parallel instrument might be constructed for fieldwork educator and facility input.

Data collection might occur throughout the fieldwork to serve formative program planning goals. For example, communication (e.g., phone calls, emails) at regular intervals throughout the placement among the AFWC, fieldwork educator, site supervisor, and student may inform fieldwork program adjustments during the student placement. In contrast, collection of SEFWE form data at the conclusion of the experience could be used to evaluate the fieldwork site in relation to desired program outcomes. Collection of SEFWE form data over time from the same fieldwork site will provide data to meet accreditation standards, demonstrating the presence of best practice indicators such as use of research evidence to guide practice and the use of therapy processes supporting client-centered and occupation-based practice.

The fieldwork facility will, in a similar way, want to evaluate the effectiveness of the fieldwork program in meeting student learning and facility goals. Student learning goals should have been identified in the MOU and facility goals identified separately by the facility. An exit interview of the on-site supervisor during the last week of the placement can be used to capture data on facility perspectives of the strengths and weaknesses of the current placement and desired changes for future placement (Exhibit 40.4). The facility

---

Exhibit 40.4. *Facility Exit Interview*

- In what ways have your expectations for this fieldwork been met?
- Are there any further expectations or preferences that you had for this fieldwork that were not met?
- In what ways have your expectations for the role of occupational therapy changed as a result of this experience?
- What supports provided by the academic program have contributed to the success of this experience? What additional supports would be desired if you were to undertake a similar experience in the future?
- What would you do similarly or differently if you were to accommodate a similar type of placement in the future?
- What, if any, further feedback or questions do you have for the academic program?

(and the academic program) may also choose to use items from the SEFWE form to provide feedback about the on-site supervisor. In addition, although the Self-Assessment Tool for Fieldwork Educator Competency (SAFECOM; AOTA, 2009; Chapter 27 in this book) is primarily used as a self-assessment tool for the occupational therapy fieldwork educator, selected items from it might be helpful to evaluate the on-site supervisor. Cumulative review of AOTA FWPE forms may help the facility identify patterns of student strengths or weaknesses. Use of the FEAT can help the facility identify the effect of the fieldwork environment, personnel variables, or learning activities on the student's learning experience.

The SAFECOM also might be used by the fieldwork educator to self-assess competencies related to his or her education role and identify goals for continuing development. In addition, the AFWC should check in with the fieldwork educator at regular intervals to see what is working, what is not, and whether timeline adjustments or further resources or education are needed. The student should also evaluate the fieldwork educator using the SEFWE form (evaluation items on the form may be revised as needed to include supervision processes that are unique to the role-emerging placement).

The student's perspective of the learning experience should be captured throughout the learning experience, and a summative perspective should be obtained at the conclusion of the fieldwork. The SEFWE form serves as the primary tool for collecting the student's summative perspective and should be used both at midterm and at the conclusion of the experience. Student perspectives should include feedback about the supervision provided, the learning experiences and assignments, the environment of the placement, and the achievement of both personal and site learning objectives. See Exhibit 40.5 for samples of formative and summative reflective questions for students.

Exhibit 40.5. *Student Formative and Summative Reflective Questions*

Formative Questions for Week 4

- What did you do over Weeks 1, 2, 3, and 4?
- Reflecting back on what you did, what did you find the most helpful to your learning? How?
- If you had known right away what you know now (at Week 4), what would you have done differently?
- How has your supervision (on-site and fieldwork educator) been helpful?
- What changes would you suggest in supervisory structures for future students?
- What contextual features of the site contribute positively to or challenge your learning?
- What do you think will be most interesting or challenging for you in the next 4 weeks?

Formative Questions for Week 8

- What did you learn from putting together the needs assessment for your site?
- In what ways were you prepared for this assignment?
- What information would you have wanted for this project that you did not have?
- Discuss the process of securing a case study at your site. How did you go about identifying appropriate assessments or interventions? What kinds of negotiations with facility staff were needed to make this happen?
- Discuss the interprofessional learning opportunities available at your site. How did you negotiate involvement in the therapy process of another discipline? What did you learn from this process?
- What ethical dilemmas have you experienced and how did you resolve them?
- What have you discovered about yourself as a learner and about participating in the supervision process?
- How have you changed in the past 4 weeks of your fieldwork?

Summative Questions for Week 12

- How did this experience help you appreciate the unique role occupational therapy plays in an emerging practice setting?
- What have you learned about working with a treatment team in the process of program planning and development?

(Continued)

Exhibit 40.5. Student Formative and Summative Reflective Questions (Cont.)

- How would you rate your comfort level in assuming indirect occupational therapy roles such as consultation, advocacy, and education? How was this placement helpful to you in exploring these roles?
- What additional support would you need?
- How did you cope with the mental complexity and emotional component of your work?
- What suggestions would you make to future students?
- Reflecting back on your experience, what content and experiences in the academic program did you find most helpful to your success?
- What suggestions do you have for your academic program to better prepare future students for the role-emerging placement?
- How do you feel about taking on program planning efforts in the future?
- In what ways do you feel prepared and what additional resources and experiences do you think would be helpful?

Summative Questions for Student Exit Interview

- Looking back, what do you view as some of the highlights of this fieldwork experience?
- What have been some challenges in participating in this placement?
- What key learning experiences and knowledge did this experience provide?
- What has helped you learn or progress during this placement?
- What might you do differently in your future practice as a result of learning from this experience?

Summary

This chapter has presented a strategic method to approaching role-emerging fieldwork. An evidence-based review of multiple factors influencing the design of the role-emerging fieldwork placement, along with a discussion of processes and structures to get started, provides a blueprint for academic programs that wish to expand in this area. The sample tools provided throughout this chapter and in Appendix 40.A further support the establishment of the infrastructure needed to sustain excellence in the student learning experience. As health care continues to change, it is the authors' hope that more academic programs will take advantage of the unique learning opportunities inherent in role-emerging fieldwork placement to help students develop the attitudes and skills needed to competently address the health care challenges of the future.

References

Accreditation Council for Occupational Therapy Education. (2012). 2011 Accreditation Council for Occupational Therapy Education (ACOTE®) standards. *American Journal of Occupational Therapy, 66,* S6–S74. http://dx.doi.org/10.5014/ajot.2012.66S6

American Occupational Therapy Association. (2001). *Fieldwork experience assessment tool (FEAT).* Retrieved July 31, 2015, from http://www.aota.org//media/Corporate/Files/EducationCareers/Accredit/FEATCHARTMidterm.pdf

American Occupational Therapy Association. (2009). *Self-assessment tool for fieldwork educator competency* (SAFECOM). Retrieved from http://www.aota.org/-/-media/Corporate/Files/EducationCareers/Educators/Fieldwork/Supervisor/Forms/Self-Assessment%20Tool%20FW%20Ed%20Competency%20(2009).pdf

Amini, D., & Gupta, J. (2012). Fieldwork level II and occupational therapy students: A position paper. *The American Journal of Occupational Therapy, 66,* S75–S77. http://dx.doi.org/10.5014/ajot.2012.66S75

Bartholomai, S., & Fitzgerald, (2007). The collaborative model of fieldwork education: Implementation of the model in a regional hospital rehabilitation setting. *Australian Occupational Therapy Journal, 54,* S23–S30.

Bonello, M. (2001). Fieldwork within the context of higher education: A literature review. *British Journal of Occupational Therapy, 64,* 93–99.

Boniface, G., Seymour, A., Polglase, T., Lawrie, C., & Clarke, M. (2012). Exploring the nature of peer and academic supervision on a role-emerging placement. *British Journal of Occupational Therapy, 75,* 196–201. http://dx.doi.org/10.4276/030802212X13336366278211

Bossers, A., Cook, J., Polatajko, H. & Laine, C. (1997). Understanding the role-emerging fieldwork placement. *Canadian Journal of Occupational Therapy, 64,* 121–134.

Clark, I. (2004). Collaboration works best. *Occupational Therapy News, 12*(10), 28.

Clarke, C., Martin, M., Sadlo, G., & de Visser, R. (2014). The development of an authentic professional identity on role-emerging placements. *British Journal of Occupational Therapy, 7,* 222–229.

Cohn, E. S., Dooley, N., & Simmons, L. A. (2002). Collaborative learning applied to fieldwork education. *Occupational Therapy in Health Care, 15,* 69–83.

Cooper, R., & Raine, R. (2009). Role-emerging placements are an essential risk for development of the occupational therapy profession: The debate. *British Journal of Occupational Therapy, 72,* 416–418.

Costa, D. (2007). *Clinical supervision in occupational therapy: A guide for fieldwork and practice.* Bethesda, MD: AOTA Press.

Dancza, K., Warren, A. Copley, J., Rodger, S., Moran, M., McKay, E., & Taylor, A. (2013). Learning experiences on role-emerging placements: An exploration from the students' perspective. *Australian Occupational Therapy Journal, 60,* 427–435. http://dx.doi.org/10.1111/1440-1630.12079

Edwards, M., & Thew, M. (2011). Models of role-emerging placements. In M. Thew, M. Edwards, S. Baptiste, & M. Molineux (Eds.), *Role-emerging occupational therapy* (pp. 15–35). West Sussex, UK: Wiley-Blackwell.

Fieldhouse, J., & Fedden, T. (2009). Exploring the learning process on a role-emerging practice placement: A qualitative study. *British Journal of Occupational Therapy, 72,* 302–307.

Fisher, A., & Savin-Baden, M., (2002). Modernising fieldwork, part 2: Realising the new agenda. *British Journal of Occupational Therapy, 65,* 275–282.

Flood, B., Haslam, L., & Hocking, C. (2010). Implementing a collaborative model of student supervision in New Zealand: Enhancing therapist and student experiences. *New Zealand Journal of Occupational Therapy, 57,* 22–26.

Fortune, T., Farnworth, L., & McKinstry, C. (2006). Project-focused fieldwork: Core business or fieldwork fillers? *Australian Occupational Therapy Journal, 53,* 233–236. http://dx.doi.org/10.1111/j.1440-1630.2006.00562x

Fortune, T., & McKinstry, C. (2012). Project-based fieldwork: Perspectives of graduate entry students and project sponsors. *Australian Occupational Therapy Journal, 59,* 265–275. http://dx.doi.org/10.1111/j.1440-1630.2012.01026x

Gregory, P., Quelch, L., & Watanabe, E. (2011). *The student experience of a role-emerging placement.* In M. Thew, M. Edwards, S. Baptiste, & M. Molineux (Eds.), *Role-emerging occupational therapy* (pp. 54–65). West Sussex, UK: Wiley-Blackwell.

Hanson, D., & DeIuliis, E. (2015). The collaborative model of fieldwork education: A blueprint for group supervision of students. *Occupational Therapy in Health Care, 29*(2), 223–239. http://dx.doi.org/10.3109/07380577.2015.1011297

Holmes, W. M., & Scaffa, M. E. (2009). An exploratory study of competencies for emerging practice in occupational therapy. *Journal of Allied Health, 38,* 81–90.

Hunt, S. G. (2006). A practice placement education model based upon a primary health care perspective used in South Australia. *British Journal of Occupational Therapy, 69,* 81–85.

Martin, M., Morris, J., Moore, A., Sadlo, G., & Crouch, V. (2004). Evaluating practice education models in occupational therapy: Comparing 1:1, 2:1, and 3:1 placements. *British Journal of Occupational Therapy, 67,* 192–200.

Molineux, M., & Baptiste, S. (2011). Emerging occupational therapy practice: Building on the foundations and seizing the opportunities. In M. Thew, M. Edwards, S. Baptiste, & M. Molineux (Eds.), *Role-emerging occupational therapy* (pp. 3–14). West Sussex, UK: Wiley-Blackwell.

Mulholland, S., & Derdall, M. (2005). A strategy for supervising occupational therapy students at community sites. *Occupational Therapy International, 12,* 28–43.

Overton, A., Clark, M., & Thomas, Y. (2009). A review of non-traditional occupational therapy practice placement education: A focus on role-emerging and project placements. *British Journal of Occupational Therapy, 72,* 294–301.

Prigg, A., & Mackenzie, L. (2002). Project placements for undergraduate occupational therapy students: Design, implementation and evaluation. *Occupational Therapy International, 9,* 210–236.

Rodger, S., Thomas, Y., Holley, S., Springfield, E., Edwards, A., Broadbridge, J., Greber, S., … Hawkins, R. (2009). Increasing the occupational therapy mental health workforce through innovative practice education: A pilot project. *Australian Occupational Therapy Journal, 56,* 409–417. http://dx.doi.org/10.1111/j.1440-1630.2009.00806.x

Smith, Y., Cornella, E., & Williams, N. (2014). Working with populations from a refugee background: An opportunity to enhance the occupational therapy educational experience. *Australian Occupational Therapy Journal, 61,* 20–27. http://dx.doi.org/10.1111/1440-1630.12037

Thew, M., Hargreaves, A., & Cronin-Davis, J. (2008). An evaluation of a role-emerging practice placement model for a full cohort of occupational therapy students. *British Journal of Occupational Therapy, 71,* 348–353.

Thomas, Y., Penman, M., & Williamson, P. (2005). Australian and New Zealand fieldwork: Charting the territory for future practice. *Australian Occupational Therapy Journal, 52,* 78–81.

Thomas, Y., & Rodger, S. (2011). Successful role-emerging placements: It is all in the preparation. In M. Thew, M. Edwards, S. Baptiste, & M. Molineux (Eds.), *Role-emerging occupational therapy* (pp. 39–53). West Sussex, UK: Wiley-Blackwell.

Wood, A. (2005). Student practice contexts: Changing face, changing place. *British Journal of Occupational Therapy, 68,* 375–378.

Appendix 40.A.
Case Example: Child Adolescent Residential Center

The following case example demonstrates the authors' application of the role-emerging fieldwork model described in Chapter 40 and illustrates how we applied each step of the model.

Stage 1: Identification of Potential Site

The site was identified through a student currently enrolled in our academic program. This residential program for children and adolescents with behavioral health issues had the goal of helping clients gain skills and behaviors for placement in the community and wanted to establish occupational therapy services. After the student request, the academic fieldwork coordinator (AFWC) arranged a meeting with the facility to discuss role-emerging fieldwork, provided documentation of fieldwork models, and described the goals of the academic program for the fieldwork. The academic program emphasized to the the residential program the coursework and Level I fieldwork experiences in the curriculum that address behavioral health needs for children and adolescents. Because program development was a desired outcome of the facility and an expected learning outcome of the academic program, the AFWC highlighted curriculum elements that supported student skills in this area. After outlining the Accreditation Council for Occupational Therapy Education (ACOTE®, 2012) guidelines for supervision of role-emerging placements, the AFWC and other academic program representatives outlined the criteria used to evaluate each student's readiness to participate responsibly in the supervisory process. Throughout this conversation, academic program representatives listened for the ability of the academic program and agency to support each other in accomplishing mutual goals.

Stage 2: Process for Securing the Site

Establishment of the memorandum of agreement was the next step in the process. In this case, the facility chose to have the university provide supervision, so a separate contract was negotiated for covering the costs of the occupational therapy supervision.

Template of Site-Specific Learning Objectives for Role-Emerging Fieldwork

A template of potential learning objectives was developed around the focus areas of the American Occupational Therapy Association (AOTA, 2002) Fieldwork Performance Evaluation as an aid for the facility and academic program to work out mutually desirable learning outcomes pertaining to both direct services and program development.

Direct Service Provision: Learning activities *involve provision of direct care to clients and might include* working collaboratively with other disciplines, such as cofacilitation of groups where occupational therapy services are not being directly billed and working directly with residents in new development programming, which would not be directly billable during the time of development.

Program Development: Learning activities are *directed toward assessment of existing programming and creation of new programs and might include* needs assessment, program planning, program implementation, and formative and summative evaluation.

Section 1: Fundamentals of Practice

Direct Service Provision and Program Development

- Adheres to ethics: Adheres consistently to the *Occupational Therapy Code of Ethics* (AOTA, 2015) and cites policies and procedures, including, when elevant, those related to human participant research.
- Adheres to safety regulations: Adheres consistently to safety regulations and anticipates potentially hazardous situations and takes steps to prevent accidents.
- Uses judgment in safety: Uses sound judgment in regards to safety of self and others during all fieldwork-related activities.

Section 2: Basic Tenets

Direct Service Provision

- Clearly and confidently articulates the values and beliefs of the occupational therapy profession to service recipients.

- Clearly, confidently, and accurately articulates the values of occupation as a method and desired outcome of occupational therapy to service recipients.
- Collaborates with the client, family, and facility throughout the occupational therapy process.
- Compares and contrasts differences between direct service in residential versus community-based settings.
- Articulates the role of occupational therapy with attention to how occupational therapy would complement versus duplicate existing services at this facility.

Program Development

- Conceptualizes and articulates potential roles for occupational therapy at this site.
- Applies occupational therapy–based conceptual models to development of programming for the site.
- Articulates to stakeholders the values, beliefs, and focus on occupation in the program development process.

Section 3: Evaluation and Screening

Direct Service Provision

- Articulates a clear and logical rationale for the evaluation process.
- Selects relevant screening and assessment methods.
- Determines the client's occupational profile and performance through appropriate assessment methods.
- Assesses client factors and contexts.
- Administers assessments and adjusts or modifies them as necessary.
- Interprets evaluation results.
- Establishes an appropriate intervention plan based on evaluation data.
- Documents the results of the evaluation process that demonstrate objective measurements of the client's occupational performance.

Program Development

- Obtains sufficient information from key stakeholders to understand the mission and vision of the facility.
- Applies skills in program planning, including completion of a needs assessment.

- Interprets needs assessment results to develop program recommendations for occupational therapy services at the facility.
- Establishes potential contributions of an occupational therapy practitioner at the site based on assessment data.
- Develops a formal written report of the needs assessment process.

Section 4: Intervention (and Program Planning)

Direct Service Provision

- Articulates a clear and logical rationale for the intervention process.
- Utilizes evidence from published research and relevant resources to make informed intervention decisions.
- Chooses occupations that motivate and challenge clients.
- Selects relevant occupations to facilitate clients meeting established goals.
- Implements intervention plans that are client-centered.
- Implements intervention plans that are occupation-based.
- Modifies task approach, occupations, and environment to maximize client performance.
- Updates, modifies, or terminates the intervention plan based on careful monitoring of the client's status.
- Documents the client's response to services in a manner that demonstrates the efficacy of interventions.
- Collaborates with other occupational therapy and occupational therapy assistant students and professionals in other disciplines in providing interdisciplinary intervention.

Program Development

- Collaborates with the facility to determine one potential area for developing occupational therapy programming.
- Develops programming based on published research and relevant resources.
- Develops programming based on an occupational therapy conceptual model to highlight engagement in occupation as a program outcome.
- Implements the programming that was developed, making modifications as indicated by formative assessment data.

- Develops a summative outcome evaluation tool for the program.
- Collects outcomes data and prepares a final report for the facility.

Section 5: Management of Occupational Therapy Services

Direct Service Provision and Program Development

- Identifies appropriate assignments or responsibilities of a potential occupational therapy assistant in this setting.
- Demonstrates understanding of costs and funding related to occupational therapy services at this site.
- Accomplishes organizational goals and fieldwork program development goals by establishing priorities, developing strategies, and meeting deadlines.
- Produces the volume of work required in the expected time frame.

Section 6: Communication

Direct Service Provision

- Clearly and effectively communicates verbally and nonverbally with clients, families, significant others, colleagues, team members, service providers, and the public. Produces clear and accurate documentation according to the site requirements.
- Ensures that all written communication is legible, using proper spelling, punctuation, and grammar.
- Uses language appropriate to the recipient of the information, including but not limited to funding agencies and regulatory agencies.

Program Development

- Clearly and effectively communicates with stakeholders in the program development process.

- Clearly and effectively expresses recommendations regarding program development to the stakeholders.
- Develops a professional, well-written report using proper spelling, punctuation, and grammar.

Section 7: Professional Behaviors

Direct Service Provision and Program Development

- Collaborates with the supervisor to maximize the learning experience.
- Takes responsibility for attaining professional competence by seeking learning opportunities and interactions with supervisors and others.
- Responds constructively to feedback.
- Demonstrates consistent work behaviors, including initiative, preparedness, dependability, and work site maintenance.
- Demonstrates effective time management.
- Demonstrates positive interpersonal skills, including but not limited to cooperation, flexibility, tact, and empathy.
- Demonstrates respect for diversity factors of others, including but not limited to sociocultural, socioeconomic, spiritual, and lifestyle choices.

Stage 3: Ready, Set, Go—Implementation

The following schedule maps the sequence for student learning of skills for direct service and program development over discrete 3-week time periods, including a description of the expected roles for the student, occupational therapy supervisor, and on-site supervisor. In addition, a sample weekly meeting guide (Exhibit 40.A.1) and descriptions of formal learning assignments corresponding with student learning objectives (Exhibit 40.A.2) are provided as additional resources.

Exhibit 40.A.1. *Occupational Therapy Student Weekly Meeting Guide*

Student Name: _____

Date: _____   **Week #** _____

Fieldwork educator should consider both direct practice and program development in review.

FUNDAMENTALS/BASIC TENETS OF PRACTICE	
Areas of Strength	**Areas of Need**

EVALUATION AND SCREENING	
Areas of Strength	**Areas of Need**

INTERVENTION	
Areas of Strength	**Areas of Need**

MANAGEMENT OF OCCUPATIONAL THERAPY SERVICES	
Areas of Strength	**Areas of Need**

COMMUNICATION/PROFESSIONAL BEHAVIORS	
Areas of Strength	**Areas of Need**

PROGRESS SUMMARY	
Direct Practice Objectives	**Program Development Objectives**

Fieldwork Schedule Revisions

Additional Student Support Needed

STUDENT LEARNING GOALS		
Student-Initiated Objectives	**Activities to Achieve Goals**	**Desired Supervisor Support**

Student Signature _____ **Date** _____

FW Educator Signature _____ **Date** _____

Exhibit 40.A.2. Formal Learning Assignments

Weekly Review of Progress

A regularly scheduled weekly meeting is set to review and clarify site-specific and student-generated learning objectives/assignments and to facilitate communication among the student, on-site supervisor, and occupational therapy supervisor. The format of the meeting should facilitate student and supervisor reflection and solidify learning goals and activities for the coming week (see Exhibit 40.A.1).

Journal and Reflective Writing Assignments

Journaling assignments are used to facilitate student reflection on a variety of subjects that might influence direct client treatment or program development process. Attention might be given to therapeutic use of self, professional presentation, and clinical or theoretical reasoning pertaining to both direct practice and program development. Specific assignments are determined collaboratively between the student and the occupational therapy supervisor at the regularly scheduled weekly meeting. Journals should be turned in 24 hours before the weekly meeting, and the occupational therapy supervisor should respond to the journaling either through written comments or during a discussion, or potentially both. (Further journaling assignments often are identified from concerns or questions students discuss in their journals.)

Interprofessional or Intraprofessional Collaboration

Collaboration experiences can include interprofessional or intraprofessional experiences. Ongoing communication and evaluation are essential to quality collaboration. The student will participate in a midterm discussion of the collaboration, identifying what is going well and what needs improvement. This discussion includes attention to interprofessional or intraprofessional communication, teams and teamwork, complementary professional roles and responsibilities, and interprofessional values and ethics. The discussion should also include the opportunity to compare and contrast occupation-based models with the models used by other disciplines in the interprofessional collaboration. The student, on-site supervisor, and occupational therapy supervisor will collaboratively design the format for a final interview or reflective summary to identify strengths, weaknesses, and suggestions for future collaboration.

Case Study

The student will prepare a final report on the evaluation and intervention process that was followed for direct intervention on a chosen client. The case study will illustrate the application of an evidence-based intervention, showing the unique role of occupational therapy as distinguished from existing occupational therapy or residential services through the application of an occupation-based model. The case study will include a theoretical orientation for services provided, research support for services, and detailed information about the client, including an occupational profile, evaluation results, occupation-based goals, and outcomes of performance collected throughout the intervention period. Although examples will be provided, the specific protocol for the case-study assignment will be negotiated between the occupational therapy supervisor and the student.

Professional Needs Assessment and Possible Program Recommendations Report

This report will be developed on the basis of the student's needs assessment using an occupation-based model. The student will use three-phase model (Witkin & Alschuld, 1995) to complete the needs assessment. This model includes (1) a preassessment to investigate what is known about the needs of the facility and to determine the focus and scope of the assessment data–gathering process; (2) an assessment to focus on identifying the issues and how they compare with the vision and to understand the magnitude of needs, with outcome needs being identified in order of priority; and (3) a postassessment to identify potential solutions to the problem or need (road map for the future of occupational therapy services). The student will develop a formal report that highlights each of these areas.

Presentation of the Needs Assessment to Key Stakeholders

This presentation will be a formal presentation of the needs assessment and possible program recommendations. This assessment will highlight key features in the report and be presented through the lens of an occupation-based model. The student should select the most pertinent information and refer to the needs assessment report.

(Continued)

Exhibit 40.A.2. Formal Learning Assignments (Cont.)

Development of One Specific Program

The student, occupational therapy supervisor, and on-site supervisor will collaborate to select one program for the student to further develop during the fieldwork experience. The student will use a program development process as determined with the occupational therapy supervisor to guide the development process. The student will apply an occupation-based model in the program development process. An example of this process is outlined by Fazio (2008), which includes developing a design, profiling the population, researching the evidence to support choices, determining staffing and personnel, finding space, estimating costs, funding the program, marketing, and evaluating the program.

Presentation of the Developed Program to Key Stakeholders

The student will present the program to key stakeholders at two points. First, the student will present the program before implementation. At this point, the student will highlight the key elements of the program as outlined by Fazio (2008) and seek feedback from the key stakeholders. The student will then implement and formatively assess the program or an element of the program. Once the program is formatively assessed and the student makes modifications, the student will again report on the changes made and the outcomes of the program in its initial implementation.

Optional Opportunities to Educate the Team About Occupational Therapy

The student, on-site supervisor, and occupational therapy supervisor will collaborate to determine whether additional presentations or opportunities to educate others about occupational therapy are necessary. These educational opportunities could take the form of a formal presentation, handout, or roundtable.

Emerging Fieldwork Schedule

This document serves as a guide and can be modified or adjusted as agreed upon by the student, on-site supervisor, and occupational therapy supervisor.

Week 1–3 Objectives

Direct Service	Program Development
Follow facility Health Insurance Portability and Accountability Act of 1996 (Pub. L. 104–191) guidelines.	Identify remaining elements needed for needs assessment.
Follow safety policies within the facility.	Identify the mission and vision of the facility.
Understand the residents' daily schedule.	Understand key stakeholders' views and ideas.
Understand the roles of the providers and staff.	Analyze facility data, such as satisfaction surveys, strategic plan, and SWOT (strengths, weakness, opportunities, threats) analysis.
Understand the documentation system.	
Identify one interprofessional collaboration and occupational therapist or occupational therapy assistant for facilitating direct intervention, and develop a plan to assist in intervention.	Understand residents' daily schedules.
	Present a preliminary needs assessment during Week 3.
Identify a resident for case study and potential evaluation tools.	

Week 1–3 Responsibilities

Student Responsibilities	On-Site Supervisor Responsibilities	Occupational Therapy Supervisor Responsibilities
Document key elements for needs assessment, including resident schedules, key stakeholder views, and facility data.	Orient to the facility policies and procedures, and inform the student and occupational therapy supervisor of any prerequisites required.	Assist the student in processing information obtained for the needs assessment, including viewing from an occupational therapy model, such as the Person–Environment–Occupation Model (Law, Cooper, & Strong 1996).
Identify and interview key stakeholders.	With the occupational therapy supervisor, establish a weekly schedule for the first week and then assist in schedule development for Weeks 2–3.	Assist the student in selecting a case study and viewing the case from an occupational therapy model perspective.
Document other disciplines' evaluations and interventions to determine how occupational therapy may complement and not duplicate a service already being provided.	Orient to documentation system and plans of care.	Assist the student in exploring resources and finalizing choices for assessment and intervention protocols for the case study client.
With supervisors, select and determine a plan for interprofessional or intraprofessional intervention collaboration.	Orient to facility schedule and resident schedules.	Assist the student in securing assessment resources as needed.
With supervisors, select a resident for the case study.	Assist the student in setting up opportunities to follow residents through programming and residential living.	Assist the student as needed to develop appropriate questions for interviewing key stakeholders.
Obtain facility data for the needs assessment.	Introduce the student to on-site staff.	Assist the student in developing the needs assessment report.
Each week, prepare a written draft of the needs assessment to review with the occupational therapy supervisor.	Process events with the student as they occur in the course of the workweek.	Provide feedback on progress toward objectives in a weekly meeting (formal form is used; see Exhibit 40.1).
Complete journal and weekly supervision sheet.	Act as a liaison in assisting the student to make connections to key stakeholders and staff for completion of objectives.	Meet weekly with student and on-site supervisor to refine learning objectives and weekly plans.
Review fieldwork objectives and identify any additional student learning objectives with the occupational and on-site supervisors (students may identify additional learning objectives specific to their interests).	Discuss and determine with the student, staff, and occupational therapy supervisor the options for interprofessional or intraprofessional collaboration that are most feasible within the center.	
Meet weekly with the occupational therapy supervisor and on-site supervisor to clarify weekly plans to ensure objectives can be accomplished.	Assist in determining facility and reimbursement regulations for documentation cosigning.	
	Meet weekly with the student and occupational therapy supervisor to clarify weekly plans to ensure objectives can be accomplished (allow approximately 1 hr).	
	Provide feedback on progress toward objectives in a weekly meeting (formal form is used; see Exhibit 40.1).	

Week 4–6 Objectives

Direct Service	Program Development
Articulate how the assessment and intervention the student provides to the identified case study client complements or adds to the existing facility services with supervisors and at a team meeting.	Review the needs assessment report with an eye toward potential occupational therapy program expansion options (i.e., a road map for the facility to look at occupational therapy in the future). All areas will not be able to be developed; the goal instead is for one area to be selected and the student learning outcome to be developing that program piece.
Complete an evaluation and report for the case study client (Week 4).	
Explain occupational profile and occupation-based goals for the case study client to the staff.	
Co-plan and provide direct interprofessional or intraprofessional intervention and ongoing assessment of effectiveness of intervention.	With supervisors, determine one area of potential occupational therapy expansion and identify the program to be developed.
Be able to analyze interprofessional or intraprofessional collaboration to identify what is going well and what could go better.	Complete research to develop the chosen program.
	Develop the program outcomes, evaluation tools, protocol/sequence, specific activities, cost estimate, billing options, and duration.
Compare and contrast occupation-based models to the models used by other disciplines in the interprofessional collaboration.	Respond to facility questions about proposed programming, educate the treatment team on one aspect of program delivery, and justify the choices made.
Complete documentation of interprofessional or intraprofessional intervention as deemed appropriate according to facility rules and regulations.	
Compare and contrast the roles of occupational therapy with other core service providers.	

Week 4–6 Responsibilities

Student Responsibilities	On-Site Supervisor Responsibilities	Occupational Therapy Supervisor Responsibilities
Prepare to discuss unique roles of team members with the occupational therapy supervisor in preparation for the team meeting, and explain how the assessment and intervention provided to the case study client complements or adds to existing occupational therapy and residential services.	Observe the student in team meetings, and note progress on objectives. Assist the student in negotiating space and time options for providing individual intervention.	Assist the student in identifying and understanding the processing unique roles of team members and the unique role occupational therapy can play by keeping the student focused on occupation-based models.
Share the evaluation report for the case study client with the on-site and occupational therapy supervisors and possibly the treatment team.	As necessary, act as a liaison for interprofessional intervention. As necessary, receive feedback from other key stakeholders in selecting an area for program development.	Provide feedback on the evaluation process and report. Oversee planning and implementation of the occupational therapy intervention used in the case study.
Present the occupational profile and occupation-based goals for the case study client to the on-site supervisor,		

(Continued)

Week 4–6 Responsibilities *(Cont.)*

Student Responsibilities	On-Site Supervisor Responsibilities	Occupational Therapy Supervisor Responsibilities
occupational therapy supervisor, and possibly staff by the end of Week 4, and begin to implement individualized and direct occupational therapy services. Continue to implement interprofessional or intraprofessional services, and participate in ongoing evaluation and dialogue about services provided with the on-site and occupational therapy supervisors and interprofessional colleagues. Co-plan and provide direct interprofessional intervention and ongoing assessment of the effectiveness of intervention. Complete a formative discussion of interprofessional collaboration at the end of Week 6 following written guidelines. Complete documentation of interprofessional intervention as deemed appropriate according to facility rules and regulations. Refine and produce the final copy of the needs assessment with recommendations (Week 4). Seek assistance as necessary when researching and developing the program (assistance could include librarian, occupational therapy supervisor, on-site supervisor, or other stakeholders). Refine the learning objective and student-directed weekly learning objectives with supervisors (i.e., the student requests to learn more about something or needs to address a skill set).	Provide feedback on the quality of the needs assessment report and recommendations. Provide feedback on progress toward objectives in the weekly meeting (formal form is used; see Exhibit 40.1).	If possible, observe interprofessional intervention and provide feedback. Review documentation as appropriate (check guidelines for signatures). Collaborate in refinement and presentation of the needs assessment. Assist the student through consultation and problem solving in developing the selected program. Provide feedback on progress toward objectives in the weekly meeting (formal form is used; see Exhibit 40.1). Collaborate with the on-site supervisor to refine learning objectives and weekly plans.

Week 7–9 Objectives

Direct Service	Program Development
Process interprofessional or intraprofessional cofacilitation, paying attention to application of models. Justify 1:1 intervention for the case study client. Communicate the case study client's occupation-based goals and progress at the team meetings. Begin providing the developed program or element of the program as a means to engage in formative evaluation and then refinement of the program (Week 8).	Refine the program through feedback from stakeholders (Week 7). Engage in formative assessment and modification of the program or element of the program as appropriate.

Week 7–9 Responsibilities

Student Responsibilities	On-Site Supervisor Responsibilities	Occupational Therapy Supervisor Responsibilities
Provide ongoing reports of client progress during team meetings. Continue to implement interprofessional or intraprofessional services and participate in ongoing dialogue with the on-site and occupational therapy supervisors and interprofessional colleagues. Prepare to discuss formative assessment data related to the new occupational therapy program being implemented; discuss implications of data in ongoing conversations with the treatment team. Initiate formal and informal means for attainment of ongoing formative assessment data from key stakeholders, and document the results. Refine and produce a summary of the formative evaluation of the program (end of Week 9). Seek assistance as necessary for continued program refinement and implementation (assistance could include the librarian, occupational therapy supervisor, on-site supervisor, or other stakeholders).	Observe the student in team meetings, and note progress on objectives. Assist the student in negotiating and responding to any challenges that arise for program implementation or individual case study intervention. As necessary, act as a liaison for interprofessional intervention. Assist in determining potential reimbursement options for the developed program. If necessary, receive feedback from other key stakeholders regarding new occupational therapy programming implementation. With the student, discuss additional opportunities for him or her to educate team members about occupational therapy. Provide feedback on the quality of the midterm program evaluation report. Provide feedback on progress toward objective identified in the learning contract through the use of the weekly meeting guide (Exhibit 40.1).	Assist student in processing formative assessment data of programming success; help student maintain focus on unique roles of team members and unique role occupational therapy can play by keeping student focused on occupation-based models. Provide feedback on means used by student to attain ongoing formative assessment data. If possible, observe interprofessional intervention and provide feedback. Discuss with student potential formats for final reflection on interprofessional experience. Review documentation as appropriate (check guidelines for signatures). Oversee planning and implementation of individual case study, occupational therapy intervention, and implementation of occupational therapy programming. Collaborate in the refinement and presentation of the midterm formative program assessment. Assist the student in identifying alternative tools or methods to address any challenges that arise in

(Continued)

Week 7–9 Responsibilities *(Cont.)*

Discuss additional opportunities for educating the team members about occupational therapy. Refine the learning objective and the student-directed weekly learning objectives with supervisors (e.g., student requests to learn more about something or needs to address a skill set).		program or individual case study implementation. Discuss with the student a format for the final case study presentation. Provide feedback on progress toward objectives in the learning contract through use of the weekly meeting guide (Exhibit 40.1). Collaborate with the on-site supervisor as needed to coordinate feedback for and resources provided to the student.

Week 10–12 Objectives

Direct Service	Program Development
Present final case study of 1:1 intervention. Plan for and implement closure of services being provided. Engage in an exit interview or discussion with the on-site supervisor and interprofessional or intraprofessional collaborators to identify strengths, weaknesses, and suggestions for future interprofessional collaboration.	Modify the program using the formative assessment data. Present the final program with additional recommendations for occupational therapy at the facility, wrapping up or adding any final details to the needs assessment and recommendations.

Week 10–12 Responsibilities

Student Responsibilities	On-Site Supervisor Responsibilities	Occupational Therapy Supervisor Responsibilities
Continue to implement 1:1 intervention for the case study client, and present the final case study of 1:1 intervention (end of Week 10). Continue to participate in the interprofessional or intraprofessional intervention; determine the format for the exit interview or reflective summary of the experience in conjunction with the on-site supervisor, occupational therapy supervisor, and interprofessional colleagues (end of Week 12). Continue to discuss with the treatment team the formative assessment data collected relative	Observe the student in team meetings, and collect data from other site sources as appropriate regarding student progress and student-initiated learning objectives. Assist the student in negotiating and responding to any challenges that arise for program or individual case study implementation or evaluation. As necessary, act as a liaison for interprofessional intervention and the final exit interview or reflective summary.	Assist the student in processing formative and summative assessment data for individual occupational therapy intervention, interprofessional intervention, and program development in view of occupational therapy models to highlight the unique contributions of occupational therapy. Oversee planning and implementation of closure of individual occupational therapy programming and the case study presentation. Observe and provide feedback to the student on interprofessional or intraprofessional intervention

(Continued)

Week 10–12 Responsibilities *(Cont.)*

to the new occupational therapy program being implemented.	Assist the student in determining the most appropriate format and audience for sharing formative and summative program assessments.	and on the exit interview or reflective summary with the on-site supervisor and interprofessional or intraprofessional colleagues.
Compile and share the formative assessment data from key stakeholders to demonstrate program modifications made in response to data obtained.	Provide feedback on the quality of final program evaluation report.	Clarify with the on-site staff any additional signatures required for documentation according to the guidelines determined at the onset of fieldwork.
Share final recommendations for future program refinement with appropriate stakeholders (end of Week 12).	Provide feedback on progress toward objectives identified in the learning contract through the use of the weekly meeting guide (Exhibit 40.A.1) and performance objectives as identified on the final AOTA (2002) Fieldwork Performance Evaluation.	Provide feedback on the means used by the student to attain formative and summative program assessment data.
Seek assistance as necessary for continued program refinement, implementation and finalprogram review, and program closure or transition.		Collaborate with the student on refinement and presentation of the final program assessment.
Refine the learning objective and student-directed weekly learning objectives with supervisors (e.g., student requests to learn more about something or needs to address a skill set).		Assist the student in identifying alternative tools or methods to address any challenges that arise in individual, interprofessional, or program implementation evaluation and closure.
		Provide feedback on weekly and final progress toward site-specific objectives identified in the learning contract.
		Collaborate with the on-site supervisor as needed to coordinate feedback and resources provided to the student and to facilitate the final student and site evaluation.

References

Accreditation Council for Occupational Therapy Education (2012). 2011 Accreditation Council for OT Education (ACOTE®) standards. *American Journal of Occupational Therapy, 66,* S6–S74. http://dx.doi.org/10.5014/ajot.2012.66S6

American Occupational Therapy Association. (2002). *AOTA Fieldwork Performance Evaluation.* Bethesda, MD: AOTA Press.

American Occupational therapy Association (in press). Occupational therapy code of ethics. *American Journal of Occupational Therapy, 69* (Suppl. 3).

Fazio, L. S. (2008). *Developing occupation-centered programs for the community.* Upper Saddle River, NJ: Pearson.

Health Insurance Portability and Accountability Act of 1996, Pub. L. 104–191, 42 U.S.C. § 300gg, 29 U.S.C § 1181-1183, and 42 USC 1320d-1320d9

Law, M., Cooper, B., & Strong, S. (1996). The Person–Environment–Occupation Model: A transactive approach to occupational performance. *Canadian Journal of Occupational Therapy, 63*(1), 9–23.

Witkin, B. R., & Altschuld, J.W. (1995). *Planning and conducting needs assessments: A practical guide.* Thousand Oaks, CA: Sage Publications.

Chapter 41.

GENERAL GUIDE FOR PLANNING INTERNATIONAL FIELDWORK

American Occupational Therapy Association Commission on Education

Purpose

Increase awareness and knowledge of subjects to be considered while planning an international fieldwork experience in relation to three types of fieldwork placements, including Level I fieldwork, Level II fieldwork, and non–Level I or II fieldwork.

Introduction

International fieldwork refers to a dual exchange. Students who are enrolled in an academic occupational therapy (OT)/occupational therapy assistant (OTA) program in the United States may complete fieldwork experiences outside the United States. If these experiences are considered part of the students' required fieldwork, placements must comply with the Accreditation Council for Occupational Therapy (ACOTE®) Standards (ACOTE, 2007a, b, & c). In addition, students enrolled in an academic OT/OTA program outside of the United States may seek fieldwork opportunities within the United States. This scenario does not require ACOTE standard compliance. While there is sensitivity to overall ACOTE fieldwork Standards for academic OT/OTA programs within the United States, this guide does not include all relevant fieldwork Standards. This document is meant to be used as a guide for planning an international fieldwork experience by raising awareness of areas to consider.

Accompanying guides and documents should be reviewed for other essential elements to consider when planning an international fieldwork.

Areas of discussion: Three major categories where the guidelines will be applied need to be identified.

Level II fieldwork	Level I fieldwork or equivalent	Non–Level I or II fieldwork*
Level II fieldwork goal: To develop competent, entry-level, generalist occupational therapists and occupational therapy assistants (ACOTE, 2007a, b, & c).	Level I fieldwork goal: To introduce students to the fieldwork experience, to apply knowledge to practice, and to develop understanding of the needs of clients (ACOTE, 2007a, b, & c).	May have broader goals and include student's professional development interests, academic OT/OTA program's social justice overtures, and student professional and personal growth.
The experience should provide the student with the opportunity to carry out professional responsibilities under supervision and for professional role modeling (ACOTE, 2007a, b, & c).	The experience may include exposure to populations and/or observations beyond occupational therapy–specific settings in relation to the academic OT/OTA program's stated objectives.	

Note: There are additional separate Standards for an experiential component required for doctoral-level-educational programs (ACOTE, 2007a).

Collaboration: A fieldwork consortium may include the academic OT/OTA program, the fieldwork educator, and the student.

Level II fieldwork	Level I fieldwork or equivalent	Non–Level I or II fieldwork*
Ensure that the academic fieldwork coordinator and faculty collaborate to design fieldwork experiences that strengthen the ties between didactic and fieldwork education. Standard B.10.2 (ACOTE, 2007a, b, & c)	Ensure that the academic fieldwork coordinator and faculty collaborate to design fieldwork experiences that strengthen the ties between didactic and fieldwork education. Standard B.10.2 (ACOTE, 2007a, b, & c)	The fieldwork site may have links with the academic OT/OTA program. An academic OT/OTA program in the receiving country may be involved in referrals to fieldwork sites.

Selection: Both the WFOT Web site and journal are good initial resources for contacts in the country of choice.

Level II fieldwork	Level I fieldwork or equivalent	Non–Level I or II fieldwork*
Document the criteria and process for selecting fieldwork sites. Ensure that the fieldwork program** reflects the sequence, depth, focus, and scope of content in the curriculum design. ACOTE Standard B.10.1 (ACOTE, 2007a & b)	Document the criteria and process for selecting fieldwork sites. Ensure that the fieldwork program** reflects the sequence, depth, focus, and scope of content in the curriculum design. ACOTE Standard B.10.1 (ACOTE, 2007c)	Wider opportunity for choices, as it does not have to meet ACOTE requirements regarding fieldwork but must meet programmatic accreditation standards.

**Fieldwork program refers to the fieldwork site's curriculum.

Communication: Disclosure and transparency are crucial in communicating among fieldwork site, academic OT/OTA program, and student. Try to access website and written documents, aiding in clarification for fieldwork site in conjunction with personal correspondences.

Level II fieldwork	Level I fieldwork or equivalent	Non–Level I or II fieldwork*
For international fieldwork, another member of the faculty may have more expertise than the academic fieldwork coordinator (AFWC). Ensure that the AFWC is responsible for advocating for the development of links between the fieldwork and didactic aspects of the curriculum, for communicating about the curriculum to fieldwork educators, and for maintaining memoranda of understanding (MOU) and site data related to fieldwork placements. ACOTE Standard B.10.4 (ACOTE, 2007a & b)	For international fieldwork, another member of the faculty may have more expertise than the AFWC. Ensure that the AFWC is responsible for advocating for the development of links between the fieldwork and didactic aspects of the curriculum, for communicating about the curriculum to fieldwork educators, and for maintaining MOU and site data related to fieldwork placements. ACOTE Standard B.10.4 (ACOTE, 2007c)	Does not have to meet ACOTE requirements regarding fieldwork but must meet programmatic accreditation standards. However, clarity in communication is crucial regarding student role, curriculum, didactic aspects, appropriate supervision, safety, etc.

Verification: Written documentation is preferred over a telephone log. Written verification enables all parties to be able to refer to the agreement over time.

Level II fieldwork	Level I fieldwork or equivalent	Non–Level I or II fieldwork*
"Documentation that a memorandum of understanding was reviewed by both parties may include a signed agreement, letter, fax, email, or other written documentation." *ACOTE Interpretative Guide* (ACOTE, 2009)	"Documentation that a memorandum of understanding was reviewed by both parties may include a signed agreement, letter, fax, email, or other written documentation." *ACOTE Interpretative Guide* (ACOTE, 2009)	Written verification is still preferred, as it ensures expectations of experience.

Duration: In addition to number of weeks, clarify length of workday and days of the week worked. For example, in some countries, a workday may be longer but include a longer lunch break. In other countries, the work week may consist of 6 shorter days or include part of the weekend. Consider discussing appropriate use of non-assigned hours with the student.

Level II fieldwork	Level I fieldwork or equivalent	Non–Level I or II fieldwork*
For OT students completing FW outside the U.S., "must not exceed 12 weeks." ACOTE Standard B.10.22 (ACOTE, 2007a & b) For OTA students completing FW outside the U.S., "must not exceed 8 weeks." ACOTE Standards B.10.22 (ACOTE, 2007c)	Try to adhere to educational program's stated objectives/requirements.	Flexible, does not have to meet ACOTE requirements regarding fieldwork but must meet programmatic accreditation standards.

Qualification: Level of qualifications for fieldwork educators for fieldwork experiences.

Level II fieldwork	Level I fieldwork or equivalent	Non–Level I or II fieldwork*
"Ensure that students attending Level II fieldwork outside the United States are supervised by an occupational therapist who graduated from a program approved by the World Federation of Occupational Therapists and has 1 year of experience in practice." ACOTE Standard B. 10.22 (ACOTE, 2007a, b, & c)	Ensure that qualified personnel supervise Level I fieldwork. Working knowledge of occupational therapy is preferred. However, the fieldwork educator does not have to be an OT or OTA.	Does not have to meet ACOTE requirements regarding fieldwork but must meet programmatic accreditation standards.

Supervision: Level of supervision differs between Level I and Level II fieldwork.

Level II fieldwork	Level I fieldwork or equivalent	Non–Level I or II fieldwork*
Decreasing supervision throughout fieldwork, ensuring that the student is working at entry-level status at end of fieldwork.	Consistent supervision, so student is able to gain exposure and observe various therapy experiences.	Not required to meet ACOTE fieldwork supervision specifications.

Legal and Pragmatic Plan: If the fieldwork will earn academic credit, there must be a plan in place for what will be accomplished during the placement.

Level II fieldwork	Level I fieldwork or equivalent	Non–Level I or II fieldwork*
Develop a memorandum of understanding (MOU). Document a policy and procedure for complying with fieldwork site health requirements and maintaining student health records in a secure setting. ACOTE Standard B.10.6 (ACOTE, 2007a, b, & c) Verify that international fieldwork will meet the requirements for state licensure.	"If a fieldtrip, observation, or service learning opportunity is used to count toward part of Level I fieldwork, then a memorandum of understanding is required." *ACOTE Interpretative Guide* (ACOTE, 2009) Document a policy and procedure for complying with fieldwork site health requirements and maintaining student health records ina secure setting. ACOTE Standard B.10.6 (ACOTE, 2007a, b, & c)	Academic OT/OTA program or university may have study abroad requirements to be met.

Accreditation: If the fieldwork will earn academic credit, there may be specific institutional or accreditation standards imposed by regional accreditors that must be met.

Level II fieldwork	Level I fieldwork or equivalent	Non-Level I or II fieldwork*
Review and meet ACOTE Fieldwork Standards (ACOTE, 2007a, b, & c).	Review and meet ACOTE Fieldwork Standards (ACOTE, 2007a, b, & c).	Verify institution's accreditation requirements regarding credit for international experiences.

Risk Management: Try to anticipate potential issues and establish preventative measures in advance.

Level II fieldwork	Level I fieldwork or equivalent	Non-Level I or II fieldwork*
Have written clarity regarding responsibilities of student, academic OT/OTA program, and fieldwork site. Contact information and procedures in emergency situations should be delineated. Ensure that liability insurance is in place as well as mechanisms for handling student health needs.	Have written clarity regarding responsibilities of student, academic OT/OTA program, and fieldwork site. Contact information and procedures in emergency situations should be delineated. Ensure that liability insurance is in place as well as mechanisms for handling student health needs.	Have written clarity regarding responsibilities of student, academic OT/OTA program, and fieldwork site. Contact information and procedures in emergency situations should be delineated. Ensure that liability insurance is in place as well as mechanisms for handling student health needs.

Evaluation of Supervision: AOTA form (Student Evaluation of Fieldwork Experience) is not specifically required.

Level II fieldwork	Level I fieldwork or equivalent	Non-Level I or II fieldwork*
Document a mechanism for evaluating the effectiveness of supervision (e.g., student evaluation of fieldwork) and for providing resources for enhancing supervision (e.g., materials on supervisory skills, continuing education opportunities, articles on theory and practice). ACOTE Standard B.10.19 (ACOTE, 2007a, b, & c)	Document a mechanism for evaluating the effectiveness of supervision (e.g., student evaluation of fieldwork) and for providing resources for enhancing supervision (e.g., materials on supervisory skills, continuing education opportunities, articles on theory and practice). ACOTE Standard B.10.19 (ACOTE, 2006)	Feedback from student regarding supervision could be provided via email, journal entry, form, or debriefing after experience.

Evaluation of Fieldwork Experience: Determine whether objectives were accomplished/expected outcomes met.

Level II fieldwork	Level I fieldwork or equivalent	Non–Level I or II fieldwork*
Fieldwork experiences should be implemented and evaluated for their effectiveness by the academic OT/OTA program. ACOTE Standard B.10.0 (ACOTE, 2007a, b, & c)	Fieldwork experiences should be implemented and evaluated for their effectiveness by the academic OT/OTA program. ACOTE Standard B.10.0 (ACOTE, 2007a, b, & c)	Evaluation is important to determine whether the experience should be repeated for future students.

Evaluation of Student Performance: AOTA form (Fieldwork Performance Evaluation for the Occupational Therapy Student) is not specifically required.

Level II fieldwork	Level I fieldwork or equivalent	Non–Level I or II fieldwork*
Document mechanisms for requiring formal evaluation of student performance on Level II fieldwork. *(AOTA, 2002a & b, or equivalent)*. ACOTE Standard B.10.21 (ACOTE, 2007a, b, & c)	Document all Level I fieldwork experiences that are provided to students, including mechanisms for formal evaluation of student performance. ACOTE Standard B.10.13 (ACOTE, 2007a, b, & c)	Although not required to meet ACOTE fieldwork specifications, feedback is helpful for guiding the student toward future experiences and future growth.

Example of Non-Level I or II fieldwork: Mission trips, research data collection, service learning, preceptorship, experiential component, volunteer organizations, team interventions, university global center overtures, clinical training application workshops, etc.

Resources

ACOTE Fieldwork Standards, including OTA, OT, and OTD standards, searching information for each country

References

Accreditation Council for Occupational Therapy Education. (2007a). Accreditation standards for a doctoral-degree-level educational program for the occupational therapist. *American Journal of Occupational Therapy, 61,* 641–651. http://dx.doi .org/10.5014/ajot.61.6.641

Accreditation Council for Occupational Therapy Education. (2007b). Accreditation standards for a master's-degree-level educational program for the occupational therapist. *American Journal of Occupational Therapy, 61,* 652–661. http://dx.doi .org/10.5014/ajot.61.6.652

Accreditation Council for Occupational Therapy Education. (2007c). Accreditation standards for an educational program for the occupational therapy assistant. *American Journal of Occupational Therapy, 61,* 662–671. http://dx.doi .org/10.5014/ajot.61.6.662

Accreditation Council for Occupational Therapy Education. (2009). *ACOTE Standards and Interpretive Guide.* Available online at: http://www.aota.org/Educate/Accredit/Standards-Review.aspx

American Occupational Therapy Association. (2002a). *Fieldwork performance evaluation form for the occupational therapy student.* Bethesda, MD: Author.

American Occupational Therapy Association. (2002b). *Fieldwork performance evaluation form for the occupational therapy assistant student.* Bethesda, MD: Author.

Prepared by:

International Fieldwork Ad Hoc Committee for the Commission on Education (1/26/09).

Patricia Crist, PhD, OTR/L, FAOTA *(Chair)— Duquesne University, PA*

Naomi Greenberg, MPH, PhD, OTR—*LaGuardia Community College, NY*

Susan K. Meyers, EdD, OTR, *Private Foundation, IN*

Susan Mullholland MSc(rehab), BScOT, OT(c)— *University of Alberta*

Patty Stutz-Tanenbaum, MS, OTR—*Colorado State University, CO*

Pamela Richardson, PhD, OTR/L, FAOTA —*San Jose University, CA*

Debra Tupe, MS, OTR—*Columbia University, NY*

Neil Harvison, PhD, OTR/L—*AOTA Staff*

Emerging Leaders Development Program Participant:
Juleen Rodakowski, OTD, OTR/L

Reprinted from http://www.aota.org/-/media/Corporate/Files/EducationCareers/Educators/International/Student%20Guide%20to%20Planning%20International%20FWfinalnh.pdf

Chapter 42.

ETHICAL CONSIDERATIONS RELATED TO INTERNATIONAL FIELDWORK

American Occupational Therapy Association Commission on Education

Purpose

1. Identify and document ethical issues, including those related to cross-cultural and practice factors that must be considered when negotiating an international placement.
2. Stimulate discussion by providing questions to ponder when evaluating the benefit/harm ratio of each placement.
3. Encourage fieldwork educators and students to articulate the value of ethical clarity in benefit of American Occupational Therapy Association members and the global connectedness of the *Centennial Vision.*

Introduction

The following is presented to generate discussion regarding ethical issues that may arise while planning international fieldwork placements. In addition, this document may be presented as issues for students to discuss or consider. Questions may trigger and promote dialogue about content and potential dilemmas. This document is meant to raise awareness of ethical issues to consider when planning for an international fieldwork experience. Accompanying guides and documents should also be reviewed for other essential elements to consider when planning an international fieldwork.

Questions to Ponder by Category

Certification Considerations

- Will the international experience prepare the student sufficiently for certification?
- Should the student's home country fieldwork assignment be specifically chosen to offer solid certification preparation to complement the international experience and offset any gaps related to requirements for certification?
- Is the academic occupational therapy (OT)/ occupational therapy assistant (OTA) program aware that international experiences are often scheduled as optional placements beyond required fieldwork?

Clarity

- Is there advance verification in writing of the type(s) of population, location, duration, credentials of fieldwork educator, supervision, contact persons, housing, hours, days of work per week, days when facility is closed for the international fieldwork placement?

- Is it clear that there will be no guaranteed replacement of the student(s) at the end of the agreed upon period of service?

Communication

- Is there clarity about availability of means for communication in the geographical location of the assignment (e.g., telephone contact, email, voice over Internet)?
- How will necessary off-site communication be handled between fieldwork educator/preceptor/coordinator and student?

Competence

- Does the student have the professional competencies to serve the population under the supervision that will be available?
- What professional competencies are expected by the fieldwork site?
- Has the academic OT/OTA program provided the titles, descriptions, and outlines of the occupational therapy courses that the student has completed?
- Is cultural sensitivity a required part of the preparation for an international experience?

Cultural Aspects

- Have the student and educational program reviewed cultural competencies significant to the population to be served?
- Will the student be able to appropriately engage with staff and clients at the international fieldwork site?
- If a student requests a placement in a culturally different environment than his or her culture of origin, does the student have the awareness, knowledge, and skills to work in the culturally different environment?
- If a key goal of international fieldwork is to expose students to varied cultures, should a request for fieldwork placement in the country of origin be pursued?
- Is the student a person who will respect the culture of the assigned site?

- Does the student demonstrate some advanced research/awareness of the cultural norms of the country to be visited?
- Is the student willing to abide by the dress code of the fieldwork site?
- Will the student be comfortable among individuals dressed according to the norms of the country?
- To what degree are religious differences a concern?

Environmental Conditions

- Will the student be able to function within the environmental conditions likely to be encountered?
- How much detail should be explored regarding insect infestation, drinking water, crime, etc., in preparation for the placement?
- What health services/alerts should the student investigate in advance?
- Are there current U.S. State Department warnings in place?

Financial Issues

- Is it ethically responsible to pursue a potential agreement before ensuring that funding will be available to implement it?
- Who (student, academic OT/OTA program) is responsible for exploring potential funding sources?
- What is the anticipated cost of travel at the time of the placement? Are Internet-based reduced-fare bookings or the equivalent an acceptable alternative to an established travel agency?
- Has the student been referred to the college's study abroad office or equivalent? Does the student need to meet specific requirements for the college?
- At what stage should the student be asked how much he or she can contribute to the expected expenses?
- Have food costs been included in the overall package so that the student will not have to choose between eating or paying for a commuter bus or needed materials?

Housing

- If the potential fieldwork educator offers to have the student stay in his or her home for a minimal fee, should the college/educational program consider the possibility?

- Are there special needs/special requirements?
- What are the merits of the various options when values and morality are considered? What is most appropriate in the host country?
- Does the student meet the criteria for on-site housing? How many students are assigned per room? Are there mixed genders?
- Is public transportation available between the housing site and the clinical service site? How long is the commute? Will there be issues regarding hitching a ride, involving staff in transportation, having to cover taxi costs?
- Is walking between housing and treatment site feasible and safe according to the standards of the host country?

Impact on Population and Beyond

- Will there be a possibility for replacement of the student when he or she leaves to carry on the services provided? Does it matter?
- What is the balance between doing good and harm if, after being provided with occupational therapy, the population has no ability to continue receiving service after the student leaves?
- Is there the possibility of even brief training of individuals in the community for carryover to maximize the value of a one-time intervention?
- Will the student's sharing of information about conditions and salaries in the United States contribute to therapists leaving that country? How can such a potentially negative impact be minimized?
- Has the student been referred to such works as F. Kronenberg's *Occupational Therapy Without Borders* (2005, 2010) to enhance use of professional nomenclature and awareness of social justice issues, such as apartheid?

Language

- What are the language requirements of the site?
- Is the student prepared to engage in language training, if required, in advance of assignment to be sufficiently proficient by the starting date?
- Is there any reason not to proceed with the placement if the student is not proficient in the language of the country, but is proficient in the language of a large segment of the population served and is, therefore, acceptable to the site?

- Will the language in which supervision is documented be understood by both student and fieldwork educator?
- Does the student or academic OT/OTA program recognize the value (cognitive/connections) of being exposed to a new language?

Legal Considerations

- Is the student aware that legal standards of the home country may not apply in the country to which the student is to be assigned?
- Is the student likely to raise concerns about laws and rights that may only apply and/or need to be posted in the home country?
- Does the student know that penalties for such violations as drug use may be much more severe in the host country than in the home country?
- Is the student sufficiently astute/informed to realize that practice carried out in the host country may well be beyond the scope of practice and supervision requirements of the state to which the student will return?

Liability

- What are the liability and risk management considerations that must be delineated and agreed upon by institutional leadership, faculty, and fieldwork educators from both the sending school and student prior to placement?
- Is the country considered a litigious society?
- Does the student's liability insurance cover an international experience?
- Will the student be registered as such in the home educational institution while completing a fieldwork placement outside of the country?
- Does the host agency provide liability coverage for students?

Respect

- Does the student already demonstrate respect for people from different ethnic backgrounds and for people of different ages and abilities?
- Is the student ready to respect the norms of the host country and the policies of the receiving agency?
- Are there safety issues within the country or fieldwork site that may compromise the student's ability to complete fieldwork at that site?

- Does the student have the self-sufficiency and emotional maturity needed to negotiate unexpected situations that might be encountered?
- Has the student been prepared to "expect the unexpected"?
- Is the fieldwork site aware that the student may be out of his or her comfort zone in the new setting?
- Is the student likely to engage in risky behaviors in the anticipated host environment?
- Is the fieldwork site located within a country of relative calm?
- What procedures are in place regarding crime, terrorism, disaster planning?

Valuing Differences

- Is the student committed to make diversity an advantage?
- Is the student eager for the learning experience offered by a different environment, different people, different equipment, different treatment approaches, and more?
- Has the student read some of the OT-related articles regarding international experiences?
- Has the student read some of the OT-related articles regarding cultural sensitivity?

Resources

U.S. Department of State. (n.d.). *Traveler's checklist.* Retrieved from www.travel.state.gov/content/passports/English/go/checklist.html

Prepared by:

International Fieldwork Ad Hoc Committee for the Commission on Education (1/26/09).

Patricia Crist, PhD, OTR/L, FAOTA *(Chair)— Duquesne University, PA*
Naomi Greenberg, MPH, PhD, OTR—*LaGuardia Community College, NY*
Susan K. Meyers, EdD, OTR, *Private Foundation, IN*
Susan Mullholland MSc (rehab), BScOT, OT(c)— *University of Alberta*
Patty Stutz-Tanenbaum, MS, OTR—*Colorado State University, CO*
Pamela Richardson, PhD, OTR/L, FAOTA—*San Jose University, CA*
Debra Tupe, MS, OTR—*Columbia University, NY*
Neil Harvison, PhD, OTR/L—*AOTA Staff*

Emerging Leaders Development Program Participant:
Juleen Rodakowski, OTD, OTR/L

References

Kronenberg, F., Algado, S. S., & Pollard, N. (2005). *Occupational Therapy Without Borders: Vol 1. Learning from the spirit of survivors.* New York: Churchill Livingstone.

Kronenberg, F., Pollard, N., & Sakellariou, D. (2010). *Occupational Therapy Without Borders: Vol 2. Twoards an ecology of occupation-based practices.* New York: Churchill Livingstone.

Reprinted from http://www.aota.org/-/media/Corporate/Files/EducationCareers/Educators/International/Ethical%20Considerations%20for%20International%20Fieldworkfinalnh.doc

Chapter 43.

EXCELLENCE IN FIELDWORK: CRITERIA FOR FIELDWORK EDUCATOR EXCELLENCE AND CRITERIA FOR FIELDWORK SITE EXCELLENCE

American Occupational Therapy Association

Excellence in Fieldwork

The American Occupational Therapy Association (AOTA) Commission on Education (COE) developed and approved the following lists of recommended criteria for fieldwork educators and fieldwork sites of excellence. In April 2007, the Representative Assembly charged the COE to develop and disseminate criteria as a resource for affiliated state associations. The criteria were developed through the work of an AOTA ad hoc committee with the goal to highlight exemplars of fieldwork that could be emulated by other sites.

The COE acknowledges that many states have already established awards for fieldwork. These lists were developed for use at your discretion in your state. They may assist you in developing new ideas for recognitions, identifying and recognizing exemplary fieldwork, or starting a discussion within your state about fieldwork.

The criteria are designed to fit the ideal type in current practice as well as prepare fieldwork for the future as the profession moves towards realizing the

Centennial Vision. The COE is engaged in a number of actions to advance fieldwork as a critical portion of our professional education. The rationale for the development of these criteria lists include:

- These awards will motivate fieldwork educators and fieldwork sites to model exemplary practices and demonstrate support of our core professional values related to fieldwork.
- Fieldwork is acknowledged as the bridge between education and practice.
- Fieldwork has the greatest potential to change practice.
- Recognizing outstanding fieldwork educators and sites will raise awareness and respect for this area of professional responsibility.

If you use any additional criteria to recognize excellence in fieldwork educators or fieldwork sites in your state, the COE is very interested in adding the criteria to this recommended list. Please send your recommended criteria to me via email at your convenience.

Thank you for your time and please feel free to contact me if I can be of any assistance.

René Padilla, PhD, OTR/L, FAOTA, *Chairperson, AOTA Commission on Education.* Email: rpadilla@creighton.edu

Reprinted from http://www.aota.org/Education-Careers/Fieldwork/Supervisor/Excellence.aspx#sthash.i2qsqrMR.dpuf

Excellence in Fieldwork Criteria: Fieldwork Educator

The following criteria are designed for recognition of current practice as well as preparing fieldwork for the future as the profession moves to realize the *Centennial Vision*. An exemplar of an excellent clinical educator demonstrates:

- AOTA and occupational therapy state association membership
- Participation in continuing education related to supervision, teaching, and evaluation of learning or mentoring
- Active engagement in ethical, evidence-based, and occupation-centered practice
- Positive evaluations from students who completed their fieldwork experiences with this clinical educator
- A 5-year history of providing consistent fieldwork education to students
- Proactive collaboration with other professionals, serving as a team member role model
- Skills at the master clinician level and presents them as a model for students
- Awareness of where his or her practice fits within the profession
- Recognition of the uniqueness of each student and adapts his or her supervisory style accordingly
- Active engagement in evaluation of his or her own effectiveness as a supervisor in addition to the fieldwork program
- Contributions to occupational therapy education beyond the fieldwork site (e.g., provides in-services, is a guest lecturer at a college, speaks at a community center, assists with admission

interviews at local occupational therapy [OT] or occupational therapy assistant [OTA] education program, serves on committees at local OT or OTA education program)
- Leadership within a professional association that promotes the values of the profession.

Reprinted from http://www.aota.org/Education-Careers/Fieldwork/Supervisor/Excellence/Fieldwork-Educator.aspx#sthash.0FfpNQyq.dpuf

Excellence in Fieldwork Criteria: Fieldwork Site

The following criteria are designed for recognition of current practice as well as preparing fieldwork for the future as the profession moves to realize the *Centennial Vision*. An exemplar of a fieldwork site of excellence demonstrates:

- 100% of occupational therapy staff with AOTA membership
- 100% of occupational therapy staff with state occupational therapy association membership
- Inclusion of the clinical educator role as a job expectation and performance standards for advancement that include effective functioning as fieldwork clinical educator
- An exemplary fieldwork manual for occupational therapists and occupational therapy assistants with an ongoing review process
- Quality assurance monitoring on some aspect of providing fieldwork education
- A reputation for exceptional occupational therapy practice in their practice area
- The delivery of ethical, evidence-based, and occupation-centered practice staff with working knowledge and use of the *Occupational Therapy Practice Framework*
- A 5-year history of providing consistent fieldwork education to occupational therapy and occupational therapy assistant students
- Good collaboration with academic institutions (e.g., site visits, participation in fieldwork-related educational activities at the academic institution)

- Staff development in the areas of teaching, assessment of learning, and supervisory skills
- Commitment to manage and adapt to challenging student placements (e.g., find alternative supervisor, assignments)
- Acceptance of both occupational therapy and occupational therapy assistant students in Level I and Level II placements
- Consistent positive evaluations from Level I and Level II students

- Institutional commitment to the occupational therapy fieldwork program and meeting students' needs for accommodations under the Americans with Disabilities Act
- Creative and innovative supervision models.

Reprinted from http://www.aota.org/Education-Careers/Fieldwork/Supervisor/Excellence/Fieldwork-Site.aspx#sthash.WbsIFCZ7.dpuf

Chapter 44.

THE MULTIPLE MENTORING MODEL OF STUDENT SUPERVISION: A FIT FOR CONTEMPORARY PRACTICE

Cherie Graves, MOT, OTR/L, and Debra Hanson, PhD, OTR/L

"I work part-time, so I can't supervise students."

"My practice is oriented around a specific specialty, so there is not enough variety in my workload for me to take a student."

"I have not yet completed training for the fieldwork educator role, so I'm not yet ready to supervise a student."

With health care advances and changing work patterns, more practicing occupational therapy practitioners are working within specialty areas and working part-time. Traditional one-to-one supervision models do not work well within these practice perimeters, leading to decreased availability of Level II fieldwork placements for a growing number of occupational therapy academic programs. The multiple mentoring supervision model offers a solution to not only increase the pool of potential fieldwork educators but also to give novice fieldwork educators the opportunity to learn from those with more experience and to give fieldwork students the opportunity to experience specialty practice areas.

What Is the Multiple Mentorship Supervision Model, and What Are the Benefits?

Multiple mentoring is not new to occupational therapy practice; it was first described by Nolinske in 1995 in an article in the *American Journal of Occupational Therapy.* It is characterized by a team of two or more fieldwork educators supervising a single student or a team of two or more students. Supporting the concept that fieldwork education is the responsibility of all occupational therapy practitioners, the model provides the opportunity to shift the responsibility for fieldwork supervision from one designated occupational therapy practitioner to any occupational therapy practitioner within an area facility who has knowledge and experience that can benefit students. Besides reducing the time spent by each individual fieldwork educator in directly supervising students, the model opens up the opportunity to supervise students for occupational therapy practitioners who work in part-time positions or in facilities with newly developing occupational therapy programs. Less experienced practitioners sharing the supervision of a student may also increase their confidence and comfort with student supervision, as reported by Copley and Nelson (2012) in the *American Journal of Occupational Therapy.*

The multiple mentoring model can expose students to multiple areas of practice as well as multiple practitioners. Because fieldwork educators who are sharing supervision responsibilities may have different practice focuses or come from different workplace environments, they learn from one another even as the student learns from them. For example, the Queensland Occupational Therapy Fieldwork Collaborative found that a shared supervision model can serve to facilitate the clinical reasoning skills of fieldwork educators, who develop common expectations for student performance by explaining to one another what they do. Students are able to draw on the expertise of a variety of practitioners, and they have reported this to be helpful in cultivating and developing their own unique approach to therapy. Having exposure to a variety of supervision styles also helps students identify their own preferred learning style.

Fieldwork sites using shared supervision models are able to offer more student placements and therefore have increased opportunity for staff recruitment due to the increased number of students who have direct experience at the site. Shared supervision may also create a more positive experience for the fieldwork educator. There is less likelihood of communication breakdowns or personality conflicts when the student's supervision is shared, according to Farrow, Gaiptman, and Rudman (2000). It may also ease the amount of pressure or strain that the fieldwork educator may feel when having sole responsibility of the student. For example, fieldwork educators have support when providing students with honest but difficult feedback or in situations where student termination is needed.

What Are the Drawbacks to Multiple Mentorship?

As with any model of student supervision, there are some challenges. Fieldwork educators and students have shared their perception that it can be difficult for students to manage the expectations and potential inconsistency of multiple supervisors. There is also a perception by fieldwork educators that more effort and time is required for supervising practitioners to work together. The need for organizing the placement prior to the arrival of students has been clearly identified and may offset the common perception that more time and effort are required when supervision is shared.

What Structures Support Multiple Mentoring Processes?

A clear orientation to the expectations of the fieldwork site and the learning model are essential to the success of multiple mentorship. To get started, it is helpful for collaborating supervisors to identify the learning opportunities available in their respective practices, including such factors as diversity of clientele, assessment procedures, intervention opportunities, and documentation requirements. This information is essential to developing site-specific learning objectives that correspond to the AOTA Fieldwork Performance Evaluation and to developing a schedule of expectations over the length of the fieldwork. A written manual that orients the student to the resources and policies of the facility, therapy expertise, teaching philosophy, and scheduling preferences of each fieldwork educator as well as the site-specific learning objectives and weekly schedule will help the student to situate him- or herself in the learning experience.

Diligent and regular communication among educators regarding their observations and evaluation of student performance throughout the placement is critical to success, according to the Queensland Occupational Therapy Fieldwork Collaborative (2007). Tracking forms and secure electronic communication venues can be helpful for fieldwork educators reviewing and discussing student work and grading expectations. Such systems can also help students and fieldwork educators communicate with one another, particularly because they may not share physical space every day.

Supervisors who openly discuss and identify clinical reasoning differences prior to student placement will find it easier to reconcile divergent expectations once a student arrives. Although individual meetings are helpful, a supervision meeting at least once a week with all supervisors present will help to ensure that expectations are clear and information is not lost. If this is not possible, other communication structures in which all supervisors contribute to identifying student strengths and weaknesses is helpful. For example, students posting questions or assignments in a shared electronic workspace, such as Google Documents, in advance of supervision meetings can help keep all supervisors apprised and ready to contribute to feedback and appropriate remediation of identified problem areas. Student learning contracts are another way for students to identify areas of concern and potential resources to address problem areas in advance of supervision meetings. Because the scheduling needs of each supervisor will vary, it is essential that a student be sensitive to supervisor schedule needs and be flexible in how he or she accesses time for each educator.

The multiple mentoring model, although it does require some upfront work, is a practical strategy for student supervision that fits the contemporary occupational therapy practice environment and provides students with new opportunities to develop and refine their practice and communication skills.

Exhibit 44.1. *Strategies for Success in Using the Multiple Mentorship Supervision Model*

- Orient students to facility resources and fieldwork educator teaching styles.
- Communicate fieldwork educator schedules and preferred communication structures.
- Set overall learning objectives and graded expectations for performance.
- Hold weekly group supervision meetings with all supervisors present or at least provide shared documentation.
- Identify clinical reasoning differences prior to supervision implementation.
- Establish structures to support regular communication between fieldwork educators and students.
- Develop forms to track student caseload and progress.
- Use learning contracts to foster student ownership of fieldwork assignment.

Resources

American Occupational Therapy Association. (2002). *Fieldwork performance evaluation for the occupational therapy student.* Bethesda, MD: Author.

Copley, J., & Nelson, A. (2012). Practice educator perspectives of multiple mentoring in diverse clinical settings. *British Journal of Occupational Therapy, 75,* 456–462. http://dx.doi.org/10.4276/030802212X13496921049662

Farrow, S., Gaiptman, B., & Rudman, D. (2000). Exploration of a group model in fieldwork education. *Canadian Journal of Occupational Therapy, 67,* 239–250. http://dx.doi.org/10.1177/000841740006700406

Nolinske, T. (1995). Multiple mentoring relationships facilitate learning during fieldwork. *American Journal of Occupational Therapy, 49*(1), 39–44. http://dx.doi.org/10.5014/ajot.49.1.39

Queensland Occupational Therapy Fieldwork Collaborative. (2007). *Clinical placement models: Clinical educators resource kit.* Retrieved from http://www.qotfc.edu.au/resource/index.html?page=65786

Cherie Graves, MOT, OTR/L, is an instructor and co-academic fieldwork coordinator for the Department of Occupational Therapy at the University of North Dakota in Grand Forks. Graves joined the university's faculty in January 2014. Prior to this, she practiced in Sioux Falls, South Dakota, for 7 years.

Debra Hanson, PhD, OTR/L, is an associate professor and a co-academic fieldwork coordinator for the Department of Occupational Therapy at the University of North Dakota in Grand Forks. Hanson has more than 25 years of experience working with fieldwork educators and students.

Part 9.

RESOURCES FOR ACADEMIC FIELDWORK EDUCATORS

OVERVIEW OF PART 9

Donna Costa, DHS, OTR/L, FAOTA

Part 9 focuses on resources for academic fieldwork coordinators (AFWCs). The role of the AFWC is complex, multifaceted, and challenging. Usually, the person who takes the job of AFWC is new to academia and finds himself or herself in an overwhelming situation. There is much to learn in this role, with often minimal support provided. Currently no training manual or course is available for AFWCs, so people in these roles must be proactive and advocate for themselves. They need to read everything about fieldwork they can and find a mentor who has successfully navigated the role and can provide support to develop their knowledge and skills.

Chapter 45, "Working Smarter in the Academic Fieldwork Coordinator Role," an outgrowth of an institute that the authors developed and presented at an American Occupational Therapy Association (AOTA) Annual Conference & Expo is the closest thing we have to a how-to manual for AFWCs. The theme "working smarter not harder" is reflected throughout the chapter. Chapter 46, "Fieldwork Councils and Consortia," lists the various U.S. fieldwork councils and consortia. If you haven't connected with one of these groups, consider doing so. If you live in an area that does not have a fieldwork consortium, consider helping to organize one. Some fieldwork consortia organize regional workshops for fieldwork educators. Others have regularly scheduled meetings for AFWCs to get together and work collaboratively.

In Chapter 47, "Maintaining Longevity in the Role of Academic Fieldwork Coordinator," experienced fieldwork educators (FWEs) discuss how to remain, and thrive professionally, in the AFWC role. AFWC positions have a relatively high turnover, with some people finding the job too difficult. Yet others remain successfully in the role for years and even decades. Therefore, the authors' insights should be helpful for AFWCs. Chapter 48, "Online Learning Resources for Academic Leadership," describes a relatively new online training program based in Australia for professions that have clinical education components (e.g., occupational therapy, physical therapy). Although this program reflects Australian policies and issues, the information is helpful to all AFWCs.

The remainder of Part 9 comprises several AOTA official documents with which AFWCs, FWEs, and students must be familiar. Chapter 49 is "Guidelines for Supervision, Roles, and Responsibilities During the Delivery of Occupational Therapy Services" on supervisory roles and responsibilities. AFWCs should read it alongside their state's practice act, which may be more or less stringent on supervisory policies. Chapter 50 contains the "Guidelines for Re-Entry Into the Field of Occupational Therapy," guidelines for occupational therapy practitioners who reenter clinical practice after having been out of the profession for a period of time. Because each state sets specific requirements for reentry, AFWCs should also read their state's practice act. Chapter 51 contains the *Occupational Therapy Code of Ethics*, revised in 2015, and Chapter 52 contains the "Enforcement Procedures for the *Occupational Therapy Code of Ethics*." Chapter 53 contains the AOTA document "Promoting Ethically Sound Practices in Occupational Therapy Fieldwork Education," which is particularly relevant to AFWCs and FWEs.

Chapter 45.

WORKING SMARTER IN THE ACADEMIC FIELDWORK COORDINATOR ROLE

Debra J. Hanson, PhD, OTR/L, FAOTA; Caryn Reichlin Johnson, MS, OTR/L, FAOTA; Camille Sauerwald, EdM, OTR; and Patricia Stutz-Tanenbaum, MS, OTR/L, FAOTA

The role of the academic fieldwork coordinator (AFWC) is unique among faculty in higher education. The AFWC is named in the Accreditation Council for Occupational Therapy Education (ACOTE®; 2012) standards as specifically responsible for the oversight of all accreditation standards related to fieldwork. Furthermore, the tasks associated with the role are complex, ranging from procedural responsibilities, such as fieldwork data management, to activities requiring relational and marketing skills, such as recruitment of fieldwork sites (Hanson, Koski, & Stutz-Tanenbaum, 2013).

Currently, most AFWCs (51.5%) have 5 or fewer years of experience in the role, according to a recent national survey (Stutz-Tanenbaum, Hanson, Koski, & Greene, 2015). The lack of available adequate training and resources to assist with role development may be a factor contributing to this statistic, because most AFWCs enter the role, despite its inherent complexity, directly from practice with less than 5 years of experience (Hanson, Stutz-Tanenbaum, & Koski, 2013). Because most academic programs employ only one academic fieldwork coordinator and that individual may not have the availability of anyone else on faculty with experience in the role, lack of available training and resources exacerbates role stress.

In 2014, the first American Occupational Therapy Association (AOTA)–sponsored institute was held to offer training for the AFWC role (Johnson, Sauerwald, Stutz-Tanenbaum, & Hanson, 2014). Those in attendance spoke to the value of having an overview of the administrative aspects of the role, learning about strategic methods for interacting with students and fieldwork educators, and aligning their scholarship and service activities to maximize professional reward. This chapter discusses five highlights from the 2014 AFWC Institute: (1) introduction to AFWC role management; (2) methods for fieldwork educator recruitment and training for fieldwork educator and site retention; (3) approaches for advising and teaching students; (4) strategies for administrative management; and (5) guidelines for maximizing professional reward through AFWC scholarship and service.

Introduction to Academic Fieldwork Coordinator Role Management

As an AFWC, you are entering a professional role that will afford many opportunities for personal and professional growth. You will stretch your skills as you learn the art of balancing personal communications with students and fieldwork educators with departmental policies and legal requirements. Management of the complexities of the AFWC role requires a strategic approach to make the most of the time and resources available. It will be important for you to streamline work tasks as much as possible, combining approaches to make the most of your work efforts. For example, you will want to create efficient data management processes that meet the immediate need for fieldwork site communications but also provide evidence to meet the requirements of one or more accreditation standards. You similarly will want to strategically choose the activities you engage in related to scholarship and service so that they also are a benefit to you in some other aspect of the AFWC role, such as recruitment of fieldwork sites or creation of resources that can be used for fieldwork educator training. As an AFWC, this strategic approach will help you avoid burnout and thrive in the role as you work smarter rather than harder.

Many skills are required for the role, ranging from knowledge of technology to facilitate data management to counseling and advisement skills for addressing students who are struggling with fieldwork. Tasks of the role are often cyclical rather than semester-based, and the AFWC is often in the position of juggling several tasks and accountability to several constituent groups simultaneously. As is the case with any complex skill, mastery of the tasks associated with the AFWC role occurs one step at a time. In this chapter, ideas, strategies, and examples are presented, followed by learning activities for you to reflect on how the information provided relates to you and your program.

Those who have longevity in the role of internship coordinator realize that it is more professionally satisfying and effective to work in collaboration with others than to work in isolation (Salzman, 2009). In addition, you can learn so much more, and more quickly, from others than you can by yourself. Therefore, an aspect of reflection throughout this chapter involves consideration of collaboration and communication opportunities with other AFWCs in your region and nationally, and with internship coordinators from other professions within your academic institution.

It is equally important to remember that the fieldwork component of any academic program is inextricably intertwined with the curriculum as a whole, and actions that you take as an AFWC must be consistent with and reflective of your overall academic program purpose and curriculum design. You will find it much more effective and rewarding and less isolating to work closely with other faculty and your program director, whether you are navigating a specific situation with a student or determining overall fieldwork policies or procedures. Therefore, this chapter includes many opportunities for you to consider the implications of fieldwork activities or initiatives as they affect the academic curriculum as a whole and the support you desire or need from other faculty within your program.

Finally, as you ponder various aspects of the AFWC role, consider your professional interests and determine where you want to expend your greatest efforts. Because the role is so diverse, many areas will demand your attention. From the educator perspective, you may be captivated by how students learn during the fieldwork experience and may choose to invest your time in exploring strategies, resources, and scholarship to enhance this process. Alternately, you may find that your skills and interests align most closely with the role's administrative aspects; therefore, you may invest your time and efforts in exploring processes for student site selection or fieldwork site retention. If your interests are in counseling and advocacy, your time and attention may be drawn to supporting and mentoring both students and fieldwork educators and your scholarship and service interests may align with supporting and investigating strategies for coaching others. Regardless of your chosen emphasis, it is important that you identify the aspects of the AFWC role that are most appealing to you so that you can derive the most satisfaction from this position.

Learning Activity 45.1.

1. Draw a picture of the aspect of the AFWC role that is most appealing to you and where you derive the most role satisfaction.
2. What activities within the AFWC role do you feel are most deserving of your time?
3. Where do you believe you can make your greatest impact on fieldwork education?
4. What do your responses to the above questions tell you about your professional role identity as an AFWC?

Fieldwork Educator Recruitment and Training and Educator and Site Retention

When working with fieldwork educators, AFWCs represent the face of the academic program in preparing students for the fieldwork site and the fieldwork site for students. Diplomacy and planning are essential to recruiting sites that are a good fit for the academic program curriculum design and for training fieldwork educators at various levels of proficiency. Most occupational therapy practitioners do not find the transition from clinician to fieldwork educator to be easy or automatic and appreciate support with preparation. Strategic planning is essential to retain fieldwork sites and maintain mutually beneficial relationships between the academic program and the fieldwork site.

Fieldwork Educator Recruitment

In your role as AFWC, you will be in touch with the clinical community more than any other member of your faculty. You are the one working with existing fieldwork sites and reaching out to new sites that have never taken your students. Before you begin, it is important to understand the reasons that motivate occupational therapy practitioners to accept fieldwork students to their organizations and the many perceived barriers that prevent them from participating in fieldwork education (Barton et al., 2013; Bondoc, Arabit, Lashgari, Finnen, & Alexander, 2009; Thomas et al., 2007). Some of the reasons practitioners work with fieldwork students include: it fulfills their sense of professional responsibility, it provides them with the opportunity to give back, and it offers a path to professional development (Hanson, 2012; Thomas et al., 2007). Barriers to accepting fieldwork students include lack of time and limited resources (Hanson, 2011). Exhibit 45.1 highlights related findings from the current literature.

Marketing your program may be an essential part of the recruitment process, particularly if you are in an environment that challenges your program to compete with other occupational therapy or occupational therapy assistant programs for a limited number of fieldwork placements. If you want fieldwork educators to appreciate the opportunities and

Exhibit 45.1. Benefits of and Barriers to Accepting Fieldwork Students

Benefits	Barriers
Keeps clinicians' skills current	Workload pressures and lack of time
Decreases workload	Low student capability
Has the potential for recruitment of occupational therapists and occupational therapy assistants	Potential difficulties with clients and consumers
Energizes and refreshes staff	Learning, supervisory, or personality style clashes
Gives students opportunities to conduct evidence-based practice activities and research projects	Limited resources (e.g., desk space, computers)
Improves staff skills and training (e.g., supervision skills)	Student or client safety and security problems
Fulfills a desire to give back to the profession	No fieldwork experience working with students
Fulfills licensure and continuing education requirements	Fieldwork educator role strain
Gives access to the academic institution's faculty and resources and prestige associated with affiliation with the academic institution	Some fieldwork sites only want students for their 2nd or 3rd placement
Gives students opportunities to research new ideas and trends and bring new ideas and creativity to the organization	New grad not yet ready to supervise students
Promotes the role of occupational therapy within the organization	Previous bad experience with student
Is a requirement for job promotion	Environment not conducive to learning

advantages that participating in fieldwork education with *your* academic program can offer them, instead of only what they can offer you, put on your "marketing hat" and show them *why*. First, you need to let them know you are there. The following are some program marketing examples to enhance your visibility within your clinical community:

- *Produce and distribute an academic program newsletter.* Champion your program by sending E-newsletters that include program, faculty, and alumni updates.
- *Attend local conferences and meetings.* Be visible in the community. Fieldwork educators are more likely to say yes and feel connected to you when you are face-to-face.
- *Use your program website.* A readily visible fieldwork section on the program website can provide useful resources and contact information.
- *Use the clinical community to teach or guest lecture.* Reach out to your clinical community when you need guest lecturers, lab assistants, or research partners. Bringing them onto your campus will help solidify your relationship.

Once you identify a new site, your attention should turn to ensuring site quality. You need to make sure that the learning experiences provided at the site meet your needs and are a good fit for your curriculum and your students. Use the questions in Exhibit 45.2, or create your own criteria, for assessing the adequacy of new fieldwork sites. These questions can be useful both initially and during periodic review.

Maximizing capacity is another consideration of site recruitment. Consider how you may be able to get more out of your existing relationships rather than looking for new sites, which require additional time for developing new contracts and training new fieldwork educators. Are there other academic programs or a fieldwork consortium you can partner with? Are you willing to consider alternate supervisory models? Can you cultivate fieldwork educators from your alumni community? The following are several possible strategies:

- *Collaborate with local occupational therapy and occupational therapy assistant programs.* Agree that each school will designate different days of the week for fieldwork experiences, thereby not competing for the same days.

Exhibit 45.2. *Questions to Determine Fieldwork Site Adequacy*

How does the site meet your location needs (i.e., within commuting distance, accessible by bus)?

How does the site meet your practice setting needs (i.e., need more pediatrics sites)?

How does the site meet your curricular needs?

- Corresponds with curricular threads and goals
- Allows students to meet fieldwork or class assignments

How does the site meet your student learning needs?

- Occupation-based
- Client-centered
- Allows hands-on participation
- Evidence-based
- Ethical environment
- Addresses psychosocial factors

How does the type of supervision meet your needs?

- Model (individual, group, multiple supervisors, or collaborative)
- Frequency of supervision (time available to process student experiences)
- Qualifications of fieldwork educators

How does the site communicate with you?

- Responsiveness to communication
- Use of email and Internet

- *Follow a collaborative supervision model.* Strong evidence supports the effectiveness of this model, which involves one fieldwork educator supervising two or more students (Dawes & Lambert, 2010; Lekkas et al., 2007; O'Connor, Cahill, & McKay, 2012; Secomb, 2008) and resources being available to support implementation of this model (Beisbier & Johnson, 2014).
- *Grow your own.* Maximize future alumni support for fieldwork education while students are still in school.

As you begin recruiting new fieldwork sites, consider whether you want to cast a wide net or target

Learning Activity 45.2.

Review the example in the table. Devise your own table, and rank the areas to target (from 1 = *most important* to 4 = *least important*) in terms of *your* program's priorities and interests. Next, indicate the potential impact each area to target could have. Finally, thinking creatively, draft some possible action plans you might take.

Area to Target	Rank Order Priorities	Rank Order Interests	Action Plan	Impact
School or program mission: Partnerships with agencies working with underserved populations are highly valued and supported.	3	4	Develop partnership with family medicine practice in underserved area to introduce developmental screening as part of its primary care services.	Aligns department activities with school mission.
Shortage of FW sites in particular practice area: OT program needs more pediatric sites.	1	2	Fieldwork students will explore the evidence to determine needs, assessment, and intervention strategies and provide developmental screening, parent education, and consultation.	Solves shortage of fieldwork sites for a particular practice area.
Faculty interests/research agenda: Faculty are interested in developing a presence in primary care.	2	1	Faculty can tie in grant and research interests with the agency.	Supports a relationship that could promote faculty research agenda.
Multisite facilities to maximize capacity and minimize contract work: There are skilled nursing facilities and hospital systems with the capacity to take students at multiple locations.	4	3	Site could provide multiple Level I and Level II placements per year. Obtain contracts with sites such as the Department of Veterans system and Genesis Rehab Services that will cover multiple locations.	Solves shortage of fieldwork sites for programs with large numbers of students.

strategically desirable fieldwork sites. By targeting and investing in key strategic relationships, you may yield more positive results for recruiting fieldwork sites that meet multiple ACOTE standards. Priorities to consider include your institution's mission, specific fieldwork needs in terms of community population or practice setting, faculty interests and your department's research agenda, and strategies to manage you own time and effort.

Fieldwork Educator Training

What makes a good fieldwork educator? It is widely recognized that "being practitioners [does] not fully prepare us for being educators" (Stutz-Tanenbaum & Hooper, 2009, p. 1). Kirke, Layton, and Sim (2007) described the qualities that make a good fieldwork educator, including outlining clear expectations, providing balanced feedback, demonstrating clinical reasoning, having strong communication skills, providing a good orientation, and fostering a flexible learning environment. The same study emphasized the responsibility of the academic program in helping to prepare fieldwork educators for taking students and recognized the need for both formal and informal training for fieldwork educators as a high priority.

ACOTE (2012) Standards C.1.3, C.1.9, and C.1.14 require academic programs to communicate and collaborate with fieldwork educators to "ensure that qualified personnel supervise" fieldwork students (ACOTE, 2012, p. S34) and that they are "adequately prepared to serve as a fieldwork educator[s]" (ACOTE, 2012, p. S36). Nowhere, however, are *qualified* and *adequately prepared* defined. Therefore, how do AFWCs know whether fieldwork educators are qualified and adequately prepared? They must decide what these terms mean to them and then, if necessary, provide training. A list of possible strategies includes:

- *Self-Assessment for Fieldwork Educator Competency* (*SAFECOM;* AOTA, 1997). This tool was developed by AOTA to allow fieldwork educators an opportunity to examine their strengths and areas of need. It is http://tinyurl.com/AOTASAFECOM
- *Fieldwork site visits.* Fieldwork site visits are not required but can be helpful in obtaining qualification information about fieldwork educators.
- *Electronic communications.* Training and informational materials can be regularly sent to fieldwork educators.
- *Information dissemination by students.* Students can help fieldwork educators develop their supervision, education skills, and evidence-based practice skills.
- *Clinical Council Days.* Clinical Council Days are continuing education events often provided by academic programs or groups of academic programs (consortia) for the clinical community. Topics should address the needs and interests the target audience (fieldwork educators). You may be able to identify one or two organizations that could potentially sponsor the event to defray costs.
- *AOTA Fieldwork Educator Certificate Program.* In 2009, AOTA trained 30 academic fieldwork coordinator–fieldwork educator teams from around the country to implement the certificate program (see http://www.aota.org/Education-Careers/Fieldwork.aspx). To date, more than 4,500 occupational therapy practitioners have attended the course and received certificates. Identify ways to offset program costs (e.g., sponsorships, institutional support), and track the number of your fieldwork educators who have participated.

Learning Activity 45.3.

This table includes the training and educational strategies targeting fieldwork educators mentioned previously in the text. In the table, identify the pros and cons for each strategy. Then identify which activities in the "Strategy Implementation" you already do and those you do not do. If you already do the activities, think of ways you can improve on their implementation. If you do not do the activities, think about whether and how you could implement them into your training program.

Training Strategy	Pros and Cons	Strategy Implementation
Fieldwork site visits	Pros: Cons:	Visit a fieldwork site to collect data to ascertain the fieldwork educator's qualifications (determine beforehand what data you need to collect).
Electronic communications	Pros: Cons:	Email training and educational materials to fieldwork educators (e.g., articles, websites, self-assessment tools, guidelines) on a regular basis.
Student input	Pros: Cons:	Have students disseminate information (through presentations and assignments while participating in the academic program or doing fieldwork) that can help fieldwork educators develop their supervision and education skills.

(Continued)

Learning Activity 45.3. *(Cont.)*		
Training Strategy	**Pros and Cons**	**Strategy Implementation**
Clinical Council Day	Pros: Cons:	Put on a Clinical Council Day that includes information on skills for the FW educator (i.e., providing balanced feedback, developing learning contracts, working with students with special needs, promoting evidence-based practice).
American Occupational Therapy Association (AOTA) Fieldwork Educator Certificate Program	Pros: Cons:	Offer the AOTA Fieldwork Educator Certificate Program.

Fieldwork Educator and Site Retention

Once you have identified quality fieldwork educators and sites and invested in their development, you want to retain them. This may be more challenging than you realize, due to the role strain that fieldwork educators might experience (Barton, Corban, Herrli-Warner, McClain, Riehle, & Tinner, 2013). Therefore, you should identify the needs of your clinical community and strategies for meeting these needs. For example, be responsive to a call for help when facility administrators question the value of fieldwork, and provide resources to justify continuing the program. On the other hand, academic programs may occasionally need to drop a site that does not live up to program expectations because of concerns about a particular fieldwork educator or about the site in general, or both. The following measures can be used to evaluate the efficacy of fieldwork educators and sites:

- *Student Evaluation of the Fieldwork Experience (SEFWE) form.* This AOTA form (available in Chapter 30) provides an opportunity for students to give feedback about the fieldwork learning experience, supervision, and environment to both the fieldwork educators and the academic program.
- *Course evaluations.* Most academic programs require students to complete course evaluations at the end of every course, including fieldwork. Because students are not always comfortable being honest on the SEFWE form, many AFWCs ask students for more specific information in their course evaluations (which may be anonymous).
- *Fieldwork educator feedback.* If issues are identified about fieldwork educator competency or site suitability, the AFWC may choose to work with the educator or site to help them develop skills in deficient areas. The efficacy of this feedback can be measured through documentation of communications or specific goal attainment.
- *Fieldwork Experience Assessment Tool.* This tool (available in Chapter 13) can be used during the fieldwork placement by both the student and fieldwork educator to identify facilitators and obstacles to student performance. Useful information can be provided by the student about the impact of the fieldwork educator's supervision on him or her.

Maintaining regular contact with your clinical community keeps you at the forefront of their minds. Many AFWCs make a habit of including information that will enhance supervisory skills with every mass communication (e.g., announcements regarding student placements) they send out. If you maintain a good database, it is easy to select the people you want to communicate with at any given time. Consider including a little bonus with each mailing that could benefit you, fieldwork educators, or students. For example, send out articles (or links to articles) related to fieldwork student education; updates about your academic program, faculty, and students; and other information of general interest. One recent study showed that occupational therapy practitioners learn important information about recent developments in the field, such as evidence-based practice and material in the *Occupational Therapy Practice Framework: Domain and Process* (3rd ed.; AOTA, 2014b), from fieldwork students (Hanson, 2011). This type of communication also helps to meet ACOTE (2012) standards related to collaboration and adequate preparation of fieldwork educators.

If you are in an area where there are other occupational therapy programs, think about the following ways you can collaborate to help your fieldwork educators be efficient and successful:

- Have all academic programs in the area send requests for fieldwork reservations on the same date.
- Design reservation forms that are similar in style and functionality.
- Use the same Level I Fieldwork Performance Evaluation form. For example, although each program may develop its own form, OT and OTA programs in the Philadelphia Region Fieldwork Consortium all use the same evaluation forms for evaluating Level I student performance, and for student evaluation of the Level I experience.
- Coordinate Level II start dates so multiple new students can be oriented at the same time.

In addition, because the array of administrative tasks and the time needed to develop a fieldwork program can be daunting, you can facilitate the process and assist fieldwork educators by providing them with the following resources:

- Fieldwork manual outline for students (see http://www.aota.org/education-careers/fieldwork/new programs/content.aspx)
- Fieldwork educator manual for training students (should address many ACOTE [2012] standards)
- Site-specific learning objectives checklist (see http://tinyurl.com/SiteLearningObjectives)
- Examples of 8- or 12-week schedules
- Links to online resources (e.g., University of Western Ontario's Preceptor Education Program: http://www.preceptor.ca/register.html).

Consider how you can give back to your fieldwork sites (see Exhibit 45.3). Many fieldwork educators enjoy training students and do it out of the goodness of their hearts or because they have a sense of professional responsibility. However, there is growing concern in the academic community about sites that want to charge the academic program for fieldwork education. It is essential that fieldwork educators and their administrators see the value in participating in fieldwork education. Giving back supports your fieldwork community and promotes the quality of fieldwork education in your clinical community.

Exhibit 45.3. *Strategies for Giving Back to Fieldwork Sites*

Strategy	Value or Benefit
Free or low-cost continuing education (e.g., student research presentations, journal clubs, recognized guest lecturers, Clinical Council Days)	Fulfills continuing education requirements for your clinical community.
American Occupational Therapy Association Fieldwork Educator Certificate Program sponsorship; consider program scholarships to sites willing to commit to taking two Level II fieldwork students and two Level I fieldwork students per year	Investment could result in 25 trained fieldwork educators, 50 Level I fieldwork reservations, and 50 Level II fieldwork reservations per year.
Library access	Supports evidence-based practice in your clinical community; online access especially is useful to fieldwork educators.
Fieldwork Educator of the Year Award	Recognition builds goodwill; this is a good event to include in your annual Clinical Council Day.
Scholarships for occupational therapy practitioners who are interested in participating in research	Creates a win-win situation by dovetailing research interests of the academic program with those of the clinical community.
Opportunities to recruit students for employment (consider a recruitment luncheon, allowing sites that have taken your fieldwork students to host a luncheon with a presentation on an approved topic and a recruitment component)	A student who has completed Level II fieldwork at a given site is ideally trained for entry-level practice at that site. Many fieldwork sites offer jobs to students who have successfully completed fieldwork in their setting.

Learning Activity 45.4.

1. List all the ways you currently give back to your fieldwork community.
2. List three no- or low-cost methods you could use in the future.
3. Identify an expensive way you could give back and how you might be able to fund it.

Advising and Teaching Students

Advising and teaching students about fieldwork before and during their placement is another pillar of the AFWC role. Fieldwork placement is an important consideration for student academic program selection and career development; therefore, the AFWC works with students to plan and implement their fieldwork education. Because Level I and Level II fieldwork are different in purpose and scope, this section discusses each separately.

Introducing Students to Fieldwork

Introducing students to fieldwork begins when they first consider applying to your academic program. Students want to know when fieldwork occurs during the curriculum, potential practice settings for placements, and previous placement locations. You can initiate the fieldwork process through the department's webpage by posting an overview of the fieldwork program, the timing for placements, and general guidelines that influence placement decisions. You should also mention some challenges related to fieldwork placements such as commuting, relocating, and expenses associated with site prerequisites (e.g., immunizations, drug screening, background checks).

Level I Fieldwork

The purpose of Level I fieldwork is to "introduce students to the fieldwork experience, to apply knowledge to practice, and to develop understanding of the needs of clients" (ACOTE, 2012, p. S34). Level I fieldwork provides a foundation for building the skills needed for Level II fieldwork. Students should understand that performance expectations evolve over time, requiring progressively higher levels of competency as students progress through the program. Student performance skills are built on a foundation of professional behavior, expected early in fieldwork—and throughout a professional career. Students should be provided with explicit expectations for their performance during Level I fieldwork so they are prepared cognitively, emotionally, and physically for the professional world, an unfamiliar realm for some students. Professional skills, such as the ability to explain occupational therapy to others, managing time, making ethical decisions, managing stress, and understanding therapeutic use of self, are valued by fieldwork educators (Hanson, 2011).

A Level I fieldwork student handbook can be a resource for clarifying expectations for both the student and the fieldwork educator. Opportunities to participate in active learning during Level I fieldwork, not just observation, help students develop the skills they need for Level II fieldwork and in the workplace (Haynes, 2011). Students should be familiar with the kinds of learning opportunities they will have on a Level I fieldwork, particularly in the area of hands-on learning. Clearly communicate with the fieldwork site about the types of hands-on learning that is appropriate for varying levels of student preparation so that the expectations you have for students and the learning experiences sites can offer are in alignment.

As an AFWC, the evaluation instrument you use for Level I fieldwork will communicate your learning expectations. However, there is no standardized tool for evaluating Level I student performance as there is

Learning Activity 45.5.

Review your program's webpage and evaluate the content (e.g., general information about Level I and II fieldwork, timing of fieldwork during the program, fieldwork locations, fieldwork prerequisites, unique characteristics about the program and fieldwork opportunities) from the perspective of students who are considering fieldwork education. Also review the websites of other occupational therapy academic programs and evaluate the content from the same student perspective. Does your webpage include information and resources that encompass the following four factors: relevant, informative, student-centered, and user friendly? If not, identify the information and resources on your page that need to be changed or added to incorporate these four factors.

for Level II (see ACOTE [2012] Standard C.1.10). Each academic program has the autonomy to develop a fieldwork performance evaluation that considers the timing in the academic program, connections with occupational therapy courses, and competencies needed for Level II fieldwork. Items in your evaluation form should clearly delineate the level of independence expected of students. Competencies included on a Level I fieldwork performance evaluation may increase in the degree of challenge from the first through the last Level I placement. For example, expectations for Level I fieldwork early in the academic program may focus on professional behaviors, whereas placements occurring later may evaluate clinical skill competencies expected for Level II (e.g., assisting with evaluations of clients, establishing goals for interventions, drafting documentation). Evaluation items may vary across practice settings. For example, items oriented toward facilitating occupational participation for adults and items pertaining to children and caregivers may differ.

Level I fieldwork also provides many opportunities for you to collaborate with faculty and fieldwork educators to integrate the academic curriculum (see ACOTE [2012] Standards C.1.1 and C.1.8). Your first step may be to work with other program faculty to develop a Level I evaluation form that reflects the academic program. Next, you may brainstorm with faculty to design fieldwork assignments that reinforce course concepts. You may also enlist the same faculty to assist with grading assignments so that they are familiar with students' ability to connect fieldwork with the classroom. This collaboration can facilitate the integration of curricular content into Level I fieldwork.

Students are not the only ones who can benefit from these experiences. Fieldwork educators also benefit from training fieldwork students (Hanson, 2012). The learning activity below will help you identify not only how fieldwork and your curriculum are integrated, but ways in which it can benefit both students and fieldwork educators.

Learning Activity 45.6.

Generate a list of the ways your academic program currently integrates Level I fieldwork into coursework; see example below to create your own. Evaluate the benefits of current assignments to students and to fieldwork educators. Work with other faculty to identify alternative Level I fieldwork assignments that might be a better fit for your curriculum and student and fieldwork educator needs.

Activities That Integrate Fieldwork and Coursework	Benefits to Students	Benefits to Fieldwork Educators
Students reflect on fieldwork experiences in a fieldwork journal	• Reinforces class concepts • Creates connections between concepts and applications in practice • Encourages self-reflection on occupational therapy practice	• Provides fieldwork educators with insight to student's clinical reasoning and the student's perspective on the fieldwork experience
Interview fieldwork educators (e.g., challenges and supports for using evidence-based practice in their setting) and incorporate the resulting data into a qualitative research project on a specific topic which the class analyzes to create common themes	• Allows students to practice interview skills • Provides students with real data to use when learning qualitative research • Provides students with a connection between their fieldwork experience and research course	• Exposes fieldwork educators to new and/or "hot" topics • Heightens understanding of the curriculum
Identify and analyze types of assessments used in the FW setting, present results to class, and recommend a new assessment to the site	• Students learn about assessment tools used in various settings, supplementing classroom learning • Students contribute to education of entire class	• Fieldwork educators learn about assessments that may benefit their clients

Level II Fieldwork

The purpose of Level II fieldwork is to "develop competent, entry-level, generalist occupational therapists. Level II fieldwork must be integral to the program's curriculum design and must include an in-depth experience in delivering occupational therapy services to clients, focusing on the application of purposeful and meaningful occupation and research, administration, and management of occupational therapy services. It is recommended that the student be exposed to a variety of clients across the lifespan and to a variety of settings" (ACOTE, 2012, p. S34). Level II fieldwork is the first opportunity for students to develop entry-level professional competence with clients through immersion in the role as an occupational therapy practitioner in the practice setting where fieldwork occurs. It is an opportunity to bridge the didactic portion of the curriculum with hands-on practical application. Level II fieldwork complements and reinforces the academic program curricular threads through hands-on learning. Students develop and practice professional behaviors expected of an entry-level OT practitioner. Students build a professional identity, embracing the philosophical roots of occupational therapy while envisioning future directions for practice.

Site Selection

AFWCs play an integral role in the site selection process. For example, students may have unrealistic expectations for completing Level II fieldwork in a specialty practice, which is beyond the scope of an entry-level program. Therefore, through the fieldwork advising and selection process, students will gain an appreciation for the kinds of foundational skills they need to be prepared for an entry-level practice in a wide array of settings.

Most academic program coursework offers limited opportunities for student choice of fieldwork selection, due to the realities of limited site choice and graduate timelines. However, students who are involved in selecting their placements take greater ownership in and are more satisfied with their fieldwork experiences; therefore, it is important to build in student choice wherever possible (Felix, Garrubba, & Devlin, 2011). In addition, you need to provide students with the resources and tools to make informed decisions about fieldwork.

Learning Activity 45.7.

Generate a list of the methods you have developed for students to reflect on and make informed decisions about Level II fieldwork placements; see example below. Identify additional resources that would further help students with these decisions.

Resource	Current Methods	Additional Resources
Description of fieldwork practice settings	• Advise a group or individual—groups may bring up questions an individual may not consider. • Post descriptions of settings on online. • Post American Occupational Therapy Association Fieldwork Data Forms online for student review (see http://www.aota.org/Education-Careers/Fieldwork/Supervisor.aspx). • Post questions for students to consider when choosing Level II fieldwork (see Appendix 45.A).	
Description of student learning experiences at fieldwork placements	• Advise a group or individual. • Post completed Student Evaluation of the Fieldwork Experience (SEFWE) forms online for students to review.	
Student reflection on own learning style and supervision needs	• Advise a group or individual. • Have students complete the Fieldwork Experience Assessment Tool or a learning style inventory to analyze their learning needs for future Level II fieldwork.	

Developing a fieldwork selection process that works for you, for the academic program, and for students may be challenging. Several factors influence how you make placement decisions, including the time and resources you have for assigning placements, the number and location of fieldwork sites available at any given time, and the relationship of your Level I and II selection processes to one another. For example, if you work alone in your role as AFWC without administrative support and you have a large number of students to place, efficiency in placement will be your greatest concern. If you are having difficulty recruiting sites, lengthen your site assignment time frame to allow for ongoing site recruitment. If a mission of your department is to support inner-city health care services, your placement process should emphasize opportunities in such facilities, which would likely include an emphasis on role-emerging placements. If your student population relies primarily on public transportation, have students identify their access and barriers to transportation as part of the selection process. If you use a same-site model (Level I and II at the same facility) of student placement, the process used to choose one placement will influence the process for the other.

Some fieldwork sites require students to interview before placement, and occasionally it is a competitive process similar to employment applications. Completion of an interview gives the site the opportunity to determine whether a student is a good fit for the site environment and the teaching/supervisory style of the fieldwork educator. The student can become acquainted with the available learning opportunities at the site and determine whether the site is a match for his or her professional goals. Opportunity to job shadow or complete a Level I fieldwork at the same-site as a Level II experience may be even more helpful to ease student anxiety and prepare both the student and fieldwork educator for the upcoming Level II experience (Evenson, Barnes, & Cohn, 2002).

Learning Activity 45.8.

Do a SWOT (strengths, weaknesses, opportunities, and threats) analysis of your fieldwork selection process; see example below. Reflect upon the current approach used to assign students to Level I and II fieldwork placements to determine its effectiveness. Decide what is working and what is not to consider new approaches that could be more effective.

Fieldwork Selection Process	Strengths	Weaknesses	Opportunities	Threats
Random assignment (i.e., lottery); no student choice	Efficient and fast	No opportunity to consider individual student strengths and learning needs Students may complain	Best use of AFWC time and energy	Greater chance of difficulties because no consideration given to student learning needs
Assignment made by academic fieldwork coordinator (AFWC) based on student choice (e.g., AFWC selects site from three student choices)	Compromise between efficiency and student choice	Student input takes AFWC time and effort to make matches Students may complain	AFWC can select options for all students balancing their interests with what is available (e.g., commuting priorities, start and end times)	Large numbers of students can be time consuming

(Continued)

Learning Activity 45.8. *(Cont.)*				
Fieldwork Selection Process	**Strengths**	**Weaknesses**	**Opportunities**	**Threats**
Assignment made by student, based on random order of choice	Student goals and needs are considered	Time consuming, less efficient for large numbers of students and for shorter placements (e.g., Level I)	A fair process, no favoritism Students have control of where fieldwork occurs	May need to separate students with Americans with Disabilities Act needs to address fieldwork accessibility and accommodations
Assignment made by collaboration between student and AFWC	Collaboration increases good fit between student and site Greater student commitment to placement	Most labor intensive for AFWC Must have a large number of possible placements in a variety of locations	Preventive model can lower incidence of problems during fieldwork	Threat to AFWC non-fieldwork responsibilities, (e.g., teaching responsibilities may be negatively affected due to time needed) Competition for placements in the region

Preparing Students for Fieldwork

Preparing students for fieldwork may be one of the AFWC's most critical tasks. Traditional academic advising is focused on helping students "understand and successfully navigate their college experience" and entails a "commitment to individual exploration and discovery," which you can use to prepare students for fieldwork (Rosenfeld, Shakespeare, & Imbriale, 2014). The art of being an AFWC involves collaborating with students to build a partnership based on shared perspectives and common goals, which can be accomplished in several ways.

An important duty for the AFWC is to prepare students for the professional behaviors expected during fieldwork. Professional behavior should be defined early and explicitly to establish the student's identity as a future occupational therapy practitioner and a representative of your academic program. You can communicate about professional behavior expectations verbally and in writing to reinforce guiding principles for success, and you can do it individually or in groups.

When done well, group advising reduces the need for individual advising and prepares students to represent your academic program well. Group advising might include practice of specific skills expected in a professional work environment, such as learning to give and receive feedback (James & Musselman, 2006).

Program-wide evaluation processes might be developed that encourage student self-reflection and faculty evaluation of student professional behavior performance (Zimmerman, Hanson, Stube, Jedlicka, & Fox, 2007). You may also develop departmental policies that apply to the fieldwork environment, such as appropriate electronic communication with fieldwork educators.

Learning Activity 45.9.

Review the table of Level II student professional behaviors and strategies to help students adopt these behaviors. Evaluate the effectiveness of each strategy in your academic program (1= *does not work,* 2 = *works for some students,* 3 = *works for all students*) and, if not effective, identify alternative strategies to help students adopt these behaviors. Identify additional professional behaviors you would like your students to adopt, and fill in the last row of the table.

Student Professional Behavior	Strategy	Strategy Effectiveness	Strategy Alternative
Has a commitment to learning	• Example: Orient students to expectations and self-responsibility during group orientation to fieldwork • Include professional behavior items in the Level I fieldwork evaluation of student	• Effective for most students • Fieldwork educator provides feedback in addition to faculty, reinforcing key professional behaviors	• Individual student meetings to reinforce student commitment to learning • AFWC reviews fieldwork educator feedback with student
Uses effective and appropriate communication styles	• Incorporate expectation in OT class performance for grade • Use role playing in class	• Generalize expectations for FW into the classroom • Practicing communication styles can support student implementation during FW	• FW communication log, students reflect upon effective and ineffective verbal and nonverbal communication, discuss reflections with AFWC
Participates in supervisory process	• Use the Fieldwork Experience Assessment Tool (FEAT) to clarify expectations	• Student is able to self-identify supervisory needs and self-advocate	• Provide more structure through written learning contract with student learning objectives addressing engagement in supervisory process
Uses effective time management and organization techniques	• Develop departmental policies for consequences if goals are not met	• Explicit expectations support compliance	• Use of auditory cues for time management • Use of smartphone calendar or daily planner to organize deadlines
Assumes the student practitioner role	• Analyze the Occupational Therapy Process Practice Model for class assignment—student analyzes FW educator evaluation, goal setting, intervention approach to translate into relevant OT practice model • Add this item to the Level I fieldwork evaluation of student	• Student links OT coursework theory and concepts with application on FW	• Fieldwork journal—student reflects upon becoming a professional, taking on the OT "mantle"

Note. AFWC = academic fieldwork coordinator; FW = fieldwork; OT = occupational therapy.

Support During Fieldwork

Many aspects of the Level II fieldwork experience may be challenging for students. For example, ethical dilemmas can challenge high standards of professional ethical conduct (AOTA, 2014a, 2015). These dilemmas can be student-related (e.g., unclear professional boundaries with clients), fieldwork educator–related (e.g., unrealistic student expectations), or related to the relationship between the student and the fieldwork educator (e.g., blurring of professional lines). Other dilemmas are related to potential threats to regulatory compliance with Medicare documentation, reimbursement, and supervision of students. Therefore, AFWCs, students, and fieldwork educators will benefit from having a framework to guide ethical decision making, such as the four-step model developed by Swisher, Arslanian, and Davis (2005). This model will help you define the scope of an ethical dilemma and identify potential strategies for solving it. AOTA also provides many tools to support ethical reasoning (see http://www.aota.org/Practice/Ethics.aspx).

Expectations for student independence increase during Level II placement as a result of the increasing demands of the health care environment (Vogel, Grice, Hill, & Moody, 2004). In addition, in the midst of time pressures, students are expected to continuously communicate with their supervisors to shape the learning process. Therefore, the AOTA Fieldwork Performance Evaluation (Chapters 58 and 59 in this book) form may be a helpful tool for student self-assessment and may also serve as a framework for student and fieldwork educator discussions regarding student progress (Atler, 2003). The SEFWE provides a format for students to give feedback to the fieldwork educator and site (see ACOTE [2012] Standard C.1.15) and can be used as a tool by the student to initiate difficult discussions in a diplomatic manner. The Fieldwork Experience Assessment Tool (Chapter 13 in this book) provides an objective format for giving and receiving feedback about the fieldwork environment; fieldwork educator engagement, teaching, and mentoring; and the student's learning behaviors and attitude. Feedback, provided diplomatically, can play a critical role in shaping the learning environment for future students.

A variety of strategies can be used to support students throughout their Level II placements. Group communication (e.g., email, chatrooms) can provide general information about occupational therapy practice, learning resources, or best practice with supervision. Individual communication is indicated for students who need additional support to be successful at their placement. Online course tools (e.g., Blackboard, Canvas) can be used as a resource to support students during fieldwork and to stimulate reflection and reasoning. You can post fieldwork documents (see the table in the next learning activity) for students to review, discuss, and share with their fieldwork educator. For example, the AFWC may post a calendar of fieldwork events for the semester with timelines and due dates for when fieldwork assignments and evaluations are due.

Learning Activity 45.10.

Review the online components of your fieldwork course and fieldwork resources for students to determine the value for students, the academic fieldwork coordinator (AFWC), and fieldwork educators and faculty (see table for recommended components and their values). Identify areas to strengthen your online course and better support students' fieldwork experience.

Online Component	Value for Students	Value for AFWC	Value for Fieldwork Educators and Faculty
Fieldwork syllabus or student handbook	Explicitly defines policies and procedures	Explicitly defines policies and procedures	NA
Fieldwork educator handbook	Makes students aware of what is communicated to the fieldwork educator (students are accountable for providing the handbook to the fieldwork educator)	Facilitates transparent communication among AFWC, fieldwork educator, and student	Information supports exchange with student about the relationship between fieldwork and current coursework

(Continued)

Learning Activity 45.10. *(Cont.)*

Online Component	Value for Students	Value for AFWC	Value for Fieldwork Educators and Faculty
Level I and II FWPE and SEFWE forms	Can be easily accessed	Saves AFWC time and paper because students can readily access forms on their own	NA
Level II fieldwork discussion board or blog (see Appendix 45.B)	Maintains connections between students and AFWC during fieldwork	Allows AFWC to keep in touch with students Makes AFWC aware of student situations	Faculty may participate or read discussion summaries, supporting classroom and fieldwork connections
Fieldwork timeline	Provides structure and organization to fieldwork	Saves AFWC time from repeating deadlines for assignments	NA
Occupational therapy–related websites (e.g., AOTA, NBCOT, OTCATS)	Creates healthy professional habits Encourages students to read and understand the value of important resources	NA	Fieldwork educators stay abreast of professional issues
Articles about fieldwork education	Supports training of students for future fieldwork educator role	Provides multiple avenues of educating students about fieldwork	Students share articles with fieldwork educators to enhance learning

Note. AFWC = academic fieldwork coordinator; AOTA = American Occupational Therapy Association; FWPE = Fieldwork Performance Evaluation; NA = not applicable; NBCOT = National Board for Certification in Occupational Therapy; OTCATs = Occupational Therapy Critically Appraised Topics; SEFWE = Student Evaluation of the Fieldwork Experience.

Administrative Management

Your administrative abilities will be crucial in the AFWC activities previously discussed. Organization and timing of tasks are critical to the administrative process, and attention to detail is required in the management of data about sites and students. In addition, you must also attend to memoranda of understanding (MOU), know the laws, regulations, and rules that affect fieldwork education, and ensure that the ACOTE (2012) standards related to fieldwork are met. However, many novice AFWCs find that they spend most of their time focusing on these administrative management tasks, at the expense of the other aspects of the AFWC role. Creating and using flexible strategies to complete these tasks will help you to expand into other aspects of the AFWC role (Smith, Burgess, & Hummell, 2010).

Organization and Time Management

Although you will do certain tasks every semester, you will find that the processes involved in moving students through their fieldwork education occur in an annual cycle. Each academic program determines when during the curriculum students perform Level I and Level II fieldwork. Those fieldwork dates will drive how and when you finish the tasks necessary to complete the cycle, but you must create deadlines and goals to effectively engage in *all* of the tasks within the AFWC role, not just those related to placements. To some extent, accomplishing your goals will be a trial-and-error process, but seeking feedback from your constituents about your process will help you use your time most wisely while responding to their needs and meeting your goals. These constituents may include administrators, other faculty, support staff, students, site student coordinators, fieldwork educators, AFWCs at nearby programs, and ACOTE as an accrediting body.

Site Data

From a practical standpoint, for you and your students, it is important to obtain and maintain accurate data about your fieldwork sites. You can work smarter if you keep that information current and easily accessible, because it is time-consuming to make updates as people move in and out of positions, companies change hands, and expectations change. Important site data include contact information for the student placement supervisor and details about hours, available transportation, and dress codes. You should also have as much information as possible about what is expected of students so that they can be prepared for their placements, and that information should be readily available to them. This information should include learning objectives for the student program at the site, information about the population served, assessment methods used, typical approaches to intervention, and other site-specific requirements. Keeping these data current will enable you to meet ACOTE (2012) standards and allow students to familiarize themselves with the site before they begin their fieldwork, which can help them be more successful.

Site data can be maintained a variety of ways. Many programs use commercially available databases to store, search, and manage information, but spreadsheets and tables can also be designed for this purpose. Some institutions use the expertise of their information technology staff to create databases specific to the occupational therapy program. Any of these solutions would consolidate information and make it easily accessible.

The AOTA Site Data Form (available at http://bit.ly/1MEfVOz), or some portion of it, is one way to collect information on fieldwork sites and determine whether site staff is sufficient to manage supervision, site frames of reference align with your curriculum, students learn site approaches to practice, and other criteria you identify as important. Information from SEFWE forms and student assignments can help you to determine whether the site continues to meet expectations. These data are also often used in annual reports to the academic institution and the accrediting body, ACOTE. Exhibit 45.4 shows ACOTE (2012) Standard C.1.2, which involves maintaining site data information and strategies for compliance.

Student Placement Data

The AFWC must maintain information about placements that have been requested, reserved, denied, or placed on hold. It may be challenging to recruit and retain sufficient numbers of placements that meet your program's needs, so you must keep track of your communications with sites to confirm them and assign students to them. Your sites will be grateful if you have a reliable way of maintaining this information, so that you minimize their work as well.

Management of student placement data will also help you demonstrate that placements conform to the

Exhibit 45.4. Strategies for Maintaining Site Data

Documenting Site Selection	Strategy
ACOTE Standard C.1.2: Maintain memoranda of understanding, comply with site requirements, maintain site objectives and site data, and communicate this information to students	• Maintain a database, available to both the AFWC and students, that includes ▪ Memoranda of understanding ▪ AOTA Site Data Form ▪ 12-week schedules ▪ Site-specific learning objectives. ▪ Site-specific SEFWE forms from former students • Develop student assignments that require students to obtain information about sites, student programs, and fieldwork educators. • Write up policies and procedures and make them available to students.

Note. ACOTE = Accreditation Council for Occupational Therapy Education; AFWC = academic fieldwork coordinator; AOTA = American Occupational Therapy Association; SEFWE = Student Evaluation of Fieldwork Experience.

philosophy of the academic program and to the curriculum, meet ACOTE (2012) standards, and ensure that students are educated as generalists. It may also be necessary to maintain this information to satisfy state regulations. As with site data, you can use a variety of methods to maintain placement information, and it makes sense to connect it to information about individual students. To work smarter, seek solutions that combine demographics, placement information, site data, and MOU status within the same database.

The AFWC is also responsible for ensuring that students are supervised by qualified and prepared fieldwork educators and that the methods of evaluating student performance are performed as expected. In addition, the academic program is required to provide resources to fieldwork educators that will enhance their ability to supervise students and evaluate their performance. See Exhibit 45.5 for ACOTE standard evaluation criteria and strategies to achieve them.

Memoranda of Understanding

MOUs delineate the responsibilities of both the academic institution and the fieldwork educator's employer regarding the education of the student. They may include student prerequisites such as health information, immunization records, background checks, and drug screens, and the duties of each party for supervising and teaching the student. The MOU also contains the liability and indemnity of both parties should there be an incident that results in legal action. The AFWC is responsible for obtaining and maintaining MOUs with a sufficient number of fieldwork sites so that students are not delayed in completing all fieldwork because of a shortage of placements.

The process of obtaining and maintaining MOUs can be time-consuming and detailed and may require legal expertise. Therefore, you should seek assistance with this process from your department or school. Typically, your institution's legal team will design an MOU to be reviewed and approved by the fieldwork site, but some affiliates will have agreements they have developed and will prefer to use. Both the affiliate and the academic institution must agree on terms of the MOU. Agreements are fully executed when signed by designated persons at the affiliate and at the academic program.

ACOTE (2012) standards require that MOUs be current for sites that are actively training fieldwork students; therefore, the AFWC needs a system to track MOU development and ensure that all MOUs are up to date. Exhibit 45.6 lists strategies for implementing ACOTE standards for MOU.

Laws and Regulations Affecting Fieldwork

Understanding the laws and regulations that affect fieldwork is necessary to ensure legal and ethical practice within the supervisory process. The federal laws and regulations that concern reimbursement for services delivered by students (Medicare), student privacy (Family Educational Rights and Privacy Act of 1974 [Pub. L. 93-380]), and patient privacy (Health Insurance Portability and Accountability Act of 1996 [Pub. L. 104–191]) will affect your handling of situations that may arise during fieldwork placements. One responsibility is to inform students and sites about the importance of observing all applicable regulations (AOTA, 2010). State regulations regarding practice will govern placement of students because of supervision requirements. In addition, state laws or regulations may influence the terms of the agreement between the academic institution and the affiliating partner.

Federal, state, and local laws or regulations are frequently introduced or amended and may affect your fieldwork program administration or the supervision requirements for students that surround reimbursement. For example, Medicare regulations regarding payment for services have shifted within the past 5 years (Chew, Fulmino, Johnson, & Russell, 2011). Other laws, regulations, or rules may affect the placement process. As an example, some states have regulations that make it difficult for programs from out-of-state to place fieldwork students (e.g., Higher Education Opportunity Act of 2008). Some sites may request reimbursement for legal processes related to executing MOUs. Some sites may adopt their own rules about how students are accepted or supervised, such as a requirement to have participated in one Level II fieldwork before being accepted for placement. As the AFWC, it is your responsibility to stay updated on these laws, regulations, and rules.

Exhibit 45.5. *Strategies for Student Performance and Fieldwork Educator Effectiveness Evaluation*

Evaluation of Student Performance and Fieldwork Educator Effectiveness	Strategy
ACOTE Standard C.1.4: Frequent assessment of student progress	• Maintain records of student evaluations. • Document communications with fieldwork educators that concern student progress. • Develop student assignments discussing supervisory experiences.
ACOTE Standard C.1.11: Promote clinical reasoning and reflective and ethical practice	• Strengthen the link between the fieldwork experience and these concepts during orientation to fieldwork, and evaluate these competencies during fieldwork through student assignments and discussions (e.g., for a student journaling assignment, have him or her write about an ethical dilemma experienced during fieldwork and how the clinical reasoning process resolved it). • Document a discussion among the student, fieldwork educator, and AFWC about these topics during midterm conferences.

ACOTE Standard C.1.14: Ensure fieldwork educators are currently licensed or otherwise regulated occupational therapists with a minimum of 1 year full-time experience and adequately prepared to serve as a fieldwork educator	• Obtain and maintain records of the following information, before or during placement, from fieldwork educators or students:
	  ▪ Years of experience
	  ▪ Active credentials
	  ▪ Participation in AOTA Fieldwork Educator Certificate Program
	  ▪ Number and level of students supervised
	  ▪ Models of supervision used.
	• Require that the fieldwork educator and AFWC sign a form verifying the previous information.
	• Maintain this information systematically.

ACOTE Standard C.1.15: Provide a mechanism for evaluating the effectiveness of supervision and enhancing supervision	• Provide a fieldwork educator handbook with information on supervision. • Review SEFWE forms to determine patterns of supervision and need for fieldwork educator support. • See additional strategies in section "Fieldwork Educator Training" of this chapter.
ACOTE Standard C.1.16: Ensure supervision provides protection of consumers and opportunities for appropriate role modeling of occupational therapy practice; progress supervision from direct to indirect	• Develop student assignments describing models of supervision they are experiencing. • Provide a fieldwork educator handbook with information about models of supervision or resources to obtain that information and development of learning objectives.
ACOTE Standard C.1.17: Where no occupational therapy services exist: • Document a plan for services and supervision • Provide a minimum of 8 hours of direct supervision each week from a qualified fieldwork educator • Ensure that an on-site supervisor designee of another profession is assigned.	• Document a progressive plan for supervision detailing responsibilities of the on-site supervisor, student, and occupational therapy supervisor. • Require students to document programs developed, interactions with the population served, and supervision sessions with the on-site supervisor. • Document occupational therapy fieldwork educator qualifications and hours that he or she is on-site.

Note. ACOTE = Accreditation Council for Occupational Therapy Education; AFWC = academic fieldwork coordinator; AOTA = American Occupational Therapy Association; SEFWE = Student Evaluation of the Fieldwork Experience.

Exhibit 45.6. Strategies for Implementing Memoranda of Understanding

Memoranda of Understanding	Strategy
ACOTE Standard C.1.5: Adequate number of MOUs	• Expand numbers of sites and MOUs by asking students where they completed observation hours or by asking for the names of sites near their homes.
ACOTE Standard C.1.6: Evidence and documentation of MOUs	• Maintain paper or electronic copies. • Track all related activities in a database that is synchronized with student placement information. • Delegate responsibilities to support staff and the legal department. • Document the system you use for MOU management.

Note. ACOTE = Accreditation Council for Occupational Therapy Education; MOU = memorandum of understanding.

Using Accreditation Standards to Promote Fieldwork Quality

You can gain a big-picture perspective about the quality of your fieldwork program by examining the methods you use to comply with ACOTE (2012) standards. Rather than devising strategies to meet these standards, consider using the standards to *guide* the development of a quality fieldwork program. The function of the accreditation council is to award "accreditation at the postsecondary level (which) performs a number of important functions, including the encouragement of efforts toward maximum educational effectiveness. The accrediting process requires institutions and programs to examine their goals, activities, and achievements; to consider the expert criticism and suggestions of a visiting team; and to determine internal procedures for action on recommendations from the accrediting agency" (AOTA, 2014b, p. 1, Section I). To a great extent, the accrediting body protects students and seeks to guarantee that the educational program is effectively preparing them for practice by requiring compliance with the standards. The standards are open to interpretation, and the council intermittently releases interpretive statements about the standards.

You must be aware of, and comply with, all of the ACOTE (2012) standards that relate to you or to fieldwork. Section C of the standards pertains directly to fieldwork and is the only section discussed in this chapter. This section describes the requirements for managing placement data and for ensuring that students' fieldwork experiences are a logical extension of the academic program and are quality fieldwork experiences. When considering how your program will comply with the standards, think about the terms used in the standards, such as *ensure, document, demonstrate, provide, require,* and *show evidence.* In addition, the standards are intentionally written to allow each program to have control over curriculum design and the means by which the standards are met.

An essential feature of a quality fieldwork program is the obvious connection between the academic program and the fieldwork site. This connection may be more readily visible in programs in which the faculty participates in fieldwork as fieldwork educators or as supplemental instructors when students are onsite. Some fieldwork experiences are designed for students to access certain populations and are associated with specific courses. Therefore, faculty who teach these courses establish the fieldwork learning objectives. However, if the AFWC is the primary liaison between the site and the academic program, the strategies he or she uses to meet ACOTE (2012) standards may be more indirect compared with those used by faculty who are personally involved with fieldwork.

Exhibit 45.7 outlines ACOTE standards, and strategies, for connecting curriculum and fieldwork content.

ACOTE (2012) standard C.1.17 is helpful in setting guidelines and procedures when establishing fieldwork in nontraditional settings where occupational therapy practitioners are not employed (Exhibit 45.8). A primary consideration is the alignment of the student's experience with the academic program's curriculum.

Exhibit 45.7. *Strategies to Connect Curriculum and Fieldwork Content*

ACOTE Standard	Strategy
C.1.1: Reflect the sequence and scope of content in the curriculum design in collaboration with faculty, maintaining strong ties between didactic and fieldwork education	• Document collaboration between fieldwork and the curriculum design through faculty meeting minutes and other communications. • Provide fieldwork educators with topical outlines of courses in which the students are engaged and ask them to match fieldwork experiences with topics. • Obtain signature pages that indicate that the site agrees with objectives set by the academic program for fieldwork.
C.1.3: Demonstrate collaboration between academic and fieldwork educators in establishing fieldwork objectives	• Train fieldwork educators in developing general learning objectives for the site and for individual students, provide templates or examples for developing objectives, and supply signature pages indicating agreement between the fieldwork site and academic program regarding established objectives. • Document communications with fieldwork educators regarding revised learning objectives for students having difficulty during fieldwork.
C.1.7: Ensure that at least one fieldwork experience (either Level I or Level II) focuses on psychological and social factors	• Focus the fieldwork experience on psychosocial development (e.g., psychosocial wellness, prevention, habilitation, rehabilitation) of the client, fieldwork educators, or the student in traditional or nontraditional settings. • Create student assignments that relate to psychosocial factors.
C.1.8: Ensure that Level I fieldwork includes experiences designed to enrich didactic coursework through directed observation and participation	• Write learning objectives for Level I fieldwork in curriculum. • Attach Level I fieldwork to a specific course in the curriculum, and state learning objectives. • Identify student assignments connecting fieldwork to coursework. • Document collaboration of the academic fieldwork coordinator with faculty to develop assignments integrating coursework with fieldwork.

Note. ACOTE = Accreditation Council for Occupational Therapy Education.

Exhibit 45.8. *Strategies for Nontraditional Settings*

Supervision in Emerging or Nontraditional Settings	Strategy
ACOTE Standard C.1.17: Where no occupational therapy services exist • Document a plan for services and supervision • Arrange a minimum of 8 hours of direct supervision each week • Designate an on-site supervisor from another profession.	• Document a progressive plan for supervision detailing responsibilities of the on-site supervisor, student, and occupational therapy supervisor. • Require students to document programs developed, interactions with population served, and supervision sessions with on-site supervisor. • Document occupational therapy fieldwork educator hours on-site.

Note. ACOTE = Accreditation Council for Occupational Therapy Education.

Maximizing Professional Rewards Through Scholarship and Service

Although given more attention in some institutional settings than others, attention to scholarship and service activities can strengthen your fieldwork program. More importantly, you will find your role as AFWC more professionally rewarding when you make the most of these opportunities. In this section, broad guidelines are provided to enhance your scholarship and service activities; however, the actual activities that you engage in will be unique to you. Therefore, a variety of thought-provoking questions are included to help you identify possibilities that are professionally rewarding and productive for you.

First, you will be encouraged to broaden your concept of scholarship and contemplate how your existing skills might be effectively used to nurture your professional role interests. Second, strategies to support evidence-based fieldwork education are considered, including collecting and applying research evidence to inform various activities of your AFWC role. Third, you will be challenged to consider how you can make the best use of the many forms of data you already collect to inform various research efforts. Finally, strategies to make the most of your service activities are explored.

Defining and Aligning Scholarship With Role Interests

Scholarship consists of a broad range of activities that include not only the creation of new knowledge but also describing, interpreting, and applying existing knowledge to fieldwork education and engaging students during fieldwork in their professional development and growth (AOTA, 2009). It is important to consider all possible applications of scholarship and to strategically choose scholarship that is a best fit for you.

Your skills in research, writing, product creation, or public speaking might influence the direction that your scholarship takes. Because only a small percentage of occupational therapy assistant and occupational therapist AFWCs hold doctoral degrees (6.3 and 29.5%, respectively), participation in research as scholarship may be particularly daunting (Hanson, Stutz-Tanenbaum, & Koski, 2013).

However, if you are interested in research, do not be dissuaded from it because of a lack of skill.

A great need exists for research in the area of fieldwork education, and particularly research on collaboration between programs rather than on projects within a particular fieldwork program (Roberts et al., 2014). This need widens the opportunities for research participation. Therefore, if you have a passion for understanding or improving an area of fieldwork education that is currently poorly understood or not working well for your program, embrace that passion. Reach out to other AFWCs, educators, or administrators and determine whether they have similar concerns. As an AFWC, you have excellent skills in fostering collaboration and communication and in tracking details, and you can use those skills as part of a research team.

Skills in practical writing and personal communications are central to the AFWC role and also play a part in many forms of scholarship. As an educator, you have skills in the use of course management systems. Because of your ongoing communication with fieldwork educators and familiarity with many practice environments, you have a good understanding of the kinds of tools that are or are not considered practical by fieldwork educators. Align these skills with your professional interests. For example, if your interest is in exploring teaching approaches *(pedagogy)* used by fieldwork educators during the first few weeks of fieldwork placement, you could design a student assignment that would allow you to collect data, with institutional review board approval, through use of a course management system. You could then use that data to create a manual of activity suggestions for fieldwork educators or an article for a research publication. Note that scholarly projects need not be a solitary activity. As in research, partnering with someone with similar interests will likely be easier and more enjoyable and create a better product.

Scholarship is most effective if it is aligned with your professional role interests. Therefore, link your scholarship to topics that are of most concern or value to you. As an AFWC, your role has many dimensions, but you will be more invested in some aspects than in others. Even if you have a variety of professional interests, if you examine them closely, you may notice that they cluster around one or two areas of focus.

Examples of scholarship pursuits that align with the educator, administrator, and counselor or adviser roles of the AFWC are given in the next Learning Activity.

Collecting Research to Inform Your Role

The direction of your scholarship starts with learning to be a consumer of research. When you begin researching the professional literature on topics of interest to you, you will find many resources for solving problems you may have been trying to figure out on your own. Consider research as a tool to help you work smarter. Many of the activities of the AFWC role explored in this chapter can be done more effectively when they are informed by research evidence. For example, as an AFWC, you likely already have developed activities and resources to effectively prepare students for their Level II fieldwork experience. Can you justify your present processes and procedures in view of research evidence? Exhibit 45.9 shows an example of how research evidence might direct your preparation of students for fieldwork.

Many aspects of fieldwork—preparing and advising students; recruiting, training, and retaining fieldwork educators; and determining administrative processes— can be explored from a research-based perspective. In addition, these activities will be more effective when they are informed by research evidence. How can you get started building a library of resources that can help you in your AFWC role? Consider the problems or issues you have encountered recently in your AFWC work, and partner with your institution librarian to find research that addresses these concerns. Create electronic or paper files on topics of interest. For example, if you are interested in administrative policies and procedures for helping students efficiently and effectively choose relevant fieldwork placements, you can collect articles related to internship site selection within the occupational therapy profession and other professions. You could expand this interest to include articles related to preparing students for fieldwork. In addition, work with the librarian to create a Scopus (Elsevier, Amsterdam, Netherlands) filing system to automatically send you articles that fit your preselected criteria.

Whether you keep an electronic file or paper documents, you can exponentially expand your resources

---

Learning Activity 45.11.

Identify a professional role in the table that represents the majority of your professional interests. After reading the scholarship pursuits for that role, think of one additional scholarship pursuit of interest to you in that category. If none of the professional roles in the table reflect your interest, identify an additional professional role that is represented in your AFWC work, a corresponding professional interest, and a scholarship pursuit that would fit this category.

Professional Role	Professional Interest	Scholarship Pursuit
Educator	The process and outcome of teaching and learning in fieldwork education	• Investigating the pedagogy used by fieldwork educators in teaching students • Measuring the effectiveness of fieldwork teaching practices
Administrator	The processes and procedures related to fieldwork education and their impact on student success	• Improving efficiency in student selection of fieldwork sites • Determining best practices for recruitment and retention of fieldwork sites
Counselor/advisor	Understanding and supporting students	• Understanding the student experience from the perspective of different ethnic groups • Developing resources or tools to support the student through various experiences

Exhibit 45.9. *Applying Research Evidence to Student Preparation for Fieldwork*

Research Evidence: Predictors for Student Success in Fieldwork (James & Musselman, 2006)	Application to Student Preparation for Fieldwork
Student asks for and uses feedback	Create opportunities to help students practice asking for and responding to feedback.
Student takes initiative in approaching supervisors with problems	Role play with students to practice approaching supervisors with problems.
Student uses coping strategies to gain a realistic perspective on a negative situation	Assign readings related to coping strategies, and then lead a discussion exploring coping strategies for specific fieldwork problems.

by sharing them with others, such as internship co-ordinators within your institution; other AFWCs within a fieldwork consortium; or the AFWC List-serv (membership in the AOTA AFWC Listserv can be explored through contacting the AOTA Education Operations Coordinator). Regardless of how the information is shared, you will inevitably hear from someone with a similar interest or collection of articles to share. Over time, you will find that you are growing your expertise in specific areas of research and are well on your way to creating a foundation for applied scholarship in fieldwork education.

Making Best Use of Data Collection

The area of fieldwork education has a strong need for research. Relatively few articles are published in the area of fieldwork education, and many of the articles published are narrative program descriptions rather than research studies. Because most studies represent one academic program, the ability to compare and contrast data or generalize findings is not often evident (Roberts, 2013). In addition, sample sizes are often small and more representative of the student perspective than that of other stakeholders, such as fieldwork educators or consumers.

There is a need for research that involves multiple constituent groups, is reflective of collaborative efforts between academic programs, and can answer timely questions that affect the fieldwork educational process. As an AFWC, you already collect much of the data from students and fieldwork educators that is needed to answer important questions about fieldwork education. For example, qualitative data are collected from students through online discussions about

learning experiences at the fieldwork site and from fieldwork sites from discussions with fieldwork advisory board members. Quantitative data are collected from students through SEFWE forms and from fieldwork sites through AOTA Site Data Forms. (Forms are available on the AOTA website. Follow prompts under education and careers, resources for fieldwork educators and fieldwork forms at www.aota.org).

How can you make the most of the data you already collect? Explore the use of all available electronic tools, such as Survey Monkey (www.surveymonkey.com) and Qualtrics (www.qualtrics.com), to summarize and analyze data from your SEFWE forms. Consider converting your AOTA Fieldwork Performance Evaluation form to an electronic format to more efficiently analyze and use its data. In addition, fieldwork data are often used to evaluate overall program or curriculum effectiveness, but they could also be used to improve your relationship with fieldwork educators. Consider how you might collect data more strategically to align with your scholarship interests. Collaborate with others in your academic program or institution who collect similar datasets to streamline your data collection efforts and to gain more data of interest. Before you collect data, think about the specific information you need for a particular presentation, research project, or product you wish to develop. Exhibit 45.10 shows examples of research studies conducted by AFWCs who collected data using focus groups and a survey that lead to resource development, positive fieldwork relationships, and research publication.

Assuming you have produced a scholarly project that is of value to you and that you want to share with others, what are your options? This work is typically presented either in person at conferences or

Exhibit 45.10. Examples of Positive Outcomes of Data Collection

Focus Groups	Survey
Purpose: Hanson (2011) conducted two online focus groups of fieldwork educators from pediatric and physical rehabilitation practice settings. Questions focused on respondents' perspectives of working with Level II fieldwork students. **Results:** Development of additional educational resources and more frequent communication with fieldwork educators resulted in improved relationships and a research publication.	**Purpose:** Working with members of a fieldwork consortium, Johnson et al. (2006) conducted a survey of Level I fieldwork sites to explore the learning activities available to students. **Results:** Data were used to develop a common list of learning activities and a Level I evaluation form appropriate for all students enrolled in the academic programs represented in the consortium.

workshops or in a publication. If you are not comfortable with public speaking, poster presentations will allow you to converse about your findings with individual conference attendees and build connections with others who have similar interests. Once a networking group is established, consider a presentation as part of a panel discussion format. Find a friend or two, develop a group presentation, and then work up to individual platform presentations.

If you are not comfortable with professional writing but have ideas and are open to feedback, consider writing in an occupational therapy practice magazine first, such as *Advance* or *OT Practice*. Article length is typically relatively short, and the editor will give you feedback and assistance in the process. If you are writing for a peer-reviewed journal, the process for acceptance is rigorous; therefore, if you are new to peer-review publishing, carefully read guidelines and requirements for submission and review to avoid rejection. Also consider getting advice about your article and the publication process from knowledgeable colleagues.

Learning Activity 45.12.

- What data do you collect that are most interesting to you?
- What research question could be addressed with these data?
- Who could you work with to expand your dataset and complement your scholarship skills?
- How could your data be used to build a stronger partnership with fieldwork sites?
- What type of presentation format would be the best fit for you?

Maximizing the Impact of Your Service

As an AFWC, you may be involved in many service activities for your academic program, institution, community, and profession. To best accomplish your professional goals, and to avoid burnout from participating in too many service activities, carefully consider your service involvement. Many aspects of service may be rewarding but may not serve your ultimate professional goals. Your service activities should be an extension of your teaching, administration, and scholarship roles and interests and should serve you and your department. Most importantly, service activities should not add more complexity or volume to your role. In this area, it is particularly important that you work smarter and not harder.

Whether it is university, departmental, professional, or community service, consider how a potential service activity promotes the mission of your department. Does it create a partnership between a facility and your program, or can it extend the impact of the curriculum into the community? For example, if your departmental mission includes serving a particular constituency, such as the poor or people in a rural area, service activities that directly affect these populations would be desirable. In addition, look for service activities that bridge the academic curriculum and fieldwork program, already a part of your responsibilities as AFWC. Other valuable endeavors involve learning more about the curriculum and helping you and other faculty understand the influence of academic learning on the student skill set. For example, if your program provides developmental screenings for low-income families in the community, you deliver a service that is consistent with your departmental

---

Learning Activity 45.13.

1. Identify at least two service activities that you engage in within your department, university, profession, or community.
2. Evaluate each service activity on a scale of 1–10 (from 1 = *not at all* to 10 = *very much*). To what degree does the activity
   - Allow you to pursue an interest aligned with your professional role?
   - Reflect your unique skills or help you learn a new skill?
   - Enhance your teaching or work with students?
   - Inform or complement your scholarship?
   - Help you recruit fieldwork sites or enhance your relationship with fieldwork sites?
   - Further the goals of your academic program?
   - Increase your understanding of your academic program?
3. Based on this evaluation, which service activities do you want to stop, expand, add, or do differently?

---

mission, you learn about the content of your curriculum in the area of pediatric assessment, and both you and other faculty members learn about your students' abilities in this area. If your service contributes to your ability to develop additional fieldwork sites, then your efforts reap yet more benefits.

Your primary consideration for service is the degree to which the activity fosters opportunity for fieldwork placement. From this perspective, you must consider how your service promotes networking opportunities and the types of partnerships your service might create between the facility and your academic program. Partnerships are important, not only for recruiting but also for retaining fieldwork sites and contributing to maintaining a consistent number of placement opportunities.

Finally, you can work smarter if you align your service and scholarship activities with each other. Is there an aspect of your service that lends itself to scholarly investigation? Is there an aspect of your scholarship that lends itself to service delivery? In addition, both your service and scholarship activities should align with your professional focus, interests, and skills. For example, in your service program providing developmental screenings for low-income families, consider how the program's scholarship applications would differ depending on whether your focus was as an administrator or as an educator. As an administrator, you would collect data from parents about how the service affects their understanding of and value for occupational therapy in their community. As an educator, you would collect data from students regarding their perceptions of how the curriculum has prepared them for this patient interaction.

Summary

The role of the academic fieldwork coordinator is unique, the activities of the role are demanding, and the rewards are great. It is our hope that this review of information relative to fieldwork educator recruitment, training, and retention; student advisement; administrative activities; and service and scholarship of the AFWC role validates your knowledge, leads to new discoveries, and assists you in creating a new vision for your role as AFWC. This chapter should also help you adopt strategies to be more efficient and effective in your work, align your scholarship and service with your professional interests, and understand the value of networking with others rather than working alone. Finally, we hope that the information provided takes you on a journey of reflection, leading to role satisfaction and maximum role potential as you take steps to move your new vision forward.

References

Accreditation Council for Occupational Therapy Education. (2012). 2011 Accreditation Council for Occupational Therapy Education (ACOTE®) standards. *American Journal of Occupational Therapy, 66,* S6–S74. http://dx.doi.org/10.5014/ajot.2012.66S6

American Occupational Therapy Association. (2009). Specialized knowledge and skills of occupational therapy educators of the future. *American Journal of Occupational Therapy, 63,* 804–818. http://dx.doi.org/10.5014/ajot.63.6.804.

American Occupational Therapy Association. (2010). *Commission on Practice and Commission on Education Joint Task Force. Practice advisory: Services provided by students in fieldwork level II settings*. Retrieved from http://www.aota.org/-/media/Corporate/Files/EducationCareers/Educators/Fieldwork/StuSuprvsn/Practice%20Advisory%20Services%20provided%20by%20students%20in%20FW%20Level%20II%20final.pdf

American Occupational Therapy Association. (2011, April). *Academic fieldwork coordinators forum*. Presented at the American Occupational Therapy Association Conference, Philadelphia.

American Occupational Therapy Association. (2012). Fieldwork level II and occupational therapy students: A position paper. *American Journal of Occupational Therapy, 66,* S75–S77. http://dx.doi.org/10.5014/ajot.2012.66S75

American Occupational Therapy Association. (2014a). *An advisory opinion for the AOTA Ethics Commission: Promoting ethically sound practices in occupational therapy fieldwork education*. Retrieved from http://www.aota.org/-/media/Corporate/Files/Practice/Ethics/Advisory/Academic-FW-Advisory.PDF

American Occupational Therapy Association. (2014b). *Occupational therapy practice framework: Domain and process* (3rd ed.). *American Journal of Occupational Therapy, 68*(Suppl. 1). http://dx.doi.org/10.5014/ajot.2014.682006

American Occupational Therapy Association. (2015, January 11). *Occupational therapy code of ethics and ethics standards*. Retrieved from http://www.aota.org/-/media/Corporate/Files/AboutAOTA/OfficialDocs/Ethics/Code%20and%20Ethics%20Standards%202010.pdf

Atler, K. (2003). *Using the Fieldwork Performance Evaluation forms: The complete guide*. Bethesda, MD: AOTA Press.

Barton, R., Corban, A., Herrli-Warner, L., McClain, E., Riehle, D., & Tinner, E. (2013). Role strain in occupational therapy fieldwork educators. *Work, 44,* 317–328. http://dx.doi.org/10.3233/WOR-121508

Beisbier, S., & Johnson, C. R. (2014, April). *Collaborative supervision: Evidence for an alternative fieldwork*. Paper presented at the American Occupational Therapy Association Annual Conference, Baltimore.

Bondoc, S., Arabit, L., Lashgari, D., Finnen, L., & Alexander, H. (2009). Fieldwork education in physical disabilities settings. *Physical Disabilities Special Interest Section Quarterly, 32*(2), 1–4.

Chew, F., Fulmino, J., Johnson, C., & Russell, L. (2011). Changes to student supervision in SNFs: Impact on fieldwork. *OT Practice, 16*(4), 15–17.

Dawes, J., & Lambert, P. (2010). Practice educators' experiences of supervising two students on allied health practice-based placements. *Journal of Allied Health, 39,* 20–27.

Evenson, M., Barnes, M. A., & Cohn, E. S. (2002). Brief Report—Perceptions of level I and level II fieldwork in the same site. *American Journal of Occupational Therapy, 56,* 103–106. http://dx.doi.org/10.5014/ajot.56.1.103

Family Educational Rights and Privacy Act of 1974, Pub. L. 93-380, 20 U.S.C. § 1232g; 34 CFR Part 99.

Felix, H., Garrubba, C., & Devlin. D. (2011). Utilization of a self-selection process for clinical rotation assignments: A report on student and clinical coordinator satisfaction. *Journal of Physician Assistant Education, 22,* 25–29.

Hanson, D. (2011). The perspectives of fieldwork educators regarding level II fieldwork students. *Occupational Therapy in Health Care, 25,* 164–177.

Hanson, D. (2012). Fieldwork Issues. Benefits for fieldwork educators in working with students. *OT Practice, 17*(20), 18.

Hanson, D., Koski, J., & Stutz-Tanenbaum, P. (2013, October). *OT/OTA academic fieldwork coordinator role and personal reward*. Poster session presented at the American Occupational Therapy Association/National Board for Certification in Occupational Therapy Education Summit, Atlanta.

Hanson, D., Stutz-Tanenbaum, P., & Koski, J. (2013, April). *OT/OTA academic fieldwork coordinator role and personal reward*. Poster session presented at the American Occupational Therapy Association Annual Conference, Indianapolis.

Haynes, C. (2011). Active participation in fieldwork level I: Fieldwork educator and student perceptions. *Occupational Therapy in Health Care, 25,* 257–269.

Health Insurance Portability and Accountability Act of 1996 (HIPAA), Pub. L. 104–191, 42 U.S.C. § 300gg, 29 U.S.C § 1181-1183, and 42 USC 1320d-1320d9.

James, K., & Musselman, L. (2006). Commonalities in level II fieldwork failure. *Occupational Therapy in Health Care, 19,* 67–81.

Johnson, C., Sauerwald, C., Stutz-Tanenbaum, P., & Hanson, D. (2014, April). *Academic Fieldwork Coordinator Institute*. Pre-conference Institute conducted at the American Occupational Therapy Association Annual Conference, Baltimore.

Kirke, P., Layton, N., & Sim, J. (2007). Informing fieldwork design: Key elements to quality in fieldwork education for undergraduate occupational therapy students. *Australian Occupational Therapy Journal, 54,* S13–S22.

Lekkas, P., Larsen, T., Kumar, S., Grimmer, K., Nyland, L., Chipchase, L.,… Finch, J. (2007). No model of clinical education for physiotherapy students is superior to another: A systematic review. *Australian Journal of Physiotherapy, 53,* 19–28.

O'Connor, A., Cahill, M., & McKay, E. A. (2012). Revisiting 1:1 and 2:1 clinical placement models: Student and clinical educator perspectives. *Australian Occupational Therapy Journal, 59,* 276–283.

Roberts, M., Hooper, B., Wood, W., & King, R. (2014). An international systematic mapping review of fieldwork education in occupational therapy. *Canadian Journal of Occupational Therapy*. Published online before print November 2014. http://dx.doi.org/10.1177/0008417414552187

Rosenfeld, M., Shakespeare, C., & Imbriale, W. (2014, May 13). A privilege or a purpose: Can higher education still afford to help students discover themselves and explore life's meaning? *Academic Advising Today*. Retrieved from http://www.nacada.ksu.edu/Resources/Academic-Advising-Today/View-Articles/A-Privilege-or-A-Purpose-Can-Higher-Education-Still-Afford-to-Help-Students-Discover-Themselves-and-Explore-Life%E2%80%99s-Meaning.aspx

Salzman, A. (2009). Portraits of persistence: Professional development of successful directors of clinical education. *Journal of Physical Therapy Education, 23,* 44–54.

Secomb, J. (2008). A systematic review of peer teaching and learning in clinical education. *Journal of Clinical Nursing, 17,* 703–716.

Smith, M., Burgess, C., & Hummell, J. (2010). Managing real world placements: Examples of good practice. In McAllister, L., Paterson, M., Higgs, L., & Bithell, C. (Eds.), *Innovations in allied health fieldwork education: A critical appraisal* (pp. 75–83). Rotterdam: Sense Publishers.

State Authorization Act. (2010). 34 CFR Parts 600, 602, 603, 668, 682, 685, 686, 690, and 691.

Swisher, L., Arslanian, L., & Davis, C. (2005). The Realm–Individual Process–Situation (RIPS) model of ethical decision making. *HPA Resource, 5*(3), 1, 3–8.

Stutz-Tanenbaum, P., & Hooper, B. (2009). Creating congruence between identities as a fieldwork educator and a practitioner. *AOTA Education Special Interest Section Quarterly, 19*(2), 1–4.

Stutz-Tanenbaum, P., Hanson, D., Koski, J. & Greene, D. (2015). Exploring the complexity of the academic fieldwork coordinator role. *Occupational Therapy in Health Care, 29*(2), 139–152.

Thomas, Y., Dickson, D., Broadbridge, J., Hopper, L., Hawkins, R., Edwards, A., & McBryde, C. (2007). Benefits and challenges of supervising occupational therapy fieldwork students: Supervisors' perspectives. *Australian Occupational Therapy Journal, 54,* S2–S12. http://dx.doi.org/10.1111/j.1440-1630.2007.00694.x

Vogel, K., Grice, K. O., Hill, S., & Moody, J. (2004). Supervisor and student expectations of level II fieldwork. *Occupational Therapy in Health Care, 18,* 5–19. http://dx.doi.org/10.1300/J003v18n01-02

Zimmerman, S., Hanson, D., Stube, J., Jedlicka, J., & Fox, L. (2007). Using the power of student reflection to enhance professional development. *The Internet Journal of Allied Health Sciences and Practice, 5*(2). Retrieved from http://ijahsp.nova.edu/articles/vol5num2/zimmerman_manuscript.pdf

Appendix 45.A. SAMPLE GUIDELINES TO CONSIDER WHEN SELECTING A LEVEL II FIELDWORK SITE—COLORADO STATE UNIVERSITY

Sample Timeline for Level II and IB fieldwork:

Tuesday, September 23/30: Level II Fieldwork Meeting overview

Monday, October 6: Out-of-state Level IIA & B FW requests can be submitted through Survey Monkey

Tuesday, October 28: Optional Fieldwork Meeting review list of recruited in-state Level IIA fieldwork

October 31 & November 4: In-state Level IIA selection process and SSM Level IB begins

Friday, November 7 @ 4:30 PM: Buyer's Remorse deadline to swap or drop in-state Level IIA fieldwork placement, student will need to work with us for a replacement site

1. **General Guidelines for Fieldwork**
   a. The summer 2015 Level II FW must occur full-time for 12 weeks between May 18 and August 21, 2015 (14-week time frame).
   b. In-state summer 2015 Level IIA fieldwork placements occur through the scheduled selection process.
   c. The fieldwork office *does ALL recruiting of ALL Level II placements.* We will work collaboratively with you to find potential fieldwork sites where you want them. Let's work together!
   d. When you sign up during the selection process or submit your request for a Level II placement to the fieldwork office, you are committing to that placement. The fieldwork office will make all reasonable attempts to secure that placement for you and then confirm it with you. It is the sign-up or request for a placement, and not the confirmation, that commits you to a fieldwork.
   e. Only one new fieldwork contract will be negotiated per student during the OT program. During the course of exploring potential fieldwork sites, if you find a new facility or site that might be covered with an existing corporate contract or receptive to using a CSU fieldwork agreement, please contact the academic fieldwork coordinator about the possibility of doing a placement at the new location.

   f. The fieldwork office will use reasonable efforts to maintain and, if necessary, negotiate fieldwork affiliation agreements. Because of legal constraints, sometimes renewal agreements at existing sites may not be approved, which may result in the cancellation of a fieldwork placement. We will work with you to schedule an acceptable alternative.
   g. When researching placements out-of-state, first try to find a site with an existing affiliation agreement/contract. There are several entities with which CSU has a multi-site "blanket" or "corporate" contracts. These contracts cover a number of sites using one legal agreement. Look at the web sites for these corporations to explore locations throughout the United States.
   h. Unexpected cancellations of fieldwork reservations may occur with confirmed reservations. These often cannot be anticipated. We ask students to be patient, flexible, and tolerant of the resulting changes. We will work with you to schedule an acceptable alternative.
   i. *Unexpected family, medical or financial crises may occur after you have confirmed* your placements. Students must document the concerns and negotiate cancellation with AFWC before another fieldwork placement is considered.
   j. Your summer Level IIA fieldwork will be with adults: inpatient acute, inpatient rehab, outpatient rehab, hands, skilled nursing, long-term acute care, mental health, or adult community.
   k. The *Level IIB fieldwork should be in a different practice setting* than Level IIA to allow exposure to a variety of settings and client characteristics. This is an ACOTE Standard.
   l. The *same-site model (SSM) for fieldwork* will be available this spring and summer. Same-site model has the same CSU OT student for a spring Level I fieldwork placement and continue with this student for a summer Level II fieldwork. This model helps students gain familiarity with the practice context, increase comfort level with the role of OT in the setting, and decrease anxiety levels during the preparation for Level II fieldwork. If the Level I FW in the SSM does not work out well for

either the student or fieldwork educator, or both, we will work with you to secure a different Level II fieldwork site.

m. If you need to *change your fieldwork dates,* please contact the fieldwork office to negotiate and notify us about the changes to ensure that your professional liability insurance and workers' compensation coverage will be in effect.

n. Full-time Level II fieldwork requires a minimum 40 hour work week plus outside readings and assignments, which can add from 5–20 hours per week additional time. Please try to limit other responsibilities (i.e., working) as much as possible. Part-time fieldwork may be possible during your second Level II fieldwork.

o. If you have concerns about the quality of your educational experiences and/or supervision during Level I or II FW with a specific fieldwork educator, *we want to know about it.* We depend on your feedback to provide the best educational learning opportunities for your FW. Please let me know how your fieldwork experiences are progressing as early as possible while there is time to do something about it.

2. **Factors for Successful Level II Fieldwork**

a. The *relationship between the student and the fieldwork educator is the single most important factor for a successful fieldwork experience,* regardless of the practice setting. You can have a fabulous experience in a setting that is not your priority if your supervisory relationship with the fieldwork educator is strong. The reverse is not true; you will not have a fabulous experience in the practice setting of your dreams if communication and support from the fieldwork educator are not positive.

b. Your similarity as a student with the fieldwork educator enhances the supervisory relationship: i.e., personality styles, learning/supervisory styles, background, culture, values, common interests, and characteristics.

c. *Do FW in a setting where you have a strong background experience and/or interest* in the practice setting. Consider doing *volunteer work to gain experience with the client population* you are most interested in.

d. *Visit, shadow, volunteer, or do Level I fieldwork placement at a site prior to requesting a Level II FW.* We encourage students to "shadow" and do site visits to become acquainted with the OT staff, the practice setting, client population, and role of OT and become more comfortable with the potential FW site. Informal visits do not need to be scheduled or approved by the fieldwork office.

3. **Personal Considerations:** *Determine your priorities when starting to consider Level II placements:* financial, timing, location, or setting (interest areas). You may need to make trade-offs of location to achieve your goal for timing and practice setting. If you have expectations to find a FW site meeting every need, we may be hard-pressed to find a fieldwork site for you.

4. **Financial**

a. Most fieldwork sites do not offer any monetary compensation. Consider the timing of your placements to maximize your financial resources during the placement.

b. A summer Level II fieldwork placement is considered part of the prior academic year financial aid package.

c. Student loans have a six (6) month grace period. The clock starts ticking when you are no longer registered as a full-time student.

d. Because you are not "on-campus" during your Level II fieldwork, *a portion of your student fees will be refunded to you.* You must pay the full amount of your student fees at the beginning of the semester, and your account will be credited after the census date of the semester.

e. You will be charged the current fee for Professional Liability Insurance through the University, once-per year.

f. There may be fees or additional costs associated with site prerequisites, including criminal background checks, basic life support training, drug screening, and immunizations.

5. **Timing for Level IIB Fieldwork**

a. Do you want to complete fieldwork and become an OTR as soon as possible? If so, do an early summer 2016 Level IIB fieldwork placement and graduate in late August.

b. Do you need a break? Do you anticipate needing a breather during the summer before doing a fall FW? Do you need the summer semester to finish your thesis? Consider taking the summer off, do FW during the fall, and graduate in December.

6. **Geographic Location**
   a. Consider doing your *fieldwork where you will have family, friends, or classmates nearby for support.* Fieldwork can be stressful and having a support system is helpful.
   b. Many OT students are offered jobs at their Level II fieldwork sites; consider where you want to live once you graduate and do at least one Level II in that region and practice area.
   c. Do you need to stay local? Can you relocate? How far can you commute?
   d. If staying local is important, you may need to be flexible with the practice setting, timing, and/or location.

7. **Interest Areas**
   a. The *curriculum prepares you to be a generalist*—seek as much diversity as possible in settings and client characteristics across Level I and II FW placements.
   b. *Consider your career goals*—in what setting do you see yourself working? Choose this practice setting for your Level IIB FW in an area of your interest.

8. **Characteristics of Settings**
   a. City and county hospitals often have more diverse client populations.
   b. University medical centers will offer an emphasis on student education, opportunities to observe surgery, attend educational lectures, a chance to work with students from other disciplines, and you may be able to participate in research conducted during your placement.

9. **Definition of Practice Settings in OT**
   a. **Inpatient adult settings:**
      1. *Acute care* settings are usually faster paced and have higher expectations of students—they expect you to "hit the ground running." The acute setting occurs in hospitals and includes ICU; there is 2–3 days length of stay (LOS) with primary focus on assessments, and discharge planning begins day one. More medically complex problems—i.e., poly-trauma, neuro, cardiac telemetry.

      2. *Acute-rehab* (also known as rehab) setting clients LOS is usually 2–3 weeks with three (3) hours of rehab per day (OT, PT, speech, and respiratory). It can occur in a general hospital setting as a rehab unit or freestanding rehab hospital. The length of stay ranges from a few weeks to a few months depending upon reimbursement source, comorbidities, and individual client circumstances.
      3. *Skilled nursing facilities* (SNF) clients' LOS is a few weeks and residents can be moved to long-term care for several months or years. SNF setting has similar client population as rehab, with usually an older adult age group neuro and orthopedic diagnoses.
      4. *Sub-acute rehab/transitional care* is usually in a hospital setting, similar client population as SNF although clients are medically unstable. There is a longer LOS, usually a couple of weeks. Clients do not have stamina for 3 hours of therapy a day. Most patients are able to be discharged home.
      5. *Long-term acute care* (LTAC) provides intensive care for 24 days or more, with variable therapy intervention according to client medical condition and stamina. People in LTAC often have traumatic injuries, usually need respiratory therapy, IV medications, or other sophisticated medical follow-up.
      6. *Acute behavioral health/psych*—adults, mostly hospital based, mostly group treatments, usually acute care inpatient, and outpatient psych/day treatment. Some sites include: adult day centers, day treatment centers, home health agencies, community rehabilitation programs, community mental health clinics, clubhouse programs, outpatient psychiatric clinics, foster care residents, sheltered workshops, group and private homes, and community support programs.
   b. **Outpatient medical**
      1. *Outpatient hand therapy:* Often supervised by a certified hand therapist (CHT) who has primary focus in hands/U/E rehab, and secondary focus with OT. Hand therapists see clients individually, although

sometimes see multiple clients, each with a unique intervention and program.

2. *Outpatient general rehab:* Adults with variety of client conditions i.e., stroke, post-surgical ortho. Clients usually seen once or twice a week.

c. **Home health:** Uncommon for Level II FW, medical model used for seeing clients in their homes to ensure safety, accessibility to bathroom, kitchen, and all parts of home, ability to care for self in home environment.

d. **Community-based placements**

1. *Community behavioral health:* Clients live in the community independently or in supported group environments. Focus of services is to support independent life skills and access to the community for work, leisure, grocery shopping, etc. May include supported employment, access to higher education, and volunteering.

2. *Adult day/older adult day:* A nonresidential program for adults/older adults providing recreational and social engagement in a community setting. The program may be provided for a specific age group, e.g., older adults, or condition: TBI.

e. **Pediatrics:** Most pediatric settings (especially medical-based pediatrics) are required by the site to be a second Level II fieldwork after another placement; often general adult medical setting is preferred.

1. *Outpatient private practice:* Private corporation owned by one person or group of professionals, may or may not have opportunity for interprofessional team work. A smaller number of therapists may be employed, may travel to provide home-based services, and to multiple clinic-based settings on contracts. Sensory integration and/or early intervention may be focus of practice.

2. *Outpatient hospital unit:* Outpatient medical pediatric unit; interprofessional team work occurs; part of a larger hospital system with referrals and resources for professional development. Children's hospitals are usually teaching facilities. Primary focus sensory integration, development approach.

3. *Early intervention:* 0–3 years children with strong family-oriented approach, often with transdisciplinary teamwork. Services provided in family home traditionally, teach caregivers strategies for managing child's feeding, personal care, and behavior. Consultation with caregivers supports caring and stimulating child's development. OT fits within IDEA federal guidelines as primary service provider with Part C for children 0–2 years.

4. *Inpatient children's hospital:* Children's hospitals are usually teaching facilities with active research and commitment to staff professional development. Medical-based environment with every staff person's focus on child's well-being and support of family. Children in inpatient are short-term; caregivers may stay in the room. Acute care is not like adult acute care, there is no Medicare guideline. Pediatric acute care is often after surgery, e.g., oncology, cardiac; pediatric rehabilitation is neuro and ortho. Similar LOS for acute and rehab.

5. *Public school settings:* OTs collaborate and consult with teachers and other education staff to provide the least restrictive environment for student's education. OT fits within IDEA federal guidelines as primary service provider with Part C for children 0–2 years (early intervention), or Part B for 3–21 years as related service provider to assist special education or speech therapist who is primary. Role of OT is to support student's educational process. FW is generally available in the fall and spring semesters. There are school holidays that add on extra time to the typical 12-week fieldwork.

f. **Emerging practice settings:**

1. Occupational justice settings are available through the NAPA-OT Guatemala Field School (must have intermediate Spanish written and verbal fluency) and at a University of Utah Refugee Resettlement location in Salt Lake City.

2. Elderhaus/Mindset: Adult and older adult day program, see above.

3. Adaptive Recreation Opportunities (ARO): OT addresses full participation in leisure and recreation type activities.

Appendix 45.B. Colorado State University Occupational Therapy Department 2014 Level II Fieldwork Discussion Board Guidelines and Topics

Fieldwork students are required to have 5 new and 5 responsive discussion board entries during the 12-week Level II fieldwork.

Confidentiality Notice: Do not name your site or use names of any people, whether they are your clients, colleagues, or fieldwork educator (make up another name). Hold fieldwork educator issues or your personal concerns for personal communication with me. Last, please respect the confidentiality and sensitivity of your peers who are writing on the discussion board. Please be diplomatic about the wording of your responses and about the vulnerability of others sharing very sensitive feelings and thoughts. Let's be tolerant of our differences and use this opportunity as a place for expanding new ideas and the learning process.

Students will be graded on a pass/fail system based upon meeting the discussion board entry criteria for a total of 10 discussion board entries as described below. There is flexibility for you to write when you feel you have something to share and to choose the topic to write about. The intent is for students to share fieldwork by reflecting with peers, faculty, and the fieldwork coordinator in order to make it a more meaningful experience.

Write a narrative story related to the topic chosen. Each new entry on the discussion board needs to include three components in order for readers to have a clear picture of the story: objective description, identification feelings/reactions, and reevaluation. It is assumed that an entry will incorporate all three components in a narrative style as opposed to separating each component. A satisfactory grade on each entry is based upon the qualities of each of three components.

Provide the following information in each new entry made:

1. An objective description: Write a description of the experience without judgments; simply recount the experience or event as it relates to the topic.
2. Identify your feelings and reactions: Describe feelings or reactions about the experience or events as it relates to the topic.

3. Reevaluate the experience: Reflect or summarize the insights gained from your experience, explain feelings, and describe what you have learned and how it affects your understanding of the problem. Reflection is not an end in itself; the purpose of reflection is to prepare you for new experiences in practice. Reevaluation of what has happened and what it means is necessary to better understand the situation and learn from it.

Some examples of reevaluation include the following; you only need to do one method of reevaluation on a new entry:

- Compare and contrast how new information based on this experience relates to current knowledge.
- Integrate current experience with additional knowledge that results in a new perspective or insight not previously held.
- Determine the authenticity of ideas (reality check) and feelings that have resulted from an outside source.
- An "Ah-ha" moment to make it your own, where knowledge leads to a different perspective on the event and changes in how to act in the future.

Sample discussion board entry:

I have had quite the fieldwork experience, from having several supervisors, many many children, and lots of different advice. I have had to formulate and learn a lot on the fly. As I began to take over therapy sessions with different children, there is one kiddo that I have thoroughly enjoyed spending time with. To begin with, I began working with this 6-year-old boy with hemiplegia CP after my 2nd week. I observed the therapist with him for two weeks before I began taking over the sessions. Having observed the sessions and reading over his goals, though I did not feel comfortable copying my therapists' sessions with him. The goals were pretty straightforward: don/doff clothes (socks and shoes) and fine motor skills, including coordination/dexterity. He would come into therapy sessions with a good sense of humor, when asked what his right hand (the affected side) was doing when it was not actively engaged in the activity, his reply would often be, "Righty's watching." The gist is that he is a very fun and imaginative kid.

My favorite session with him was when we started with some gross motor activities to engage his scapula and try to get some stability and range into his right side. We began our session as bears crawling over bolsters and reaching for our "food" (bug-shaped puzzle pieces) and rolling back over the bolster to "eat" our food by placing them into the puzzle. Afterward, we bear-walked over to the table because the bears were going to have a party and we beaded our party necklaces before we made our party favors, which were coloring, cutting, and gluing a craft. Then it was time for the bears to snack again and he had to reach for the rubber fruit with his right side and place the one-inch pieces into the bear canister. He got to choose where his snack was found; for example, grapes were found in the air, while bananas and apples he scavenged from the ground.

I'm not sure why this was my favorite session of all of my fieldwork. I think that for the first time I felt that I had really been "myself" in a therapy session. I was able to utilize all of his goals into 1 hour of fun while tapping into this 6-year-old's imaginative world. He loved it, I enjoyed being a bear and having a bear party while addressing the skills my therapist really wanted to do. I think that it was also refreshing to work with an individual who was particularly trying to improve his deficits. He knew that his right hand should be involved and when cued, he would engage it, when he wasn't utilizing it, he still had the sense of humor to joke about it. This session allowed me to see that I can address many goals with creativity and I didn't necessarily need to break the therapy session into "Goal 1: fine motor dexterity; activity," etc. It was just a very memorable experience that I wanted to share.

Discussion Board Topics:

1. *Select transitions in fieldwork*
   Describe your experiences in the first few weeks of your Level II fieldwork. What surprises you about this fieldwork? What were your expectations prior to starting compared with what you discovered when you started? How do you feel about being there, how do you fit into this group of OTs?

2. *Self-advocacy*
   Describe your challenges and successes with self-advocacy during your fieldwork experience. What have you learned about yourself, others, and the OT profession through the advocacy process?

3. *Professional identity*
   As you continue the process toward becoming an occupational therapist, describe what you have learned about yourself as a professional. How has your view of yourself changed as a person and a professional? How do you feel about this new role? What has felt comfortable to do and what are your challenges?

4. *Professional habits*
   Describe habits of an effective professional in this OT practice area. Share habits you have acquired and comment on a specific new habit you are developing. How did the habit materialize (was it role modeled, was it a coping strategy) and why has it become important for you to become a professional?

5. *Onward and upward*
   You are approaching the end of your OT academic and fieldwork training and it is time to move into the next chapter of becoming an occupational therapist. Describe the emotions you are feeling and the process of leaving this phase of your life and moving into the real working world of OT.

6. *Intervention ideas*
   One of the hardest things when you are getting started as an OT is coming up with creative intervention ideas. Share some of your own ideas for interventions or ideas you have seen other OTs use. If you are in a brain blackout for interventions, tell us about your client and we will brainstorm with you.

7. *Evidence-based practice*
   Describe how the OTs in your FW setting make decisions about interventions. Do you see evidence-based practice used to guide decision-making for the OT process in your setting? What are the barriers and supports? How are you using evidence-based practice with your clients?

8. *Documentation*

How will you measure and document progress to reflect occupational improvement? What are supports and barriers in this setting and with using this documentation system?

9. *Cultural/lifestyle/values*

Describe how the client's cultural, lifestyle, and/or values have influenced your client-centered approach toward intervention. Explain the communication process for you to understand where they are coming from and how you were able to relate.

10. *Creating a therapeutic relationship*

What are your strategies for creating a therapeutic relationship, especially with challenging, difficult-to-reach clients? Describe a situation that has been particularly challenging for you. What did you do to build a relationship?

11. *Select best practice in fieldwork education*

Compare effective with ineffective supervisory strategies during your fieldwork. Describe

teaching strategies, learning experiences, structuring learning, reflective feedback, etc. Describe what makes it work for you, or what could be more effective.

12. *Assessments*

Describe the types of assessments you are using in your fieldwork and what kind of information you gain from the established assessments. How do you find out about a client's occupation? What a person does/did with their time prior to this and the meaning behind it? Describe how you were able to modify procedures for an assessment with a challenging client.

Copyright © Colorado State University. Reprinted with permission.

Chapter 46.

FIELDWORK COUNCILS AND CONSORTIA

American Occupational Therapy Association

Contact information current as of 2013.

COUNCIL OR CONSORTIUM	SCHOOLS INVOLVED	CONTACTS
NORTHEAST		
Metropolitan Occupational Therapy Education Council of NY/NJ (MOTEC)	• Columbia University, NY (OT) • Dominican College, NY (OT) • Kean University, NJ (OT) • LaGuardia Community College, NY (OTA) • Long Island University, NY (OT) • Mercy College, NY (OT and OTA) • New York Institute of Technology (OT) • New York University (OT) • Seton Hall University, NJ (OT) • SUNY Downstate, NY (OT) • Stony Brook University, NY (OT) • Touro College, NY (OT and OTA) • York College of City University of New York (OT)	Marge Boyd, MPH, OTR/L, Co-Chair Dominican College 845-848-6033 marge.boyd@dc.edu Kristina Vilonen, MA, OTR, Co-Chair Dominican College 845-848-6038 kristina.vilonen@dc.edu
New England Occupational Therapy Education Council (NEOTEC)	• American International College (OT) • Bay Path College (OT) • Boston University (OT) • Bristol Community College (OTA) • Community College of Rhode Island (OTA) • Housatonic Community College (OTA) • Manchester Community College (OTA) • New England Institute of Technology (OTA and Applicant OT) • North Shore Community College (OTA)	Contact one of the FW coordinators at the affiliated schools for information

(Continued)

COUNCIL OR CONSORTIUM	SCHOOLS INVOLVED	CONTACTS
NORTHEAST		
	• Quinnipiac University (OT) • Quinsigamond Community College (OTA) • Sacred Heart University (OT) • Salem State College (OT) • Springfield College (OT) • Tufts University (OT) • University of New Hampshire (OT) • Worcester State College (OT)	
Occupational Therapy Educators' Alliance	• Husson University (OT) • Kennebec Valley Technical College (OTA) • University of New England (OT) • University of Southern Maine/ Lewiston–Auburn College (OT)	Betsy DeBrakeleer, COTA/L, AP, ROH University of New England 207-283-0171 ext. 2188 Fax: 207-294-5963 BdeBrakeleer@une.edu
Upstate NY Region Clinical Counsel	• Ithaca College (OT) • Keuka College (OT) • Maria College (OTA) • The Sage Colleges (OT) • Utica College (OT)	Cora Bruns Utica College cbruns@utica.ucsu.edu
Metro-Buffalo OT Fieldwork Council	• University at Buffalo, SUNY (OT) • D'Youville College (OT) • Erie Community College (OTA)	Metro-Buffalo OT Fieldwork Council www.OTfieldwork.net
MID-ATLANTIC		
Philadelphia Region Fieldwork Consortium	• Harcum College, PA (OTA) • Philadelphia University, PA (OT & OTA) • Richard Stockton College of New Jersey (OT) • Temple University, PA (OT) • Thomas Jefferson University, PA (OT) • University of the Sciences in Philadelphia, PA (OT and Developing OTD)	Caryn Johnson Thomas Jefferson University 215-503-9607 caryn.johnson@mail.tju.edu
Pittsburgh Fieldwork Council	• Community College of Allegheny County (OTA) • Chatham University (OT) • Duquesne University (OT) • Kaplan Career Institute-ICM (OTA) • University of Pittsburgh (OT)	Lisa Hopkins, OTR/L The Western Pennsylvania Hospital 4800 Friendship Ave. Pittsburgh, PA 15224 lhopkins@wpahs.org
Virginia Fieldwork Council	• James Madison University (OT) • Jefferson College of Health Sciences (OT and OTA) • Radford University (developing OT) • Shenandoah University (OT) • Southwest Virginia Community College (OTA) • Tidewater Community College (OTA) • Virginia Commonwealth University (OT)	Laura Evans, OTR/L Chippenham Medical Center 804-323-8766 laura.evans@hcahealthcare.com

(Continued)

COUNCIL OR CONSORTIUM	SCHOOLS INVOLVED	CONTACTS
MID-ATLANTIC		
North Carolina Occupational Therapy Fieldwork Education Consortium (NCOTFWEC)	• Cabarrus College of Health Sciences (OTA) • Cape Fear Community College (OTA) • Durham Technical Community College (OTA) • East Carolina University (OT) • Lenoir-Rhyne University (OT) • Pitt Community College (OTA) • University of North Carolina at Chapel Hill (OT) • Winston-Salem State University (OT)	
MIDWEST		
Wiscouncil (Wisconsin Council on Occupational Therapy Education)	• Concordia University Wisconsin (OT) • Fox Valley Technical College (OTA) • Madison Area Technical College (OTA) • Milwaukee Area Technical College (OTA) • Mount Mary College (OT) • University of Wisconsin–La Crosse (OT) • University of Wisconsin–Madison (OT) • University of Wisconsin–Milwaukee (OT) • Western Technical College (OTA) • Wisconsin Indianhead Technical College–Ashland (OTA)	Contact one of the FW coordinators at the affiliated schools for information
Minn-Dak Fieldwork Consortium	• Anoka Technical College (OTA) • College of St. Scholastica (OT) • Lake Area Technical Institute (OTA) • Northland Community & Technical College (OTA) • North Dakota State College of Science (OTA) • St. Catherine University (OT and OTA) • University of Mary (OT) • University of Minnesota (OT) • University of North Dakota (OT) • University of South Dakota (OT)	Deb Hanson University of North Dakota 701-777-2218 dhanson@medicine.nodak.edu Cindy Anderson University of Mary 701-355-8112 canderson@umary.edu
Michigan Occupational Therapy Education Consortium (MOTEC)	• Baker College of Allen Park (OTA) • Baker College Center for Graduate Studies (OT) • Baker College of Muskegon (OTA) • Eastern Michigan University (OT) • Grand Rapids Community College (OTA) • Grand Valley State University (OT) • Macomb Community College (OTA) • Mott Community College (OTA) • Saginaw Valley State University (OT) • Wayne County Community College (OTA) • Wayne State University (OT) • Western Michigan University (OT)	Juliane Chreston, MSHEd, OTR Baker College Center for Graduate Studies 810-766-2130 juliane.chreston@baker.edu Jean Prast, OTD, OTR Saginaw Valley State University 989-964-4153 jekruege@svsu.edu

(Continued)

COUNCIL OR CONSORTIUM	SCHOOLS INVOLVED	CONTACTS
MIDWEST		
Illinois Fieldwork Consortium	• Chicago State University (OT) • Governors State University (OT) • Illinois Central College (OTA) • Lewis & Clark Community College (OTA) • Lincoln Land Community College (OTA) • Midwestern University (OT) • Parkland College (OTA) • Rush University (OT) • South Suburban College of Cook County (OTA) • Southern Illinois Collegiate Common Market (OTA) • University of Illinois at Chicago (OT) • Wright College (OTA)	Kathy Preissner University of Illinois at Chicago 312-996-5220 kpreiss@uic.edu Sharon Ogg Rush University Medical Center 312-942-6988 sharon_Ogg@rsh.net
Gateway Occupational Therapy Education Council (Missouri)	• Lewis and Clark Community College (OTA) • Maryville University (OT) • St. Charles Community College (OTA) • St. Louis University (OT) • St. Louis Community College, Meramec (OTA) • University of Missouri, Columbia (OT) • Washington University, St. Louis (OT & OTD)	Jeanenne Dallas, MA, OTR/L Academic Fieldwork Coordinator Washington University in St. Louis Program in OT dallasj@wustl.edu Office: 314-286-1623 Fax: 314-286-0631 Francie Woods, MA, OTR/L OTA Program Coordinator St. Charles Community College Telephone: 636-922-8638 fwoods@stchas.edu Website: www.midwestgotec.org
Ohio Academic Fieldwork Coordinators Consortium	• Cincinnati State Technical and Community College (OTA) • Cleveland State University (OT) • Cuyahoga Community College (OTA) • Kent State University (OTA) • North Central State College (OTA) • Ohio State University (OT) • Owens Community College (OTA) • Rhodes State College (OTA) • Shawnee State University (OT & OTA) • Sinclair Community College (OTA) • Stark State College of Technology (OTA) • University of Findlay (OT) • University of Toledo (OT) • Xavier University (OT) • Zane State College (OTA)	Georganna Joary Miller, MEd, OTR/L Xavier University 513-745-3104 millerg@xavier.edu Dennis S. Cleary, MS, OTR/L The Ohio State University 614-292-5824 cleary.26@osu.edu Cindy A. Kief, ND, COTA/L Cincinnati State Technical and Community College 513-569-1691 Fax: 513-569-1659 Cindy.kief@cincinnatistate.edu
Heartland Occupational Therapy Fieldwork Alliance (HOTFA)	• Metropolitan Community College–Penn Valley, MO (OTA) • Newman University, KS (OTA) • Ozarks Technical Community College, MO (OTA) • Rockhurst University, MO (OT) • University of Kansas Medical Center (OT)	Liz Zayat MS, OTR/L Rockhurst University OT Education Program 816-501-4129 liz.zayat@rockhurst.edu

(Continued)

COUNCIL OR CONSORTIUM	SCHOOLS INVOLVED	CONTACTS
MIDWEST		
Midwest Regional Fieldwork Consortium	• Central Community College, Grand Island Campus (OTA) • College of St. Mary (OT) • Creighton University (OT & OTD) • Kirkwood Community College (OTA) • St. Ambrose University (OT)	Andrea Thinnes, OTD, OTR/L Occupational Therapy Program Creighton University School of Pharmacy and Health Professions 402-280-5929 andreathinnes@creighton.edu
Indiana Fieldwork Consortium	• Brown Mackie College–South Bend (OTA) • Brown Mackie College–Indianapolis (OTA) • Indiana University/IUPUI (OT) • University of Indianapolis (OT) • University of Southern Indiana (OT & OTA)	Sue Vanage, MS, OTR 317-554-8329 svanage@brownmackie.edu Margaret (Peg) Coffey, MA, COTA, ROH 574-323-2740 mcoffey@brownmackie.edu Sharon Pape, MS, OTR 317-274-8006 shbpape@iupui.edu Becky Barton, DHS, OTR 317-788-3511 rbarton@uindy.edu Mary Kay Arvin, OTR/L, CHT 812-465-1103 mkarvin@usi.edu Janet Kilbane, MEd, OTR 812-465-1177 jkilbane@usi.edu
SOUTHEAST		
Florida Fieldwork Consortium	• Barry University (OT) • Daytona State College (OTA) • Florida Agricultural and Mechanical University (OT) • Florida Gulf Coast University (OT) • Florida Hospital College of Health Sciences (OTA) • Florida International University (OT) • Keiser University (OTA) • State College of Florida (OTA) • Nova Southeastern University (OT & Developing OTD) • Polk Community College (OTA) • University of Florida (OT) • University of St. Augustine (OT)	Contact one of the FW coordinators at the affiliated schools for information. http://floteceducation.org/

(Continued)

COUNCIL OR CONSORTIUM	SCHOOLS INVOLVED	CONTACTS
SOUTHEAST		
Louisiana and East Texas Fieldwork Alliance	• Bossier Parish Community College (OTA) • Delgado Community College (OTA) • Louisiana State University Health Sciences Center–New Orleans (OT) • Louisiana State University Health Sciences Center–Shreveport (OT) • Panola College (OTA) • University of Louisiana at Monroe (OTA)	Gretchen Reeks, MA, LOTR Louisiana State University–Shreveport 318-813-2953 Fax: 318-813-2957 Greeks@lsuhsc.edu
WEST		
Rocky Mountain Fieldwork Consortium	• Casper College, WY (OTA) • Colorado State University (OT) • College of Southern Nevada (OTA) • Eastern New Mexico University–Roswell (OTA) • Idaho State University (OT) • Pima Medical Institute, Denver Campus, CO (Developing OTA) • Pueblo Community College, CO (OTA) • Salt Lake Community College, UT (OTA) • Touro University Nevada (OT) • University of New Mexico (OT) • University of North Dakota (OT) • University of North Dakota @ Casper College, WY (OT) • University of Utah (OT) • Western New Mexico University (OTA & Developing OT)	Patricia Stutz-Tanenbaum, MS, OTR 970-491-7795 Fax: 970-491-6290 tanenbaum@cahs.colostate.edu Website: http://www.ot.cahs.colostate.edu/
California Occupational Therapy Fieldwork Council	• California State University Dominguez Hills (OT) • Dominican University of California (OT) • Loma Linda University, CA (OT) • Sacramento City College, Sacramento (OTA) • San Jose State University (OT) • Santa Ana College (OTA) • Samuel Merritt College (OT) • University of Southern California, Los Angeles (OT)	Ruth Jeffries, OTR Loma Linda University 909-558-4948, ext. 41340 Fax: 909-558-0239 ruth-jeffries@sahp.llu.edu Diane Mayfield, MA, OTR Santa Ana College 714-564-6684 Fax: 714-564-6158 mayfield_diane@rsccd.org

Last updated March 2013.

Reprinted from http://www.aota.org/-/media/Corporate/Files/EducationCareers/Educators/Fieldwork/Supervisor/Fieldwork%20Consortiums%2032013.pdf

Chapter 47.

MAINTAINING LONGEVITY IN THE ROLE OF ACADEMIC FIELDWORK COORDINATOR

Jaynee Taguchi Meyer, OTD, OTR/L; Jeanenne Dallas, MA, OTR/L; Mary Evenson, OTD, MPH, OTR/L, FAOTA, FNAP; and Debra J. Hanson, PhD, OTR/L, FAOTA

Becoming an academic fieldwork coordinator (AFWC) may not be a career goal that many aspire to, but it can be very rewarding and fulfilling (Exhibit 47.1). Being an AFWC is a very complex role requiring skills in marketing and multifaceted

---

Exhibit 47.1. *Reflections of Academic Fieldwork Coordinators on Taking on the Role*

- I was not specifically thinking about the [AFWC] role, but I did know that I wanted to be a faculty member. —*Debra Hanson*
- This was a position that I did not seek out, but my program chair offered it to me in 2006. I am happy to report . . . it has worked out. —*Jeanenne Dallas*
- I was first a fieldwork educator, fieldwork site coordinator, and then consultant, and conducted a research study about fieldwork as part of a master's thesis. Becoming an AFWC was the next logical step for me. —*Jaynee Taguchi Meyer*
- I can honestly say that I have never found myself feeling bored in the position of being an AFWC. —*Mary Evenson*

---

organization and top-notch negotiation and interpersonal abilities, including tact and compassion. An understanding of the complexities of practice, administration, and education is critical. Knowledge of educational pedagogy and an understanding of classroom and clinical practice environments are essential.

In this chapter, four AFWCs with a total of 64 years of practice in our positions share experiences, insight, and advice about thriving in the role of AFWC in occupational therapy. What are our secrets to longevity in this role? What are the rewards and lessons we learned along the way? What advice do we offer new AFWCs?

Who Are AFWCs?

AFWCs serve as the primary liaison between the academic program and the clinical practice community of fieldwork sites and educators. The role involves extensive administrative responsibilities (e.g., knowledge of legal contract negotiations; liability insurance; Health Insurance Portability and

Accountability Act of 1996 [HIPAA; Pub. L. 104–191] and educational confidentiality or Family Education Rights and Privacy Act [FERPA] issues; student eligibility conditions for placement, including, but not limited to, background checks, health and immunization requirements, drug testing, and orientation). Accreditation standards require meticulous record-keeping and reporting to document communication and collaboration with faculty, students, and fieldwork educators, along with learning outcomes and program evaluation. Being in the AFWC position for many years enables mastery development and competency in this role and the development of a unique set of skills that are critical to and valued by the academic program.

Longevity

AFWCs may have both teaching and administrative roles and responsibilities or work solely in fieldwork coordination. Some inherit developed programs, and others build from the ground up. Among our group of AFWCs, longevity seems to come from having (1) networks of AFWC colleagues for support, collaboration, and resource and knowledge exchange; (2) program director support and administrative staff to handle high volumes of information, record-keeping, and communication; (3) freedom and flexibility to develop scholarship and teaching; (4) expansive practice community connections; (5) effective and efficient organizational systems and policies; and (6) flexible ways of working.

Networks

Participating in supportive networks increases AFWC longevity. According to Mary Evenson, "The specificity of the [AFWC] role and responsibilities creates a small group of professionals who have developed and possess advanced knowledge and skills related to academic fieldwork education. AFWC colleagues [are] an open and supportive network of fieldwork specialists who generously share their experience and recommendations." Connecting with an AFWC network and having AFWC mentors in the same state and across the country validate daily dilemmas and challenges faced, according to Jaynee Taguchi Meyer. Networks and mentors help AFWCs develop systems

to manage the enormous amounts of information processed in this position and teach valuable lessons not otherwise found in research literature.

Academic fieldwork education consortia (see Chapter 46) consist of AFWCs from occupational therapy and occupational therapy assistant programs organized by state or geographic areas. Networking and mutual support are strengthened through participation in these consortia. Missouri, for example, has a very active consortium, according to Jeanenne Dallas. "We work well with each other and share resources. If I need help with an issue, I can turn to them for advice. We also mentor new AFWCs, and I believe that helps me feel successful." Involvement in consortia promotes feelings of community and success. Evenson shares that "I have been an active member in a regional education consortium, the New England Occupational Therapy Education Council (NEOTEC), a regional educational consortium... [that promotes] fieldwork education and offers mutual support to all members." Consortia can offer innovative collaborative projects, such as the design and implementation of templates for fieldwork data forms and site-specific learning objectives. Some consortia sponsor free educational conferences for local fieldwork educators.

"Being the only faculty in the AFWC position can be isolating," Debra Hanson notes. Precious time is saved by corresponding with a colleague rather than trying to figure out each problem by yourself. AFWCs share issues that are universal and across programs. Talking to other AFWCs, you realize that your students are no worse or no better than other students. Visiting with colleagues and collaborating on projects of mutual interest can be helpful. Service and scholarship projects with key colleagues in the AFWC role may be achieved.

The American Occupational Therapy Association (AOTA) offers invaluable support, including the AFWC Forum and other events at the Annual Conference & Expo, biennial joint AFWC and Academic Leadership Council meetings, and AOTA's AFWC email list. Using these resources fosters staying abreast of national issues and events. Networking with others across the nation is especially helpful and expands collegial networks of AFWCs. Hanson recently had the opportunity to serve as AFWC representative to the AOTA Commission on Education, and that "helped me to gain a more national perspective on fieldwork issues in our profession."

Program Director and Administrative Staff Support

A critical key to longevity as an AFWC is having a program director and faculty who understand and support your role and work. This position entails a lot of responsibility; therefore, success in this position would be difficult without an administration that supports, assists, and stands by your decisions.

"Having sufficient administrative staff assistance, made possible by a supportive program director, is another key to longevity in the role of AFWC," according to Taguchi Meyer. Some AFWCs have administrative staff support, and others do not. Dallas said, "I do not think I could handle the amount of work that this job entails without my [administrative assistant]." An administrative fieldwork assistant can be a point person for Level I and II student placements. Other tasks that administrative support staff could coordinate include but are not limited to

- Contract negotiation and maintenance
- Site-specific and college or university prerequisite completion (onboarding) and record-keeping
- Fieldwork site and student database management
- Communication with sites
- Mail and reservation request organization.

Administrative responsibilities may feel tedious and less satisfying than teaching students and fieldwork educators, collaborating with colleagues, and engaging in scholarship for your own professional development. Administrative support staff who carry out detailed aspects of everyday work afford an AFWC freedom to pursue tasks more representative of his or her abilities, and can be key to AFWCs continuing in this role, affirms Hanson. The AFWC may then devote increased time and effort toward

- Advising and coaching students and fieldwork educators
- Evaluating and developing fieldwork sites and educators
- Facilitating development of students' clinical reasoning
- Counseling students and fieldwork educators during fieldwork when issues or problems arise
- Taking on other supervisory and teaching responsibilities and developing these abilities.

"Developmentally, the organizational components of the role, the administrative details, and working with struggling students made up the lion's share of work during the early years [in this role]," according to Hanson. Over time, as AFWCs become more strategic, other people can set up systems to make the process more manageable. In addition, procedures for division of labor can be drawn up and inherited from previous AFWCs when assuming this role.

Scholarship, Teaching, and Professional Development

Scholarly work such as writing and publishing on fieldwork-related topics enhances longevity and satisfaction. Researching literature related to fieldwork and then writing short briefs for the "Fieldwork Issues" column for *OT Practice* were a source of learning for Hanson. For Taguchi Meyer, "Presenting at local, state, national, and international conferences contributes to AFWC career satisfaction and professional growth and development while promoting the professional development of fieldwork educators, other AFWCs, faculty, and students." These scholarly activities should translate into a higher quality of fieldwork experiences.

Evenson finds attendance at World Federation of Occupational Therapy Congresses to be enriching learning experiences. Learning about fieldwork education in the international community promotes creative and innovative ideas for designing emerging and population-based fieldwork experiences.

Having the opportunity to teach courses contributes to longevity in the AFWC role. Hanson draws from her own practice experience and expertise and explores growing professional interests in other areas in teaching. She taught mental health courses, which was motivating and gratifying. Teaching other courses such as qualitative and quantitative research and occupational therapy theory courses enabled her professional expertise to grow.

Pursuing doctoral coursework and degrees offers opportunities to explore fieldwork as a phenomenon of study, and many underdeveloped areas for research in fieldwork exist. When doctoral projects are related to fieldwork, professional development as an AFWC is enhanced. As Hanson described it,

It was exciting, for example, to catch up on the research literature related to fieldwork and to apply this literature to my practice as an AFWC. It was interesting to dream about potential research projects and to try out a few in independent study coursework and then pursue publication of same. All of this helped me to align my professional identify as an AFWC.

Completing a doctoral degree had the greatest impact on Evenson, whose position is in an entry-level doctor of occupational therapy (OTD) program. Advanced professional skills developed through doctoral study, application of evidence, and dissemination of scholarship outcomes were later applied in her teaching and collaboration with faculty colleagues, contributing to curriculum development.

Expansive Practice Community Connections

For longevity, it is important to have connections with fieldwork sites and practitioners and a good fieldwork database, according to Dallas. When an AFWC steps into an established academic program, he or she should inherit an organized fieldwork program with an ample number of sites locally and throughout the country. Many academic programs admit students from all over the United States and other countries, so a wide range of practice community connections and fieldwork sites to offer students is helpful.

AFWCs in new programs need to build fieldwork collaborations from the ground up, likely starting with their own practice contacts and those of the faculty. According to Taguchi Meyer, "Maximizing the use of organizational software and technology (fieldwork site and student databases, Word documents, spreadsheets, and online tools) helps AFWCs and fieldwork coordination teams manage the enormous amount of information that need to be catalogued, stored, and utilized in a fieldwork database."

Effective and Efficient Organizational Systems and Policies

A fieldwork program that has effective and efficient organizational systems and policies is paramount to longevity. Such policies and procedures are usually developed over time. For example, fieldwork program manuals helped Dallas learn the

job, and a written procedure manual was helpful for accreditation. Finding creative ways to solve complex dilemmas makes processes more effective and efficient.

Evenson found that investigating and being open to research from interprofessional colleagues, especially nursing and physical and speech therapy, can be important sources of evidence for clinical education and fieldwork. Furthermore, learning about and understanding how other professions' and disciplines' academic programs use different systems and approaches to evaluate student performance, solicit placement reservations, and schedule and assign students provides valuable insights to managing fieldwork within our profession.

Flexible Ways of Working

Flexibility in the work schedule and workplace is paramount to longevity in the AFWC role. For example, going off campus to visit and develop fieldwork sites is critical to establishing and maintaining good relations with fieldwork sites and practitioners, according to Taguchi Meyer. "Working remotely can increase productivity by minimizing interruptions."

Rewards of Being an AFWC

Serving as the "bridge between education and practice is one of the most rewarding aspects of being an AFWC," says Evenson. "With this role comes a responsibility to stay up-to-date with changes in practice, health care policy and regulations, and reimbursement and payment in both the public and private sectors of health care services." Supporting all stakeholders involved with fieldwork education by "sharing this knowledge and expertise with faculty colleagues, students, and fieldwork educators is essential," advises Evenson. "I strive to be a role model and offer advice grounded in my own practice experience and in having supported numerous students to be successful during fieldwork." When AFWCs advise students about fieldwork, students' feelings and interests should be considered when developing realistic fieldwork education experience goals.

Advising and facilitating the growth and development of students is another rewarding aspect of the role. Dallas believes she gets to "know the students better than any other faculty member" through time spent together preparing for and during fieldwork. "I don't just teach them one semester and then never see them again. I am with them from Day 1 to Day 1,001 . . . that's what I tell them. I get to enter that last grade of their time with us, and I can honestly say that I know them and wish them well," Dallas shares. "I get to see them grow from being a terrified-looking first-year student to the last day of Level II fieldwork when they are eager and ready to go out in the occupational therapy world." AFWCs get to see the fruits of the efforts of many.

Helping struggling Level II fieldwork students identify problem areas and obstacles to learning to develop a practical plan to overcome problems and maximize professional and clinical strengths and become successful is rewarding for AFWCs. Taguchi Meyer states,

> Working with a student who failed a fieldwork experience to help him or her try again (and succeed) is particularly rewarding. In these situations, the AFWC usually separately engages both the fieldwork educator and the student in a reflective review to identify underlying issues and ways to recover from the difficulty and improve in the future. It's really tough work, but so rewarding when practitioners become better educators, students become practitioners, and I somehow had a hand in making that happen! As I've told students who failed a fieldwork, "Some of the best practitioners and fieldwork educators, for that matter, are those who failed a Level II fieldwork themselves!"

It is exciting when students realize and express connections that they are making from applications of classroom knowledge to contexts of fieldwork and practice. On the most basic level, helping students find their own therapeutic use of self while focusing on the occupational therapy process—evaluation and screening, intervention planning, interventions, and outcomes—is an approach to fieldwork advising that focuses on the foundation of occupational therapy, according to Evenson. "The AFWC plays a pivotal role in supporting this learning through actively collaborating with faculty and fieldwork educators to

design meaningful learning experiences aligning with the curricular goals of the academic program and the service delivery initiatives of various practice settings."

Another reward for AFWCs is promoting the growth of fieldwork sites and fieldwork educators. Taguchi Meyer noted, "I like the transformative aspects of fostering the growth and development of new and established fieldwork educators and sites." AFWCs can help practitioners, facilities, and organizations establish new student programs or further develop existing programs. In addition, with the help of AFWCs, practitioners, who may be novices, may develop into proficient fieldwork educators, and fieldwork sites may become highly sought-after facilities and organizations among students.

Training practitioners about the importance and influence of their role as fieldwork educators in the preparation of future occupational therapy practitioners is one of Taguchi Meyer's favorite parts of being an AFWC. "Collaborating to find ways to 'make it work,' and challenging myself to find some aspect of fieldwork that piques my curiosity and thirst for knowledge and professional growth, are what make it worthwhile to me."

Most Important Thing Learned

The most important thing that Evenson learned, and one of the most challenging aspects of this work, was supporting and working with occupational therapy students with special needs and personal circumstances that might contribute to their struggle in fieldwork. "In my experience, the profession can offer a great deal of flexibility in designing non-traditional Level II fieldwork experiences, frequently on a part-time fieldwork basis, to support students who need accommodations in order to be successful in completing the fieldwork portion of the curriculum and transitioning into the practice arena."

Some students struggle greatly in fieldwork but do not fail because they listen to and accept feedback, respond to it by modifying their behavior, and do not give up. Others do fail Level II fieldwork. It is hoped that these students then embark on a "journey of self-discovery and self-acceptance" of their individual strengths and challenges or limitations, according to Evenson. Failing fieldwork can be a devastating experience for students. The students who do not let it define them learn to listen to and accept feedback, do the hard work of making changes, and grow, says Hanson. The best outcomes occur when, with AFWC support, the student takes responsibility and ownership for developing personal and professional strategies to enable him or her to succeed and enter professional practice.

According to Dallas, "Sometimes I have to be the mediator and impartial party when fieldwork performance issues arise." Listening well and understanding the perspectives of both the student and the fieldwork educator, which can be very different, helps the AFWC appreciate both sides of the story before coming to any conclusions, according to Hanson. In addition, Hanson says, it is important for the AFWC to recognize "the impact of the practice setting—social, physical, and cultural—on each student's learning experience." Students cannot be treated in one uniform way. Issues need to be addressed on a case-by-case basis, and fairness to all students is a must. In describing the importance of helping struggling students, Dallas stated, "I have the students' futures in my hands. I am the person who passes them on to a career in occupational therapy, and I take that seriously."

Greatest Influences on Professional Career as an AFWC

At one point in Hanson's development, she began to view her primary identity as the AFWC as opposed to a member of the teaching faculty.

> Once I made that shift, I was able to more strategically align my teaching, scholarship, and service (as is required for the promotion and tenure process at my university) to support my fieldwork efforts. It was not uncommon for me, prior to this realization, to follow the same pattern as my colleagues with highlighting courses that I taught, rather than finding a unique way to highlight my AFWC role. Seeing my contributions on paper helped me recognize the various aspects of my AFWC role and in doing so recognize the value of that role.

Dallas appreciates talking to other AFWCs to get ideas about how they handle their positions. She stated,

> We tend to talk about the "problem" students, but there are so many [wonderful] students who also make this a worthwhile position. I am very proud that I am one of the first people students contact when they drop by the school. They thank me for being there for them and for all the work that I have put into their education. When a student who struggled with fieldwork comes back or emails me a heartfelt thank you, that is the biggest effect on my professional development.

The professional journey *before* becoming an AFWC had the greatest effect on Taguchi Meyer's career as an AFWC. She became a fieldwork educator 1 year after school and sought continuing education and literature on fieldwork. She mentored occupational therapy staff in clinical teaching at a large urban acute care hospital and presented on fieldwork at state, national, and international conferences before and after becoming an AFWC. Volunteering for AOTA increased her understanding of national fieldwork issues.

Taguchi Meyer's master's thesis research found that the mission and vision of a clinical facility or organization, and the complexity of a practitioner's life as a whole, highly influenced whether or not a practitioner educated fieldwork students. She oversaw clinical training in physical therapy and speech–language pathology, consulted remotely with occupational therapy fieldwork educators in skilled nursing facilities, and saved her non-revenue-generating consultant position using evidence demonstrating the cost-effectiveness of clinical education. All these experiences prepared her to be a successful and enduring AFWC.

Advice for New AFWCs

Before moving into the AFWC role, Evenson recommends asking "specific questions about workload and how the academic program allocates time to accomplish teaching, service, scholarship, and administrative responsibilities." She found that "the challenge of managing multiple roles and heavy workload responsibilities" to be a continuous endeavor throughout her 20 years as an AFWC. Various personal and professional strategies can help you thrive and counter burnout. In addition, when moving into the AFWC position, it is important to have a great administrative assistant who knows the work well and can make the transition into the position much easier. Dallas stated, "I knew this person and that she had been in the position for 8 years with three other AFWCs. I knew that she could train me. I [made] sure she was staying, so that relieved my mind."

Personal Strategies

Some personal strategies to use to succeed in your job are to know and take care of yourself, take vacations, and realize the job is never done.

Know and Take Care of Yourself

The following are ways to promote physical and mental well-being:

- Be aware of lifestyle choices that enable you to manage stress and strive for balance. For example, yoga, meditation, and mindfulness support may support you.
- Participate in health-promoting occupations to maintain your own health and well-being.
- Have a solid support system, daily fitness routine, and nutritious diet to help counter stressful work demands. "I can be effective in my job to the degree that I also take the time to nurture myself and to have fun," shares Hanson.
- Do not take yourself too seriously or make more of a situation than it actually is. Let go of the things you do not have control of to focus better on the things you can influence.

Take Vacations

Take vacations, and arrange coverage while you are away. "Unplug from email to avoid always being on call," advises Evenson. Working longer hours is not the answer.

Realize That the Job Is Never Done

"The work will wait for you to get to it, sooner or later. In some instances, 'letting things set' can be advantageous in arriving at an ultimate solution," suggests Evenson.

Professional Strategies

Many professional strategies will help you succeed in your job.

Set and Communicate Boundaries

Being clear about when you are and are not available to students and colleagues is important in avoiding burnout. You cannot be available to them all the time and get your other work done. "Stick to your office hours, and discourage them popping in for 'one quick question'" urges Taguchi Meyer. "Post office hours and appointment availability for students to meet with you. Maintaining and sticking to posted office hours helps decrease interruption, enabling an AFWC to do the necessary development and academic work."

Most fieldwork issues are not emergencies unless there is a medical or safety situation that requires immediate attention, according to Evenson. An instant response from you is not necessary except in emergencies. Other tactics in setting boundaries are

- Close your door when working to decrease interruptions.
- Carefully consider the pros and cons of giving your cell phone number to students and fieldwork educators.
- Allow cell phone calls only during available hours, and set rules for leaving messages and returning calls, recommends Dallas.
- Block off time for answering email and other responsibilities.
- "Maintain a healthy work–life balance, whatever that means for you (e.g., not checking or responding to email after hours or over weekends)," encourages Taguchi Meyer.
- Do not schedule meetings on evenings or weekends unless it is critically necessary (and not just convenient).
- Carefully consider student access to you on social media.

Be Organized and a Master of Time Management

AFWCs can do the following to be organized and effectively manage their time:

- Be mindful of your time. "There may be a perception that you have more time to fill in for substitute teaching or that you need to be available at all times for any faculty member, student, or fieldwork educator," cautions Hanson.

- Map out a timetable, being careful to schedule in paperwork or administrative responsibilities and on- and off-campus meetings.
- Do not undersell what you do; it is an important role, and you need time to do it well.
- "Continually evaluate your workload and health and well-being, and do not lose sight of them," advises Taguchi Meyer.

Be Flexible and Open to Feedback

Because situations always change, be flexible and open to feedback by taking the following advice from Hanson and Evenson:

- Once processes and policies are in place, do not get too attached.
- If someone else's idea will streamline or eliminate unnecessary steps, listen to him or her. Colleagues can help you step back and objectively evaluate what you are doing.
- Learn to see change as a good thing. This attitude helps you stay fresh and responsive to the needs of your students and fieldwork educators.
- Listen and be humble in accepting feedback from faculty, students, fieldwork site coordinators, and fieldwork educators. Although you might not agree, what they share is important and warrants your consideration.

Be Compassionate

Evenson advises, "Find compassionate and adept ways to share feedback that might be hard for others to hear, whether with students who are having difficulty or failing or with your academic and fieldwork educator colleagues in conveying feedback and comments that may be perceived as criticism."

Develop Strong Faculty Connections

You can develop strong connections with your faculty by collaborating and consulting with them on fieldwork decisions and consulting them about dilemmas that arise in fieldwork.

Understand Your Academic Program's Curriculum Design Thoroughly

It is important to understand your curriculum design because "the more you understand the academic curriculum design and philosophy, the better position you are in to foster connections between coursework and fieldwork," according to Hanson. You will inevitably field questions from both fieldwork educators and faculty such as "Why isn't more research evidence applied in practice? How will students learn how to apply theory to practice if fieldwork educators never talk about theory? Why don't students have less theory and more practical skills when they come to fieldwork?" You should have ready answers. However, understand that questions and dilemmas about the curriculum are not just yours to answer; "they belong to the entire faculty and curriculum," says Hanson.

Develop Strong Connections With Other AFWCs

Taguchi Meyer and Dallas suggest developing strong connections with other AFWCs by

- Using AOTA's closed email list for AFWCs to post questions, ask advice, and connect with others.
- Finding an AFWC mentor who has experience in this role.
- Getting perspective about your workload from the AFWC community.
- Becoming involved in a fieldwork consortium to share resources.

Develop Strong Connections With Your College or University's Resources

Taguchi Meyer recommends getting to know the following people and organizations on your campus:

- Legal counsel
- Student health center
- Student counseling center
- Office of students with disabilities
- Office of overseas studies or international students' office
- Biosafety officers (with Occupational Safety and Health Administration training)
- Clinical education coordinators from related disciplines, such as physical therapy, speech therapy, social work, and medicine.

Become an Expert at Networking

Keep in contact with former students. When a special need arises, you will have numerous people to contact for help. It is also a great way to get new fieldwork sites and contracts. "Seeing and hearing from former students keeps up enthusiasm for this position," shares Dallas.

Educate Yourself About Fieldwork

Learn about all aspects of fieldwork by

- Reading everything you can about fieldwork and clinical education in occupational therapy and in other health disciplines in the United States and elsewhere.
- Taking the AOTA Fieldwork Educator Certificate Program course.
- "Attending AFWC programs at AOTA conferences and other educational sections to gather knowledge about what other programs and people are doing and increase your knowledge of not only fieldwork but also academic curriculum development," urges Taguchi Meyer.

Understand Your Position and Role

To understand your position and role as an AFWC, Hanson advises you to do the following:

- Make a chart or visual aid that helps you understand the complexity of your role (a whiteboard in your office will help you track details needing follow-up and activities to be accomplished at various points of the year).
- Resist the urge to change everything right away.
- Before you make changes, follow the processes that are in place for 1 year (much of your work will be annual).
- Keep notes as you go along, recording what works well or what changes are needed.
- Make decisions as objectively as possible rather than reactively as you go along (be mindful that the AFWC role has many layers of complexity, and often one layer will influence others).
- Be patient as you develop systems that work for you, whether it is setting up a fieldwork database to enable data management or implementing policies and procedures for students to choose placements.

Focus on Successes

"There is always something you can complain about in the area of fieldwork, but there are also successes and things to celebrate. Focus on the successes, and take time regularly to give yourself a pat on the back and the rest of the fieldwork team, too!" shares Hanson.

Recognize Your Own Expertise

You are in a unique position, Hanson continues, "which requires a balance of attention to detail and to the big picture and a balance of administrative and communication skills. Give yourself credit for having the skills to navigate this unique position."

Have a Sense of Humor

Resist the urge to take things too seriously or personally, advises Dallas.

Summary

Becoming and being an AFWC may be a road less traveled in occupational therapy, but it can be worthwhile, gratifying, and satisfying. Although it is rigorous and detail-oriented work, for a creative, enthusiastic, resourceful, and compassionate person with a heart for students, practitioners, and clinical training, it can be a rewarding and fulfilling career.

References

Family Educational Rights and Privacy Act of 1974, 20 U.S.C. § 1232g.

Health Insurance Portability and Accountability Act of 1996, Pub. L. 104–191, 42 U.S.C. § 300gg, 29 U.S.C § 1181-1183, and 42 USC 1320d-1320d9.

Chapter 48.

ONLINE LEARNING RESOURCES FOR ACADEMIC LEADERSHIP

Donna Costa, DHS, OTR/L, FAOTA

Academic fieldwork coordinators (AFWCs) bridge the academic and clinical environments and are responsible for the coordination of all activities related to student fieldwork placements. Other health care disciplines have similar positions but may use other terms to refer to them. Similarly, other health care disciplines refer to *clinical education* by other terms such as *practicum, professional experience, internship, extramural placement, field education, sandwich course, service learning,* or *clinical placement.*

An important element of fieldwork coordination is fostering productive and reciprocal partnerships among fieldwork sites, the university, and the students. However, there is a lack of structured training for AFWCs to learn the roles and responsibilities of the position. In addition, the person recruited into the AFWC role frequently has limited academic experience, and without a systematic training program, the roles and responsibilities may feel overwhelming to the AFWC (Stutz-Tanenbaum, Hanson, Koski, & Green, 2015).

Moreover, the AFWC is a key role in occupational therapy academic programs, but it differs greatly from traditional faculty roles because of its more varied workload. The AFWC has more administrative responsibilities compared with other faculty and is frequently in the field representing the program to community partners. Although no published data exist on

how long an AFWC holds that position, anecdotal evidence suggests that it is often just a few years.

This situation is not unique to the United States or to the profession of occupational therapy. For example, several academic and health industry partners in Australia collaborated to develop the Leading Fieldwork project, which has resulted in a comprehensive and cohesive academic leadership development program specifically designed for AFWCs across disciplines. The design of this Academic Leadership for Fieldwork Coordinator Program has been informed by the literature on work-integrated learning leadership and an online survey of AFWCs at the two partner universities involved in the project: Curtin University (Perth, Australia) and Charles Sturt University (campuses across Australia). The term *work-integrated learning* refers to educational programs that combine a workplace-based component with classroom learning within an individual's program of study. The term has been adopted by universities around the globe to identify programs that add a practical employment-based learning component to school-based learning (Jones et al., 2012). In Australia, fieldwork is classified as a type of work-integrated learning.

According to the final report on the program (Jones et al., 2012),

Data collected during the project suggest that [AFWCs] are dedicated staff who are committed to their students. However, workload, resourcing issues, and a lack of development opportunities have resulted in a tendency for fieldwork educators to focus on operational roles and "getting the job done" rather than the crucial strategic areas of innovation and relationship building with placement providers and industry. (p. ii)...

The aim of the project was to develop and trial an academic leadership development program designed to enhance the leadership capabilities of [AFWCs] (those academic staff responsible for the management and co-ordination of a practicum, professional experience, internships, extra mural placements or clinical placements) to enable them to improve student learning experiences whilst on fieldwork placement. The leadership program can be adapted for professional staff also working in fieldwork administration and management. (p. iii)

The following products were developed during the project (Jones et al., 2012):

- Final report (Jones et al., 2012), which includes evaluation data on the program pilots and project findings
- Academic Leadership for Fieldwork Coordinators Program, which includes seven online modules that can be adapted to different university contexts and staff with clinical or practice-based education responsibilities and a guide for running the program
- Statement about AFWC roles
- Leadership survey tool for AFWCs
- Package of program resources

- Three websites with available project resources:
  - Curtin University (http://academicleadership.curtin.edu.au/ALFCP/)
  - The Australian Collaborative Education Network (http://acen.edu.au), and
  - Charles Sturt University's Education for Practice Institute (https://www.csu.edu.au/efpi).

Sophisticated leadership skills are required to manage fieldwork education programs to maximize benefits for students, the university, and fieldwork sites. AFWCs must have a working knowledge of pedagogy to help fieldwork sites create quality fieldwork experiences for students. In addition, they must be familiar with ever-changing legislation and legal issues related to contract management and risk management, and they must possess advanced communication and negotiation skills.

The AFWC role requires a diverse set of leadership capabilities, and it is important to recognize that this role is a leadership position. Until a formalized training program for AFWCs is created in the United States, AFWCs should use all currently available resources, including the Academic Leadership for Fieldwork Educators Program, and should find an experienced AFWC to serve as a mentor.

References

Jones, S., Ladyshewsky, R., Smith, M., Trede, F., Flavell, H., & Chapman, R. (2012). *Leading fieldwork: Academic leadership for fieldwork coordinators*. Retrieved from http://academicleadership.curtin.edu.au/local/docs/fieldwork/FCReport.pdf

Stutz-Tanenbaum, P., Hanson, D., Koski, J., & Greene D. (2015). Exploring the complexity of the academic fieldwork coordinator role. *Occupational Therapy in Health Care, 29*, 139–152.

Chapter 49.

GUIDELINES FOR SUPERVISION, ROLES, AND RESPONSIBILITIES DURING THE DELIVERY OF OCCUPATIONAL THERAPY SERVICES

American Occupational Therapy Association

This document is a set of guidelines describing the supervision, roles, and responsibilities of occupational therapy practitioners. Intended for both internal and external audiences, it also provides an outline of the roles and responsibilities of occupational therapists, occupational therapy assistants, and occupational therapy aides during the delivery of occupational therapy services.

General Supervision

These guidelines provide a definition of supervision and outline parameters regarding effective supervision as it relates to the delivery of occupational therapy services. The guidelines themselves cannot be interpreted to constitute a standard of supervision in any particular locality. Occupational therapists, occupational therapy assistants, and occupational therapy aides are expected to meet applicable state and federal regulations, adhere to

relevant workplace and payer policies and to the *Occupational Therapy Code of Ethics and Ethics Standards* (American Occupational Therapy Association [AOTA], 2010), and participate in ongoing professional development activities to maintain continuing competency.

Within the scope of occupational therapy practice, *supervision* is a process aimed at ensuring the safe and effective delivery of occupational therapy services and fostering professional competence and development. In addition, in these guidelines, supervision is viewed as a cooperative process in which two or more people participate in a joint effort to establish, maintain, and/or elevate a level of competence and performance. Supervision is based on mutual understanding between the supervisor and the supervisee about each other's competence, experience, education, and credentials. It fosters growth and development, promotes effective utilization of resources, encourages creativity and innovation, and provides education and support to achieve a goal.

Supervision of Occupational Therapists and Occupational Therapy Assistants

Occupational Therapists

Based on education and training, occupational therapists, after initial certification and relevant state licensure or other governmental requirements, are autonomous practitioners who are able to deliver occupational therapy services independently. Occupational therapists are responsible for all aspects of occupational therapy service delivery and are accountable for the safety and effectiveness of the occupational therapy services and service delivery process. Occupational therapists are encouraged to seek peer supervision and mentoring for ongoing development of best practice approaches and to promote professional growth.

Occupational Therapy Assistants

Based on education and training, occupational therapy assistants, after initial certification and meeting state regulatory requirements, must receive supervision from an occupational therapist to deliver occupational therapy services. Occupational therapy assistants deliver occupational therapy services under the supervision of and in partnership with occupational therapists. Occupational therapists and occupational therapy assistants are equally responsible for developing a collaborative plan for supervision. The occupational therapist is ultimately responsible for the implementation of appropriate supervision, but the occupational therapy assistant also has a responsibility to seek and obtain appropriate supervision to ensure proper occupational therapy is being provided.

General Principles

1. Supervision involves guidance and oversight related to the delivery of occupational therapy services and the facilitation of professional growth and competence. It is the responsibility of the occupational therapy assistant to seek the appropriate quality and frequency of supervision to ensure safe and effective occupational therapy service delivery. It is the responsibility of the occupational therapist to provide adequate and appropriate supervision.

2. To ensure safe and effective occupational therapy services, it is the responsibility of occupational therapists to recognize when they require peer supervision or mentoring that supports current and advancing levels of competence and professional growth.

3. The specific frequency, methods, and content of supervision may vary and are dependent on the
   a. Complexity of client needs,
   b. Number and diversity of clients,
   c. Knowledge and skill level of the occupational therapist and the occupational therapy assistant,
   d. Type of practice setting,
   e. Requirements of the practice setting, and
   f. Other regulatory requirements.

4. Supervision of the occupational therapy assistant that is more frequent than the minimum level required by the practice setting or regulatory requirements may be necessary when
   a. The needs of the client and the occupational therapy process are complex and changing,
   b. The practice setting provides occupational therapy services to a large number of clients with diverse needs, or
   c. The occupational therapist and occupational therapy assistant determine that additional supervision is necessary to ensure safe and effective delivery of occupational therapy services.

5. There are a variety of types and methods of supervision. Methods can include but are not limited to direct, face-to-face contact and indirect contact. Examples of methods or types of supervision that involve direct face-to-face contact include observation, modeling, client demonstration, discussions, teaching, and instruction. Examples of methods or types of supervision that involve indirect contact include phone conversations, written correspondence, and electronic exchanges.

6. Occupational therapists and occupational therapy assistants must abide by facility and state requirements regarding the documentation of a supervision plan and supervision contacts. Documentation may include the
   a. Frequency of supervisory contact,
   b. Methods or types of supervision,
   c. Content areas addressed,
   d. Evidence to support areas and levels of competency, and
   e. Names and credentials of the persons participating in the supervisory process.

7. Peer supervision and mentoring related to professional growth, such as leadership and advocacy skills development, may differ from the peer supervision mentoring needed to provide occupational therapy services. The person providing this supervision, as well as the frequency, method, and content of supervision, should be responsive to the supervisee's advancing levels of professional growth.

Supervision Outside the Delivery of Occupational Therapy Services

The education and expertise of occupational therapists and occupational therapy assistants prepare them for employment in arenas other than those related to the delivery of occupational therapy. In these other arenas, supervision may be provided by non–occupational therapy professionals.

1. The guidelines of the setting, regulatory agencies, and funding agencies direct the supervision requirements.
2. The occupational therapist and occupational therapy assistant should obtain and use credentials or job titles commensurate with their roles in these other employment arenas.
3. The following can be used to determine whether the services provided are related to the delivery of occupational therapy:
   a. State practice acts;
   b. Regulatory agency standards and rules;
   c. *Occupational Therapy Practice Framework: Domain and Process* (3rd ed., AOTA, 2014) and other AOTA official documents; and
   d. Written and verbal agreement among the occupational therapist, the occupational therapy assistant, the client, and the agency or payer about the services provided.

Roles and Responsibilities of Occupational Therapists and Occupational Therapy Assistants During the Delivery of Occupational Therapy Services

Overview

The focus of occupational therapy is to assist the client in "achieving health, wellness, and participation in life through engagement in occupation" (AOTA, 2014, p. S2).

Occupational therapy addresses the needs and goals of the client related to engaging in areas of occupation and considers the performance skills, performance patterns, context and environment, and client factors that may influence performance in various areas of occupation.

1. The occupational therapist is responsible for all aspects of occupational therapy service delivery and is accountable for the safety and effectiveness of the occupational therapy service delivery process. The occupational therapy service delivery process involves evaluation, intervention planning, intervention implementation, intervention review, and targeting of outcomes and outcomes evaluation.
2. The occupational therapist must be directly involved in the delivery of services during the initial evaluation and regularly throughout the course of intervention, intervention review, and outcomes evaluation.
3. The occupational therapy assistant delivers safe and effective occupational therapy services under the supervision of and in partnership with the occupational therapist.
4. It is the responsibility of the occupational therapist to determine when to delegate responsibilities to an occupational therapy assistant. It is the responsibility of the occupational therapy assistant who performs the delegated responsibilities to demonstrate service competency and also not to accept delegated responsibilities that go beyond the scope of an occupational therapy assistant.
5. The occupational therapist and the occupational therapy assistant demonstrate and document service competency for clinical reasoning and judgment during the service delivery process as well as for the performance of specific techniques, assessments, and intervention methods used.
6. When delegating aspects of occupational therapy services, the occupational therapist considers the following factors:
   a. Complexity of the client's condition and needs;
   b. Knowledge, skill, and competence of the occupational therapy assistant;
   c. Nature and complexity of the intervention;

d. Needs and requirements of the practice setting; and

e. Appropriate scope of practice of an occupational therapy assistant under state law and other requirements.

Roles and Responsibilities

Regardless of the setting in which occupational therapy services are delivered, occupational therapists and occupational therapy assistants assume the following general responsibilities during evaluation; intervention planning, implementation, and review; and targeting and evaluating outcomes.

Evaluation

1. The occupational therapist directs the evaluation process.
2. The occupational therapist is responsible for directing all aspects of the initial contact during the occupational therapy evaluation, including
   a. Determining the need for service,
   b. Defining the problems within the domain of occupational therapy to be addressed,
   c. Determining the client's goals and priorities,
   d. Establishing intervention priorities,
   e. Determining specific further assessment needs, and
   f. Determining specific assessment tasks that can be delegated to the occupational therapy assistant.
3. The occupational therapist initiates and directs the evaluation, interprets the data, and develops the intervention plan.
4. The occupational therapy assistant contributes to the evaluation process by implementing delegated assessments and by providing verbal and written reports of observations, assessments, and client capacities to the occupational therapist.
5. The occupational therapist interprets the information provided by the occupational therapy assistant and integrates that information into the evaluation and decision-making process.

Intervention Planning

1. The occupational therapist has overall responsibility for the development of the occupational therapy intervention plan.

2. The occupational therapist and the occupational therapy assistant collaborate with the client to develop the plan.
3. The occupational therapy assistant is responsible for being knowledgeable about evaluation results and for providing input into the intervention plan, based on client needs and priorities.

Intervention Implementation

1. The occupational therapist has overall responsibility for intervention implementation.
2. When delegating aspects of the occupational therapy intervention to the occupational therapy assistant, the occupational therapist is responsible for providing appropriate supervision.
3. The occupational therapy assistant is responsible for being knowledgeable about the client's occupational therapy goals.
4. The occupational therapy assistant in collaboration with the occupational therapist selects, implements, and makes modifications to occupational therapy interventions, including, but not limited to, occupations and activities, preparatory methods and tasks, client education and training, and group interventions consistent with demonstrated competency levels, client goals, and the requirements of the practice setting.

Intervention Review

1. The occupational therapist is responsible for determining the need for continuing, modifying, or discontinuing occupational therapy services.
2. The occupational therapy assistant contributes to this process by exchanging information with and providing documentation to the occupational therapist about the client's responses to, and communications during, intervention.

Targeting and Evaluating Outcomes

1. The occupational therapist is responsible for selecting, measuring, and interpreting outcomes that are related to the client's ability to engage in occupations.

2. The occupational therapy assistant is responsible for being knowledgeable about the client's targeted occupational therapy outcomes and for providing information and documentation related to outcome achievement.
3. The occupational therapy assistant may implement outcome measurements and provide needed client discharge resources.

Supervision of Occupational Therapy Aides[1]

An *aide,* as used in occupational therapy practice, is an individual who provides supportive services to the occupational therapist and the occupational therapy assistant. Aides do not provide skilled occupational therapy services. An aide is trained by an occupational therapist or an occupational therapy assistant to perform specifically delegated tasks. The occupational therapist is responsible for the overall use and actions of the aide. An aide first must demonstrate competency to be able to perform the assigned, delegated client and nonclient tasks.

1. The occupational therapist must oversee the development, documentation, and implementation of a plan to supervise and routinely assess the ability of the occupational therapy aide to carry out nonclient- and client-related tasks. The occupational therapy assistant may contribute to the development and documentation of this plan.
2. The occupational therapy assistant can supervise the aide.
3. *Nonclient-related tasks* include clerical and maintenance activities and preparation of the work area or equipment.
4. *Client-related tasks* are routine tasks during which the aide may interact with the client. The following factors must be present when an occupational therapist or occupational therapy assistant delegates a selected client-related task to the aide:
   a. The outcome anticipated for the delegated task is predictable.
   b. The situation of the client and the environment is stable and will not require that the aide make judgment, interpretations, or adaptations.
   c. The client has demonstrated some previous performance ability in executing the task.
   d. The task routine and process have been clearly established.
5. When performing delegated client-related tasks, the supervisor must ensure that the aide
   a. Is trained and able to demonstrate competency in carrying out the selected task and using equipment, if appropriate;
   b. Has been instructed on how to specifically carry out the delegated task with the specific client; and
   c. Knows the precautions, signs, and symptoms for the particular client that would indicate the need to seek assistance from the occupational therapist or occupational therapy assistant.
6. The supervision of the aide needs to be documented. Documentation includes information about frequency and methods of supervision used, the content of supervision, and the names and credentials of all persons participating in the supervisory process.

Summary

These guidelines about supervision, roles, and responsibilities are to assist in the appropriate utilization of occupational therapists, occupational therapy assistants, and occupational therapy aides and in the appropriate and effective provision of occupational therapy services. It is expected that occupational therapy services are delivered in accordance with applicable state and federal regulations, relevant workplace policies, the *Occupational Therapy Code of Ethics and Ethics Standards* (AOTA, 2010), and continuing competency and professional development guidelines. For information regarding the supervision of occupational therapy students, please refer to *Fieldwork Level II and Occupational Therapy Students: A Position Paper* (AOTA, 2012; see Chapter 12).

---

[1]Depending on the setting in which service is provided; aides may be referred to by various names. Examples include, but are not limited to, *rehabilitation aides, restorative aides, extenders, paraprofessionals,* and *rehab techs* (AOTA, 2009).

References

American Occupational Therapy Association. (2009). Guidelines for supervision, roles, and responsibilities during the delivery of occupational therapy services. *American Journal of Occupational Therapy, 63,* 797–803. http://dx.doi.org/10/5014/ajot.63.6.797

American Occupational Therapy Association. (2010). Occupational therapy code of ethics and ethical standards (2010). *American Journal of Occupational Therapy, 64*(Suppl.), S17–S26. http://dx.doi.org/10.5014/ajot.2010.64S17

American Occupational Therapy Association. (2012). Fieldwork level II and occupational therapy students: A position paper. *American Journal of Occupational Therapy, 66,* S75–S77. http://dx.doi.org/10.5014/ajot.2012.66S75

American Occupational Therapy Association. (2014). Occupational therapy practice framework: Domain and process (3rd ed.). *American Journal of Occupational Therapy, 68*(Suppl. 1). http://dx.doi.org/10.5014/ajot.2014.682005

Additional Reading

American Occupational Therapy Association. (2010). Standards of practice for occupational therapy. *American Journal of Occupational Therapy, 64*(Suppl.), S106–S111. http://dx.doi.org/10.5014/ajot.2010.64S106

Authors

Sara Jane Brayman, PhD, OTR/L, FAOTA

Gloria Frolek Clark, MS, OTR/L, FAOTA

Janet V. DeLany, DEd, OTR/L

Eileen R. Garza, PhD, OTR, ATP

Mary V. Radomski, MA, OTR/L, FAOTA

Ruth Ramsey, MS, OTR/L

Carol Siebert, MS, OTR/L

Kristi Voelkerding, BS, COTA/L

Patricia D. LaVesser, PhD, OTR/L, *SIS Liaison*

Lenna Aird, *ASD Liaison*

Deborah Lieberman, MHSA, OTR/L, FAOTA, *AOTA Headquarters Liaison*

for

The Commission on Practice
Sara Jane Brayman, PhD, OTR/L, FAOTA, *Chairperson*

Adopted by the Representative Assembly 2004C24

Edited by the Commission on Practice 2014
Debbie Amini, EdD, OTR/L, CHT, FAOTA, *Chairperson*

Adopted by the Representative Assembly Coordinating Council (RACC) for the Representative Assembly, 2014.

Note. This document replaces the 2009 document *Guidelines for Supervision, Roles, and Responsibilities During the Delivery of Occupational Therapy Services,* previously published and copyrighted in 2009 by the American Occupational Therapy Association in the *American Journal of Occupational Therapy, 63,* 797–803. http://dx.doi.org/10.5014/ajot.63.6.797

Chapter 50.

GUIDELINES FOR REENTRY INTO THE FIELD OF OCCUPATIONAL THERAPY

American Occupational Therapy Association

Purpose of the Guidelines

These guidelines are designed to assist occupational therapists and occupational therapy assistants who have left the field of occupational therapy for 24 months or more and have chosen to return to the profession and deliver occupational therapy services. The guidelines represent minimum recommendations only and are designed to support practitioners in meeting their ethical obligation to maintain high standards of competence.

It is expected that practitioners will identify and meet requirements outlined in applicable state and federal regulations, relevant workplace policies, the *Occupational Therapy Code of Ethics (2015)* (American Occupational Therapy Association [AOTA], 2015a), and continuing competence and professional development guidelines prior to reentering the field.

Clarification of Terms

Reentry—For the purpose of this document, reentering occupational therapists and occupational therapy assistants are individuals who

- Have practiced in the field of occupational therapy; and
- Have not engaged in the practice of occupational therapy (may include direct intervention, supervision, teaching, consultation, administration, case or care management, community programming, or research) for a minimum of 24 months; and
- Wish to return to the profession in the capacity of delivering occupational therapy services to clients.

Formal Learning—This term refers to any learning that has established goals and objectives that are measureable. It may include activities such as

- Attending workshops, seminars, lectures, and professional conferences;
- Auditing or participating in formal academic coursework;
- Participating in external self-study series (e.g., AOTA Self-Paced Clinical Courses); or
- Participating in independent distance learning, either synchronous or asynchronous (e.g., continuing education articles; video, audio, or online courses) with established goals and objectives that are measurable.

Supervised Service Delivery—For this document, *supervised service delivery* refers to provision of occupational therapy services under the supervision of a qualified occupational therapist. The *Guidelines for Supervision, Roles, and Responsibilities During the Delivery of Occupational Therapy Services* (AOTA, 2014a) state that

> within the scope of occupational therapy practice, *supervision* is a process aimed at ensuring the safe and effective delivery of occupational therapy services and fostering professional competence and development. [It is] a cooperative process in which two or more people participate in a joint effort to establish, maintain, and/or elevate a level of competence and performance. (p. S16)

Specific Guidelines for Reentry

Practitioners who are seeking reentry must abide by state licensure and practice regulations and any requirements established by the workplace. In addition, the following suggested guidelines are recommended:

1. Engage in a formalized process of self-assessment (e.g., self-assessment tools, such as AOTA's [2003] *Professional Development Tool*), and complete a professional development plan that addresses the *Standards for Continuing Competence* (AOTA, 2015b).
2. Attend a minimum of 10 hours of formal learning related to occupational therapy service delivery for each 12 consecutive months out of practice. At least 20 hours of the formal learning must have occurred within the past 24 months of reentry.
3. Attain relevant updates to core knowledge of the profession of occupational therapy and the responsibilities of occupational therapy practitioners that are consistent with material found in AOTA official documents such as the *Occupational Therapy Practice Framework: Domain and Process* (3rd ed.; AOTA, 2014b), the *Occupational Therapy Code of Ethics (2015)* (AOTA, 2015a), *Standards for Continuing Competence* (AOTA, 2015b), *Standards of Practice for Occupational Therapy* (AOTA, 2010), and *Guidelines for Supervision, Roles, and Responsibilities During the Delivery of Occupational Therapy Services* (AOTA, 2014a).

4. Complete of a minimum of 30 hours of documented supervised service delivery in occupational therapy, which is recommended for practitioners who have been out of practice for 3 or more years.
   a. The supervised service delivery should be completed between the 12 months prior to anticipated reentry and the first 30 days of employment.
   b. The reentering practitioner, in conjunction with the supervising occupational therapy practitioner(s), should establish specific goals and objectives for the 30 hours. Goals, objectives, and related assessment of performance may be developed or adapted from a variety of sources, including competency and performance review resources existing within the setting as well as AOTA resources such as the *Fieldwork Performance Evaluation for the Occupational Therapy Student* forms (AOTA, 2002a, 2002b).
   c. The supervised service delivery experience should focus on the area of practice to which the practitioner intends to return.
   d. Supervised service delivery should occur with a practitioner at the same or greater professional level (i.e., an occupational therapist, not an occupational therapy assistant, supervises a returning therapist).
   e. Supervision should be direct face-to-face contact, which may include observation, modeling, cotreatment, discussions, teaching, and instruction (AOTA, 2014a) and may be augmented by indirect methods such as electronic communications.

Ongoing Continuing Competence

Once practitioners have successfully returned to the delivery of occupational therapy services, they are encouraged to engage in activities that support them in their ongoing continuing competence, such as

- Seeking mentoring, consultation, or supervision—especially during the first year of return to practice;
- Engaging in relevant AOTA Special Interest Section forums to build a professional network and facilitate opportunities for practice guidance;

- Exploring relevant AOTA Board and Specialty Certifications and using the identified criteria as a blueprint for ongoing professional development; and
- Joining and becoming active in both AOTA and the state occupational therapy association to stay abreast of practice trends and increase opportunities for networking.

References and Resources

American Occupational Therapy Association. (2002a). *Fieldwork performance evaluation for the occupational therapy assistant student.* Bethesda, MD: AOTA Press.

American Occupational Therapy Association. (2002b). *Fieldwork performance evaluation for the occupational therapy student.* Bethesda, MD: AOTA Press.

American Occupational Therapy Association. (2003, May). *Professional development tool.* Retrieved October 12, 2014, from http://www1.aota.org/pdt/index.asp

American Occupational Therapy Association. (2010). Standards of practice for occupational therapy. *American Journal of Occupational Therapy, 64*(6, Suppl.), S106–S111. http://dx.doi.org/10.5014/ajot.2010.64S106

American Occupational Therapy Association. (2014a). Guidelines for supervision, roles, and responsibilities during the delivery of occupational therapy services. *American Journal of Occupational Therapy, 68*(Suppl. 3), S16–S22. http://dx.doi.org/10.5014/ajot.2014.686S03

American Occupational Therapy Association. (2014b). Occupational therapy practice framework: Domain and process (3rd ed.). *American Journal of Occupational Therapy, 68*(Suppl. 1). http://dx.doi. org/10.5014/ajot.2014.682006

American Occupational Therapy Association. (2015a). Occupational therapy code of ethics (2015). *American Journal of Occupational Therapy, 69*(Suppl. 3), 6913410030. http://dx.doi.org/10.5014/ajot.2015.696S03

American Occupational Therapy Association. (2015b). Standards for continuing competence. *American Journal of Occupational Therapy, 69*(Suppl. 3), 6913410055. http://dx.doi.org/10.5014/ajot.2015.696S16

Authors

Melisa Tilton, BS, COTA/L ROH, *Chair*
Clare Giuffrida, PhD, MS, OTR/L, FAOTA
Christy L. A. Nelson, PhD, OTR/L, FAOTA
Winifred Schultz-Krohn, PhD, OTR/L, BCP, FAOTA, *Chairperson*
Maria Elena E. Louch, *AOTA Staff Liaison for the Commission on Continuing Competence and Professional Development*

Adopted by the Representative Assembly 2010CApr11

Revisions adopted 2015Apr16

Note. This revision replaces the 2010 document *Guidelines for Re-Entry Into the Field of Occupational Therapy,* previously published and copyrighted in 2010 by the American Occupational Therapy Association in the *American Journal of Occupational Therapy, 64*(6, Suppl.), S27–S29. http://dx.doi.org/10.5014/ajot.2010.64S27

Chapter 51.

OCCUPATIONAL THERAPY CODE OF ETHICS (2015)

American Occupational Therapy Association

Preamble

The 2015 *Occupational Therapy Code of Ethics* (Code) of the American Occupational Therapy Association (AOTA) is designed to reflect the dynamic nature of the profession, the evolving health care environment, and emerging technologies that can present potential ethical concerns in research, education, and practice. AOTA members are committed to promoting inclusion, participation, safety, and well-being for all recipients in various stages of life, health, and illness and to empowering all beneficiaries of service to meet their occupational needs. Recipients of services may be individuals, groups, families, organizations, communities, or populations (AOTA, 2014b).

The Code is an AOTA Official Document and a public statement tailored to address the most prevalent ethical concerns of the occupational therapy profession. It outlines Standards of Conduct the public can expect from those in the profession. It should be applied to all areas of occupational therapy and shared with relevant stakeholders to promote ethical conduct.

The Code serves two purposes:

1. It provides aspirational Core Values that guide members toward ethical courses of action in professional and volunteer roles.

2. It delineates enforceable Principles and Standards of Conduct that apply to AOTA members.

Whereas the Code helps guide and define decision-making parameters, ethical action goes beyond rote compliance with these Principles and is a manifestation of moral character and mindful reflection. It is a commitment to benefit others, to virtuous practice of artistry and science, to genuinely good behaviors, and to noble acts of courage. Recognizing and resolving ethical issues is a systematic process that includes analyzing the complex dynamics of situations, weighing consequences, making reasoned decisions, taking action, and reflecting on outcomes. Occupational therapy personnel, including students in occupational therapy programs, are expected to abide by the Principles and Standards of Conduct within this Code. Personnel roles include clinicians (e.g., direct service, consultation, administration); educators; researchers; entrepreneurs; business owners; and those in elected, appointed, or other professional volunteer service.

The process for addressing ethics violations by AOTA members (and associate members, where applicable) is outlined in the Code's Enforcement Procedures (AOTA, 2014a).

Although the Code can be used in conjunction with licensure board regulations and laws that guide standards of practice, the Code is meant to be a freestanding document, guiding ethical dimensions of professional behavior, responsibility, practice, and decision making. This Code is not exhaustive; that is, the Principles and Standards of Conduct cannot address every possible situation. Therefore, before making complex ethical decisions that require further expertise, occupational therapy personnel should seek out resources to assist in resolving ethical issues not addressed in this document. Resources can include, but are not limited to, ethics committees, ethics officers, the AOTA Ethics Commission or Ethics Program Manager, or an ethics consultant.

Core Values

The profession is grounded in seven longstanding Core Values: (1) Altruism, (2) Equality, (3) Freedom, (4) Justice, (5) Dignity, (6) Truth, and (7) Prudence. *Altruism* involves demonstrating concern for the welfare of others. *Equality* refers to treating all people impartially and free of bias. *Freedom* and personal choice are paramount in a profession in which the values and desires of the client guide our interventions. *Justice* expresses a state in which diverse communities are inclusive; diverse communities are organized and structured such that all members can function, flourish, and live a satisfactory life. Occupational therapy personnel, by virtue of the specific nature of the practice of occupational therapy, have a vested interest in addressing unjust inequities that limit opportunities for participation in society (Braveman & Bass-Haugen, 2009).

Inherent in the practice of occupational therapy is the promotion and preservation of the individuality and *Dignity* of the client by treating him or her with respect in all interactions. In all situations, occupational therapy personnel must provide accurate information in oral, written, and electronic forms (*Truth*). Occupational therapy personnel use their clinical and ethical reasoning skills, sound judgment, and reflection to make decisions in professional and volunteer roles (*Prudence*).

The seven Core Values provide a foundation to guide occupational therapy personnel in their interactions with others. Although the Core Values are not themselves enforceable standards, they should be considered when determining the most ethical course of action.

Principles and Standards of Conduct

The Principles and Standards of Conduct that are enforceable for professional behavior include (1) Beneficence, (2) Nonmaleficence, (3) Autonomy, (4) Justice, (5) Veracity, and (6) Fidelity. Reflection on the historical foundations of occupational therapy and related professions resulted in the inclusion of Principles that are consistently referenced as a guideline for ethical decision making.

Beneficence

Principle 1. Occupational therapy personnel shall demonstrate a concern for the well-being and safety of the recipients of their services.

Beneficence includes all forms of action intended to benefit other persons. The term *beneficence* connotes acts of mercy, kindness, and charity (Beauchamp & Childress, 2013). Beneficence requires taking action by helping others, in other words, by promoting good, by preventing harm, and by removing harm. Examples of beneficence include protecting and defending the rights of others, preventing harm from occurring to others, removing conditions that will cause harm to others, helping persons with disabilities, and rescuing persons in danger (Beauchamp & Childress, 2013).

Related Standards of Conduct

Occupational therapy personnel shall

A. Provide appropriate evaluation and a plan of intervention for recipients of occupational therapy services specific to their needs.
B. Reevaluate and reassess recipients of service in a timely manner to determine whether goals are being achieved and whether intervention plans should be revised.
C. Use, to the extent possible, evaluation, planning, intervention techniques, assessments, and therapeutic equipment that are evidence-based,

current, and within the recognized scope of occupational therapy practice.

D. Ensure that all duties delegated to other occupational therapy personnel are congruent with credentials, qualifications, experience, competency, and scope of practice with respect to service delivery, supervision, fieldwork education, and research.

E. Provide occupational therapy services, including education and training, that are within each practitioner's level of competence and scope of practice.

F. Take steps (e.g., continuing education, research, supervision, training) to ensure proficiency, use careful judgment, and weigh potential for harm when generally recognized standards do not exist in emerging technology or areas of practice.

G. Maintain competency by ongoing participation in education relevant to one's practice area.

H. Terminate occupational therapy services in collaboration with the service recipient or responsible party when the services are no longer beneficial.

I. Refer to other providers when indicated by the needs of the client.

J. Conduct and disseminate research in accordance with currently accepted ethical guidelines and standards for the protection of research participants, including determination of potential risks and benefits.

Nonmaleficence

Principle 2. Occupational therapy personnel shall refrain from actions that cause harm.

Nonmaleficence "obligates us to abstain from causing harm to others" (Beauchamp & Childress, 2013, p. 150). The Principle of *Nonmaleficence* also includes an obligation to not impose risks of harm even if the potential risk is without malicious or harmful intent. This Principle often is examined under the context of due care. The standard of *due care* "requires that the goals pursued justify the risks that must be imposed to achieve those goals" (Beauchamp & Childress, 2013, p. 154). For example, in occupational therapy practice, this standard applies to situations in which the client might feel pain from a treatment intervention; however, the acute pain is justified by potential longitudinal, evidence-based benefits of the treatment.

Related Standards of Conduct

Occupational therapy personnel shall

A. Avoid inflicting harm or injury to recipients of occupational therapy services, students, research participants, or employees.

B. Avoid abandoning the service recipient by facilitating appropriate transitions when unable to provide services for any reason.

C. Recognize and take appropriate action to remedy personal problems and limitations that might cause harm to recipients of service, colleagues, students, research participants, or others.

D. Avoid any undue influences that may impair practice and compromise the ability to safely and competently provide occupational therapy services, education, or research.

E. Address impaired practice and, when necessary, report it to the appropriate authorities.

F. Avoid dual relationships, conflicts of interest, and situations in which a practitioner, educator, student, researcher, or employer is unable to maintain clear professional boundaries or objectivity.

G. Avoid engaging in sexual activity with a recipient of service, including the client's family or significant other, student, research participant, or employee, while a professional relationship exists.

H. Avoid compromising the rights or well-being of others based on arbitrary directives (e.g., unrealistic productivity expectations, falsification of documentation, inaccurate coding) by exercising professional judgment and critical analysis.

I. Avoid exploiting any relationship established as an occupational therapy clinician, educator, or researcher to further one's own physical, emotional, financial, political, or business interests at the expense of recipients of services, students, research participants, employees, or colleagues.

J. Avoid bartering for services when there is the potential for exploitation and conflict of interest.

Autonomy

Principle 3. Occupational therapy personnel shall respect the right of the individual to self-determination, privacy, confidentiality, and consent.

The Principle of *Autonomy* expresses the concept that practitioners have a duty to treat the client according to the client's desires, within the bounds of accepted standards of care, and to protect the client's confidential information. Often, respect for Autonomy is referred to as the *self-determination principle*. However, respecting a person's autonomy goes beyond acknowledging an individual as a mere agent and also acknowledges a person's right "to hold views, to make choices, and to take actions based on [his or her] values and beliefs" (Beauchamp & Childress, 2013, p. 106). Individuals have the right to make a determination regarding care decisions that directly affect their lives. In the event that a person lacks decision-making capacity, his or her autonomy should be respected through involvement of an authorized agent or surrogate decision maker.

Related Standards of Conduct

Occupational therapy personnel shall

A. Respect and honor the expressed wishes of recipients of service.

B. Fully disclose the benefits, risks, and potential outcomes of any intervention; the personnel who will be providing the intervention; and any reasonable alternatives to the proposed intervention.

C. Obtain consent after disclosing appropriate information and answering any questions posed by the recipient of service or research participant to ensure voluntariness.

D. Establish a collaborative relationship with recipients of service and relevant stakeholders to promote shared decision making.

E. Respect the client's right to refuse occupational therapy services temporarily or permanently, even when that refusal has potential to result in poor outcomes.

F. Refrain from threatening, coercing, or deceiving clients to promote compliance with occupational therapy recommendations.

G. Respect a research participant's right to withdraw from a research study without penalty.

H. Maintain the confidentiality of all verbal, written, electronic, augmentative, and nonverbal communications, in compliance with applicable laws, including all aspects of privacy laws and exceptions thereto (e.g., Health Insurance Portability and Accountability Act [Pub. L. 104–191], Family Educational Rights and Privacy Act [Pub. L. 93–380]).

I. Display responsible conduct and discretion when engaging in social networking, including but not limited to refraining from posting protected health information.

J. Facilitate comprehension and address barriers to communication (e.g., aphasia; differences in language, literacy, culture) with the recipient of service (or responsible party), student, or research participant.

Justice

Principle 4. Occupational therapy personnel shall promote fairness and objectivity in the provision of occupational therapy services.

The Principle of *Justice* relates to the fair, equitable, and appropriate treatment of persons (Beauchamp & Childress, 2013). Occupational therapy personnel should relate in a respectful, fair, and impartial manner to individuals and groups with whom they interact. They should also respect the applicable laws and standards related to their area of practice. Justice requires the impartial consideration and consistent following of rules to generate unbiased decisions and promote fairness. As occupational therapy personnel, we work to uphold a society in which all individuals have an equitable opportunity to achieve occupational engagement as an essential component of their life.

Related Standards of Conduct

Occupational therapy personnel shall

A. Respond to requests for occupational therapy services (e.g., a referral) in a timely manner as determined by law, regulation, or policy.

B. Assist those in need of occupational therapy services in securing access through available means.

C. Address barriers in access to occupational therapy services by offering or referring clients to financial aid, charity care, or pro bono services within the parameters of organizational policies.

D. Advocate for changes to systems and policies that are discriminatory or unfairly limit or prevent access to occupational therapy services.

E. Maintain awareness of current laws and AOTA policies and Official Documents that apply to the profession of occupational therapy.

F. Inform employers, employees, colleagues, students, and researchers of applicable policies, laws, and Official Documents.

G. Hold requisite credentials for the occupational therapy services they provide in academic, research, physical, or virtual work settings.

H. Provide appropriate supervision in accordance with AOTA Official Documents and relevant laws, regulations, policies, procedures, standards, and guidelines.

I. Obtain all necessary approvals prior to initiating research activities.

J. Refrain from accepting gifts that would unduly influence the therapeutic relationship or have the potential to blur professional boundaries, and adhere to employer policies when offered gifts.

K. Report to appropriate authorities any acts in practice, education, and research that are unethical or illegal.

L. Collaborate with employers to formulate policies and procedures in compliance with legal, regulatory, and ethical standards and work to resolve any conflicts or inconsistencies.

M. Bill and collect fees legally and justly in a manner that is fair, reasonable, and commensurate with services delivered.

N. Ensure compliance with relevant laws, and promote transparency when participating in a business arrangement as owner, stockholder, partner, or employee.

O. Ensure that documentation for reimbursement purposes is done in accordance with applicable laws, guidelines, and regulations.

P. Refrain from participating in any action resulting in unauthorized access to educational content or exams (including but not limited to sharing test questions, unauthorized use of or access to content or codes, or selling access or authorization codes).

Veracity

Principle 5. Occupational therapy personnel shall provide comprehensive, accurate, and objective information when representing the profession.

Veracity is based on the virtues of truthfulness, candor, and honesty. The Principle of *Veracity* refers to comprehensive, accurate, and objective transmission of information and includes fostering understanding of such information (Beauchamp & Childress, 2013). Veracity is based on respect owed to others, including but not limited to recipients of service, colleagues, students, researchers, and research participants.

In communicating with others, occupational therapy personnel implicitly promise to be truthful and not deceptive. When entering into a therapeutic or research relationship, the recipient of service or research participant has a right to accurate information. In addition, transmission of information is incomplete without also ensuring that the recipient or participant understands the information provided.

Concepts of veracity must be carefully balanced with other potentially competing ethical principles, cultural beliefs, and organizational policies. Veracity ultimately is valued as a means to establish trust and strengthen professional relationships. Therefore, adherence to the Principle of Veracity also requires thoughtful analysis of how full disclosure of information may affect outcomes.

Related Standards of Conduct

Occupational therapy personnel shall

A. Represent credentials, qualifications, education, experience, training, roles, duties, competence, contributions, and findings accurately in all forms of communication.

B. Refrain from using or participating in the use of any form of communication that contains false, fraudulent, deceptive, misleading, or unfair statements or claims.

C. Record and report in an accurate and timely manner and in accordance with applicable regulations all information related to professional or academic documentation and activities.

D. Identify and fully disclose to all appropriate persons errors or adverse events that compromise the safety of service recipients.

E. Ensure that all marketing and advertising is truthful, accurate, and carefully presented to avoid misleading recipients of service, research participants, or the public.

F. Describe the type and duration of occupational therapy services accurately in professional contracts, including the duties and responsibilities of all involved parties.

G. Be honest, fair, accurate, respectful, and timely in gathering and reporting fact-based information regarding employee job performance and student performance.

H. Give credit and recognition when using the ideas and work of others in written, oral, or electronic media (i.e., do not plagiarize).

I. Provide students with access to accurate information regarding educational requirements and academic policies and procedures relative to the occupational therapy program or educational institution.

J. Maintain privacy and truthfulness when using telecommunication in the delivery of occupational therapy services.

Fidelity

Principle 6. Occupational therapy personnel shall treat clients, colleagues, and other professionals with respect, fairness, discretion, and integrity.

The Principle of Fidelity comes from the Latin root *fidelis,* meaning loyal. *Fidelity* refers to the duty one has to keep a commitment once it is made (Veatch, Haddad, & English, 2010). In the health professions, this commitment refers to promises made between a provider and a client or patient based on an expectation of loyalty, staying with the client or patient in a time of need, and compliance with a code of ethics. These promises can be implied or explicit. The duty to disclose information that is potentially meaningful in making decisions is one obligation of the moral contract between provider and client or patient (Veatch et al., 2010).

Whereas respecting Fidelity requires occupational therapy personnel to meet the client's reasonable expectations, the Principle also addresses maintaining respectful collegial and organizational relationships (Purtilo & Doherty, 2011). Professional relationships are greatly influenced by the complexity of the environment in which occupational therapy personnel work. Practitioners, educators, and researchers alike must consistently balance their duties to service recipients, students, research participants, and other professionals as well as to organizations that may influence decision making and professional practice.

Related Standards of Conduct

Occupational therapy personnel shall

A. Preserve, respect, and safeguard private information about employees, colleagues, and students unless otherwise mandated or permitted by relevant laws.

B. Address incompetent, disruptive, unethical, illegal, or impaired practice that jeopardizes the safety or well-being of others and team effectiveness.

C. Avoid conflicts of interest or conflicts of commitment in employment, volunteer roles, or research.

D. Avoid using one's position (employee or volunteer) or knowledge gained from that position in such a manner as to give rise to real or perceived conflict of interest among the person, the employer, other AOTA members, or other organizations.

E. Be diligent stewards of human, financial, and material resources of their employers, and refrain from exploiting these resources for personal gain.

F. Refrain from verbal, physical, emotional, or sexual harassment of peers or colleagues.

G. Refrain from communication that is derogatory, intimidating, or disrespectful and that unduly discourages others from participating in professional dialogue.

H. Promote collaborative actions and communication as a member of interprofessional teams to facilitate quality care and safety for clients.

I. Respect the practices, competencies, roles, and responsibilities of their own and other professions to promote a collaborative environment reflective of interprofessional teams.

J. Use conflict resolution and internal and alternative dispute resolution resources as needed to resolve organizational and interpersonal conflicts, as well as perceived institutional ethics violations.

K. Abide by policies, procedures, and protocols when serving or acting on behalf of a professional organization or employer to fully and accurately represent the organization's official and authorized positions.

L. Refrain from actions that reduce the public's trust in occupational therapy.

M. Self-identify when personal, cultural, or religious values preclude, or are anticipated to negatively affect, the professional relationship or provision of services, while adhering to organizational policies when requesting an exemption from service to an individual or group on the basis of conflict of conscience.

References

American Occupational Therapy Association. (2014a). Enforcement procedures for the *Occupational therapy code of ethics and ethics standards. American Journal of Occupational Therapy, 68*(Suppl. 3), S3–S15. http://dx.doi.org/10.5014/ajot.2014.686S02

American Occupational Therapy Association. (2014b). Occupational therapy practice framework: Domain and process. (3rd ed.). *American Journal of Occupational Therapy, 68*(Suppl. 1). http://dx.doi.org/10.5014/ajot.2014.682006

Beauchamp, T. L., & Childress, J. F. (2013). *Principles of biomedical ethics* (7th ed.). New York: Oxford University Press.

Braveman, B., & Bass-Haugen, J. D. (2009). Social justice and health disparities: An evolving discourse in occupational therapy research and intervention. *American Journal of Occupational Therapy, 63,* 7–12. http://dx.doi.org/10.5014/ajot.63.1.7

Purtilo, R., & Doherty, R. (2011). *Ethical dimensions in the health professions* (5th ed.). Philadelphia: Saunders/Elsevier.

Veatch, R. M., Haddad, A. M., & English, D. C. (2010). *Case studies in biomedical ethics.* New York: Oxford University Press.

Ethics Commission

Yvette Hachtel, JD, OTR/L, *Chair (2013–2014)*
Lea Cheyney Brandt, OTD, MA, OTR/L, *Chair (2014–2015)*
Ann Moodey Ashe, MHS, OTR/L *(2011–2014)*
Joanne Estes, PhD, OTR/L *(2012–2015)*
Loretta Jean Foster, MS, COTA/L *(2011–2014)*
Wayne L. Winistorfer, MPA, OTR *(2014–2017)*
Linda Scheirton, PhD, RDH *(2012–2015)*
Kate Payne, JD, RN *(2013–2014)*
Margaret R. Moon, MD, MPH, FAAP *(2014–2016)*
Kimberly S. Erler, MS, OTR/L *(2014–2017)*
Kathleen McCracken, MHA, COTA/L *(2014–2017)*
Deborah Yarett Slater, MS, OT/L, FAOTA, *AOTA Ethics Program Manager*

Adopted by the Representative Assembly 2015AprilC3.

Note. This document replaces the 2010 document *Occupational Therapy Code of Ethics and Ethics Standards (2010),* previously published and copyrighted in 2010 by the American Occupational Therapy Association in the *American Journal of Occupational Therapy, 64,* S17–S26. http://dx.doi.org/10.5014/ajot.2010.64S17

Chapter 52.

ENFORCEMENT PROCEDURES FOR THE *OCCUPATIONAL THERAPY CODE OF ETHICS*

American Occupational Therapy Association

1. Introduction

The principal purposes of the *Occupational Therapy Code of Ethics* (hereinafter referred to as the Code) are to help protect the public and to reinforce its confidence in the occupational therapy profession rather than to resolve private business, legal, or other disputes for which there are other more appropriate forums for resolution. The Code also is an aspirational document to guide occupational therapists, occupational therapy assistants, and occupational therapy students toward appropriate professional conduct in all aspects of their diverse professional and volunteer roles. It applies to any conduct that may affect the performance of occupational therapy as well as to behavior that an individual may do in another capacity that reflects negatively on the reputation of occupational therapy.

The *Enforcement Procedures for the Occupational Therapy Code of Ethics* have undergone a series of revisions by the Association's Ethics Commission (hereinafter referred to as the EC) since their initial adoption. This public document articulates the procedures that are followed by the EC as it carries out its duties to enforce the Code. A major goal of these *Enforcement Procedures* is to ensure objectivity and fundamental fairness to all individuals who may be parties in an ethics complaint. The *Enforcement Procedures* are used to help ensure compliance with the Code which delineates enforceable Principles and Standards of Conduct that apply to Association members.

Acceptance of Association membership commits individuals to adherence to the Code and cooperation with its *Enforcement Procedures*. These are established and maintained by the EC. The EC and Association's Ethics Office make the *Enforcement Procedures* public and available to members of the profession, state regulatory boards, consumers, and others for their use.

The EC urges particular attention to the following issues:

1.1 Professional Responsibility—All occupational therapy personnel have an obligation to maintain the Code of their profession and to promote and support these ethical standards among their colleagues. Each Association member must be alert to practices that undermine these standards and is obligated to take action that is appropriate in the circumstances. At the same time, members must carefully weigh their judgments as to potentially unethical practice to ensure that they are based on objective evaluation and not on personal bias or prejudice, inadequate information, or simply differences of professional viewpoint. It is recognized that individual occupational therapy personnel may not have the authority or ability to address or correct all situations of concern. Whenever feasible and appropriate, members should first pursue other corrective steps within the relevant institution or setting and discuss ethical concerns directly with the potential Respondent before resorting to the Association's ethics complaint process.

1.2. Jurisdiction—The Code applies to persons who are or were Association members at the time of the conduct in question. Later nonrenewal or relinquishment of membership does not affect Association jurisdiction. The *Enforcement Procedures* that shall be utilized in any complaint shall be those in effect at the time the complaint is initiated.

1.3. Disciplinary Actions/Sanctions (Pursuing a Complaint)—If the EC determines that unethical conduct has occurred, it may impose sanctions, including reprimand, censure, probation (with terms) suspension, or permanent revocation of Association membership. In all cases, except those involving only reprimand (and educative letters), the Association will report the conclusions and sanctions in its official publications and also will communicate to any appropriate persons or entities. If an individual is on either the Roster of Fellows (ROF) or the Roster of Honor (ROH), the EC Chairperson (via the EC Staff Liaison) shall notify the VLDC Chairperson and Association Executive Director (ED) of their membership suspension or revocation. That individual shall have their name removed from either the ROF or the ROH and no longer has the right to use the designated credential of FAOTA or ROH during the period of suspension or permanently, in the case of revocation.

The EC Chairperson shall also notify the Chairperson of the Board for Advanced and Specialty Certification (BASC) (via Association staff liaison, in writing) of final disciplinary actions from the EC in which an individual's membership has been suspended or revoked. These individuals are not eligible to apply for or renew certification.

The potential sanctions are defined as follows:

1.3.1. Reprimand—A formal expression of disapproval of conduct communicated privately by letter from the EC Chairperson that is nondisclosable and noncommunicative to other bodies (e.g., state regulatory boards [SRBs], National Board for Certification in Occupational Therapy® [NBCOT®]). Reprimand is not publicly reported.

1.3.2. Censure—A formal expression of disapproval that is publicly reported.

1.3.3. Probation of Membership Subject to Terms—Continued membership is conditional, depending on fulfillment of specified terms. Failure to meet terms will subject an Association member to any of the disciplinary actions or sanctions. Terms may include but are not limited to

  a. Remedial activity, applicable to the violation, with proof of satisfactory completion, by a specific date; and

  b. The corrected behavior which is expected to be maintained.

Probation is publicly reported.

1.3.4. Suspension—Removal of Association membership for a specified period of time. Suspension is publicly reported.

1.3.5. Revocation—Permanent denial of Association membership. Revocation is publicly reported.

1.4. Educative Letters—If the EC determines that the alleged conduct may or may not be a true breach of the Code but in any event does not warrant any of the sanctions set forth in Section 1.3. or is not completely in keeping with the aspirational nature of the Code or within the prevailing standards of practice or professionalism, the EC may send a private letter to educate the Respondent about relevant standards of practice and/or appropriate professional behavior. In addition, a different private educative letter, if appropriate, may be sent to the Complainant.

1.5. Advisory Opinions—The EC may issue general advisory opinions on ethical issues to inform and educate the Association membership. These opinions shall be publicized to the membership and are available in the *Reference Guide to the Occupational Therapy Code of Ethics* as well as on the Association website.

1.6. Rules of Evidence—The EC proceedings shall be conducted in accordance with fundamental fairness. However, formal rules of evidence that are used in legal proceedings do not apply to these *Enforcement Procedures*. The Disciplinary Council (see Section 5) and the Appeal Panel (see Section 6) can consider any evidence that they deem appropriate and pertinent.

1.7. Confidentiality and Disclosure—The EC develops and adheres to strict rules of confidentiality in every aspect of its work. This requires that participants in the process refrain from any communication relating to the existence and subject matter of the complaint other than with those directly involved in the enforcement process. Maintaining confidentiality throughout the investigation and enforcement process of a formal ethics complaint is essential in order to ensure fairness to all parties involved. These rules of confidentiality pertain not only to the EC but also apply to others involved in the complaint process. Beginning with the EC Staff Liaison and support staff, strict rules of confidentiality are followed. These same rules of confidentiality apply to Complainants, Respondents and their attorneys, and witnesses involved with the EC's investigatory process. Due diligence must be exercised by everyone involved in the investigation to avoid compromising the confidential nature of the process. Any Association member who breaches these rules of confidentiality may become subject to an ethics complaint/investigatory process himself or herself. Non–Association members may lodge an ethics complaint against an Association member, and these individuals are still expected to adhere to the Association's confidentiality rules. The Association reserves the right to take appropriate action against non–Association members who violate confidentiality rules, including notification of their appropriate licensure boards.

1.7.1. Disclosure—When the EC investigates a complaint, it may request information from a variety of sources. The process of obtaining additional information is carefully executed in order to maintain confidentiality. The EC may request information from a variety of sources, including state licensing agencies, academic councils, courts, employers, and other persons and entities. It is within the EC's purview to determine what disclosures are appropriate for particular parties in order to effectively implement its investigatory obligations. Public sanctions by the EC, Disciplinary Council, or Appeal Panel will be publicized as provided in these *Enforcement Procedures*. Normally, the EC does not disclose information or documentation reviewed in the course of an investigation unless the EC determines that disclosure is necessary to obtain additional, relevant evidence or to administer the ethics process or is legally required.

Individuals who file a complaint (i.e., *Complainant*) and those who are the subject of one (i.e., *Respondent*) must not disclose to anyone outside of those involved in the complaint process their role in an ethics complaint. Disclosing this information in and of itself may jeopardize the ethics process and violate the rules of fundamental fairness by which all parties are protected. Disclosure of information related to any case under investigation by the EC is prohibited and, if done, will lead to repercussions as outlined in these *Enforcement Procedures* (see Section 2.2.3.).

2. Complaints

2.1. Interested Party Complaints

2.1.1. Complaints stating an alleged violation of the Code may originate from any individual, group, or entity within or outside the Association. All complaints must be in writing, signed by the Complainant(s), and submitted to the Ethics Office at the Association headquarters. Complain- ants must complete the Formal Statement of Complaint Form at the end of this document. All complaints shall identify the person against whom the complaint is directed (the Respondent), the ethical principles that the Complainant believes have been violated, and the key facts and date(s) of the alleged ethical violations. If lawfully available, supporting documentation should be attached. Hard-copy complaints must be sent to the address indicated on the complaint form.

Complaints that are emailed must be sent as a pdf attachment, marked "Confidential" with "Complaint" in the subject line to ethics@aota.org and must include the complaint form and supporting documentation.

2.1.2. Within 90 days of receipt of a complaint, the EC shall make a preliminary assessment of the complaint and decide whether it presents sufficient questions as to a potential ethics violation that an investigation is warranted in accordance with Section 3. Commencing an investigation does not imply a conclusion that an ethical violation has in fact occurred or any judgment as to the ultimate sanction, if any, that may be appropriate. In the event the EC determines at the completion of an investigation that the complaint does rise to the level of an ethical violation, the EC may issue a decision as set forth in Section 4 below. In the event the EC determines that the complaint does not rise to the level of an ethical violation, the EC may direct the parties to utilize other conflict resolution resources or authorities via an educative letter. This applies to all complaints, including those involving Association elected/volunteer leadership related to their official roles.

2.2. Complaints Initiated by the EC

2.2.1. The EC itself may initiate a complaint (a *sua sponte* complaint) when it receives information from a governmental body, certification or similar body, public media, or other source indicating that a person subject to its jurisdiction may have committed acts that violate the Code. The Association will ordinarily act promptly after learning of the basis of a *sua sponte* complaint, but there is no specified time limit.

If the EC passes a motion to initiate a *sua sponte* complaint, the Association staff liaison to the EC will complete the Formal Statement of Complaint Form (at the end of this document) and will describe the nature of the factual allegations that led to the complaint and the manner in which the EC learned of the matter. The Complaint Form will be signed by the EC Chairperson on behalf of the EC. The form will be filed with the case material in the Association's Ethics Office.

2.2.2. *De Jure* Complaints—Where the source of a *sua sponte* complaint is the findings and conclusions of another official body, the EC classifies such *sua sponte* complaints as *de jure*. The procedure in such cases is addressed in Section 4.2.

2.2.3. The EC shall have the jurisdiction to investigate or sanction any matter or person for violations based on information learned in the course of investigating a complaint under Section 2.2.2.

2.3. Continuation of Complaint Process—If an Association member relinquishes membership, fails to renew membership, or fails to cooperate with the ethics investigation, the EC shall nevertheless continue to process the complaint, noting in its report the circumstances of the Respondent's action. Such actions shall not deprive the EC of jurisdiction. All correspondence related to the EC complaint process is in writing and sent by mail with signature and proof of date received. In the event that any written correspondence does not have delivery confirmation, the Association Ethics Office will make an attempt to search for an alternate physical or electronic address or make a second attempt to send to the original address. If the Respondent does not claim correspondence after two attempts to deliver, delivery cannot be confirmed or correspondence is returned to the Association as undeliverable, the EC shall consider that it has made good-faith effort and shall proceed with the ethics enforcement process.

3. EC Review and Investigations

3.1. Initial Action—The purpose of the preliminary review is to decide whether or not the information submitted with the complaint warrants opening the case. If in its preliminary review of the complaint the EC determines that an investigation is not warranted, the Complainant will be so notified.

3.2. Dismissal of Complaints—The EC may at any time dismiss a complaint for any of the following reasons:

3.2.1. Lack of Jurisdiction—The EC determines that it has no jurisdiction over the Respondent (e.g., a complaint against a person who is or was not an Association member at the time of the alleged incident or who has never been a member).

3.2.2. Absolute Time Limit/Not Timely Filed—The EC determines that the violation of the Code is alleged to have occurred more than 7 years prior to the filing of the complaint.

3.2.3. Subject to Jurisdiction of Another Authority—The EC determines that the complaint is based on matters that are within the authority of and are more properly dealt with by another governmental or nongovernmental body, such as an SRB, NBCOT®, an Association component other than the EC, an employer, educational institution, or a court.

3.2.4. No Ethics Violation—The EC finds that the complaint, even if proven, does not state a basis for action under the Code (e.g., simply accusing someone of being unpleasant or rude on an occasion).

3.2.5. Insufficient Evidence—The EC determines that there clearly would not be sufficient factual evidence to support a finding of an ethics violation.

3.2.6. Corrected Violation—The EC determines that any violation it might find already has been or is being corrected and that this is an adequate result in the given case.

3.2.7. Other Good Cause.

3.3. Investigator and EC (Avoidance of Conflict of Interest)—The investigator chosen shall not have a conflict of interest (i.e., shall never have had a substantial professional, personal, financial, business, or volunteer relationship with either the Complainant or the Respondent). In the event that the EC Staff Liaison has such a conflict, the EC Chairperson shall appoint an alternate investigator who has no conflict of interest. Any member of the EC with a possible conflict of interest must disclose and may be recused.

3.4. Investigation—If an investigation is deemed warranted, the EC Chairperson shall do the following within thirty (30) days: Appoint the EC Staff Liaison at the Association headquarters to investigate the complaint and notify the Respondent by mail (requiring signature and proof of date of receipt) that a complaint has been received and an investigation is being conducted. A copy of the complaint and supporting documentation shall be enclosed with this notification. The Complainant also will receive notification by mail (requiring signature and proof of date of receipt) that the complaint is being investigated.

3.4.1. Ordinarily, the Investigator will send questions formulated by the EC to be answered by the Complainant and/or the Respondent.

3.4.2. The Complainant shall be given thirty (30) days from receipt of the questions (if any) to respond in writing to the investigator.

3.4.3. The Respondent shall be given thirty (30) days from receipt of the questions to respond in writing to the Investigator.

3.4.4. The EC ordinarily will notify the Complainant of any substantive new evidence adverse to the Complainant's initial complaint that is discovered in the course of the ethics investigation and allow the Complainant to respond to such adverse evidence. In such cases, the Complainant will be given a copy of such evidence and will have fourteen (14) days in which to submit a written response. If the new evidence clearly shows that there has been no ethics violation, the EC may terminate the proceeding. In addition, if the investigation includes questions for both the Respondent and the Complainant, the evidence submitted by each party in response to the investigatory questions shall be provided to the Respondent and available to the Complainant on request. The EC may request reasonable payment for copying expenses depending on the volume of material to be sent.

3.4.5. The Investigator, in consultation with the EC, may obtain evidence directly from third parties without permission from the Complainant or Respondent.

3.5. Investigation Timeline—The investigation will be completed within ninety (90) days after receipt of notification by the Respondent or his or her designee that an investigation is being conducted, unless the EC determines that special circumstances warrant additional time for the investigation. All timelines noted here can be extended for good cause at the discretion of the EC, including the EC's schedule and additional requests of the Respondent. The Respondent and the Complainant shall be notified in writing if a delay occurs or if the investigational process requires more time.

3.6. Case Files—The investigative files shall include the complaint and any documentation on which the EC relied in initiating the investigation.

3.7. Cooperation by Respondent—Every Association Respondent has a duty to cooperate reasonably with enforcement processes for the Code. Failure of the Respondent to participate and/or cooperate with the investigative process of the EC shall not prevent continuation of the ethics process, and this behavior itself may constitute a violation of the Code.

3.8. Referral of Complaint—The EC may at any time refer a matter to NBCOT®, the SRB, ACOTE®, or other recognized authorities for appropriate action. Despite such referral to an appropriate authority, the EC shall retain jurisdiction. EC action may be stayed for a reasonable period pending notification of a decision by that authority, at the discretion of the EC (and such delays will extend the time periods under these *Procedures*). A stay in conducting an investigation shall not constitute a waiver by the EC of jurisdiction over the matters. The EC shall provide written notice by mail (requiring signature and proof of date of receipt) to the Respondent and the Complainant of any such stay of action.

4. EC Review and Decision

4.1. Regular Complaint Process

4.1.1. Decision—If at the conclusion of the investigation the EC determines that the Respondent has engaged in conduct that constitutes a breach of the Code, the EC shall notify the Respondent and Complainant by mail with signature and proof of date received. The notice shall describe in sufficient detail the conduct that constitutes a violation of the Code and indicate the sanction that is being imposed in accordance with these *Enforcement Procedures.*

4.1.2. Respondent's Response—Within 30 days of notification of the EC's decision and sanction, if any, the Respondent shall

4.1.2.1. Accept the decision of the EC (as to both the ethics violation and the sanction) and waive any right to a Disciplinary Council hearing, or

4.1.2.2. Accept the decision that he/she committed unethical conduct but within thirty (30) days, submit to the EC a statement (with any supporting documentation) setting forth the reasons why any sanction should not be imposed or reasons why the sanction should be mitigated or reduced.

4.1.2.3. Advise the EC Chairperson in writing that he or she contests the EC's decision and sanction and requests a hearing before the Disciplinary Council.

Failure of the Respondent to take one of these actions within the time specified will be deemed to constitute acceptance of the decision and sanction. If the Respondent requests a Disciplinary Council hearing, it will be scheduled. If the Respondent does not request a Disciplinary Council hearing but accepts the decision, the EC will notify all relevant parties and implement the sanction. Correspondence with the Respondent will also indicate that public sanctions may have an impact on their ability to serve in Association positions, whether elected or appointed, for a designated period of time.

4.2. *De Jure* Complaint Process

4.2.1. The EC Staff Liaison will present to the EC any findings from external sources (as described above) that come to his or her attention and that may warrant *sua sponte* complaints pertaining to individuals who are or were Association members at the time of the alleged incident.

4.2.2. Because *de jure* complaints are based on the findings of fact or conclusions of another official body, the EC will decide whether or not to act based on such findings or conclusions and will not ordinarily initiate another investigation, absent clear and convincing evidence that such findings and conclusions were erroneous or not supported by substantial evidence. Based on the information presented by the EC Staff Liaison, the EC will determine whether the findings of the public body also are sufficient to demonstrate an egregious violation of the Code and therefore warrant taking disciplinary action.

4.2.3. If the EC decides that a breach of the Code has occurred, the EC Chairperson will notify the Respondent in writing of the violation and the disciplinary action that is being taken. Correspondence with the Respondent will also indicate that public sanctions may have an impact on their ability to serve in Association positions, whether elected or appointed, for a designated period of time. In response to the *de jure sua sponte* decision and sanction by the EC, the Respondent may

4.2.3.1. Accept the decision of the EC (as to both the ethics violation and the sanction) based solely on the findings of fact and conclusions of the EC or the public body, and waive any right to a Disciplinary Council hearing;

4.2.3.2. Accept the decision that the Respondent committed unethical conduct but within thirty (30) days submit to the EC a statement (with any supporting documentation) setting forth the reasons why any sanction should not be imposed or reasons why the sanction should be mitigated or reduced; or

4.2.3.3. Within thirty (30) days, present information showing the findings of fact of the official body relied on by the EC to impose the sanction are clearly erroneous and request reconsideration by the EC. The EC may have the option of opening an investigation or modifying the sanction in the event they find clear and convincing evidence that the findings and the conclusions of the other body are erroneous.

4.2.4. In cases of *de jure* complaints, a Disciplinary Council hearing can later be requested (pursuant to Section 5 below) only if the Respondent has first exercised Options 4.2.3.2 or 4.2.3.3.

4.2.5. Respondents in an ethics case may utilize Options 4.2.3.2 or 4.2.3.3 (reconsideration) once in responding to the EC. Following one review of the additional information submitted by the Respondent, if the EC reaffirms its original sanction, the Respondent has the option of accepting the violation and proposed sanction or requesting a Disciplinary Council hearing. Repeated requests for reconsideration will not be accepted by the EC.

5. Disciplinary Council

5.1. Purpose—The purpose of the Disciplinary Council (hereinafter to be known as the Council) hearing is to provide the Respondent an opportunity to present evidence and witnesses to answer and refute the decision and/or sanction and to permit the EC Chairperson or designee to present evidence and witnesses in support of his or her decision. The Council shall consider the matters alleged in the complaint; the matters raised in defense as well as other relevant facts, ethical principles, and federal or state law, if applicable. The Council may question the parties concerned and determine ethical issues arising from the factual matters in the case even if those specific ethical issues were not raised by the Complainant. The Council also may choose to apply Principles or other language from the Code not originally identified by the EC. The Council may affirm the decision of the EC or reverse or modify it if it finds that the decision was clearly erroneous or a material departure from its written procedure.

5.2. Parties—The parties to a Council Hearing are the Respondent and the EC Chairperson.

5.3. Criteria and Process for Selection of Council Members

5.3.1. Criteria

5.3.1.1. Association Administrative Standard Operating Procedures (SOP) and Association Policy 2.6 shall be considered in the selection of qualified potential candidates for the Council, which shall be composed of qualified individuals and Association members drawn from a pool of candidates who meet the criteria outlined below. Members ideally will have some knowledge or experience in the areas of activity that are at issue in the case. They also will have experience in disciplinary hearings and/or general knowledge about ethics as demonstrated by education, presentations, and/or publications.

5.3.1.2. No conflict of interest may exist with either the Complainant or the Respondent (refer to Association Policy A.13—Conflict of Interest for guidance).

5.3.1.3. No individual may serve on the Council who is currently a member of the EC or the Board of Directors

5.3.1.4. No individual may serve on the Council who has previously been the subject of an ethics complaint that resulted in a public EC disciplinary action within the past three (3) years.

5.3.1.5. The public member on the Council shall have knowledge of the profession and ethical issues.

5.3.1.6. The public member shall not be an occupational therapist or occupational therapy assistant (practitioner, educator, or researcher.)

5.4. Criteria and Process for Selection of Council Chairperson

5.4.1. Criteria

5.4.1.1. Must have experience in analyzing/reviewing cases.

5.4.1.2. May be selected from the pool of candidates for the Council or a former EC member who has been off the EC for at least three (3) years.

5.4.1.3. The EC Chairperson shall not serve as the Council Chairperson.

5.4.2. Process

5.4.2.1. The Representative Assembly (RA) Speaker (in consultation with EC Staff Liaison) will select the Council Chairperson.

5.4.2.2. IIf the RA Speaker needs to be recused from this duty, the RA Vice Speaker will select the Council Chairperson.

5.5. Process

5.5.1. Potential candidates for the Council pool will be recruited through public postings in official publications and via the electronic forums. Association leadership will be encouraged to recruit qualified candidates. Potential members of the Council shall be interviewed to ascertain the following:

    a. Willingness to serve on the Council and availability for a period of three (3) years and

    b. Qualifications per criteria outlined in Section 5.3.1.

5.5.2. The President and EC Staff Liaison will maintain a pool of no fewer than six (6) and no more than twelve (12) qualified individuals.

5.5.3. The President, with input from the EC Staff Liaison, will select from the pool the members of each Council within thirty (30) days of notification by a Respondent that a Council is being requested.

5.5.4. Each Council shall be composed of three (3) Association members in good standing and a public member.

5.5.5. The EC Staff Liaison will remove anyone with a potential conflict of interest in a particular case from the potential Council pool.

5.6. Notification of Parties (EC Chairperson, Complainant, Respondent, Council Members)

5.6.1. The EC Staff Liaison shall schedule a hearing date in coordination with the Council Chairperson.

5.6.2. The Council (via the EC Staff Liaison) shall notify all parties at least forty-five (45) days prior to the hearing of the date, time, and place.

5.6.3. Case material will be sent to all parties and the Council members by national delivery service or mail with signature required and/or proof of date received.

5.7. Hearing Witnesses, Materials, and Evidence

5.7.1. Within thirty (30) days of notification of the hearing, the Respondent shall submit to the Council a written response to the decision and sanction, including a detailed statement as to the reasons that he or she is appealing the decision and a list of potential witnesses (if any) with a statement indicating the subject matter they will be addressing.

5.7.2. The Complainant before the Council also will submit a list of potential witnesses (if any) to the Council with a statement indicating the subject matter they will be addressing. Only under limited circumstances may the Council consider additional material evidence from the Respondent or the Complainant not presented or available prior to the issuance of their proposed sanction. Such new or additional evidence may be considered by the Council if the Council is satisfied that the Respondent or the Complainant has demonstrated the new evidence was previously unavailable and provided it is submitted to all parties in writing no later than fifteen (15) days prior to the hearing.

5.7.3. The Council Chairperson may permit testimony by conference call (at no expense to the participant), limit participation of witnesses in order to curtail repetitive testimony, or prescribe other reasonable arrangements or limitations.

The Respondent may elect to appear (at Respondent's own expense) and present testimony. If alternative technology options are available for the hearing, the Respondent, Council members, and EC Chairperson shall be so informed when the hearing arrangements are sent.

5.8. Counsel—The Respondent may be represented by legal counsel at his or her own expense. Association Legal Counsel shall advise and represent the Association at the hearing. Association Legal Counsel also may advise the Council regarding procedural matters to ensure fairness to all parties. All parties and the Association Legal Counsel (at the request of the EC or the Council) shall have the opportunity to question witnesses.

5.9. Hearing

5.9.1. The Council hearing shall be recorded by a professional transcription service or telephone recording transcribed for Council members and shall be limited to two (2) hours.

5.9.2. The Council Chairperson will conduct the hearing and does not vote.

5.9.3. Each person present shall be identified for the record, and the Council Chairperson will describe the procedures for the Council hearing. An oral affirmation of truthfulness will be requested from each participant who gives factual testimony in the Council hearing.

5.9.4. The Council Chairperson shall allow for questions.

5.9.5. The EC Chairperson shall present the ethics complaint, a summary of the evidence resulting from the investigation, and the EC decision and disciplinary action imposed against the Respondent.

5.9.6. The Respondent may present a defense to the decision and sanction after the EC presents its case.

5.9.7. Each party and/or his or her legal representative shall have the opportunity to call witnesses to present testimony and to question any witnesses including the EC Chairperson or his or her designee. The Council Chairperson shall be entitled to provide reasonable limits on the extent of any witnesses' testimony or any questioning.

5.9.8. The Council Chairperson may recess the hearing at any time.

5.9.9. The Council Chairperson shall call for final statements from each party before concluding the hearing.

5.9.10. Decisions of the Council will be by majority vote.

5.10. Disciplinary Council Decision

5.10.1. An official copy of the transcript shall be sent to each Council member, the EC Chairperson, the Association Legal Counsel, the EC Staff Liaison, and the Respondent and his or her counsel as soon as it is available from the transcription company.

5.10.2. The Council Chairperson shall work with the EC Staff Liaison and the Association Legal Counsel in preparing the text of the final decision.

5.10.3. The Council shall issue a decision in writing to the Association ED within thirty (30) days of receiving the written transcription of the hearing (unless special circumstances warrant additional time). The Council decision shall be based on the record and evidence presented and may affirm, modify, or reverse the decision of the EC, including increasing or decreasing the level of sanction or determining that no disciplinary action is warranted.

5.11. Action, Notification, and Timeline Adjustments

5.11.1. A copy of the Council's official decision and appeal process (Section 6) is sent to the Respondent, the EC Chairperson, and other appropriate parties within fifteen (15) business days via mail (with signature and proof of date received) after notification of the Association ED.

5.11.2. The time limits specified in the *Enforcement Procedures for the Occupational Therapy Code of Ethics* may be extended by mutual consent of the Respondent, Complainant, and Council Chairperson for good cause by the Chairperson.

5.11.3. Other features of the preceding *Enforcement Procedures* may be adjusted in particular cases in light of extraordinary circumstances, consistent with fundamental fairness.

5.12. Appeal—Within thirty (30) days after notification of the Council's decision, a Respondent upon whom a sanction was imposed may appeal the decision as provided in Section 6. Within thirty (30) days after notification of the Council's decision, the EC also may appeal the decision as provided in Section 6. If no appeal is filed within that time, the Association ED or EC Staff Liaison shall publish the decision in accordance with these procedures and make any other notifications deemed necessary.

6. Appeal Process

6.1. Appeals—Either the EC or the Respondent may appeal. Appeals shall be written, signed by the appealing party, and sent by mail requiring signature and proof of date of receipt to the Association ED in care of the Association Ethics Office. The grounds for the appeal shall be fully explained in this document. When an appeal is requested, the other party will be notified.

6.2. Grounds for Appeal—Appeals shall generally address only the issues, procedures, or sanctions that are part of the record before the Council. However, in the interest of fairness, the Appeal Panel may consider newly available evidence relating to the original complaint only under extraordinary circumstances.

6.3. Composition and Leadership of Appeal Panel—The Vice-President, Secretary, and Treasurer shall constitute the Appeal Panel. In the event of vacancies in these positions or the existence of a conflict of interest, the Vice President shall appoint replacements drawn from among the other Board of Directors members. If the entire Board has a conflict of interest, the Board Appeal process (Attachment C of EC SOP) shall be followed. The President shall not serve on the Appeal Panel. No individual may serve on the Council who has previously been the subject of an ethics complaint that resulted in a specific EC disciplinary action.

The Appeal Panel Chairperson will be selected by its members from among themselves.

6.4. Appeal Process—The Association ED shall forward any letter of appeal to the Appeal Panel within fifteen (15) business days of receipt. Within thirty (30) days after the Appeal Panel receives the appeal, the Panel shall determine whether a hearing is warranted. If the Panel decides that a hearing is warranted, timely notice for such hearing shall

be given to the parties. Participants at the hearing shall be limited to the Respondent and legal counsel (if so desired), the EC Chairperson, the Council Chairperson, the Association Legal Counsel, or others approved in advance by the Appeal Panel as necessary to the proceedings.

6.5. Decision

6.5.1. The Appeal Panel shall have the power to (a) affirm the decision; (b) modify the decision; or (c) reverse or remand to the EC, but only if there were procedural errors materially prejudicial to the outcome of the proceeding or if the Council decision was against the clear weight of the evidence.

6.5.2. Within thirty (30) days after receipt of the appeal if no hearing was granted, or within thirty (30) days after receipt of the transcript of an Appeal hearing if held, the Appeal Panel shall notify the Association ED of its decision. The Association ED shall promptly notify the Respondent, the original Complainant, appropriate Association bodies, and any other parties deemed appropriate (e.g., SRB, NBCOT®). For Association purposes, the decision of the Appeal Panel shall be final.

7. Notifications

All notifications referred to in these *Enforcement Procedures* shall be in writing and shall be delivered by national delivery service or mail with signature and proof of date received.

8. Records and Reports

At the completion of the enforcement process, the written records and reports that state the initial basis for the complaint, material evidence, and the disposition of the complaint shall be retained in the Association Ethics Office for a period of five (5) years.

9. Publication

Final decisions will be publicized only after any appeal process has been completed.

10. Modification

The Association reserves the right to (a) modify the time periods, procedures, or application of these *Enforcement Procedures* for good cause consistent with fundamental fairness in a given case and (b) modify its *Code* and/or these *Enforcement Procedures,* with such modifications to be applied only prospectively.

Adopted by the Representative Assembly 2015Nov-CO13 as Attachment A of the Standard Operating Procedures (SOP) of the Ethics Commission.

Reviewed by BPPC 1/04, 1/05, 9/06, 1/07, 9/09, 9/11, 9/13, 9/15

Adopted by RA 4/96, 5/04, 5/05, 11/06, 4/07, 11/09, 12/13

Revised by SEC 4/98, 4/00, 1/02, 1/04, 12/04, 9/06

Revised by EC 12/06, 2/07, 8/09, 9/13, 9/15

This document replaces the 2014 document *Enforcement Procedures for the Occupational Therapy Code of Ethics and Ethics Standards,* previously published and copyrighted in 2014 by the American Occupational Therapy Association in the *American Journal of Occupational Therapy, 68*(Suppl. 3), S3–S15. http://dx.doi.org/10.5014/ajot.2014.686S02

AMERICAN OCCUPATIONAL THERAPY ASSOCIATION
ETHICS COMMISSION

Formal Complaint of Alleged Violation of the
Occupational Therapy Code of Ethics

If an investigation is deemed necessary, a copy of this form will be provided to the individual against whom the complaint is filed.

Date: _____

Complainant: (Information regarding individual filing the complaint)

NAME: _____   SIGNATURE: _____

ADDRESS: _____   TELEPHONE: _____

_____   EMAIL ADDRESS: _____

Respondent: (Information regarding individual against whom the complaint is directed)

NAME: _____   SIGNATURE: _____

ADDRESS: _____   TELEPHONE: _____

_____   EMAIL ADDRESS: _____

1. **Summarize** in a written attachment the **facts and circumstances, including dates and events,** that support a violation of the *Occupational Therapy Code of Ethics* and this complaint. Include steps, if any, that have been taken to resolve this complaint before filing.

2. **Please sign and date all documents you have written and are submitting.** *Do not include confidential documents such as patient or employment records.*

3. **If you have filed a complaint about this same matter with any other agency (e.g., NBCOT®; SRB; academic institution; any federal, state, or local official), indicate to whom it was submitted, the approximate date(s) and resolution if known.**

I certify that the statements/information within this complaint are correct and truthful to the best of my knowledge and are submitted in good faith, not for resolution of private business, legal, or other disputes for which other appropriate forums exist.

_____

Signature

Send completed form, with accompanying documentation, **IN AN ENVELOPE MARKED** *CONFIDENTIAL* **to**

Ethics Commission
American Occupational Therapy Association, Inc.
Attn: Ethics Program Manager/Ethics Office
4720 Montgomery Lane, Suite 200
Bethesda, MD 20814-3449

OR email all material in pdf format to
ethics@aota.org with "Complaint" in subject line

Office Use Only:
Membership Verified?   ❏ Yes   ❏ No
By: _____

Chapter 53.

PROMOTING ETHICALLY SOUND PRACTICES IN OCCUPATIONAL THERAPY FIELDWORK EDUCATION

American Occupational Therapy Association

An Advisory Opinion for the AOTA Ethics Commission

Occupational therapy education, at both the professional and the technical level, helps shape and ensure the future of the profession. Toward this end, occupational therapists and occupational therapy assistants may assume roles in academic settings as faculty or academic fieldwork coordinators (AFWCs) or fieldwork educators (FWEs), sometimes also known as *clinical instructors (CIs)*. Practitioners in these roles aim to provide students with an educational experience culminating in their graduation as competent and ethical practitioners.

This dynamic triad (i.e., faculty/AFWCs, FWEs, students) works together to produce the next generation of occupational therapy practitioners. Faculty design and implement curricular-based programs to facilitate student development of knowledge, skills, values, and behaviors necessary for entry-level practice. FWEs complement the academic portion of students' education by providing them with an opportunity to observe, apply, and practice academic-based knowledge and skills in a "real-life" clinical setting.

During fieldwork, students develop and must demonstrate knowledge, skills, and professional behaviors at progressively higher levels of responsibility (American Occupational Therapy Association [AOTA], 2009). Throughout the educational process, faculty, AFWCs, FWEs, and students are responsible for maintaining high standards of ethical conduct.

Academic Fieldwork Coordinator and Fieldwork Educator Responsibilities

The *AFWC* is an individual employed by educational institutions to implement the fieldwork education program. This individual is responsible for the program's compliance with Accreditation Council for Occupational Therapy Education (ACOTE®) standards related to fieldwork education. An *FWE* is a clinician who agrees to supervise students' fieldwork experiences. AFWCs collaborate with FWEs to develop fieldwork education objectives and experiences and to make sure that student supervision is effective and ensures the safety and well-being of all stakeholders (ACOTE, 2012).

Ethical Issues in AFWC and FWE Roles

AFWCs and FWEs meet professional responsibilities related to their multiple roles while at the same time negotiating demands stemming from current societal trends and health care delivery environments. Cost containment measures, diminishing reimbursement, and expectations for higher staff productivity levels are pressuring clinicians to do more with fewer resources (Hanson, 2011; Weinstein & Nesbitt, 2007). Contemporary business-oriented health care practice environments can affect the development and implementation of fieldwork education programs in various ways (Barton et al., 2013; Thomas et al., 2007; see Case Scenario 53.1).

AFWCs

ACOTE (2012) accreditation standards direct AFWCs to develop and place fieldwork students at clinical sites that will provide them with an appropriate fieldwork experience. These standards include, but are not limited to, ensuring that

- Settings meet curricular goals and provide experiences related to the academic program,
- Supervisors are adequately prepared and can effectively meet students' learning needs,
- Fieldwork experiences promote ethical practice and develop professionalism, and
- Supervision processes protect consumers and provide for appropriate role modeling.

However, AFWCs are increasingly challenged to meet these expectations. Multiple demands on their time lead to FWEs taking fewer students (Vogl, Grice, Hill, & Moody, 2004), thus diminishing the availability of fieldwork clinical sites.

Dilemmas can arise for AFWCs who are ethically obligated to meet these standards yet may be tempted to place students in suboptimal clinical settings in order to provide enough sites for everyone in the class. Applying sound critical reasoning and professional judgment will determine whether a clinical site can provide appropriate and positive

fieldwork experiences that meet ACOTE standards. In situations in which this is not the case, AFWCs must demonstrate moral courage by refraining from placing students at such clinical sites or by removing them when it becomes evident that the site no longer is providing appropriate educational experiences or meeting the learning needs of students.

FWEs

FWEs are ethically obligated to provide appropriate supervision despite challenges created by current practice demands, including having less time allocated to this responsibility (Casares et al., 2003). With a primary duty to their clients, FWEs must simultaneously balance their own daily clinical work demands with responsibilities for student supervision. Of utmost importance is FWEs' responsibility to ensure the safety and well-being of their clients. Doing so requires FWEs to honestly appraise students' capabilities to be certain they are competent to provide safe and effective interventions.

Honest appraisals may lead to the determination that some students do not meet competency standards and thus should fail their fieldwork rotation. FWEs may struggle with the decision as to whether to fail a student. FWEs may believe that a student who successfully completes the academic portion of his or her education should be able to demonstrate the competency level needed to pass fieldwork. Unfortunately, this is not always the case. It is possible for a student to successfully meet academic standards yet not be able to competently apply his or her academic knowledge in a real-life practice setting. When this occurs, FWEs have an ethical obligation to accurately and objectively appraise a student's abilities and draw on their moral courage in making a determination that a student should fail his or her fieldwork rotation.

Ethical fieldwork student supervision requires transparent, clear, and open verbal and written communication. FWEs should provide ongoing and objective feedback to students to keep them informed of their progress or of areas that require improvement. In addition, precise documentation related to supervisory activities will enable the supervisor to more fairly evaluate student performance and ultimately support the final evaluation. These strategies should prevent student misunderstanding related to the performance evaluation and ultimately to the evaluation grade. In situations in which a student is struggling to meet fieldwork expectations, the FWE should initiate

Case Scenario 53.1

Fieldwork Educator and Coordinator Ethical Considerations: Sara, Julie, and Michael

Sara is an occupational therapist and fieldwork educator (FWE) who works on a well-known orthopedic unit of a large medical center. Julie, an academic fieldwork coordinator (AFWC) at a local university, contacted Sara at the last minute and asked her to accept a Level II student whose fieldwork site had canceled his rotation. Sara, who was very busy, hurriedly agreed to supervise the student with the stipulation that he had successfully completed course requirements related to physical agent modalities (PAMs), as student use of PAMs is legal in this state, and PAMs are widely used on the unit. Julie quickly assured Sara that Michael did meet course objectives related to PAMs.

During the first weeks of his rotation, Michael quickly adapted to the demands of the facility. At a meeting to discuss his progress, Sara gave Michael positive feedback about his performance and told him she felt he was ready to assume his own caseload. Michael told Sara that he was enjoying this rotation and hoped to work at this facility. As they were leaving the meeting, Sara casually said to Michael, "Julie told me that you successfully met course objectives related to PAMs; this is good, because as you know, we do a lot of PAMs here," Michael smiled and nodded his head as Sara walked away.

However, Michael failed to inform Sara that he did not actually have any training in applying hot packs because the equipment used by his academic program was broken the semester they covered PAMs. He decided not to tell Sara because he was afraid of appearing incompetent.

The next week, Michael received a physician's referral to treat Mrs. Brown, an elderly woman who had had rotator cuff surgery. The referral directed the occupational therapist to increase shoulder range of motion using hot packs as indicated in preparation for occupation-based activities involving shoulder motion. After completing an initial evaluation, Michael placed hot packs on Mrs. Brown's shoulder and proceeded to document his evaluation findings. After a while, Mrs. Brown began to cry and told Michael that the hot packs were hurting her. When he removed the packs, Michael saw a red burn on Mrs. Brown's shoulder.

Because student use of PAMs is not legal in all states, AFWCs, FWEs, and students should always be knowledgeable about state licensure regulations to ensure that duties assigned to students are in compliance with state law. As previously noted, Sara was able to have Michael apply the hot packs, as it was aligned with regulations in that state's licensure law. However, violation of several ethical principles led to Mrs. Brown's highly preventable burn injury.

First, Sara was ultimately responsible for protecting Mrs. Brown from harm (Principle 2A, Nonmaleficence). Michael was neither trained nor competent in administering thermal agent modalities (Principle 1E, Beneficence), and it was Sara's responsibility to provide appropriate supervision and personally verify his level of competency before allowing him to apply the hot packs (Principles 5G and 5H, Procedural Justice). In keeping with client safety as her primary duty, Sara should have administered the hot packs to Mrs. Brown. Furthermore, the parties involved should have openly and honestly represented Michael's lack of training in PAMs. Julie violated Principle 6B (Veracity) by misrepresenting Michael's training and competency. Michael violated the same principle when his failure to communicate his lack of training misled Sara into believing that he was competent. Open, honest communication, along with meeting ethical responsibilities related to protecting client safety and effective student supervision, could have prevented Mrs. Brown's painful injury and the potential liability that resulted from it.

prompt communication with the AFWC. FWEs and AFWCs should maintain ongoing, clear, and open communication about student performance issues. Doing so will keep a student who is struggling informed of his or her progress toward passing the fieldwork rotation and minimize feelings that he or she has been treated unfairly.

FWEs, as supervisors, are also responsible for ensuring that students are provided with an appropriate and effective educational experience. As part of the educational experience, FWEs should serve as exemplary role models by adhering to high standards of ethical and professional behaviors. In addition, FWEs must ensure that students function according to their role expectations. For example, students should not be expected to perform as if they are substitutes for regular employees in order to address staff shortages or demands for high productivity. Similarly, occupational therapy assistants who are completing fieldwork as part of their educational requirements to become occupational therapists should function in the role of an occupational therapy–level fieldwork student and not be expected to perform assistant-level job responsibilities.

With an increase in the number of laddering programs for occupational therapy assistants, it may be tempting to meet staffing needs by having an occupational therapist Level II fieldwork student who is an occupational therapy assistant provide assistant-level intervention services. Doing so, however, denies the occupational therapy student his or her rights to an appropriate fieldwork education experience.

Another area of ethical concern relates to billing and reimbursement for services provided by fieldwork students. FWEs are responsible for ensuring that billing for such services meets local, state, federal, and payer standards and regulations. Furthermore, billing for services provided by fieldwork students must accurately reflect who provided the services and the actual services provided. Doing otherwise constitutes insurance fraud.

Application of Ethical Principles

Principle 1. Beneficence

Several principles of the *Occupational Therapy Code of Ethics and Ethics Standards (2010)* (Code and Ethics Standards; AOTA, 2010) guide the ethical conduct of AFWCs and FWEs. Principle 1, Beneficence, requires taking action toward the good of others (AOTA, 2010). For AFWCs and FWEs, doing this good could mean educating students about the Code and Ethics Standards, including procedures for reporting unresolved issues (Principle 1K). Furthermore, AFWCs and FWEs whose conduct is consistent with high standards of ethical behavior serve as role models and provide a valuable influence on students' professional socialization.

Principle 1 also directs those providing occupational therapy education and training to do so within their area of expertise and level of competency (Principle 1J). Through ongoing professional development activities, AFWCs and FWEs develop knowledge and skills related to best practice in fieldwork education. For example, an FWE could develop and document expertise by participating in continuing education such as an AOTA-sponsored Fieldwork Educator's Certificate Workshop.

Principle 2. Nonmaleficence

A primary responsibility related to Principle 2, Nonmaleficence (AOTA, 2010) requires protecting service recipients and students (among others) from harm (Principle 2A). AFWCs and FWEs have a duty to make sure students are competent in providing safe and effective interventions to ensure both client and student safety. Principle 2 also directs those working with students to establish and maintain professional boundaries to avoid harming or exploiting them. Students may be vulnerable to exploitation due to the inherent power imbalance created by AFWCs' and FWEs' advanced experience and evaluative responsibilities (Estes & Brandt, 2011; Pettifor, McCarron, Schoepp, Stark, & Stewart, 2011). AFWCs and FWEs should avoid conflicts of interest with students by refraining from forming friendships with them via online social networking sites (Estes & Brandt, 2010).

Principle 3. Autonomy and Confidentiality

Principle 3, Autonomy and Confidentiality (AOTA, 2010), promotes transparent and meaningful communication with students. AFWCs and FWEs should fully inform students about both programmatic and facility or organizational policies and procedures related to their progression through and retention in fieldwork (Principle 3D). According to Principle 3G, AFWCs and FWEs are ethically bound to "ensure that confidentiality and the right to privacy are respected and maintained regarding all information obtained about… students…. Laws and regulations may require disclosure to appropriate authorities without consent" (AOTA, 2010, p. S21).

Two federal statutes provide boundaries for sharing information from students' academic records— the Health Insurance Portability and Accountability Act (HIPAA; 1996) and the Family Educational Rights and Privacy Act (FERPA; 1974). Specifically, the HIPAA privacy rule requires that an individual provide written permission for others to share his or her protected health information. Thus, to comply with HIPAA regulations, an AFWC may not share information about a student's health or disability status with a fieldwork site without the student's written permission.

FERPA protects the privacy of information contained in students' academic records. Generally, students ages 18 years or older must give permission for academic personnel to share information contained in the students' academic records.

However, FERPA does allow sharing of information without students' permission between academic officials with legitimate educational interests. According to FERPA,

> An educational agency or institution may disclose personally identifiable information from an academic record of a student without the consent required... if the disclosure meets one or more of the following conditions: (1) (i) (A) The disclosure is to other school officials, including teachers, within the agency or institution whom the agency or institution has determined to have legitimate educational interests. (B) A contractor, consultant, volunteer, or other party to whom an agency or institution has outsourced institutional services or functions may be considered a school official. (FERPA, 1974)

Thus, AFWCs and FWEs may legally share information contained in students' academic records (without students' permission) with those who have legitimate educational interests, including those under contractual agreement with a university. (Additional information about FERPA can be accessed at www .ed.gov/policy/gen/guid/fpco/ferpa.)

AFWCs and FWEs must balance the legal boundaries afforded by FERPA with their ethical responsibilities. Before sharing information from a student's academic records without the student's permission, AFWCs and FWEs should determine that sharing the information will be in the student's best interest. That is, the goal of sharing information should be to support a student's success in fieldwork. It is unethical to share information not relevant to a student's fieldwork experience that could negatively bias relevant parties toward that student. It is ethical to share only information that is relevant to

promoting a student's successful completion of his or her fieldwork experience. For example, an AFWC may choose to share with an FWE that, on the basis of a particular student's academic performance, he or she may need initial support in developing strategies to successfully manage multiple demands of a fast-paced environment in a timely manner. On the other hand, it would be unethical for an AFWC to share with a student's FWE that the student had to repeat several courses in order to attain the minimum GPA required for retention in the occupational therapy program. Doing so could send the message that the student's academic performance was poor, leading the FWE to expect that the student will perform poorly in fieldwork.

AFWCs and FWEs who are unsure as to whether sharing students' academic information is within legal or ethical boundaries should seek university or facility legal counsel. In the event that legal counsel is not available, they should err on the side of caution and not share the information.

Principle 5. Procedural Justice

Complying with the broad spectrum of laws, institutional policies, and AOTA documents applicable to occupational therapy practice is mandated by Principle 5, Procedural Justice (AOTA, 2010). AFWCs and FWEs should model professional and ethical behavior for students by adhering to the Code and Ethics Standards (Principle 5A), resolving conflicts between institutional policies and ethical practice (Principle 5B), holding appropriate state or national credentials (Principle 5E), maintaining continuing competence (Principle 5F), advocating for employees with disabilities (Principle 5M), and assisting in facility policy development to promote ethical compliance (Principle 5N) (AOTA, 2010). Specifically related to student supervision, FWEs are ethically bound to provide appropriate and effective supervision to students, consistent with all sources of laws, rules, regulations, policies, standards, and guidelines (Principles 5G and 5H), especially those related to billing and reimbursement [Principle 5O] (AOTA, 2010).

Principle 6. Veracity

AFWCs and FWEs are ethically bound to be truthful in fulfilling all aspects of their professional duties.

Principle 6, Veracity (AOTA, 2010), provides the means for establishing trusting relationships. Related to fieldwork education, this translates to accurately representing student competencies (Principle 6A); avoiding any form of communication that is false, fraudulent, or unfair (Principle 6B); accurately recording and reporting information in a timely manner (Principle 6C); and being accurate, honest, fair, and respectful when reporting information about student performance (Principle 6H; AOTA, 2010). To these ends, AFWCs and FWEs should maintain accurate and timely documentation of activities and interactions related to student fieldwork performance and supervision.

Student Responsibilities

Students are expected to work under the direction of their supervisors to meet fieldwork expectations at progressively increasing levels of responsibility.

They are to adhere to the same legal and ethical standards expected of occupational therapy practitioners in meeting client intervention duties and other responsibilities while on fieldwork (see Case Scenario 53.2).

In addition, some principles of the Code and Ethics Standards are particularly pertinent to the student role. Like clinicians, students have a primary duty to protect the safety and well-being of their clients. Doing so requires students to be transparent in communicating with their clients and supervisors. Specifically, students have a duty to divulge their status as students to their clients.

Protecting the safety and well-being of clients also might require students to share concerns about their own levels of competence and confidence with their supervisors. This is especially important for students who are asked to provide interventions for which they may not feel adequately prepared or have the competence to provide. Finally, students can promote clients' well-being and update therapists at the

---

Case Scenario 53.2

Fieldwork Student Ethical Considerations: Abby, Maxine, and Gail

Abby is in the 8th week of her second occupational therapy Level II fieldwork rotation at a large, university-based hospital. She did so well at her first rotation that they offered her a position. She has also done well on this rotation, receiving a glowing midterm evaluation from Gail, her supervisor. Abby, however, does not share the same positive assessment about the supervision she is receiving from Gail. It seems that Gail is rarely around when Abby has questions about her clients, and Abby has the impression that Gail leaves early, especially on Fridays.

On a particularly busy Friday afternoon, Gail approached Abby, asking her to pick up 3 clients that Gail could not treat that day. Gail shared that she was going out of town for the weekend with her boyfriend and wanted to leave early to get ready. On her way out the door, Gail added, "And, can you please document treatment notes in the charts of the 3 clients I saw this morning? I jotted down what I did with each one; just write them as if you did the treatments, sign your name, and I will co-sign on Monday when I return. Have a great weekend!" Abby, shocked by what Gail asked her to do, immediately called Maxine, her academic fieldwork coordinator, and asked her what she should do.

Abby is right to be concerned about what Gail asked her to do and to seek advice from Maxine. In doing this, Abby is adhering to Principle 2I (Nonmaleficence) of the Code and Ethics Standards in that she exercised professional judgment in response to an administrative directive that could cause harm to clients. In general, Gail is not meeting her ethical responsibility to provide appropriate supervision to Abby, thus violating Principle 5H (Procedural Justice) of the Code and Ethics Standards. Specifically, Gail's directive asked Abby to violate not only ethical but legal standards.

Of major concern is that Gail asked Abby to produce fraudulent documentation that the facility will submit to a third party for reimbursement and thus constitutes insurance fraud. Doing so would violate several ethical principles, particularly those under Principle 6 (Veracity) of the Code and Ethics Standards. Specifically, Abby's documentation of Gail's intervention sessions is in violation of Principles 6B (participating in written communication that contains false and fraudulent statements) and 6D (submitting fraudulent documentation).

Abby's course of action deems her to be well on her way to becoming an ethical occupational therapist.

facility by sharing evidence-based practice resources related to clinical interventions they have learned about in their recent academic studies.

Students also need to protect clients' privacy and confidentiality. They may find themselves in a position of sharing their fieldwork experiences with faculty or classmates in the context of teaching–learning environments. This sharing could be in the form of classroom discussions, written assignments, or virtual discussion boards. In all of these situations, students must discern what, if any, information they can communicate about clients, and how to do that to maintain compliance with HIPAA regulations. Students must protect client privacy and confidentiality and be respectful in the information they share about their supervisor and the clinical site and its employees (Estes & Brandt, 2011). Students should not share information related to their fieldwork experiences through online social networking sites (e.g., Facebook, LinkedIn).

Students also have duties related to promoting ethical practice during their fieldwork experiences. This requires that they be knowledgeable about the Code and Ethics Standards as well as policies and procedures for handling concerns about situations or issues that may challenge those Principles. Like practitioners, students are expected to "discourage, prevent, expose, and correct any breaches of the Code and Ethics Standards, and report any breaches of the former to appropriate authorities" (Principle 7C; AOTA, 2010, p. S25). Students who find themselves in this difficult situation should promptly discuss their concerns with their AFWC to minimize the chance of unpleasant consequences later in the fieldwork rotation. The AFWC can assist the student by helping him or her analyze the situation to define the issues, explore potential strategies, and determine the most appropriate course of action.

The AFWC and student should maintain an ongoing communication throughout the situation so that the AFWC can continue to advise and support the student. While communicating concerns about a possible breach of the Code and Ethics Standards, students must represent the situation in an honest, fair, objective, and respectful manner.

Ethical Issues for Students

Meeting these ethical responsibilities may not always be easy for students. Fieldwork can be a stressful experience for many students as they transition from academic learning to real-life application of theory and techniques in clinical settings. Findings of a study exploring ethical tensions encountered by occupational therapy fieldwork students indicated that students' experiences were generally ethical in nature but also described four areas of concern (Kinsella, Park, Appiagyei, Chang, & Chow, 2008). Students struggled with systemic restraints (e.g., lack of time or appropriate assessment tools), conflicting values (e.g., among practitioners, clients, team members, other students), witnessing questionable behaviors by practitioners (e.g., disrespectful attitudes, inappropriate language, breach of confidentiality), and experiences related to students themselves failing to speak up (e.g., advocating for clients, responding assertively when witnessing unethical behavior).

The power differential between students and AFWCs, FWEs, or clinicians may dissuade students from meeting their ethical obligations. This issue may create fear of repercussions such as not being taken seriously, retribution in the form of delaying completion of or failing their fieldwork rotation, being labeled a troublemaker, or limiting future job opportunities.

A final issue some students face relates to whether or not they should disclose to AFWCs or FWEs that they have a nonevident disability (Estes & Brandt, 2011). Statutory law (e.g., ADA, 1990; FERPA, 1976; HIPAA, 1996) protects the confidentiality of students' disability status, leaving to students the decision of whether to share this information with fieldwork sites (Estes & Brandt, 2011). Students who would like to receive accommodations for a qualified disability are responsible for initiating a request for the accommodations and providing supporting documentation. Students who choose not to share this information must understand that they will not receive accommodations for which they may otherwise be qualified for under the ADA. More important, though, students who choose not to share this information must ensure that they are able to provide safe and effective client interventions without accommodations (Estes & Brandt, 2011).

Strategies for Meeting Ethical Responsibilities

Several strategies may help students meet their ethical responsibilities when dealing with difficult fieldwork situations. Students must first pay attention to situations in which their moral sensitivity (Kirsch, 2009) produces feelings of discomfort in reaction to events that may have ethical ramifications. For example, a student who witnesses a supervisor complaining about his or her patients to a colleague in a crowded elevator will likely have a "gut feeling" that the supervisor's behavior is inappropriate. When feelings such as this occur, students should discuss the situation with their AFWC, who can help them analyze the situation, define inherent issues, and develop strategies for effectively dealing with it. Such strategies may include a student discussing the situation with his or her supervisor (or other relevant players such as another team member), either alone or with the AFWC present.

Students should approach such discussions in a professional manner, being sure to communicate their concerns in an honest, objective, and respectful manner. Citing relevant policies, guidelines, regulations, or statutes in support of his or her concerns can strengthen a student's position. With ongoing guidance from the AFWC, a student can better navigate difficult situations in ways that minimize the chance of negative consequences while maintaining ethical obligations.

Summary and Conclusion

Fieldwork education is a critical component of educating competent and ethical practitioners. As such, key stakeholders (i.e., AFWCs, FWEs, students) must work to ensure the ethical development and implementation of fieldwork education programs that meet professional standards for developing knowledge and skills as well as appropriate professional, ethical conduct. The *Occupational Therapy Code of Ethics and Ethics Standards (2010)* (AOTA, 2010) provides guidance for promoting ethically sound fieldwork education experiences.

Of primary concern for all of the stakeholders is protecting the safety and well-being of clients served. Beyond this, AFWCs and FWEs are responsible for adhering to the multiple sources of guidelines, standards, regulations, and legal statutes related to fieldwork education. They are also responsible for demonstrating high standards of ethical and professional conduct in their communications and actions, especially because doing so provides positive role modeling for students. Meeting these standards may be challenging given the nature of the current health care environment.

Students, too, must be held to the same ethical standards during their fieldwork experiences. However, an inherent power imbalance in the supervisory relationship may result in student vulnerability and lead to unique ethical challenges for them. In successfully navigating these ethical challenges, AFWCs, FWEs, and students work together to generate competent and caring occupational therapy practitioners of the future.

References

Accreditation Council for Occupational Therapy Education. (2012). 2011 Accreditation Council for Occupational Therapy Education (ACOTE®) standards. *American Journal of Occupational Therapy, 66*(6 Suppl.), S6–S74. http://dx.doi.org/10.5014/ajot.2012.66S6

Aiken, F., Menaker, L., & Barsky, L. (2001). Fieldwork education: The future of occupational therapy depends on it. *Occupational Therapy International, 8*(2), 86–95. http://dx.doi.org/10.1002/oti.135

American Occupational Therapy Association. (2009). Occupational therapy fieldwork education: Value and purpose. *American Journal of Occupational Therapy, 63*(6), 821–822. http://dx.doi.org/10.5014/ajot.63.6.821

American Occupational Therapy Association. (2010). Occupational Therapy Code of Ethics and Ethics Standards (2010). *American Journal of Occupational Therapy, 64*(6 Suppl.), S17–S26. http://dx.doi.org/10.5014/ajot.2010.64S17

Americans With Disabilities Act of 1990, Pub L. No. 101-336, 101 Stat. 327.

Barton, R., Corban, A., Herrrli-Warner, L., McClain, E., Riehle, D., & Tinner, E. (2013). Role strain in occupational therapy fieldwork educators. *Work, 44*, 317–328. http://dx.doi.org/10.3233/WOR-121508

Casares, G.S., Bradley, K.P., Jaffe, L.E., & Lee G.P. (2003). Impact of the changing health care environment on fieldwork education. *Journal of Allied Health, 32*, 246–251.

Estes, J., & Brandt, L. C. (2010). On-line social networking: Advisory opinion. In D. Slater (Ed.), *Reference guide to Occupational Therapy Code of Ethics and Ethics Standards (2010)* (pp. 213–217). Bethesda, MD: AOTA Press.

Estes, J., & Brandt, L. C. (2011). Navigating fieldwork's ethical challenges. *OT Practice, 16*(7), 7–15.

Family Educational Rights and Privacy Act, 20 U.S.C. §1232g, 34 CFR Part 99 (1974).

Friedland, J., Polatajko, H., & Gage, M. (2001). Expanding the boundaries of occupational therapy practice through student fieldwork experiences: Description of a provincially-funded community development project. *Canadian Journal of Occupational Therapy, 68*(5), 301–309.

Hanson, D. J. (2011). The perspectives of fieldwork educators regarding level II fieldwork students. *Occupational Therapy in Health Care, 25*(2–3), 164–177. http://dx.doi.org/10.3109/07380577.2011.561420

Health Insurance Portability and Accountability Act of 1996, Pub. L. No. 104-191, §2, 110 Stat. 1936.

Kinsella, E. A., Park, A. J., Appiagyei, J., Chang, E., & Chow, D. (2008). Through the eyes of students: Ethical tensions in occupational therapy practice. *Canadian Journal of Occupational Therapy, 75*(3), 176–183.

Kirsch, N. R. (2009). Ethical decision-making: Application of a problem-solving model. *Topics in Geriatric Rehabilitation, 25*(4), 285–291.

Pettifor, J., McCarron, M. C. E., Schoepp, G., Stark, C., & Stewart, D. (2011). Ethical supervision in teaching, research, practice, and administration. *Canadian Psychology, 52*(3), 198–205. http://dx.doi.org/10.1037/a0024549

Thomas, Y., Dickson, D., Broadbridge, J., Hopper, L., Hawkins, R., Edwards, A., & McBryde, C. (2007). Benefits and challenges of supervising occupational therapy fieldwork students: Supervisors' perspectives. *Australian Occupational Therapy Journal, 54,* S2–S12. http://dx.doi.org/10.1111/j.1440-1630.2007.00694.x

Vogl, K. A., Grice, K. O., Hill, S., & Moody, J. (2004). Supervisor and student expectations of level II fieldwork. *Occupational Therapy in Health Care, 18*(1/2), 5–19. http://dx.doi.org/10.1080/J003v18n01_02

Weinstein, M., & Nesbitt, J. (2007). Ethics in health care: Implications for education and practice. *Home Health Care Management and Practice, 19*(2), 112–117. http://dx.doi.org/10.1177/1084822306294453

Joanne Estes, MS, OTR/L

Education Representative, Ethics Commission (2009–2012, 2012–2015)

The author acknowledges the contributions of Rachel Clark, Emily Freytag, Kellie Tekulve, and Stephanie Vorherr to this paper.

Part 10.

CONTINUING COMPETENCY

OVERVIEW OF PART 10

Donna Costa, DHS, OTR/L, FAOTA

Students and practitioners are constantly being told they need to be lifelong learners—and for good reason. The field of occupational therapy, as is the case for all health professions, is advancing at a rapid rate thanks to new developments in science and medicine. All practitioners must keep abreast of new developments in clinical practice to provide the best evidence-based care to patients and clients.

The same is true in the fields of professional education and fieldwork education. It is not enough to graduate from an occupational therapy program, pass the National Board for Certification in Occupational Therapy (NBCOT®) exam, and get a job. Fieldwork educators must continue to meet continuing competency requirements by taking continuing education courses, returning to school, or reading professional journals. Therefore, continued competence as it applies to fieldwork education is addressed in Part 10. Chapter 54, "Continuing Competency as a Fieldwork Educator," discusses ways that fieldwork educators can maintain their knowledge and skills, some of which can lead to earning continuing education units (CEUs) that can be used toward state licensure. Chapter 55, "NBCOT® and Continuing Competency," discusses NBCOT requirements to maintain OTR or COTA credentials. In addition, it discusses several fieldwork-related activities that count toward the professional development units (PDUs) needed for recertification—fieldwork educators can fulfill their professional responsibilities by supervising fieldwork students and earn CEUs and PDUs in the process.

Just as constant developments occur in areas of clinical practice, changes constantly occur in academic and clinical education. Part of the commitment to being a fieldwork educator means maintaining competence in the role. Fieldwork educators can take the American Occupational Therapy Fieldwork Educator Certificate Program Workshop, read books and articles related to fieldwork education, become involved with a local fieldwork consortium, and attend fieldwork education workshops at state and local conferences. Not only will they benefit from the new knowledge and skills, but the students they supervise will benefit from this skillset.

Chapter 54.

CONTINUING COMPETENCY AS A FIELDWORK EDUCATOR

Donna Costa, DHS, OTR/L, FAOTA

In 2015, the occupational therapy profession reached a milestone: All 50 states now license the practice of occupational therapy. Each state's individual licensing board determines the elements of its state practice acts; these are statutes enacted by each state that define the scope of practice of occupational therapy within the state and outline licensing requirements. The Regulatory Affairs Division of the American Occupational Therapy Association (AOTA) maintains an up-to-date listing of the practice acts for each state, which you can find at http://bit.ly/1DL1LZb.

Practice Acts and Guidelines

Each state practice act includes a requirement for continuing competency, usually in the form of continuing education. In addition, most, but not all, states have requirements for continuing education. The AOTA website maintains an up-to-date listing of all states' continuing education requirements that you can find at http://bit.ly/1N48qAk.

According to AOTA (2003) continuing competence guidelines,

It is the responsibility of each licensee to design and implement his or her own strategy for developing and demonstrating continuing competence. Each licensee has current and/or anticipated roles and responsibilities that require specific knowledge, attitude, abilities, and skills. It is incumbent upon each licensee to examine his or her unique responsibilities, assess his or her continuing competence needs related to these responsibilities, and develop and implement a plan to meet those needs. (p. 9)

Fieldwork educators have no formal requirements for maintaining competence. The current Accreditation Council for Occupational Therapy Education (ACOTE®) standards state that for the Level II fieldwork experience, "the student is supervised by a currently licensed or otherwise regulated occupational therapist (or occupational therapy assistant for the occupational therapy assistant student) who has a minimum of 1 year full-time of practice experience subsequent to initial certification and who is adequately prepared to serve as a fieldwork educator" (ACOTE, 2012, p. S63). The standards do not define the meaning of "adequately prepared to serve as a fieldwork educator." Standard C.1.15 states that a mechanism must be in place to evaluate the effectiveness of supervision provided to fieldwork students and to provide resources for enhancing supervision (ACOTE, 2012). These resources include materials on supervisory skills, continuing education opportunities, and articles on theory and practice.

Continuing Education and Resources

Fieldwork educators who would like to advance their knowledge and skills in the area of student supervision and education should consider enrolling in the AOTA Fieldwork Educators Certificate Program workshop (see Chapter 69, "AOTA Fieldwork Educators Certificate Program Workshop"). During the workshop, participants complete the Self-Assessment of Fieldwork Educator Competency form (Chapter 27) to evaluate their strengths and weaknesses. This form also can be used to periodically assess fieldwork educator knowledge and skills and to devise a professional development plan (see p. 8 of the form) to support continued competency of fieldwork educators. Fieldwork educators list strengths, areas to develop, and competency areas to address with goal statements. The means to achieve professional development goals are listed as independent study, academic coursework, workshops and continuing education, student feedback, consultation with the academic fieldwork coordinator, presentations, publications, research activities, mentorship, peer review, and shared supervision of students.

A small but steady increase has occurred in the number of fieldwork education articles appearing in the occupational therapy literature, with several focused on research. Therefore, to enhance knowledge and skills of best practice in fieldwork education, groups of fieldwork educators could form, or fieldwork consortia could host, journal clubs to read, review, and discuss these articles.

Another resource for fieldwork educators to gain continuing competency is the *Specialized Knowledge and Skills of Occupational Therapy Educators of the Future* document (AOTA, 2009), which has replaced previous role competencies documents. The purpose of this document is to aid the creation of professional development plans for academic program directors, occupational therapy and occupational therapy assistant program faculty, academic fieldwork coordinators, and fieldwork educators. The document includes tables, each of which presents a desired attribute and lists competencies for the attribute at the novice, intermediate, and advanced level.

Conclusion

Because the goal of fieldwork education is to prepare students to become competent, entry-level occupational therapy practitioners, the onus is on fieldwork educators to provide the teaching, mentoring, role modeling, and supervision required to meet that goal. Just as the practice of occupational therapy is continually changing, the practice of fieldwork education is continually evolving. Continuing competency as a fieldwork educator should be taken just as seriously as that required for clinical practice.

References

Accreditation Council for Occupational Therapy Education. (2012). 2011 Accreditation Council for Occupational Therapy Education (ACOTE®) standards and interpretive guide. *American Journal of Occupational Therapy, 66*(Suppl.), S6–S74. http://dx.doi.org/10.5014/ajot.2012.66S6

American Occupational Therapy Association. (2003). *Model continuing competence guidelines for occupational therapists and occupational therapy assistants: A resource for state regulatory boards.* Bethesda, MD: Author.

American Occupational Therapy Association. (2009). Specialized knowledge and skills of occupational therapy educators of the future. *American Journal of Occupational Therapy, 63*, 804–818. http://dx.doi.org/10.5014/ajot.636.804

Chapter 55.

NBCOT® AND CONTINUING COMPETENCY

Donna Costa, DHS, OTR/L, FAOTA

The National Board for Certification of Occupational Therapy (NBCOT®) recognizes many types of professional activities that can count toward the number of professional development units (PDUs) needed for recertification (see www.nbcot.org for more information). For fieldwork supervision, the following three professional development categories can earn occupational therapy practitioners PDUs:

1. **Level I fieldwork direct supervision.** This must not be your primary work role. In other words, you must work for the agency as a direct provider of services seeing patients or clients. For each Level I student you supervise (occupational therapist or occupational therapy assistant), you can earn 1 PDU for each week of supervision, for a maximum of 18 units per 3-year certification period. You need to have a letter of verification or certificate from the occupational therapy or occupational therapy assistant academic program with the dates the supervision was provided and the student's name.

2. **Level II fieldwork direct supervision.** This cannot be your primary work role. For each Level II student you supervise (occupational therapist

or occupational therapy assistant), you can earn 1 PDU for each week of supervision you provide, for a maximum of 18 units per 3-year certification period. You need to obtain a letter of verification or certificate from the occupational therapy or occupational therapy assistant academic program that has the dates of the fieldwork assignment and the student's name. It is possible to get PDUs if you co-supervise a student, but you have to keep a record of the dates and times of the supervision you provided. It is possible to earn PDUs for supervising more than one student at a time, but you need to keep records of the dates and times you provided supervision.

3. **Entry-level or postdoctoral advanced fieldwork direct supervision.** This cannot be your primary work role. For each doctoral-level student you supervise, you can earn 1 PDU for each week of supervision you provide, up to a maximum of 18 units per 3-year certification period. A letter of verification or certificate from the school is required that lists the dates the supervision was provided and the student's name. As with the Level II fieldwork supervision, co-supervision is allowed; keep a record of dates and times when you provided the supervision.

Figure 55.1. Certificate for verification of fieldwork supervision.

Verification of Fieldwork Supervision

ID 26 rev020910

NBCOT® National Board for Certification in Occupational Therapy

Clinical Fieldwork Supervisor:

NBCOT Certification Number:

has provided the following fieldwork supervision:

Fieldwork Level: ☐ Level I ☐ Level II

Number of OTR Students Supervised:

Number of COTA Students Supervised:

Name of Facility:

Dates of Supervision:

Signature, Academic Fieldwork Coordinator

Print Name

Date

Reprinted with permission of the National Board for Certification in Occupational Therapy.

Occupational practitioners can earn PDUs for other professional development activities related to fieldwork education while also increasing their own competency as a fieldwork educator. Attending the 2-day American Occupational Therapy Association (AOTA) Fieldwork Educator Certificate Program gives participants 15 contact hours of continuing education—1.25 PDUs for each hour attended, for a total of 18.75 PDUs. Documentation of attendance is required from AOTA with the dates, time, attendee name, agenda, and indication of successful completion of the course. Reading professional journal articles about fieldwork or a book such as this one on fieldwork education provides 1 PDU for each two articles or two book chapters read. In this case, you would need to create an annotated bibliography and a report stating how the articles or book chapters have assisted you in improving skills in your role. Forms are available at www.nbcot.org.

Figure 55.1 is an example of the certificate that can be found on the NBCOT website at http://tinyurl.com/NBCOTfwcert and downloaded.

Part 11.

ASSESSMENT OF STUDENT COMPETENCIES

OVERVIEW OF PART 11

Donna Costa, DHS, OTR/L, FAOTA

During Level II fieldwork, students are guided toward the attainment of entry-level competencies. Part 11 covers the job of the fieldwork educator to formally and informally assess a student's progress toward meeting these competencies. Chapter 56, "Using the AOTA Fieldwork Performance Evaluation Forms," describes the current American Occupational Therapy Association Fieldwork Performance Evaluation (FWPE) forms for the occupational therapist and occupational therapy assistant student. The forms, found in Chapters 58 and 59, were designed to be used in a variety of practice settings.

However, to make the items on the FWPE forms more specific and objective, the fieldwork educator needs to write site-specific objectives for each of the items on the FWPE, which is addressed in Chapter 57, "The Importance of Site-Specific Objectives and Sample Objectives." For the FWPE forms to be a valid, objective measure of a student's level of competency, it is critical that fieldwork educators understand the intent of the forms, become familiar with item scoring, and recognize the importance of making each item measurable based on the specifics of the fieldwork site.

Chapter 56.

USING THE AOTA FIELDWORK PERFORMANCE EVALUATION FORMS

Donna Costa, DHS, OTR/L, FAOTA

The Fieldwork Performance Evaluation for the Occupational Therapy Student form (see Chapter 59; American Occupational Therapy Association [AOTA], 2002b) and the Fieldwork Performance Evaluation for the Occupational Therapy Assistant Student form (see Chapter 58; AOTA, 2002a) were developed and copyrighted by AOTA in 2002 and must be purchased from AOTA. At the time of publication of this book, the AOTA Commission on Education is working on new evaluation forms, and AOTA is investigating the possibility of making these forms available electronically.

These two documents were developed as companion documents for the profession and have identical formats. For fieldwork educators providing concurrent fieldwork opportunities to both occupational therapist and occupational therapy assistant students, having companion documents makes evaluating performance easier. The purpose of evaluating the student is to provide feedback on his or her entry-level competence in a particular practice setting (i.e., how this student measures up to what is expected of someone newly hired into an occupational therapist or occupational therapy assistant position in

this setting). The focus of the items in both forms is on occupation-based practice, and the forms were intended to be used in a wide variety of practice settings. If you are an academic fieldwork coordinator or new to the role of fieldwork educator, consider accessing AOTA's Inservice in a Box "Understanding the OT/OTA Fieldwork Performance Evaluations" (http://www.aota.org/education-careers/fieldwork/supervisor/inservice.aspx), which is available for free.

The cover page of the forms specifies important information relative to the fieldwork experience, including start and end dates of placement, number of hours completed, whether or not the student passed, fieldwork educator name, and spaces for signatures of both the fieldwork educator and student. The second page describes the purpose of the forms and has clearly described instructions for scoring to ensure that the fieldwork educator completes the forms accurately and avoids overinflating scores.

Performance items start on the third page of the forms (25 items for occupational therapy assistant students and 42 for occupational therapy students). Because they are companion documents, items on both forms are identical or similar in content. These items are presented in the order they occur in the occupational therapy process. Ethics and safety items are intentionally listed first to emphasize the importance of ensuring consumer safety. Every student must pass all items in this section to complete the fieldwork experience successfully. Space is provided for comments at the bottom of the cover page and at the end of each section. This space allows for inclusion of specific written examples to clarify the rating of the items and to give the student detailed information about performance areas of strength and those that require further development. The items are divided into categories on both forms, and the categories and the number of items in each one are listed in Exhibit 56.1.

Each performance item on the forms is graded on a 4-point scale, with 4 being the maximum score

(i.e., the student has demonstrated remarkable skill and capability beyond that of an entry-level practitioner in the setting or has exceeded the fieldwork site's expectations). However, it is critical that fieldwork educators understand the rating scale and use it as it is intended. A rating of 4 should be given only to the top 5% of students that the fieldwork educator has ever supervised. If this is the fieldwork educator's first student, he or she has no 5% reference. The understanding is that a score of 4 represents exceptional performance and should be rarely given. The description for each score on the 4-point scale is listed in Exhibit 56.2.

The forms' seventh page, the Performance Rating Summary Sheet, provides an "at-a-glance" numerical overview of the student's performance for each item at midterm and final evaluations. This sheet can be helpful in identifying possible patterns in student

Exhibit 56.1. *Performance Item Categories and Numbers*

Occupational Therapist Student Form Category (number of items)	Occupational Therapy Assistant Student Form Category (number of items)
Fundamentals of practice (3)	Fundamentals of practice (3)
Basic tenets of occupational therapy (4)	Basic tenets of occupational therapy (3)
Evaluation and screening (10)	Evaluation and screening (5)
Intervention (9)	Intervention (6)
Communication (4)	Communication (2)
Professional behaviors (7)	Professional behaviors (6)
Management of services (5)	
Total 42	**Total** 25

Exhibit 56.2. *Performance Item Scoring*

Score	Description of Performance
4 = *exceeds standards*	Performance is highly skilled and self-initiated. This rating is rarely given and should represent the top 5% of all the students you have supervised.
3 = *meets standards*	Performance is consistent with entry-level practice. This rating is infrequently given at midterm and is a strong rating at final.
2 = *needs improvement*	Performance is progressing but still needs improvement for entry-level practice. This is a realistic rating of performance at midterm, and some ratings of 2 may be reasonable at final.
1 = *unsatisfactory*	Performance is below standards and requires development for entry-level practice. This rating is given when there is concern about performance.

scores and areas of strength or concern. Minimum passing scores, which are objective ratings of the student's competency, are listed at the bottom of the page. References used in the documents and definitions of the terms used in the documents are defined on the last page of the forms to ensure uniformity across fieldwork educators.

For the occupational therapy student, a midterm score of 90 and above indicates satisfactory performance, whereas a score of 89 and below indicates unsatisfactory performance. At the final evaluation, the occupational therapy student must have a score of 122 or above to earn a passing score; a score of 121 or below means the student did not pass.

For the occupational therapy assistant student, a midterm score of 54 or above indicates satisfactory performance, where as a score of 53 or below indicates unsatisfactory performance. At the final evaluation, the occupational therapy assistant student must earn a score of 70 or above to pass; a score of 69 or below means the student did not pass.

Note several important considerations in scoring these forms. First, every item must be scored. If a fieldwork educator finds that an item does not apply in his or her setting, it is the responsibility of the fieldwork educator to create an assignment or learning activity that will permit evaluation of that competency. Second, each score given must be in whole numbers; fractions are not permitted.

When completed, the forms are returned to the college or university, and it is the responsibility of the academic institution to issue the grade for academic credit on the student's transcripts. The fieldwork educator is making a recommendation to the academic institution whether or not to pass a student and certifies student performance for the academic program. It is the responsibility of the academic program to determine the pass criterion level, grade, and eligibility for graduation. In most cases, the academic program abides by the recommendation of the fieldwork educator, but it does have the prerogative to modify it when it is deemed necessary. Most colleges and universities use a pass or fail grading system for fieldwork experiences; however, some academic institutions convert the numerical scores into letter grades. Regardless, this knowledge should not influence the fieldwork educator in assigning numerical scores.

References

American Occupational Therapy Association. (2002a). *Fieldwork Performance Evaluation for the Occupational Therapy Assistant Student.* Bethesda, MD: Author.

American Occupational Therapy Association. (2002b). *Fieldwork Performance Evaluation for the Occupational Therapy Student.* Bethesda, MD: Author.

Chapter 57.

THE IMPORTANCE OF SITE-SPECIFIC OBJECTIVES AND SAMPLE OBJECTIVES

Donna Costa, DHS, OTR/L, FAOTA

The American Occupational Therapy Association (AOTA) Fieldwork Performance Evaluation (FWPE) forms for occupational therapy (see Chapter 59) and occupational therapy assistant (see Chapter 58) students were created in 2002 to objectively measure student performance during Level II fieldwork experiences across practice settings. However, to individualize them to their specific practice setting, fieldwork educators must create site-specific learning objectives for each of the items on the forms. These learning objectives are then used by the student and fieldwork educator to guide learning activities, assignments, case studies, and supervision throughout the fieldwork experience and to guide the midterm and final evaluation process.

Site-specific objectives are required to accurately measure entry-level competence in a particular practice setting. These objectives are essential because students must understand how each item on the FWPE form will be measured and what the expectations are for their performance to successfully complete the fieldwork experience. Atler (2003) notes that "developing site-specific objectives allows fieldwork educators to (a) identify the specific competencies that students must demonstrate to pass the fieldwork

rotation and (b) clarify how students will demonstrate competencies for objectives that may not be part of the daily activities in the setting" (p. 22). Site-specific objectives should be written in the same manner as patient or client treatment goals, using the RUMBA framework (Atler & Wimmer, 2003):

- *R.* Is the site-specific objective relevant to the practice setting, and is it something that is considered an essential entry-level skill for the practice setting?
- *U.* Is the site-specific objective understandable to the student?
- *M.* Is the site-specific objective measurable? Can the performance be measured?
- *B.* Is the site-specific objective behavioral? Can the objective be clearly observed?
- *A.* Is the site-specific objective achievable within the desired time frame, given the demands and resources of the site?

The first step in writing site-specific objectives is for the fieldwork educator to identify entry-level competencies for the fieldwork site. He or she can look at job descriptions for occupational therapy and occupational therapy assistant staff to start and then have a series of discussions with team members during which the following questions are asked:

- What is the domain of occupational therapy at your facility? What specific services, treatments, and programs does the occupational therapy department provide?
- What is the purpose of the occupational therapy evaluation process at your facility? What specific assessments are utilized?
- What intervention approaches do you utilize at your facility? What specific treatments, groups, and protocols are used?
- How would you describe safe and ethical practice at your facility? What specific safety precautions must staff adhere to?

Next, the fieldwork educator selects one item from the FWPE form and writes an objective using the RUMBA framework (Atler & Wimmer, 2003). He or she quantifies the item by adding the level of independence expected of the student and the frequency the student is expected to perform the tasks in the objective and then specifies the quality of performance expected. Some examples of objectives from Wimmer (2003) are

- FWPE (occupational therapy student; Item 16): "Establishes an accurate and appropriate plan based on evaluation results" (Atler & Wimmer, 2003, Slide 29).
  - *School setting.* Provides behavior-based measurable occupational therapy goals during the individualized education program (IEP) meeting that reflect the student's needs and priorities.
  - *Acute care hospital setting.* Develops within 24 hours after evaluation an intervention plan that is achievable during the client's length of stay.
- FWPE (occupational therapy student; Item 18): "Articulates a clear and logical rationale for the intervention process" (Wimmer, 2004, Slide 33).
  - *Mental health setting.* Clearly explains the rationale for the intervention activities selected using the Model of Human Occupation (Wimmer, 2004).
  - *School setting.* Clearly describes why a student requires pull-out occupational therapy

interventions versus classroom occupational therapy interventions (Wimmer, 2004).
  - *Rehab setting.* Discusses rationale of intervention choices using motor learning principles (Wimmer, 2004).
  - *Community setting.* Consistently explains to various team members and community agencies the purpose of community-based occupational therapy services in clearly understood language (Wimmer, 2004).
- FWPE (occupational therapy assistant student; Item 8): "Establishes service competency in assessment methods, including, but not limited to, interview, observations, assessment tools, and chart reviews within the context of the service delivery setting" (Wimmer, 2004, Slide 35).
  - *Mental health setting.* Accurately administers the Allen Cognitive Level Screen and a structured intake interview after establishment of service competency (Wimmer, 2004, Slide 35).
  - *Rehab setting.* Accurately completes the activities of daily living and mobility assessments using the Functional Independence Measure (Keith, Granger, Hamilton, & Sherwin, 1987) after establishment of service competency.
- FWPE (occupational therapy assistant student; Item 16): "Effectively interacts with clients to facilitate accomplishment of established goals" (Wimmer, 2004, Slide 38).
  - *Mental health setting:* Consistently maintains nonjudgmental, firm, consistent approach while conveying respect for the client.
  - *School setting:* Uses a variety of effective interaction styles during individual and group sessions to facilitate students' engagement in activities and progress toward IEP goals (Wimmer, 2004).
  - *Rehab setting:* Engages in effective "in the moment" interactions during intervention sessions to ensure safety and maximize functional outcomes of clients (Wimmer, 2004).

The AOTA website has numerous examples of site-specific objectives (see http://www.aota.org/Education-Careers/Fieldwork/SiteObj.aspx) written for the following settings: adult acute care, adult outpatient, adult rehab, early childhood intervention, geriatrics, mental health, pediatrics, physical disabilities, and school. It can be helpful to review these examples before writing objectives. In some cases, they may exactly describe a particular settings' entry-level competence; in others, they may need only a minor modification to fit the setting.

References

Atler, K. (2003). *Using the Fieldwork Performance Evaluations: The complete guide*. Bethesda, MD: AOTA Press.

Atler, K., & Wimmer, R. (2003). *Understanding the OT/OTA Fieldwork Performance Evaluations*. Retrieved from http:// www.aota.org/Education-Careers/Fieldwork/Supervisor/Inservice.aspx

Keith, R. A., Granger, C. V., Hamilton, B. B., & Sherwin, F. S. (1987). The Functional Independence Measure: A new tool for rehabilitation. *Advances in Clinical Rehabilitation, 1,* 6–18.

Wimmer, R. (2004). *Writing site-specific objectives for the FWPE forms*. Presentation at the 2004 AOTA Annual Conference in Mineapolis, MN. Available at http://www.aota.org/Education-Careers/Fieldwork/SiteObj.aspx

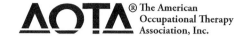® The American
Occupational Therapy
Association, Inc.

Chapter 58.

FIELDWORK PERFORMANCE EVALUATION FORM FOR THE OCCUPATIONAL THERAPY ASSISTANT STUDENT

American Occupational Therapy Association

MS./MR. _____

NAME: (LAST)   (FIRST)   (MIDDLE)

_____

COLLEGE OR UNIVERSITY

FIELDWORK SETTING:

_____

NAME OF ORGANIZATION/FACILITY

_____

ADDRESS: (STREET OR PO BOX)

_____

CITY   STATE   ZIP

_____

TYPE OF FIELDWORK

ORDER OF PLACEMENT: 1 2 3 4   OUT OF   1 2 3 4

FROM: _____ TO: _____
DATES OF PLACEMENT

_____

NUMBER OF HOURS COMPLETED

_____

FINAL SCORE

PASS: _____   NO PASS: _____

SUMMARY COMMENTS:
(ADDRESSES STUDENT'S CLINICAL COMPETENCE)

SIGNATURES:

I HAVE READ THIS REPORT.

_____

SIGNATURE OF STUDENT

_____

NUMBER OF PERSONS CONTRIBUTING TO THIS REPORT

_____

SIGNATURE OF RATER #1

_____

PRINT NAME/CREDENTIALS/POSITION

_____

SIGNATURE OF RATER #2 (IF APPLICABLE)

_____

PRINT NAME/CREDENTIALS/POSITION

This evaluation form is a revision of the 1983 American Occupational Therapy Association, Inc. (AOTA) Fieldwork Evaluation Form for the Occupational Therapy Assistant and was produced by a committee of the Commission on Education.

Purpose

The primary purpose of the Fieldwork Performance Evaluation for the Occupational Therapy Assistant Student is to measure entry-level competence of the occupational therapy assistant student. The evaluation is designed to differentiate the competent student from the incompetent student and is not designed to differentiate levels above entry-level competence. For further clarification on entry-level competency, refer to the Standards of Practice for Occupational Therapy (AOTA, 1998).

The evaluation is designed to measure the performance of the occupational therapy process and was not designed to measure the specific occupational therapy tasks in isolation. This evaluation reflects the 1998 Accreditation Council for Occupational Therapy Education Standards (ACOTE®, 1999) and the National Board for Certification in Occupational Therapy, Inc. Practice Analysis results (NBCOT®, 1997). In addition, this evaluation allows students to evaluate their own strengths and challenges in relation to their performance as an occupational therapy assistant.

Use of the Fieldwork Performance Evaluation for the Occupational therapy Student

The Fieldwork Performance Evaluation is intended to provide the student with an accurate assessment of his/her competence for entry-level practice. Both the student and fieldwork educator should recognize that growth occurs over time. **The midterm and final evaluation scores will reflect development of student competency and growth.** In order to effectively use this evaluation to assess student competence, site-specific objectives need to be developed. Utilize this evaluation as a framework to assist in ensuring that all key performance areas are reflected in the site-specific objectives.

Using this evaluation at midterm and final, it is suggested that the student complete a self-evaluation of his/her own performance. During the midterm review process, the student and fieldwork educator should collaboratively develop a plan, that would enable the student to achieve entry-level competence by the end of the fieldwork experience. This plan should include specific objectives and enabling activities to be used by the student and fieldwork educator in order to achieve the desired competence.

The Fieldwork Educator must contact the Academic Fieldwork Coordinator when: (1) a student exhibits unsatisfactory behavior in a substantial number of tasks or (2) a student's potential for achieving entry-level competence by the end of the affiliation is in question.

Directions for Rating Student Performance

- There are 25 performance items.
- Every item must be scored, using the 1- to 4-point rating scale (see below).
- **The rating scales should be carefully studied prior to using this evaluation.** Definitions of the scales are given at the top of each page.
- Circle the number that corresponds to the description that best describes the student's performance.
- **The ratings for the Ethics and Safety items must be scored at 3 or above on the final evaluation for the student to pass the fieldwork experience.** If the ratings are below 3, continue to complete the Fieldwork Performance Evaluation to provide feedback to the student on her/his performance.
- Record midterm and final ratings on the Performance Rating Summary Sheet.
- Compare overall midterm and final score to the scale below.

Overall Midterm Score

Satisfactory Performance .... 54 and above

Unsatisfactory Performance .... 53 and below

Overall Final Score

Pass .... 70 points and above

No Pass .... 69 points and below

Rating Scale for Student Performance

4—**Exceeds Standards:** Performance is highly skilled and self-initiated. This rating is **rarely given** and **would represent the top 5% of all the students** you have supervised.

3—**Meets Standards:** Performance is consistent with **entry-level** practice. This rating is **infrequently given at midterm** and is a **strong rating at final.**

2—**Needs Improvement:** Performance **is progressing but** still needs improvement for entry-level practice. This is a **realistic rating of performance at midterm,** and some ratings of 2 may be reasonable at the final.

1—**Unsatisfactory:** Performance is **below standards** and requires development for entry-level practice. This rating is given when **there is a concern about performance.**

I. Fundamentals of Practice

All items in this area must be scored at a #3 or above on the final evaluation in order to pass fieldwork.

1. **Ethics:** Adheres consistently to the American Occupational Therapy Association Code of Ethics (AOTA, 2000) and site's policies and procedures.

   Midterm   1   2   3   4
   Final   1   2   3   4

2. **Safety:** Adheres consistently to safety regulations. Anticipates potentially hazardous situations and takes steps to prevent accidents.

   Midterm   1   2   3   4
   Final   1   2   3   4

3. **Safety:** Uses sound judgment in regard to safety of self and others during all fieldwork-related activities.

   Midterm   1   2   3   4
   Final   1   2   3   4

Comments on strengths and areas for improvement:
- **Midterm**

- **Final**

II. Basic Tenets of Occupational Therapy

4. **Occupational Therapy Philosophy:** Clearly communicates the values and beliefs of occupational therapy, highlighting the use of occupation to clients, families, significant others, and service providers.

   Midterm   1   2   3   4
   Final   1   2   3   4

5. **Occupational Therapist/Occupational Therapy Assistant Roles:** Communicates the roles of the occupational therapist and occupational therapy assistant to clients, families, significant others, and service providers.

   Midterm   1   2   3   4
   Final   1   2   3   4

6. **Evidence-Based Practice:** Makes informed practice decisions based on published research and relevant informational resources.

   Midterm   1   2   3   4
   Final   1   2   3   4

Comments on strengths and areas for improvement:
- **Midterm**

- **Final**

III. Evaluation/Screening

(Includes daily evaluation of interventions)

7. **Gathers Data:** Under the supervision of and in cooperation with the occupational therapist or occupational therapy assistant, accurately gathers relevant information regarding a client's occupations of self-care, productivity, leisure, and the factors that support and hinder occupational performance.

   Midterm   1   2   3   4
   Final   1   2   3   4

8. **Administers Assessments:** Establishes service competency in assessment methods, including but not limited to interviews, observations, assessment tools, and chart reviews within the context of the service delivery setting.

   Midterm   1   2   3   4
   Final   1   2   3   4

9. **Interprets:** Assists with interpreting assessments in relation to the client's performance and goals in collaboration with the occupational therapist.

   Midterm   1   2   3   4
   Final   1   2   3   4

10. **Reports:** Reports results accurately in a clear, concise manner that reflects the client's status and goals.

    Midterm   1   2   3   4
    Final   1   2   3   4

11. **Establish Goals:** Develops client-centered and occupation-based goals in collaboration with the occupational therapist.

    Midterm   1   2   3   4
    Final   1   2   3   4

Comments on strengths and areas for improvement:
- **Midterm**

- **Final**

IV. Intervention

12. **Plans Intervention:** In collaboration with the occupational therapist, establishes methods, duration, and frequency of interventions that are client-centered and occupation-based. Intervention plans reflect context of setting.

    Midterm   1   2   3   4
    Final   1   2   3   4

13. **Selects Intervention:** Selects and sequences relevant interventions that promote the client's ability to engage in occupations.

    Midterm   1   2   3   4
    Final   1   2   3   4

14. **Implements Intervention:** Implements occupation-based interventions effectively in collaboration with clients, families, significant others, and service providers.

    Midterm   1   2   3   4
    Final   1   2   3   4

15. **Activity Analysis:** Grades activities to motivate and challenge clients in order to facilitate progress.

    Midterm   1   2   3   4
    Final   1   2   3   4

16. **Therapeutic Use of Self:** Effectively interacts with clients to facilitate accomplishment of established goals.

    Midterm   1   2   3   4
    Final   1   2   3   4

17. **Modifies Intervention Plan:** Monitors the client's status in order to update, change, or terminate the intervention plan in collaboration with the occupational therapist.

    Midterm   1   2   3   4
    Final   1   2   3   4

Comments on strengths and areas for improvement:
- **Midterm**

- **Final**

V. Communication

18. **Verbal/Nonverbal Communication:** Clearly and effectively communicates verbally and non-verbally with clients, families, significant others, colleagues, service providers, and the public.

    Midterm   1   2   3   4

    Final   1   2   3   4

19. **Written Communication:** Produces clear and accurate documentation according to site requirements. All writing is legible, using proper spelling, punctuation, and grammar.

    Midterm   1   2   3   4

    Final   1   2   3   4

Comments on strengths and areas for improvement:

- **Midterm**

- **Final**

VI. Professional Behaviors

20. **Self-Responsibility:** Takes responsibility for attaining professional competence by seeking learning opportunities and interactions with supervisor(s) and others.

    Midterm   1   2   3   4

    Final   1   2   3   4

21. **Responds to Feedback:** Responds constructively to feedback.

    Midterm   1   2   3   4

    Final   1   2   3   4

22. **Work Behaviors:** Demonstrates consistent work behaviors including initiative, preparedness, dependability, and worksite maintenance.

    Midterm   1   2   3   4

    Final   1   2   3   4

23. **Time Management:** Demonstrates effective time management.

    Midterm   1   2   3   4

    Final   1   2   3   4

24. **Interpersonal Skills:** Demonstrates positive interpersonal skills, including but not limited to cooperation, flexibility, tact, and empathy.

    Midterm   1   2   3   4

    Final   1   2   3   4

25. **Cultural Competence:** Demonstrates respect for diversity factors of others, including but not limited to sociocultural, socioeconomic, spiritual, and lifestyle choices.

    Midterm   1   2   3   4

    Final   1   2   3   4

Comments on strengths and areas for improvement:
- **Midterm**

- **Final**

PERFORMANCE RATING SUMMARY SHEET

Performance Items	Midterm Ratings	Final Ratings
I. FUNDAMENTALS OF PRACTICE		
1. Ethics		
2. Safety (adheres)		
3. Safety (judgment)		
II. BASIC TENETS OF OCCUPATIONAL THERAPY		
4. OT philosophy		
5. OT/OTA roles		
6. Evidence-based practice		
III. EVALUATION/SCREENING (includes daily evaluation of interventions)		
7. Gathers data		
8. Administers assessments		
9. Interprets		
10. Reports		
11. Establishes goals		
IV. INTERVENTION		
12. Plans intervention		
13. Selects intervention		
14. Implements intervention		
15. Activity analysis		
16. Therapeutic use of self		
17. Modifies intervention plan		
V. COMMUNICATION		
18. Verbal/nonverbal communication		
19. Written communication		
VI. PROFESSIONAL BEHAVIORS		
20. Self-responsibility		
21. Responds to feedback		
22. Work behaviors		
23. Time management		
24. Interpersonal skills		
25. Cultural competence		
TOTAL SCORE		

MIDTERM:

Satisfactory Performance . . . . 54 and above

Unsatisfactory Performance . . . . 53 and below

FINAL:

Pass . . . . 70 points and above

No Pass . . . . 69 points and below

References

Accreditation Council for Occupational Therapy Education. (1999). Standards for an accredited educational program for the occupational therapy assistant. *American Journal of Occupational Therapy, 53,* 583–589. http://dx.doi.org/10.5014/ajot.53.6.583

American Occupational Therapy Association. (1993). Occupational therapy roles. *American Journal of Occupational Therapy, 47,* 1087–1099. http://dx.doi.org/10.5014/ajot.47.12.1087

American Occupational Therapy Association. (1998). Standards of practice for occupational therapy. *American Journal of Occupational Therapy, 52,* 866–869. http://dx.doi.org/10.5014/ajot.52.10.866

American Occupational Therapy Association. (2000). Occupational therapy code of ethics. (2000). *American Journal of Occupational Therapy, 54,* 614–616. http://dx.doi.org/10.5014/ajot.54.6.614

American Occupational Therapy Association. (2002). Occupational therapy practice framework: Domain and process. *American Journal of Occupational Therapy, 56,* 606–639. http://dx.doi.org/10.5014/ajot.56.6.606

Law, M. (2000). Evidence-based practice: What can it mean for me? *OT Practice,* 5(Aug 28), 16–17.

National Board for Certification in Occupational Therapy. (1997). *National Study of Occupational Therapy Practice, Executive Summary.* Gaithersburg, MD: Author.

Neistadt, M. E., & Crepeau, E. B. (1998). *Willard and Spackman's occupational therapy* (9th ed.). Philadelphia: Lippincott Williams & Wilkins.

Sackett, D. L., Richardson, W. S., Rosenberg, W., & Haynes, R. B. (1997). *Evidence-based medicine: How to practice and teach EBM.* New York: Churchill Livingstone.

Townsend, E. (Ed.). (1997). *Enabling occupation: An occupational therapy perspective.* Ottawa, Ontario: CAOT.

Code of Ethics: Refer to http://www.aota.org/about-occupational-therapy/ethics.aspx

Collaborate: To work together with a mutual sharing of thoughts and ideas (ACOTE, 1999)

Competency: Adequate skills and abilities to practice as an entry-level occupational therapist or occupational therapy assistant

Entry-Level Practice: Refer to AOTA, 1993

Evidence-Based Practice: "Conscientious, explicit, and judicious use of current best evidence in making decisions about the care of individual patients. The practice of evidence-based [health care] means integrating individual clinical expertise with the best available external clinical evidence from systematic research" (Law, 2000; Sackett, Richardson, Rosenberg, & Haynes, 1997, p. 2).

Occupation: Groups of activities and tasks of everyday life, named, organized, and given value and meaning by individuals and a culture; occupation is everything people do to occupy themselves, including looking after themselves (self-care), enjoying life (leisure), and contributing to the social and economic fabric of their communities (productivity); the domain of concern and the therapeutic medium of occupational therapy. (Townsend, 1997, p. 181).

Occupational Performance: The result of a dynamic, interwoven relationship between persons, environment, and occupation over a person's lifespan; the ability to choose, organize, and satisfactorily perform meaningful occupations that are culturally defined and age appropriate for looking after oneself, enjoying life, and contributing to the social and economic fabric of a community. (Townsend, 1997, p. 181).

Spiritual: (a context) The fundamental orientation of a person's life; that which inspires and motivates that individual. (AOTA, 2002)

Glossary

Activity Analysis: "A way of thinking used to understand activities, the performance components to do them, and the cultural meanings typically ascribed to them" (Neistadt & Crepeau, 1998, p. 135).

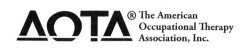® The American
Occupational Therapy
Association, Inc.

Chapter 59.

FIELDWORK PERFORMANCE EVALUATION FORM FOR THE OCCUPATIONAL THERAPY STUDENT

American Occupational Therapy Association

MS./MR. _____

NAME: (LAST)   (FIRST)   (MIDDLE)

_____

COLLEGE OR UNIVERSITY

FIELDWORK SETTING:

_____

NAME OF ORGANIZATION/FACILITY

_____

ADDRESS: (STREET OR PO BOX)

_____

CITY   STATE   ZIP

_____

TYPE OF FIELDWORK

ORDER OF PLACEMENT: 1 2 3 4 OUT OF 1 2 3 4

FROM: _____   TO: _____

DATES OF PLACEMENT

_____

NUMBER OF HOURS COMPLETED

FINAL SCORE

PASS: _____   **NO PASS:** _____

SUMMARY COMMENTS:
(ADDRESSES STUDENT'S CLINICAL COMPETENCE)

SIGNATURES:

I HAVE READ THIS REPORT.

_____

SIGNATURE OF STUDENT

_____

NUMBER OF PERSONS CONTRIBUTING TO THIS REPORT

_____

SIGNATURE OF RATER #1

_____

PRINT NAME/CREDENTIALS/POSITION

_____

SIGNATURE OF RATER #2 (IF APPLICABLE)

_____

PRINT NAME/CREDENTIALS/POSITION

This evaluation form is a revision of the 1987 American Occupational Therapy Association, Inc. (AOTA) Fieldwork Evaluation Form for the Occupational Therapist and was produced by a committee of the Commission on Education.

Purpose

The primary purpose of the Fieldwork Performance Evaluation for the Occupational Therapy Student is to measure entry-level competence of the occupational therapy student. The evaluation is designed to differentiate the competent student from the incompetent student and is not designed to differentiate levels above entry-level competence. For further clarification on entry-level competency, refer to the Standards of Practice for Occupational Therapy (AOTA, 1998).

The evaluation is designed to measure the performance of the occupational therapy process and was not designed to measure the specific occupational therapy tasks in isolation. This evaluation reflects the 1998 Accreditation Council for Occupational Therapy Education Standards (ACOTE®, 1999) and the National Board for Certification in Occupational Therapy, Inc. Practice Analysis results (NBCOT®, 1997). In addition, this evaluation allows students to evaluate their own strengths and challenges in relation to their performance as an occupational therapist.

Use of the Fieldwork Performance Evaluation for the Occupational Therapy Student

The Fieldwork Performance Evaluation is intended to provide the student with an accurate assessment of his/her competence for entry-level practice. Both the student and fieldwork educator should recognize that growth occurs over time. **The midterm and final evaluation scores will reflect development of student competency and growth.** In order to effectively use this evaluation to assess student competence, site-specific objectives need to be developed. Utilize this evaluation as a framework to assist in ensuring that all key performance areas are reflected in the site-specific objectives.

Using this evaluation at midterm and final, it is suggested that the student complete a self-evaluation of his/her own performance. During the midterm review process, the student and fieldwork educator should collaboratively develop a plan, which would enable the student to achieve entry-level competence by the end of the fieldwork experience. This plan should include specific objectives and enabling activities to be used by the student and fieldwork educator in order to achieve the desired competence.

The Fieldwork Educator must contact the Academic Fieldwork Coordinator when: (1) a student exhibits unsatisfactory behavior in a substantial number of tasks or (2) a student's potential for achieving entry-level competence by the end of the affiliation is in question.

Directions for Rating Student Performance

- There are 42 performance items.
- Every item must be scored, using the 1- to 4-point rating scale (see below).
- **The rating scales should be carefully studied prior to using this evaluation.** Definitions of the scales are given at the top of each page.
- Circle the number that corresponds to the description that best describes the student's performance.
- **The ratings for the Ethics and Safety items must be scored at 3 or above on the final evaluation for the student to pass the fieldwork experience.** If the ratings are below 3, continue to complete the Fieldwork Performance Evaluation to provide feedback to the student on her/his performance.
- Record midterm and final ratings on the Performance Rating Summary Sheet.
- Compare overall midterm and final score to the scale below.

Overall Midterm Score

Satisfactory Performance . . . . 90 and above
Unsatisfactory Performance . . . . 89 and below

Overall Final Score

Pass. . . . . 122 points and above
No Pass. . . . . 121 points and below

Rating Scale for Student Performance

4—**Exceeds Standards:** Performance is highly skilled and self-initiated. This rating is **rarely given** and **would represent the top 5% of all the students** you have supervised.

3—**Meets Standards:** Performance is consistent with **entry-level** practice. This rating is **infrequently given at midterm and is a strong rating at final.**

2—**Needs Improvement:** Performance **is progressing but** still needs improvement for entry-level practice. This is a **realistic rating of performance at midterm,** and some ratings of 2 may be reasonable at the final.

1—**Unsatisfactory:** Performance is **below standards** and requires development for entry-level practice. This rating is given when **there is a concern about performance.**

I. Fundamentals of Practice

All items in this area must be scored at a #3 or above on the final evaluation in order to pass fieldwork.

1. **Adheres to ethics:** Adheres consistently to the American Occupational Therapy Association Code of Ethics (AOTA, 2000) and site's policies and procedures including, when relevant, those related to human subject research.

Midterm	1	2	3	4
Final	1	2	3	4

2. **Adheres to safety regulations:** Adheres consistently to safety regulations. Anticipates potentially hazardous situations and takes steps to prevent accidents.

Midterm	1	2	3	4
Final	1	2	3	4

3. **Uses judgment in safety:** Uses sound judgment in regard to safety of self and others during all fieldwork-related activities.

Midterm	1	2	3	4
Final	1	2	3	4

Comments on strengths and areas for improvement:
• **Midterm**

• **Final**

II. Basic Tenets of Occupational Therapy

4. Clearly and confidently **articulates the values and beliefs** of the occupational therapy profession to clients, families, significant others, colleagues, service providers, and the public.

Midterm	1	2	3	4
Final	1	2	3	4

5. Clearly, confidently, and accurately **articulates the value of occupation** as a method and desired outcome of occupational therapy to clients, families, significant others, colleagues, service providers, and the public.

Midterm	1	2	3	4
Final	1	2	3	4

6. Clearly, confidently, and accurately **communicates the roles of the occupational therapist and occupational therapy assistant** to clients, families, significant others, colleagues, service providers, and the public.

Midterm	1	2	3	4
Final	1	2	3	4

7. **Collaborates with** client, family, and significant others throughout the occupational therapy process.

Midterm	1	2	3	4
Final	1	2	3	4

Comments on strengths and areas for improvement:

• **Midterm**

• **Final**

III. Evaluation/Screening:

8. **Articulates a clear and logical rationale** for the evaluation process.

Midterm	1	2	3	4
Final	1	2	3	4

9. **Selects relevant screening and assessment methods** while considering such factors as client's priorities, context(s), theories, and evidence-based practice.

Midterm	1	2	3	4
Final	1	2	3	4

10. **Determines client's occupational profile** and performance through appropriate assessment methods.

Midterm	1	2	3	4
Final	1	2	3	4

11. **Assesses client factors and context(s)** that support or hinder occupational performance.

Midterm	1	2	3	4
Final	1	2	3	4

12. **Obtains sufficient and necessary information** from relevant resources such as client, families, significant others, service providers, and records prior to and during the evaluation process.

Midterm	1	2	3	4
Final	1	2	3	4

13. **Administers assessments** in a uniform manner to ensure findings are valid and reliable.

Midterm	1	2	3	4
Final	1	2	3	4

14. **Adjusts/modifies the assessment procedures** based on client's needs, behaviors, and culture.

Midterm	1	2	3	4
Final	1	2	3	4

15. **Interprets evaluation results** to determine client's occupational performance strengths and challenges.

Midterm	1	2	3	4
Final	1	2	3	4

16. **Establishes an accurate and appropriate plan** based on the evaluation results, through integrating multiple factors such as client's priorities, context(s), theories, and evidence-based practice.

Midterm	1	2	3	4
Final	1	2	3	4

17. **Documents the results of the evaluation** process that demonstrates objective measurement of client's occupational performance.

Midterm	1	2	3	4
Final	1	2	3	4

Comments on strengths and areas for improvement:
• **Midterm**

• **Final**

IV. Intervention

18. **Articulates a clear and logical rationale** for the intervention process.

Midterm	1	2	3	4
Final	1	2	3	4

19. **Utilizes evidence** from published research and relevant resources to make informed intervention decisions.

Midterm	1	2	3	4
Final	1	2	3	4

20. **Chooses occupations** that motivate and challenge clients.

Midterm	1	2	3	4
Final	1	2	3	4

21. **Selects relevant occupations** to facilitate clients meeting established goals.

Midterm	1	2	3	4
Final	1	2	3	4

22. **Implements intervention plans that are client-centered.**

    Midterm   1   2   3   4
    Final   1   2   3   4

23. **Implements intervention plans that are occupation-based.**

    Midterm   1   2   3   4
    Final   1   2   3   4

24. **Modifies task approach, occupations, and the environment** to maximize client performance.

    Midterm   1   2   3   4
    Final   1   2   3   4

25. **Updates, modifies, or terminates the intervention plan** based upon careful monitoring of the client's status.

    Midterm   1   2   3   4
    Final   1   2   3   4

26. **Documents client's response** to services in a manner that demonstrates the efficacy of interventions.

    Midterm   1   2   3   4
    Final   1   2   3   4

Comments on strengths and areas for improvement:

• **Midterm**

• **Final**

V. Management of Occupational Therapy Services

27. **Demonstrates through practice or discussion the ability to assign** appropriate responsibilities to the occupational therapy assistant and occupational therapy aide.

    Midterm   1   2   3   4
    Final   1   2   3   4

28. **Demonstrates through practice or discussion the ability to actively collaborate** with the occupational therapy assistant.

    Midterm   1   2   3   4
    Final   1   2   3   4

29. **Demonstrates understanding of the costs and funding** related to occupational therapy services at this site.

    Midterm   1   2   3   4
    Final   1   2   3   4

30. **Accomplishes organizational goals** by establishing priorities, developing strategies, and meeting deadlines.

    Midterm   1   2   3   4
    Final   1   2   3   4

31. **Produces the volume of work** required in the expected time frame.

    Midterm   1   2   3   4
    Final   1   2   3   4

Comments on strengths and areas for improvement:

• **Midterm**

• **Final**

VI. Communication

32. **Clearly and effectively communicates verbally and nonverbally** with clients, families, significant others, colleagues, service providers, and the public.

    Midterm   1   2   3   4
    Final   1   2   3   4

33. **Produces clear and accurate documentation** according to site requirements.

    Midterm   1   2   3   4
    Final   1   2   3   4

34. All written communication is legible, using proper spelling, punctuation, and grammar.

Midterm	1	2	3	4
Final	1	2	3	4

35. Uses language appropriate to the recipient of the information, including but not limited to funding agencies and regulatory agencies.

Midterm	1	2	3	4
Final	1	2	3	4

Comments on strengths and areas for improvement:

• **Midterm**

• **Final**

VII. Professional Behaviors

36. Collaborates with supervisor(s) to maximize the learning experience.

Midterm	1	2	3	4
Final	1	2	3	4

37. Takes responsibility for attaining professional competence by seeking out learning opportunities and interactions with supervisor(s) and others.

Midterm	1	2	3	4
Final	1	2	3	4

38. Responds constructively to feedback.

Midterm	1	2	3	4
Final	1	2	3	4

39. Demonstrates consistent work behaviors including initiative, preparedness, dependability, and worksite maintenance.

Midterm	1	2	3	4
Final	1	2	3	4

40. Demonstrates effective time management.

Midterm	1	2	3	4
Final	1	2	3	4

41. Demonstrates positive interpersonal skills including but not limited to cooperation, flexibility, tact, and empathy.

Midterm	1	2	3	4
Final	1	2	3	4

42. Demonstrates respect for diversity factors of others including but not limited to socio-cultural, socioeconomic, spiritual, and lifestyle choices.

Midterm	1	2	3	4
Final	1	2	3	4

Comments on strengths and areas for improvement:

• **Midterm**

• **Final**

PERFORMANCE RATING SUMMARY SHEET

Performance Items	Midterm Ratings	Final Ratings
I. FUNDAMENTALS OF PRACTICE		
1. Adheres to ethics 2. Adheres to safety regulations 3. Uses judgment in safety		
II. BASIC TENETS OF OCCUPATIONAL THERAPY		
4. Articulates values and beliefs 5. Articulates value of occupation 6. Communicates role of occupational therapist 7. Collaborates with clients		
III. EVALUATION/SCREENING		
8. Articulates clear rationale for evaluation 9. Selects relevant methods 10. Determines occupational profile 11. Assesses client and contextual factors 12. Obtains sufficient and necessary information 13. Administers assessments 14. Adjusts/modifies assessment procedures 15. Interprets evaluation results 16. Establishes accurate plan 17. Documents results of evaluation		
IV. INTERVENTION		
18. Articulates clear rationale for intervention 19. Utilizes evidence to make informed decisions 20. Chooses occupations that motivate and challenge 21. Selects relevant occupations 22. Implements client-centered interventions 23. Implements occupation-based interventions 24. Modifies approach, occupation, and environment 25. Updates, modifies, or terminates intervention plan 26. Documents client's response		
V. MANAGEMENT OF OT SERVICES		
27. Demonstrates ability to assign through practice or discussion 28. Demonstrates ability to collaborate through practice or discussion 29. Understands costs and funding 30. Accomplishes organizational goals 31. Produces working expected time frame		
VI. COMMUNICATION		
32. Communicates verbally and nonverbally 33. Produces clear documentation 34. Written communication is legible 35. Uses language appropriate to recipient		

(Continued)

Performance Items	Midterm Ratings	Final Ratings
VII. PROFESSIONAL BEHAVIORS		
36. Collaborates with supervisor 37. Takes responsibility for professional competence 38. Responds constructively to feedback 39. Demonstrates consistent work behaviors 40. Demonstrates time management 41. Demonstrates positive interpersonal skills 42. Demonstrates respect for diversity		
TOTAL SCORE		

MIDTERM:

Satisfactory Performance . . . . .90 and above
Unsatisfactory Performance . . . . . . .89 and below

FINAL:

Pass. . . . . 122 points and above
No Pass. . . . . 121 points and below

References

Accreditation Council for Occupational Therapy Education. (1999). Standards for an accredited educational program for the occupational therapist. *American Journal of Occupational Therapy, 53,* 575–582. http://dx.doi.org/10.5014/ajot.53.6.5875

American Occupational Therapy Association. (1993). Occupational therapy roles. *American Journal of Occupational Therapy, 47,* 1087–1099. http://dx.doi.org/10.5014/ajot.47.12.1087

American Occupational Therapy Association. (1998). Standards of practice for occupational therapy. *American Journal of Occupational Therapy, 52,* 866–869. http://dx.doi.org/10.5014/ajot.52.10.866

American Occupational Therapy Association. (2000). Occupational therapy code of ethics (2000). *American Journal of Occupational Therapy, 54,* 614–616. http://dx.doi.org/10.5014/ajot.54.6.614

American Occupational Therapy Association. (2002). Occupational therapy practice framework: Domain and process. *American Journal of Occupational Therapy, 56,* 606–639. http://dx.doi.org/10.5014/ajot.56.6.606

American Occupational Therapy Association. (2004). Role competencies for an academic fieldwork coordinator (Roles document) (2003). *American Jarnal of occupational Therapy, 58,* 653-654. http://dx.doi.org/10.5014/ajot.58.6.653

Law, M. (2000). Evidence-based practice: What can it mean for me? *OT Practice, 5*(Aug 28), 16–17.

National Board for Certification in Occupational Therapy. (1997). *National Study of Occupational Therapy Practice, Executive Summary.*

Neistadt, M. E., & Crepeau, E. B. (1998). *Willard and Spackman's occupational therapy* (9th ed.). Philadelphia: Lippincott Williams & Wilkins.

Sackett, D. L., Richardson, W. S., Rosenberg, W., & Haynes, R. B. (1997). *Evidence-based medicine: How to practice and teach EBM.* New York: Churchill Livingstone.

Townsend, E. (Ed.). (1997). *Enabling occupation: An occupational therapy perspective.* Ottawa, Ontario: CAOT.

World Health Organization. (2001). *International classification of functioning, disability and health (ICF).* Geneva, Switzerland: Author.

Glossary

Client Factors: Those factors that reside within the client and that may affect performance in areas of occupation. Client factors include body functions and body structures (AOTA, 2002).

- Body functions (a client factor, including physical, cognitive, psychosocial aspects)—"the physiological function of body systems (including psychological functions)" (WHO, 2001, p. 10).
- Body structures—"anatomical parts of the body such as organs, limbs and their components [that support body function]" (WHO, 2001, p. 10).

Code of Ethics: Refer to http://www.aota.org/about-occupational-therapy/ethics.aspx

Collaborate: To work together with a mutual sharing of thoughts and ideas. (ACOTE Glossary)

Competency: Adequate skills and abilities to practice as an entry-level occupational therapist or occupational therapy assistant

Context: Refers to a variety of interrelated conditions within and surrounding the client that influence performance. Contexts include cultural, physical, social, personal, spiritual, temporal, and virtual (AOTA, 2002).

Efficacy: Having the desired influence or outcome (Neistadt & Crepeau, 1998).

Entry-Level Practice: Refer to "Occupational Therapy Roles" (AOTA, 2004).

Evidence-Based Practice: "Conscientious, explicit and judicious use of current best evidence in making decisions about the care of individual patients. The practice of evidence-based [health care] means integrating individual clinical expertise with the best available external clinical evidence from systematic research" (Law, 2000; Sackett, Richardson, Rosenberg, & Haynes, 1997, p. 2).

Occupation: Groups of activities and tasks of everyday life, named, organized, and given value and meaning by individuals and a culture; occupation is everything people do to occupy themselves, including looking after themselves (self-care), enjoying life (leisure), and contributing to the social and economic fabric of their communities (productivity); the domain of concern, and the therapeutic medium of occupational therapy (Townsend, 1997, p. 181).

Occupational Performance: The result of a dynamic, interwoven relationship between persons, environment, and occupation over a person's lifespan; the ability to choose, organize, and satisfactorily perform meaningful occupations that are culturally defined and age appropriate for looking after oneself, enjoying life, and contributing to the social and economic fabric of a community (Townsend, 1997, p. 181).

Occupational Profile: A profile that describes the client's occupational history, patterns of daily living, interests, values, and needs (AOTA, 2002).

Spiritual: (a context) The fundamental orientation of a person's life; that which inspires and motivates that individual (AOTA, 2002).

Theory: "An organized way of thinking about given phenomena. In occupational therapy the phenomenon of concern is occupational endeavor. Theory attempts to (1) define and explain the relationships between concepts or ideas related to the phenomenon of interest, (2) explain how these relationships can predict behavior or events, and (3) suggest ways that the phenomenon can be changed or controlled. Occupational therapy theory is concerned with four major concepts related to occupational endeavor: person, environment, health, and occupation" (Neistadt & Crepeau, 1998, p. 521).

Part 12.

CHALLENGING FIELDWORK SITUATIONS

OVERVIEW OF PART 12

Donna Costa, DHS, OTR/L, FAOTA

Fieldwork educators can expect that sometimes they will experience challenging fieldwork situations in the same way that they experience challenging patients. Part 12 addresses these challenging situations and suggests strategies to deal with them. Chapter 60, "Working With Marginal Students—Remediation or Failure?" focuses on marginal students who may be at risk of failing the fieldwork experience. Chapter 61, "The Challenges of Working With Advanced Students," focuses on working with advanced students who achieve entry-level competencies at an earlier stage than expected. Regardless of whether a student is average, advanced, or marginal, fieldwork educators must provide the just-right challenge to students throughout their Level I or II experience, which is the focus of Chapter 62, "Progression in Fieldwork Supervision—Providing the Just-Right Challenge."

Because more students with disabilities are entering academic programs, Chapter 63, "Working With Occupational Therapy and Occupational Therapy Assistant Students With Disabilities," discusses working with students with disabilities. Fieldwork educators need to know the laws and protections afforded to these students and how to maximize the learning environment for student success. Chapter 64 contains the "Advisory Opinion on Ethical Considerations for Professional Education of Students With Disabilities," which addresses ethical considerations for the professional education of students with disabilities.

Chapter 60.

WORKING WITH MARGINAL STUDENTS—REMEDIATION OR FAILURE?

Donna Costa, DHS, OTR/L, FAOTA

This chapter focuses on some strategies you can use with students often labelled as *marginal*, meaning that the student has been unable to achieve the benchmarks fieldwork educators have established toward entry-level competency. It is imperative that the fieldwork educator recognize the warning signs indicating unsatisfactory performance and notify the academic fieldwork coordinator (AFWC) as soon as possible so that action can be taken. There is nothing worse than an AFWC being notified for the first time that the student is in danger of failing the fieldwork experience in the final weeks of the fieldwork performance. Inherent in the job of being a fieldwork educator is being a gatekeeper for the profession, that is, ensuring that the students who complete Level II fieldwork have met or exceeded entry-level competencies.

Reasons Why Students Fail Fieldwork

The reasons why students are not successful during fieldwork can be divided into three categories: academic reasons, personal reasons, and supervisory reasons.

Academic Reasons

Academic reasons for failure can include any or all of the following: a weak knowledge base, difficulty with demonstration of clinical skills, underdeveloped clinical skills, a limited ability to engage in problem-solving strategies, slowness to learn, poor retention of material, and poor learning strategies. The strategies the fieldwork educator uses to help students in this situation are: help the student pinpoint the nature of the academic difficulty, support the student, ensure patient safety, document behaviors, identify areas of weakness, provide feedback to the student, and help the student learn skills and knowledge required for entry-level practice.

Personal Reasons

Personal reasons for failure tend to be the most commonly discussed in the literature (James & Musselman, 2005; Lew, Cara, & Richardson, 2007). The student may exhibit any or all of the following: poor insight; lack of motivation; a negative attitude toward the fieldwork educator, site, patients, or colleagues; a display of overconfidence or underconfidence; demonstration of impolite, angry, or rude behavior; ongoing occurrences of lateness or absence; inappropriate personal appearance (grooming, dress, or hygiene); argumentative interactions with the fieldwork educator; time management issues; failure to accept feedback from the fieldwork educator and then modify performance; disorganization; symptoms of anxiety or depression; manifestation of a learning disability; ineffective interpersonal skills; lack of insight into self; difficulty with viewing the "big picture"; and failure to take responsibility for own behavior.

Supervisory Reasons

Supervisory reasons for failure warrant the fieldwork educator taking stock of him- or herself and asking whether anything in the supervisory relationship is adversely affecting the student's performance. It has been repeatedly cited in the literature (Christie, Joyce, & Moeller, 1985; Costa, 2014; Kautzmann, 1990; Rodger et al., 2014) that the relationship between the fieldwork educator and the student is a critical element in the fieldwork experience. Some of the issues that may negatively affect a student's performance on fieldwork include the fieldwork educator using a teaching style that is rigid and does not adapt to the student's individual learning needs; expectations not being clearly articulated for the student's performance; not enough time spent observing the student's performance; insufficient role modeling, precluding the student from the opportunity to see ideal performance; a mismatch between the personalities of the student and the fieldwork educator; barriers in the fieldwork site such as not enough time for the student; insufficient orientation to the fieldwork site at the start of the assignment; and failure to provide feedback to the student on a regular basis from the beginning.

Using the American Occupational Therapy Association (AOTA) Fieldwork Education Assessment Tool (see Chapter 13; also available at http://tinyurl.com/FEATMidterm) is recommended as a way to assess how the fieldwork experience is progressing and what will emerge as the areas that need to be adapted to maximize student learning. Keeping accurate records on the student's performance from the start of fieldwork and updating them weekly is key to avoiding last-minute problems.

Possible Barriers to Identifying Warning Signs of Failure

McCreedy and Graham (1997) offered a list of some potential roadblocks that may occur during fieldwork. Sometimes fieldwork educators state that they do not know a student is failing until they write out the midterm or final evaluation. This situation is more likely to occur when two or more fieldwork educators oversee one student and do not communicate with each other. The result is that the student often gets caught in the middle. In addition, the primary fieldwork educator may have taken time off and the new supervisor is not aware of any problems. The student may have previously failed a fieldwork experience. This may result in his or her coming to the next Level II fieldwork experience with lowered self-confidence, increased stress, and an inability to stop using ineffective strategies (Gutman, McCreedy, & Heisler, 1998).

Other barriers include the fieldwork educator having limited or no experience with supervising students and the fieldwork site going through internal issues (e.g., preparing for accreditation, being sold to another health care organization). Additional issues may include expectations or learning objectives not in place at the start of the fieldwork experience and the fieldwork educator not wanting to hurt the student's feelings.

Strategies to Be Used With Marginal Students

Fieldwork educators can and should use numerous strategies when working with marginal students, such as

- *Keeping accurate supervision logs.* Each time you meet with a student, complete an entry that includes the date and time you met with the student and what was discussed. Keep copies of all documentation submitted by the student if discussed.
- *Writing weekly summaries of the student's progress.* Summaries provide an ongoing record of progress made, goals established, and other learning activities. A copy is given to the student so that he or she has written feedback on progress or lack thereof.

- *Involving the AFWC as soon as possible.* Involving the AFWC is critical and will provide both you and the student with additional supports. Contact the AFWC when you have concerns about student safety, patient safety, or the quality of the fieldwork experience.
- *Spelling out consequences for lack of progress.* The student needs to be made aware of what will happen if he or she fails to make progress toward the established learning goals. These are not idle threats; they are specific consequences for a student's behavior.
- *Creating a learning contract for the student.* A learning contract provides the student with specific learning objectives that must be met and target dates clearly established. Just as with writing a treatment plan for a patient or client, this document needs to be specific. It is not sufficient to write "Student will improve." The fieldwork educator needs to specify the behavior that needs improvement in quantifiable terms.

The learning contract for a student is similar to a treatment plan developed for a patient or client because it is developed collaboratively. The Self-Assessment for Fieldwork Educator Competency document (AOTA, 2009; Chapter 27) specifies that learning contracts are collaboratively developed to support the student's occupation-based fieldwork experience (with outcome-based measurable learning objectives). Learning contracts increase each student's responsibility for his or her own learning and specify what needs to be learned, the methods to be used to learn it, what evidence will be used to demonstrate acquired knowledge, and target dates. The learning contract is usually developed between the fieldwork educator and the student, but with a marginal student at risk for failing fieldwork, it is helpful for the AFWC also to be involved in developing the contract. All parties sign and keep a copy of the learning contract and put into place a plan to review it on a particular date. The steps involved in developing the learning contract with specific examples are listed in Exhibit 60.1.

Exhibit 60.1. Steps in Creating the Learning Contract

Outcome	Identify the learning outcome in specific terms (e.g., Student will complete initial evaluation report).
Measurement	Be specific about the details of each learning activity (e.g., The initial evaluation report will be completed within 24 hours of seeing a patient and with no more than 2 errors).
Resources	List the available resources the student could use in meeting each learning objective (e.g., Reading other initial evaluation reports. Talking with other therapists or students).
Process, Procedures, and Strategies	List the steps the student will take to meet the learning objective, such as • Become familiar with evaluation form by reviewing it and identifying source of information for each section. • Read initial evaluation documentation completed by other therapists. • Observe other therapists conducting evaluations and read their documentation. • Find a quiet environment for completing documentation.
Evidence of Learning	Specify what proof will be used to demonstrate that the student has achieved this learning objective (e.g., Initial evaluation report submitted to fieldwork educator within 24 hours of seeing patient).
Target Date	Identify the date by when this learning objective must be met. These are short-term goals and so the usual parameters are just a few days.
Initials	Ensure all parties involved (i.e., student, fieldwork educator, academic fieldwork coordinator) sign the learning contract and all receive copies of it.

Terminating a Placement

Despite the best efforts of fieldwork educators, AFWCs, and students, sometimes a student will fail to meet learning objectives and termination of the fieldwork experience needs to be initiated. This process is usually very difficult for all parties involved. Termination of a student should never come as a surprise to anyone because there should have been ongoing communication and learning contracts. The termination process has three steps: preparation, implementation, and follow-up.

Preparation

Contact the AFWC to discuss the decision to terminate, and submit any necessary documentation to the AFWC. Schedule a time when all parties can meet. Consider the timing of this carefully: It may be beneficial to schedule this first thing in the morning or at the end of the day. Make sure to schedule sufficient time to fully discuss all aspects of the termination. Find a place to hold the meeting that is free from distractions. Gather all copies of documentation you have related to the fieldwork experience. Talk with the AFWC about who will start speaking and what parts of the conversation you or the AFWC will lead. Consider who has the best relationship with the student; that is the person who should say the words "You have failed this Level II fieldwork experience."

Because this meeting is usually upsetting for all parties involved, you need to prepare yourself emotionally. There may be tears shed and other strong emotions expressed. When the termination meeting is about to start, it is important for the ground rules for the meeting to be communicated. State that everyone will have a chance to speak. Start with identifying the student's accomplishments and strengths. Then discuss the limitations in performance and how the student has not been able to achieve entry-level competencies. Following that, the AFWC should specify the consequences for termination of the placement. These consequences are specific to each academic program. The student may want to know what his or her grade will be and sometimes will ask whether it is possible to withdraw from the placement. The student is likely to have other

questions related to academic standing and what will happen in the future.

Implementation

Allow the student to leave in a way that preserves his or her dignity. The student may or may not want to say goodbye to staff, other students, or patients. Discuss in advance with the AFWC how this situation will be handled. If the student wants to make a quick exit, you may want to ask how he or she wants his or her departure explained to others.

Follow-up

What happens after the termination meeting is often critical to a successful outcome for the student. He or she has invested a great deal, emotionally, personally, and financially. A plan must be developed for the rest of the student's academic career and, again, must be specific to each student.

Policies are developed by each academic program that spell out these procedures in a student manual, generally given to students at the program orientation. Most academic programs allow for one Level II fieldwork failure, but generally a second termination during Level II fieldwork will result in dismissal from the academic program. Remember that the student always has a right to appeal these decisions, which is why maintaining written documentation throughout the fieldwork experience is so important. The AFWC will follow up with the student and assess whether he or she has any mental health issues that require intervention.

The follow-up for the fieldwork educator is a more reflective process. Fieldwork educators have often said that failing a student is the most difficult task encountered. The fieldwork educator may have to complete a formal written report to the academic program or complete the AOTA Fieldwork Performance Evaluation for the OTA or OT Student (Chapters 58 and 59). To assist in preparing for the next fieldwork student, discuss what happened with colleagues and other supportive people and consider gaining more knowledge and skills related to being a fieldwork educator, such as taking a course or reading relevant literature.

Failure to Fail

Sometimes, despite documentation of unsatisfactory performance during fieldwork, a fieldwork site or a fieldwork educator will decide to pass a marginal student. The reasons for this decision are varied and include the following:

- Fieldwork educators who are novices may be uncertain about their roles and can be reluctant to fail students because they are unsure of the legitimacy of their judgments and their ultimate decision about the student's skills (Scanlon, Care, & Gessler, 2001).
- Fieldwork educators may be focused on the concern that students have encountered financial debt related to their education and that the majority of students have jobs and family commitments (Duffy, 2003).
- The fieldwork educator might not have kept adequate documentation about the student's performance throughout the fieldwork experience.
- Fieldwork educators may not want to cause students to experience distress or may not want to deal with the emotions likely to be experienced during a termination.
- Fieldwork educators may believe that failing a student is a personal failure on their part; they think, "If only I had done something differently." This thought is second-guessing oneself, not a personal failure. The student has failed to achieve the entry-level competencies you presented at the outset of the fieldwork experience.
- The fieldwork educator may be new to this role and not have any training or preparation for what to expect or administrative support.
- The fieldwork educator has waited too long to provide negative feedback about a student's performance, and now there is insufficient time to address the issues.
- The fieldwork educator has become close to the student and is concerned about the student's personal situation; therefore, the focus is on how this failure will affect the student's future career path.

References

American Occupational Therapy Association. (2009). *The American Occupational Therapy Association Self-Assessment Tool for Fieldwork Educator Competency.* Bethesda, MD: Author. Retrieved from http://www.aota.org/-/media/Corporate/Files/EducationCareers/Educators/Fieldwork/Supervisor/Forms/Self-Assessment%20Tool%20FW%20Ed%20Competency%20(2009).pdf

Christie, B., Joyce, P., & Moeller, P. (1985). Fieldwork experience, Part II: The supervisor's dilemma. *American Journal of Occupational Therapy, 39*(10), 675–681. http://dx.doi.org/10.5014/ajot.39.10.675

Costa, D. (2014). Supervision module. In *Fieldwork Educator Certificate Program.* Bethesda, MD: American Occupational Therapy Association.

Duffy, K. (2003). *Failing students: A qualitative study of factors that influence the decisions regarding assessment of students' competence in practice.* Glasgow, UK: Glasgow Caledonian University. Retrieved from http://www.nmc.uk.org/aFrameDisplay.aspx?DocumentID=1330

Gutman, S., McCreedy, P., & Heisler, P. (1998). Student Level II fieldwork failure: Strategies for intervention. *American Journal of Occupational Therapy, 52,* 143–149. http://dx.doi.org/10.5014/ajot.52.2.143

James, K., & Musselman, L. (2005). Commonalities in Level II fieldwork failure. *Occupational Therapy in Health Care, 19,* 67–81.

Kautzmann, L. (1990). Clinical teaching: Fieldwork supervisors' attitudes and values. *American Journal of Occupational Therapy, 44*(9), 835–838. http://dx.doi.org/10.5014/ajot.44.9.835

Lew, N., Cara, E., & Richardson, P. (2007). When fieldwork takes a detour. *Occupational Therapy in Health Care, 21,* 105–122.

McCreedy, P., & Graham, G. (1997). *Strategies to resolve issues surrounding student fieldwork failure.* Workshop presented at AOTA Annual Conference in Orlando, FL.

Rodger, S., Thomas, Y., Greber, C., Broadbridge, J., Edwards, A., Newton, J., & Lyons, M. (2014). Attributes of excellence in practice educators: The perspectives of Australian occupational therapy students. *Australian Occupational Therapy Journal, 61,* 159–167.

Scanlon, J., Care, W., & Gessler, S. (2001). Dealing with the unsafe student in clinical practice. *Nurse Educator, 26,* 23–27.

Chapter 61.

THE CHALLENGES OF WORKING WITH ADVANCED STUDENTS

Donna Costa, DHS, OTR/L, FAOTA

Every once in a while, fieldwork educators have the opportunity to work with a student who is more advanced on the continuum of entry-level competence. This kind of student does not need a lot of prodding, is a self-starter, is able to complete required documentation quickly, and is able to handle the caseload assigned to him or her. The advanced student catches on quickly to what is expected of him or her and uses supervision sessions to raise questions, issues, and concerns. This student often reaches the benchmarks for entry-level competence by midterm or shortly thereafter and, as a result, may express feeling "done" with the fieldwork placement.

Challenge of Advanced Students

Advanced students can present as much of a challenge and require as much attention as marginal students. They often finish tasks quickly and then have time on their hands. Advanced students may start to appear bored or actually voice concerns that there isn't anything else for them to learn. Sometimes, their performance can actually start to deteriorate. Therefore, creating a just-right challenge is a key strategy to be used with this kind of student.

In addition, using the American Occupational Therapy Association (AOTA) Fieldwork Experience Assessment Tool (see Chapter 13) can be useful in identifying what parts of the fieldwork experience are not challenging enough for the advanced student. Extra assignments and opportunities must be created for these students that do not lead them to think they are being penalized for getting work done early or achieving competencies early. It is important to meet with the student to collaborate on additional learning opportunities that are of interest to the student.

Strategies to Use

The following strategies may be helpful to fieldwork educators in working with advanced students:

- *Identify the situation.* Meet with and tell the student that he or she is doing very well and has met most of the entry-level competencies. Have the student tell you why he or she is appearing bored.
- *Determine what the student is interested in learning more about.* Perhaps the student needs or wants to work with clients with conditions that have

not been presented yet, would like to experience some additional rotations or site visits to other similar practice settings, or would like to shadow another health professional or another occupational therapy practitioner who uses different modalities or interventions.

- *Identify the just-right challenge for the student.* Have the student develop a proactive learning contract. You can use the same format as the remedial learning contract, but give the student more responsibility in writing it. The components of the learning contract are as follows:
  - Learning objectives: What are the learning objectives and how are they measured?
  - Learning resources and strategies: How will the student learn the objectives?
  - Evidence: How will the student demonstrate this new learning?
  - Validation (optional): How will the student's competency in this area be measured?
  - Time frame: What is the target date for completion?
- *Provide more independence, if possible.* Depending on the statutes and regulations that govern fieldwork supervision in your state and the type of practice setting, it may be possible to give the student more independence in carrying out daily responsibilities. Consider giving this student some responsibility for working with Level I or II students if they are present at your site.
- *Document additional responsibilities given.* When it comes time to complete the AOTA Fieldwork Performance Evaluation form (Chapters 59 and 58) for this student, include in your narrative description of performance the additional responsibilities given to the student and indicate how well they were done. This way, the student receives recognition for meeting and exceeding entry-level competencies.

Summary

Working with the advanced student should be a memorable success experience for both the fieldwork educator and the student. You will have provided the just-right challenge to this student, and the fieldwork experience will be influential in shaping the direction of this student's career choice as an occupational therapy practitioner.

Chapter 62.

PROGRESSION IN FIELDWORK SUPERVISION—PROVIDING THE JUST-RIGHT CHALLENGE

Donna Costa, DHS, OTR/L, FAOTA

Students come to fieldwork education armed with a great deal of knowledge that they have learned in the classroom. They may have had few opportunities, however, to either see this knowledge in practice or to apply skills learned. By the time the occupational therapy or occupational therapy assistant student leaves the Level II fieldwork experience, he or she is expected to have achieved entry-level competency in the practice area covered in the experience. What happens between the start and end of the fieldwork experience is a complex interaction among the fieldwork educator, student, and practice environment.

Providing a Road Map

Fieldwork educators sometimes expect that there will be a steady progression in students' knowledge and skills. The reality is that it is often a bumpy road, filled with accomplishments and setbacks. As a fieldwork educator, you are guiding the fieldwork experience for the student, providing learning activities and assignments that will lead to progression toward entry-level competency. To this end, the fieldwork educator needs to create and provide the student with a "road map" to guide the process. This road map needs to be dynamic and flexible because no two students will progress in the same way and at the same rate.

I suggest calling this road map what it is: Level II Fieldwork Student Progression. Start with a description of where the student needs to be by the time his or her fieldwork experience is over. You can use your entry-level occupational therapist job description to start because that is entry-level competency. Be specific about the following elements of the road map:

- Number of patients on caseload
- Number of screenings and evaluations
- Time frame to complete evaluation reports (e.g., within 24 hours of patient evaluation session)
- Time frame for other kinds of documentation required (e.g., progress notes, discharge summaries)
- Attendance and active participation at treatment meetings
- Evidence of good interprofessional team member skills (i.e., positive relationships with other team members)
- In-service presentations to team.

Once you complete this document, you can establish benchmarks for each week of the student's fieldwork experience. This document should be described to students at the beginning of the fieldwork so they know they will be held accountable for progressing toward entry-level competence.

The Just-Right Challenge

The concept of the just-right challenge was originally conceived by Ayres (2006) to describe the practitioner's choice of treatment activities that are neither too easy nor too difficult for a child. Allen, Blue, and Earhart (1998) also used this concept when describing treatment for clients with cognitive dysfunction issues, advocating for the practitioner to select treatment activities that are just slightly above the client's current level of cognitive functioning. The concept of the just-right challenge is described more fully in the conceptual framework for therapeutic occupation (Nelson & Jepsen-Thomas, 2003), which defined a *challenge* as the balance between the inherent level of difficulty in the occupation and the client's level of developmental competencies. A task has to be difficult enough to provide a challenge to the person attempting it, but not so difficult that the person gives up in frustration. Nelson and Jepsen-Thomas (2003) discussed how both too much challenge and too little challenge result in an imbalance, inhibiting successful performance by the client. A task with too much challenge is too difficult, and a task with too little challenge is too easy, and they both lead to failure. The problem is not with the client, but with the assigned task.

How does the just-right challenge apply to fieldwork education? Students are assigned a variety of tasks by their fieldwork educators, designed to promote learning and the development of clinical reasoning. Just as occupational therapy practitioners grade treatment activities for clients to meet the just-right challenge, so, too, do fieldwork educators grade assignments for students that will lead to eventual mastery of entry-level practice competencies. However, assigning and grading tasks requires ongoing vigilance to the responses of the students to the tasks. Fieldwork educators must evaluate whether the assignment is too hard or too easy for a particular student at a particular point in his or her professional development. Both will lead to increasing frustration for the student, who will become bored if the tasks are too easy or feel increasingly incompetent if the tasks are too difficult.

Several elements might need to be adjusted to provide the just-right challenge in fieldwork education, including

- Pace of the treatment setting
- Institutional environment and the amount of distractions and support in the clinic
- Number of clients treated per day
- Whether clients are seen individually or in groups
- Acuity of clients' or patients' conditions, diagnoses, or injuries and whether the cases are complex, requiring advanced problem solving or routine requiring long-term care
- Types of treatment interventions at your facility and whether they are the same for all clients or individualized and occupation-based in design
- Time-intensive documentation required by the facility
- Number and complexity of written fieldwork assignments given by the supervisor
- Frequency and length of supervision, whether it is provided individually or in groups, and whether it is conducted "on the run" between client encounters or at scheduled times.

One way to formally assess all of these elements is to use the American Occupational Therapy Association Fieldwork Experience Assessment Tool (see Chapter 27). The data collected through this instrument will provide fieldwork educators with valuable information about the level of challenge inherent in the fieldwork experience. It is also a valuable self-assessment for a student to complete to develop a self-directed plan for future learning. Just as therapeutic activities are either graded up or down for patients and clients, the same can be done for fieldwork students.

Collaboration to Achieve the Just-Right Challenge

The burden for determining the difficulty of assignments is ideally shared between the student and the fieldwork educator. Initially, the fieldwork educator takes the lead in directing the course of the fieldwork experience. However, as the student becomes more comfortable and feels more competent, he or she should begin to provide input during the supervisory process, identifying needed experiences to enhance learning. Having regularly scheduled supervision sessions between the fieldwork educator and the student can facilitate this collaborative process.

Open-ended questions can be asked of the student, such as "Tell me how difficult or easy it has been for you to work with your assigned patients this past week?" and "Tell me how you have experienced the pace here in the past few weeks?" The student should feel empowered to ask the fieldwork educator to step up the pace if it is too slow or ask for time to catch up if it is difficult to keep up. To help the student reach this point of empowerment, the fieldwork educator has to establish a tone of acceptance and collaboration. All too often I hear students tell their "war stories" about fieldwork educators who did not listen, did not invite their feedback, or rejected their input. This attitude can sometimes lead to a student learning to be passive and only doing what they are told to do—no more and no less.

Fieldwork educators are mentors for the students they supervise. They lead by example, provide inspiration, challenge students to think on their feet, encourage when the going gets tough, and demonstrate their commitment to professional excellence and lifelong learning. Christie (1999) described the supervision provided by fieldwork educators as

a dynamic, empowering process that fosters the integration of theoretical knowledge and

application of therapeutic principles with the conscious use of self to enhance the effectiveness of our practice. However, I believe we need to educate ourselves more about supervision, what it means and how to conduct effective supervision using a conceptual model to ensure safe practice. (p. 57)

References

Allen, C., Blue, T., & Earhart, C. (1998) *Understanding cognitive performance modes.* Ormond Beach, FL: Allen Conferences.

Ayres, J. (2006). *Sensory integration and the child: Understanding hidden sensory challenges. 25th anniversary edition.* Los Angeles: Western Psychological Services.

Christie, A. (1999). A meaningful occupation: The just right challenge. *Australian Occupational Therapy Journal, 46,* 52–68.

Nelson, D., & Jepsen-Thomas, J. (2003). Occupational form, occupational performance, and a conceptual framework for therapeutic occupation. In P. Kramer, J. Hinojosa, & C. Royeen (Eds.), *Perspectives on human occupation: Participation in life* (pp. 87–155). Philadelphia: Lippincott.

Note. Part of this chapter is excerpted from "The Just-Right Challenge in Fieldwork," by D. Costa, 2008, *OT Practice, 13*(16), pp. 10–11, 24. Reprinted with permission.

Chapter 63.

WORKING WITH OCCUPATIONAL THERAPY AND OCCUPATIONAL THERAPY ASSISTANT STUDENTS WITH DISABILITIES

Donna Costa, DHS, OTR/L, FAOTA

The *Centennial Vision* of the American Occupational Therapy Association (AOTA; 2007) includes having a diverse workforce. This diversity includes having occupational therapy practitioners with a broad range of abilities and disabilities (Taguchi-Meyer, 2014). Increased numbers of students with disabilities of all types are pursuing higher education, with the proportion of college freshman increasing threefold between 1978 and 1998 (Cook, Rumrill, & Tankersley, 2009). The National Center for Educational Statistics (2011) reported that for the academic year 2009–2010, 88% of 2- and 4-year academic institutions admitted students with disabilities. This number reflects only the students with disabilities who disclosed their disability. Many students, for a variety of reasons, choose not to disclose their disability. The report also stated that this number is expected to rise by 14% in the future. These increases are due in part to legislation such as the American with Disabilities Act of 1990 (ADA; Pub. L. 101–336) and Section 504 of the Rehabilitation Act of 1973 (Pub. L. 93–112) that provide protection for people with disabilities. In addition, newer medical treatments and medications for people with disabilities have diminished symptoms or

helped improve functional ability, making college attendance a possibility for them.

College students most often disclose the conditions of learning disabilities and psychiatric disorders (Sharby & Roush, 2009). However, despite the increasing prevalence of disability disclosure overall, a corresponding increase in educators' understanding of the challenges of students with disabilities has not occurred (Sharby & Roush, 2009). Many students manage the stresses and demands of academic coursework throughout elementary and secondary education but have increased difficulty with the rigor associated with postsecondary education. According to AOTA (2010), "It is not unusual for a disability to be discovered after a student enters professional school or even as late as Level II fieldwork. Sometimes students with learning or emotional disabilities have succeeded up to the point of professional school through extremely hard work and dedication. However, the demands of professional school and fieldwork can push such a student past his or her ability to compensate" (p. 5).

Cook and colleagues (2009) noted that "the success of any college student, particularly in the academic realm, is to some degree determined by the type and quality of interactions that he or she has with his or her instructors" (p. 84). Because occupational therapy professional education comprises both academic and clinical coursework, this statement relates to both occupational therapy college professors and fieldwork educators. Fieldwork educators, as much as the faculty in the academic programs, must understand the legal requirements of working with students with disabilities. It is important to remember that the laws enacted regarding disability (ADA and Section 504 of the Rehabilitation Act of 1973) were intended to be antidiscrimination acts; they are not entitlement acts (AOTA, 2010). In addition, the responsibility for disclosing a disability lies with the student.

Most occupational therapy programs conduct orientation sessions at the beginning of coursework and cover the issues of disabilities. Students are encouraged to disclose a disability to the academic institution's office for students with disabilities. However, many students fail to disclose disabilities for multiple reasons, such as not wanting to be treated differently, having shame about or avoiding stigma attached to the diagnosis or condition, fearing judgment or discrimination, not wanting to be labeled, fearing rejection, having concern about alienation from peers, and believing he or she can manage it on their own. Even after a student makes the decision to disclose to the academic program, he or she may be reluctant to disclose to the fieldwork site for similar reasons. Note that the Family Educational Rights and Privacy Act of 1974 (Pub. L. 93-380) regulations preclude an academic program from sharing information with fieldwork sites without the student's express written consent.

The primary issue for fieldwork educators is how to proceed after a student discloses a disability while on fieldwork. This disclosure is often made after the student has encountered substantial difficulty with fieldwork challenges or after negative feedback about his or her performance. Because fieldwork is considered an extension of the academic program, it includes academic credit. Therefore, when the student discloses to the fieldwork educator that he or she has a disability, the academic fieldwork coordinator must be contacted, who, in turn, must involve the office that handles disability issues. Note that giving the student accommodations is not retroactive to the start of the fieldwork experience, only to the time that the disclosure has been made.

At that point, all parties must discuss what accommodations can be provided at the fieldwork site. According to Scott, Wells, and Hannebrink (1997),

> The institution is always responsible for students who are participating in its programs whether on or off campus. The question is whether the institution has primary or secondary responsibility. The [academic] institution has the ultimate responsibility for the provision of reasonable accommodation. The intern site generally assumes the duty for providing accommodation on site; the [academic] institution, however, must monitor what happens in that environment to ensure that its students are not discriminated against and are provided necessary accommodations. (p. 44)

Scott and colleagues also stated that "students with disabilities have a right under ADA (Title II) to be seen first as capable people with marketable skills and only secondarily as people who happen to have disabilities" (p. 46).

Kornblau (1995) articulated the following DIALOGUE system of prevention, which was suggested as a process to prevent problems from developing between fieldwork educators and students with disabilities:

- *D.* Provide fieldwork educators with information regarding the legal issues related to working with students with disabilities.
- *I.* Identify students with disabilities who might request accommodations on fieldwork and meet with them to discuss the decision to disclose their condition to the fieldwork site and the types of reasonable accommodations that might be requested of the fieldwork site.
- *A.* Assess the advantages and disadvantages of disclosing a disability with students who are reluctant to tell a potential fieldwork site.
- *L.* List accommodations given in school and discuss what types of accommodations will be needed during fieldwork (this topic must be discussed in light of the site requirements given by the fieldwork site to the academic program).
- *O.* Open lines of communication are critical, and the student needs to understand that the disclosure of disability is best made before the fieldwork experience begins.

- *G.* Go to the fieldwork site before the fieldwork experience begins, and schedule a meeting with the student, the academic fieldwork coordinator, and the fieldwork educator. Seeing the environmental demands of the fieldwork site is the optimal way to explore workable solutions to challenges that may arise during the fieldwork experience.
- *U.* Undertake all of the necessary steps for complying with the laws related to disability.
- *E.* Encourage all parties to keep the lines of communication open between themselves so that any challenges that arise during fieldwork can be addressed before they develop into bigger problems.

Sharby and Roush (2009) proposed the following six-step analytical decision-making model to assess students' needs and provide reasonable accommodations:

1. *Positive climate.* Faculty, staff, and fieldwork educators must have a positive attitude when working with students with disabilities. In the occupational therapy literature, students with disabilities have reported that the attitudes of other occupational therapy practitioners are a barrier for them (Collins, 1997; Hirneth & Mackenzie, 2004; Jung et al., 2014; Velde, Chapin, & Wittman, 2005).

2. *Identify essential functions or technical standards.* A fieldwork site cannot refuse to accept a student unless the student cannot perform the essential job functions with or without reasonable accommodations. *Essential job functions,* or *technical standards,* are descriptions of job duties or requirements that are fundamental to a particular position. Occupational therapy education programs are increasingly defining these technical standards and making them available to students as part of the application process. Fieldwork sites should also develop these standards.

3. *Identify students' challenges and strengths.* Faculty in the academic program should meet with students who have disclosed disabilities and identify the challenges that may arise during fieldwork and the strengths the students will bring to fieldwork. Identifying strengths is important because it helps to articulate the compensatory strategies student use.

4. *Analyze learning activities.* During discussions with students, all the different types of learning activities that will be assigned, in the classroom and while on fieldwork, should be reviewed. Each learning activity may need a different accommodation, depending on the nature of the student's disability.

5. *Determine reasonable accommodations.* The same kinds of reasonable accommodations granted in the academic program will need to be granted in the fieldwork site. Academic fieldwork coordinators and fieldwork educators may find the resources available on the Job Accommodation Network (http://askjan.org/) very useful for determining fieldwork site accommodations.

6. *Implement and assess reasonable accommodations.* Reasonable accommodations should be implemented in a consistent way in the classroom and at the fieldwork site. Keeping open lines of communication between all parties is most helpful in this situation.

In summary, "occupational therapy faculty and fieldwork educators must remain mindful of their obligations both to their occupational therapy students and to the clients those students will someday serve. Patient safety is always paramount. However, there will be students who can become competent occupational therapists despite their disabilities if given reasonable accommodations" (AOTA, 2010, p. 9).

References

American Occupational Therapy Association. (2007). AOTA's *Centennial Vision* and executive summary. *American Journal of Occupational Therapy, 61,* 613–614. http://dx.doi.org/10.5014/ajot.61.6.613

American Occupational Therapy Association. (2010). *Ethical considerations for the professional education of students with disabilities.* Available from http://www.aota.org/-/media/Corporate/Files/Practice/Ethics/Advisory/Students-Disabilities-Advisory.pdf

Americans with Disabilities Act of 1990, Pub. L. 101–336, 42 U.S.C. §§ 12101–12213 (2000).

Collins, L. (1997). Students and the ADA: Decreasing boundaries, not standards. *OT Practice, 2*(9), 20–29.

Cook, L., Rumrill, P., & Tankersley, M. (2009). Priorities and understanding of faculty members regarding college students with disabilities. *International Journal of Teaching and Learning in Higher Education, 21,* 84–96.

Family Educational Rights and Privacy Act of 1974, Pub. L. 93-380, 20 U.S.C. § 1232g; 34 CFR Part 99.

Hirneth, M., & Mackenzie, L. (2004). The practice education of occupational therapy students with disabilities: Practice educators' perspectives. *British Journal of Occupational Therapy, 67,* 396–402.

Jung, B., Baptiste, S., Dhillion, S., Kravchenko, T., Stewart, D., & Vanderkaay, S. (2014). The experience of student occupational therapists with disabilities in Canadian universities. *International Journal of Higher Education, 3,* 146–154.

Kornblau, B. (1995). Fieldwork education and students with disabilities: Enter the Americans with Disabilities Act. *American Journal of Occupational Therapy, 49,* 139–145. http://dx.doi.org/10.5014/ajot.49.2.139

National Center for Educational Statistics. (2011). *Students with disabilities at degree-granting postsecondary institutions.* Retrieved from http://nces.ed.gov/search/?q=college+students+with+disabilities

Rehabilitation Act of 1973, Pub. L. 93–112, 29 U.S.C. §§ 701-796l.

Scott, S. S., Wells, S. A., & Hannebrink, S. (1997). *Educating students with disabilities: What academic and fieldwork educators need to know.* Bethesda, MD: American Occupational Therapy Association.

Sharby, N., & Roush, S. (2009). Analytical decision-making model for addressing the needs of allied health students with disabilities. *Journal of Allied Health, 38,* 54–62.

Taguchi-Meyer, J. (2014). Ensuring a diverse workforce: Fieldwork success for occupational therapy students with disabilities. *OT Practice, 19*(2), 18–19.

Velde, B., Chapin, M., & Wittman, P. (2005). Working around "it": The experience of occupational therapy students with a disability. *Journal of Allied Health, 34,* 83–89.

Chapter 64.

ADVISORY OPINION ON ETHICAL CONSIDERATIONS FOR THE PROFESSIONAL EDUCATION OF STUDENTS WITH DISABILITIES

American Occupational Therapy Association

An Advisory Opinion for the AOTA Ethics Commission

Introduction

Assisting individuals with disabilities and valuing diversity are core tenets of the profession of occupational therapy. According to the American Occupational Therapy Association (AOTA, 2009b),

> The occupational therapy profession affirms the right of every individual to access and fully participate in society.... We maintain that society has an obligation to provide the reasonable accommodations necessary to allow individuals access to social, educational, recreational, and vocational opportunities. (pp. 819–820)

Most often the individual with a disability is a client, but sometimes the individual is a student in an occupational therapy educational program. Regardless of whether the student has a disability, educational programs must balance the needs of their students with their obligations to the future clients that program graduates will serve. Educators must treat students fairly and act in accordance with the *AOTA Occupational Therapy Code of Ethics and Ethics Standards (2010)* (referred to as the Code and Ethics Standards; AOTA, 2010a) and federal and state laws.

This Advisory Opinion discusses ethical issues that may arise during the classroom and fieldwork portions of the educational process of occupational therapy students who have disabilities. First, a brief background of key legislation is provided, including the Americans with Disabilities Act (ADA), Section 504 of the Rehabilitation Act of 1973, and the Family Educational Rights and Privacy Act (FERPA). Next, the Code and Ethics Standards is applied to two case studies that describe situations that may arise in the classroom and in fieldwork education. Last, the Advisory Opinion summarizes key issues. When the term *educational program* is used, it applies to both the academic and fieldwork portion of the educational program unless otherwise stated.

Background

The ADA (1990) extended civil rights to individuals with disabilities. Similarly, the Rehabilitation Act of 1973, and specifically Section 504, defined exactly how services must be provided to people with disabilities who request assistance. These legislative mandates pertain to all aspects of American life, from housing and education to employment, recreation, and religion. In any situation where an otherwise qualified person might be prevented from achieving his or her potential due to a disability, ADA and the Rehabilitation Act demand assurances that opportunities be available for all.

The ADA and Section 504 of the Rehabilitation Act of 1973 are antidiscrimination acts, not entitlement acts. As such, they are outcome-neutral, and the responsibility for initiating accommodation rests with the student. The ADA and Section 504 require that individuals, such as those entering higher education, receive the opportunity to participate in educational and vocational endeavors for which they are otherwise qualified. An equal opportunity to participate does not mean that there will be equal outcomes. Just like their non-disabled peers, some students with disabilities will fail coursework and fieldwork. The ADA focuses on whether students with disabilities in higher education have equal access to an education. It is not intended to optimize academic success: "The intent of the law, again, was to level the playing field, not to tilt it" (Gordon & Keiser, 1998, p. 5).

Because the ADA's intention is to protect against discrimination based on a disability, a student can receive such protection only if he or she has substantial impairments that affect major life activities and he or she is found to be disabled relative to the general population (Gordon & Keiser, 1998). Some conditions warrant intervention but may not rise to the level of impairment as defined by the ADA. Furthermore,

> Documentation of a specific disability does not translate directly into specific accommodations. Reasonable accommodations are individually determined and should be based on the functional impact of the condition and its likely interaction with the environment (course assignments, program requirements, physical design, etc.). As such, accommodation recommendations may vary from individual to individual with the "same" disability diagnosis and from environment to environment for the same individual. (Association on Higher Education and Disability, 2004b)

There are specific requirements for diagnosis and documentation in order to qualify for protection under the ADA as an individual with a disability. The diagnosis must be made and documented by a qualified professional, such as a physician, neuropsychologist, or educational psychologist, among others: "The general expectation is that people conducting evaluations have terminal degrees in their profession and are fully trained in differential diagnosis" (Gordon & Keiser, 1998, p. 13). The Association on Higher Education and Disability (2004a) provides additional information on best practices in documentation of a disability in higher education. The report based on the evaluator's findings must also be sufficient to allow for careful administrative review.

The coordination of the documentation and services for students with disabilities is usually managed through an administrative office at the college or university. This office is frequently called the Office of Disability Accommodations (ODA). The ODA determines if the student qualifies for accommodations and what accommodations are allowable by disability law and regulations.

The above process assumes that the student is aware of his or her disability and self-identifies. If a student chooses not to self-identify, he or she is within individual rights to pursue postsecondary education. However, such a student is not protected by the law. Simply stated, unless a student self-identifies as being eligible for protections under the ADA and Section 504, no associated privileges are afforded.

Because occupational therapy practitioners in their professional role assist people with impairments in their efforts to be successful, it is sometimes difficult for a faculty member to refrain from making special arrangements for a student who appears to have a disability but who has not self-identified or who has not completed the process to qualify for accommodations. However, educators must consider fundamental fairness to all students, including those who may struggle for a variety of other reasons but who do not qualify for special treatment.

It is not unusual for a disability to be discovered after a student enters professional school or even as late as Level II fieldwork. Sometimes students with learning or emotional disabilities have succeeded up to the point of professional school through extremely hard work and dedication. However, the demands of professional school and fieldwork can push such a student past his or her ability to compensate.

If the student is otherwise qualified, the educational program must determine if the student can perform the essential job function of being an occupational therapy student with or without reasonable accommodation. For a more complete discussion of essential job functions and reasonable accommodations in academic and practice settings, see Gupta, Gelpi, and Sain (2005). A variety of documents exist that contribute to understanding the essential job functions of an occupational therapist or occupational therapy assistant (AOTA, 2009a, 2010b, 2010c; U.S. Department of Labor, National O*NET Consortium, 2003, 2004).

In the field of health education, essential job functions are generally referred to as *technical standards.* Many occupational therapy programs include the technical standards as part of the admissions process (e.g., Medical College of Georgia, 2008; Samuel Merritt College, n.d.; Stony Brook University, 2004; University of Kansas, 2003; University of Tennessee, n.d.).

The last federal law relevant to this advisory opinion is the Family Educational Rights and Privacy Act, which protects the privacy of all students' educational records. Generally, "institutions must have written permission from the student in order to release any information from a student's educational record" (Van Dusen, 2004, p. 4). This protection of privacy applies to all students, regardless of disability.

Protection of confidential information is part of FERPA, the ADA, and Section 504. The Association on Higher Education and Disability (1996) stated that "disability-related information should be treated as medical information and handled under the same strict rules of confidentiality as is other medical information" (p. 1). The student alone determines whether to share information, decides what information to share, and selects which faculty members may receive information: "The Department of Justice has indicated that a faculty member generally does not need to know what the disability is, only that it has been appropriately verified by the individual (or office) assigned this responsibility on behalf of the institution" (Association on Higher Education and Disability, 1996, p. 1).

Application to Practice: Case Studies

Two case studies illustrate how to apply ethical reasoning to students with disabilities.

Case 1

Ashley is an occupational therapy student with a learning disability. Ashley is your advisee and in the first semester in the occupational therapy program. She makes an appointment with you and tells you about her learning disability and the difficulties she has had, shows you a psychological report describing her disability, and asks to be given extra time to complete exams and assignments. You advise her to go to the university's Office of Disability Accommodations. Ashley does not want to go to the ODA because she thinks that the university would label her as a student with a disability. You inform Ashley of the risks of not seeking accommodations and encourage her to reconsider. She leaves your office undecided.

You do not hear from Ashley again until after midterm exams, when she discovers she has a failing grade in two classes. She admits that she did not go to the ODA and states she thought she could make it on her own. Ashley says that one of her instructors gave her more time, and she can't understand why the other occupational therapy instructors did not. Ashley finally agrees to go to the ODA, but she also wants to be able to retake her midterm exams in the two courses she is failing. She wants more time for taking exams and turning in assignments. The ODA determines that Ashley does qualify as a student with learning disabilities and that her accommodations can include time and a half for exams, but she must turn in assignments on the dates they are due in the syllabi. She is also not allowed to retake the two midterm exams.

Your behavior as Ashley's advisor demonstrates understanding, caring, and responsiveness (core value: altruism) to Ashley's situation. By requiring Ashley to go to the ODA, you followed procedures (Code and Ethics Standards Principle 5, Procedural Justice), which requires that you are familiar with and comply with institutional rules and federal laws, in this case the ADA and Section 504. The instructor who gave Ashley more time on the exam before accommodations were in place demonstrated altruism but violated Principle 5 of the Code and Ethics Standards because university procedures stipulate that accommodations should not be given until the ODA determines that the student is entitled to them and specifies what the accommodations should be. Making accommodations without consulting the ODA may result in an unfair disadvantage for other students who may have extenuating circumstances affecting their performance by denying them an equal opportunity for extra time.

Principle 1 of the Code and Ethics Standards (Beneficence) applies to all faculty involved in this case. Specifically, Principle 1J reads, "Occupational therapy personnel shall provide occupational therapy education, continuing education, instruction, and training that are within the instructor's subject area of expertise and level of competence." Although academic and fieldwork educators may typically think of competence in terms of educating students without disabilities, knowledge of laws related to educating students with disabilities is also required.

Case 2

Tanisha is preparing for her first Level II fieldwork experience. She has a diagnosis of anxiety disorder for which she has received accommodations during the academic portion of her education. As the academic fieldwork coordinator, you encourage Tanisha to contact the ODA to determine what accommodations she would qualify for during clinical education. Tanisha states that she does not want to reveal to the fieldwork site that she has a disability because she plans to apply for jobs in this city after graduation. She says she feels more confident now and wants to prove to herself that she can perform without assistance. After you explain the risks and benefits of disclosure, Tanisha decides not to disclose or ask for accommodations from her clinical site. You contact Tanisha after Week 2

to review her progress. Tanisha says things are OK. At Week 4, Jeremy, Tanisha's clinical educator, calls you to say that he is concerned about Tanisha's difficulty with time management and turning in documentation on time. He says that Tanisha's level of knowledge appears solid but that she sometimes "shuts down" in stressful situations. Jeremy asks if Tanisha has some learning or emotional issues that he should know about. He wants your advice on how to help Tanisha be more successful.

As the academic fieldwork coordinator, you must consider the ethical principle of Autonomy and Confidentiality (Principle 3). Principle 3G is especially applicable to this case:

> Occupational therapy personnel shall ensure that confidentiality and the right to privacy are respected and maintained regarding all information obtained about.... students.... The only exceptions are when a practitioner or staff member believes than an individual is in serious foreseeable or imminent harm. Laws and regulations may require disclosure to appropriate authorities without consent. (p. S21)

In a similar fashion, Fidelity (Principle 7B) requires that "occupational therapy personnel shall preserve, respect, and safeguard private information about employees, colleagues, and students unless otherwise mandated by national, state, or local laws or permission to disclose is given by the individual" (p. S24). Veracity (Principle 6E) also applies to this case: "Occupational therapy personnel shall accept responsibility for any action that reduces the public's trust in occupational therapy" (p. S24). Principle 6E creates tension between your duty to your student and your duty to consumers of occupational therapy services. However, you realize that you have a greater obligation to avoid breaching confidentiality with Tanisha, as you do not have evidence at this point that Tanisha's behavior is putting clients at risk. If you had information to indicate that clients were at risk, you would have a greater obligation to protect the clients and to focus on Tanisha's lack of competence in the area of client safety.

You must also consider Procedural Justice (Principle 5), which requires you to be familiar and comply with institutional rules and federal laws, which in this case are the ADA, Section 504, and

FERPA. Last, you consider Principle 1K, which states that "occupational therapy personnel shall provide students and employees with information about the Code and Ethics Standards, opportunities to discuss ethical conflicts, and procedures for reporting unresolved ethical conflicts" (p. S19). It is important that you model ethical conduct for Jeremy and Tanisha.

A more thorough discussion of ethical dilemmas involving confidentiality of students with disabilities during fieldwork education can be found in an article by Brown and Griffiths (2000). AOTA's website also provides useful information on this topic, including the following question and answer:

> Does the academic program have to tell the fieldwork setting that the student has a disability? The academic program is not required to, nor should it, inform the fieldwork site of a student's disability without the student's permission. It is the student's decision whether or not to disclose a disability. The academic fieldwork coordinator will counsel students on the pros and cons of sharing this type of information prior to beginning fieldwork. If a student decides not to disclose this information, the academic fieldwork coordinator is legally not allowed to share that information with the fieldwork setting.
>
> A fieldwork setting cannot refuse to place a student with a disability unless that student is unable to perform the essential job functions with or without reasonable accommodations. To refuse placement solely on the student's disability is discriminatory and illegal. (AOTA, 2000)

After considering the Code and Ethics Standards and other documents, you decide you cannot directly answer Jeremy's question about a disability, but you could brainstorm with Jeremy about strategies that might help Tanisha be more successful. You could encourage Jeremy to document Tanisha's difficulties and to give her frequent and specific feedback. If these suggestions don't correct the problems, a learning contract or site visit could be considered. You could contact Tanisha to assist her with making an informed decision by providing her with the potential risks of nondisclosure. However, as an autonomous person with freedom to exercise

choice and self-direction, Tanisha must make the final decision. Autonomous persons can and do take risks. Tanisha may be risking failure of her first Level II fieldwork, but taking the risk is her choice. Wells and Hanebrink (2000) noted that

> The decision to disclose or not to disclose as well as when and how to disclose is solely the right of the student. The fieldwork site can be held accountable only from the point in which they are informed or receive a request for accommodation. (p. 9)

Education programs should provide clinical sites with information about educating students with disabilities and the requirements of the ADA and Section 504 in regard to education and encourage sites to call the academic fieldwork coordinator when questions arise. The AOTA Self-Assessment Tool for Fieldwork Educator Competency (AOTA, n.d.; Chapter 27) is a potential resource for educating fieldwork educators in general. Under Administration Competencies, Item 11 is pertinent to this discussion: "The fieldwork educator defines essential functions and roles of a fieldwork student, in compliance with legal and accreditation standards (e.g., ADA, Family Educational Rights and Privacy Act, fieldwork agreement, reimbursement mechanism, state regulations, etc.)" (p. 7).

Discussion

Occupational therapy faculty and fieldwork educators must remain mindful of their obligations both to their occupational therapy students and to the clients those students will someday serve. Patient safety is always paramount. However, there will be students who can become competent occupational therapists despite their disabilities if given reasonable accommodations. Although the student has rights and responsibilities, so do the academic and clinical sites:

> The institution is always responsible for students who are participating in its programs whether on or off campus. The question is whether the institution has primary or secondary responsibility. The institution has the ultimate responsibility for the provision of reasonable accommodation. The intern

site generally assumes the duty for providing accommodation on site; the institution, however, must monitor what happens in that environment to ensure that its students are not discriminated against and are provided necessary accommodations.... Students with disabilities have a right under ADA (Title II) to be seen first as capable people with marketable skills and only secondarily as people who happen to have disabilities. (Scott, Wells, & Hanebrink, 1997, pp. 44, 46)

According to the Northeast Technical Assistance Center (1999), faculty should not make assumptions about a student's ability to work in a particular field. Most often, concerns that students may not be able to "cut it" are based on fears and assumptions, not facts. Remember, too, that employers are also required to comply with the ADA.

References

American Occupational Therapy Association. (2000). *Answers to your fieldwork questions.* Retrieved from http://www.aota.org/EducationCareers/Educators/Fieldwork/Answers.aspx

American Occupational Therapy Association. (2009a). Guidelines for supervision, roles, and responsibilities during the delivery of occupational therapy services. *American Journal of Occupational Therapy, 58,* 797–803. http://dx.doi.org/10.5014/ajot.63.6.797

American Occupational Therapy Association. (2009b). Occupational therapy's commitment to nondiscrimination and inclusion. *American Journal of Occupational Therapy, 63,* 819– 820. http://dx.doi.org/10.5014/ajot.63.6.819

American Occupational Therapy Association. (2010a). Occupational therapy code of ethics and ethics standards (2010). *American Journal of Occupational Therapy, 64*(6 Suppl.), S17– S26. http://dx.doi.org/10.5014/ajot.2010.64S17

American Occupational Therapy Association. (2010b). Scope of practice. *American Journal of Occupational Therapy, 64*(6 Suppl.), S70–S77. http://dx.doi.org/10.5014/ajot.2010.64S70

American Occupational Therapy Association. (2010c). Standards of practice for occupational therapy. *American Journal of Occupational Therapy, 64*(6 Suppl.), S106–S111. http://dx.doi.org/10.5014/ajot.2010.64S106

American Occupational Therapy Association.(n.d.). *The American Occupational Therapy Association self-assessment tool for fieldwork educator competency.* Retrieved from http://www.aota.org/-/media/Corporate/Files/EducationCareers/Educators/Fieldwork/Supervisor/Forms/Self-Assessment%20Tool%20FW%20Ed%20Competency%20(2009).ashx

Americans With Disabilities Act of 1990, Pub. L.101–336, 42 U.S.C. § 12101.

Association on Higher Education and Disability. (1996). *Confidentiality & disability issues in higher education* [Brochure]. Huntersville, NC: Author.

Association on Higher Education and Disability. (2004a). *Best practices resources.* Retrieved May 21, 2010, from http://www.ahead.org/resources/best-practices-resources

Association on Higher Education and Disability. (2004b). *Principles: Foundation principles for the review of documentation and the determination of accommodations.* Retrieved May 21, 2010, from http://www.ahead.org/resources/best-practices-resources/principles

Brown, K., & Griffiths, Y. (2000). Confidentiality dilemmas in clinical education. *Journal of Allied Health, 29,* 13–17.

Family Educational Rights and Privacy Act, 20 U.S.C. § 1232g; 34 CFR Part 99 (1974).

Gordon, M., & Keiser, S. (1998). *Accommodations in higher education under the Americans With Disabilities Act (ADA): A no-nonsense guide for clinicians, educators, administrators, and lawyers.* DeWitt, NY: GSI Publications.

Gupta, J., Gelpi, T., & Sain, S. (2005, August). Reasonable accommodations and essential job functions in academic and practice settings. *OT Practice,* pp. CE1–CE7.

Medical College of Georgia. (2008). *Technical standards for occupational therapy.* Retrieved November 21, 2010, from http://www.mcg.edu/sah/ot/standards.html

Northeast Technical Assistance Center. (1999). *Nondiscrimination in higher education.* Retrieved January 21, 2007, from http://www.netac.rit.edu/publication/tipsheet/ADA.html

Rehabilitation Act of 1973, Pub. L. 93–112, 29 U.S.C. § 701 et seq.

Samuel Merritt College. (n.d.). *Occupational therapy technical standards.* Retrieved July 3, 2007, from http://www.samuelmerritt.edu/occupational_therapy/technical_standards

Scott, S. S., Wells, S., & Hanebrink, S. (1997). *Educating college students with disabilities: What academic and fieldwork educators need to know.* Bethesda, MD: AOTA Press.

Stony Brook University. (2004). *Technical standards for admission and continuation in the occupational therapy program.* Retrieved from http://www.hsc.stonybrook.edu/shtm/ot/tech-standards.cfm

University of Kansas. (2003). *Occupational therapy education department policy: Technical standards and essential functions for occupational therapy students.* Retrieved November 24, 2007, from http://alliedhealth.kumc.edu/programs/ot/documents/PDF/techstds_preadm.pdf

University of Tennessee.(n.d.). *Technical standards for students in occupational therapy.* Retrieved July 3, 2007, from http://www.uthsc.edu/allied/ot/tech_standards.php

U.S. Department of Labor, National O*NET Consortium. (2003). *Summary report for occupational therapists.* Retrieved January 14, 2008, from http://online.onetcenter.org/link/summary/29-1122.00

U.S. Department of Labor, National O*NET Consortium. (2004). *Summary report for occupational therapy assistants.* Retrieved January 14, 2008, from http://online.onetcenter.org/link/summary/31-2011.00

Van Dusen, W. R. (2004). *FERPA: Basic guidelines for faculty and staff: A simple step-by-step approach for compliance.* Retrieved January 21, 2007, http://www.nacada.ksu.edu/Resources/FERPA-Overview.htm

Wells, S. A., & Hanebrink, S. (2000). Lesson 11: Students with disabilities and fieldwork. In *Meeting the fieldwork challenge: AOTA self-paced clinical course.* Bethesda, MD: AOTA Press.

Linda Gabriel, PhD, OTR/L
Education Representative, Ethics Commission (2003–2009)

Betsy DeBrakeleer, COTA/L, ROH
OTA Representative Ethics Commission (2005–2008)

Lorie J. McQuade, MEd, CRC
Public Member, Ethics Commission (2004–2007)

Part 13.

PROFESSIONAL BEHAVIOR

OVERVIEW OF PART 13

Donna Costa, DHS, OTR/L, FAOTA

During fieldwork education, students are expected to be able to apply the knowledge and skills learned in the classroom to the patients and clients they serve. However, the process of becoming an entry-level practitioner also includes the development of professional behaviors, which is the focus of Part 13.

Chapter 65 contains the American Occupational Therapy Association's "Advisory Opinion on Patient Abandonment." Because documentation is a large part of the daily work done by occupational therapy practitioners, fieldwork students must learn and master the process. Although documentation formats vary widely across clinical practice settings, they have common elements, which are presented in the AOTA official document in Chapter 66, "Guidelines for Documentation of Occupational Therapy." Chapter 67, "Professional Dress and Appearance," addresses professional dress and appearance for fieldwork sites and how to teach students the importance of this professional behavior. Chapter 68, "A Fieldwork Educator's Guide to Social Networking," focuses on social networking from a fieldwork education perspective. Fieldwork educators should read this chapter carefully before developing policies and procedures for their fieldwork site.

Chapter 65.

ADVISORY OPINION ON PATIENT ABANDONMENT

American Occupational Therapy Association

An Advisory Opinion for the AOTA Ethics Commission

Introduction

According to Dictionary.com (2011), *abandon* is defined as "to leave completely and finally." A legal definition clarifies what abandonment means in the health care setting: "withdrawal from treatment of a patient without giving reasonable notice or providing a competent replacement" (USLegal.com, n.d.).

One should note that according to this second definition, a health care professional can indeed "abandon" a patient appropriately, as long as some notice has been given. Tangential to withdrawing from a case in which treatment has already begun is the refusal to initiate treatment, which many patients also take as an act of abandonment. This "right" (as it is sometimes called) of health care professionals to withdraw from the treatment of a patient or to refuse to initiate treatment is supported by the American Medical Association's (AMA's) Principles of Medical Ethics, Principle VI: "A physician shall, in the provision of appropriate patient care, except in emergencies, be free to choose whom to serve, with whom to associate, and the environment in which to provide medical services" (AMA, 1994, p. 101). Similarly, the Comprehensive Accreditation Manual for

Hospitals (Joint Committee on the Accreditation of Healthcare Organizations [JCAHO], 1998) calls for the development of policies and procedures within health care facilities governing "how staff may request to be excused from participating in an aspect of patient care on grounds of conflicting cultural values, ethics, or religious beliefs…." (p. HR-21).

Belief in this "right" of health care professionals to refuse to treat can be found throughout the health care system in this country, because it flows out of the strong value Americans place on freedom of choice. As biomedical ethicist Albert R. Jonsen (1995) explained,

> There has long been, in the United States, a reluctance to force one person to provide services to another against his or her will.…The right to refuse to care for a particular patient, either by not accepting that person as a patient or by discharging oneself from responsibility in a recognized way, is deeply embedded in the ethos of American medicine. (p. 100)

The issue of patient abandonment versus the health care professional's rights is one of several problems that contribute to the growing tension between patients and medical personnel. Finding and maintaining a balance between patient needs and the personal rights of those involved with health care delivery on this issue of abandonment would go far toward easing such tensions as we move into the next millennium.

Clarifying "Patient Abandonment"

We must recognize that there are legitimate reasons across all fields of health care to cease providing treatment to a patient. Some of these are clear-cut. First, when treatment needs exceed the ability and expertise of a health care professional, the patient is best served by having care transferred to a more qualified practitioner. Because the goal of health care is the well-being of the patient, withdrawing from a case when one's skill can no longer be of benefit is justified, even though claims of abandonment may be raised by the patient. However, the manner in which one presents the need for a transfer of care and the degree to which the patient is made aware of this need and involved in the choice of a new practitioner are important factors in lessening the patient's perception of abandonment.

Second, it is commonly agreed that a health care practitioner may withdraw from the care of a patient who acts inappropriately within the health care setting. The most common situation discussed is when a patient becomes violent or acts in ways that endanger the practitioner, other patients, or staff. However, this would also include inappropriate sexual advances from a patient (or possibly from a patient's guardian, spouse, parent, and so forth). In such cases, a practitioner may, if necessary, withdraw from the treatment of the patient without abandoning the patient, as the health care relationship has already been severed and the bond of trust damaged.

A third area, but one that involves more difficulty, arises from issues regarding the cultural and religious values of health care practitioners. As noted in the Comprehensive Accreditation Manual for Hospitals (JCAHO, 1998), in the delivery of health care there should be respect for a health care practitioner's "cultural values, ethics, and religious beliefs and the impact these may have on patient care" (p. HR-21). The Accreditation Manual emphasizes that to respect all staff members, a health care institution

(or practice) should establish policies for how staff members can make requests to discontinue care for ethical, religious, and cultural reasons, as well as policies for ensuring that patient care will not be negatively affected. It is further noted that addressing such issues in advance, even at the time of hiring or contracting, will be the most helpful for maintaining an appropriate level of patient care.

What makes these issues difficult is the subjective nature of "personal values." Who is to say what represents a cultural value? What if one's culture is in the minority—do minority values still have weight? Religious values might also be difficult to determine, as not all members of the same religion hold the same values. Should those making the decisions recognize only mainstream values of the staff member's religion? And, of course, ethical values flow from the individual's own conscience. How should a manager or a supervisor regard a staff member's ethical claims? Should all expressed values carry the same weight, simply because someone claims they are important? The Accreditation Manual goes on to note that if an appropriate (in the judgment of the manager or supervisor) request has been made, accommodations should be made when possible and cites the following "Examples of Implementation" to support Standard HR.6:

> There will be an understanding that if events prevent the accommodation at a specific point because of an emergency situation, the employee will be expected to perform assigned duties so he or she does not negatively affect the delivery of care or services.
>
> If an employee does not agree to render appropriate care or services in an emergency situation because of personal beliefs, the employee will be placed on a leave of absence from his or her current position and the incident will be reviewed. (JCAHO, 1998, p. HR-21)

Such cases will surely be difficult for all involved, especially if they have not been addressed prior to the emergent situation. The issue here is further complicated by the fact that even though health care is becoming more diverse, when we work with each other we are not always aware of each other's diverse beliefs, nor are we always open and understanding about such differences. Supervisors and employers need to become more aware of their staff's values, and staff members need to continue to keep patient care at the focus of their work during times of personal conflict.

Beyond the above reasons for discontinuing patient care, disagreement begins to arise. What about refusing to treat a noncompliant patient? What if that patient is extremely noncompliant, rather than only occasionally noncompliant? In another vein, what about the patient who does not pay his or her bills? Is refusing to treat such a patient justifiable? What if the patient is unable to pay the bills? Would this make a difference? Or one might consider an especially demanding patient. If a patient takes time away from the care of others and continually calls the practitioner beyond normal care hours, is withdrawal from the care of such a patient acceptable? Yet another problematic case might involve a patient whose appearance or manners disgust a practitioner. If a practitioner is so put off by a patient that it impedes his or her ability to be an effective therapist, would withdrawing from the case be an act of abandonment or patient benefit? Finally, perhaps the most-addressed cases involve persons with AIDS. Does the fear of contagion validate withdrawal from treating such a patient? Across the literature, there is little agreement as to what constitutes abandonment in such situations. Legal cases have not added much clarity (Southwick, 1988, pp. 37–41).

The Duty to Treat

Although there is disagreement about the issue of abandonment and the duty of health care professionals to treat patients, even in the face of personal inconvenience or risk, some helpful insights can be gained from the thought of bioethicist Edmund D. Pellegrino. In his chapter "Altruism, Self-Interest, and Medical Ethics," Pellegrino (1991) addressed the particular case of physicians and the treatment of persons with AIDS. To begin, the author questioned the notion that "medicine is an occupation like any other, and the physician has the same 'rights' as the businessman or the craftsman" (Pellegrino, 1991, p. 114). As a counter to this notion, Pellegrino drew out three things specific to the nature of medicine that he argued establish a duty of physicians to treat the sick, even in the face of personal risk. Pellegrino first pointed out the uniqueness of the medical relationship, in that it

involves a vulnerable and dependent person who is at risk of exploitation who must trust another to be restored to health. As Pellegrino explained, "Physicians invite that trust when offering to put knowledge at the service of the sick. A medical need in itself constitutes a moral claim on those equipped to help." Next, the author points out that, in short, medical education is a privilege. Societies make special allowances for people to study medicine for the good of the society, thereby establishing a covenant with future health care professionals. Based on this, Pellegrino concluded, "The physician's knowledge, therefore, is not individually owned and ought not be used primarily for personal gain, prestige, or power. Rather, the profession holds this knowledge in trust for the good of the sick." Finally, Pellegrino pointed to the oath that physicians take before practicing medicine: "That oath—whichever one is taken—is a public promise that the new physician understands the gravity of this calling and promises to be competent and to use that competence in the interests of the sick." Although the debate continues, several have asserted that Pellegrino made a strong case for the duty to treat (Arras, 1991; Jonsen, 1995). And although Pellegrino's comments were directed toward physicians, his reasoning cuts across all fields of medical practice.

The Duty to Treat, Patient Abandonment, and Occupational Therapy

The points presented by Pellegrino (1991) have direct bearing on the profession of occupational therapy. The Preamble to the *Occupational Therapy Code of Ethics and Ethics Standards (2010)* (referred to as the Code and Ethics Standards; American Occupational Therapy Association [AOTA], 2010) recognizes the vulnerability of the people who seek occupational therapy services and are aware of the trust that is required in the healing relationship. Even though the recipient of treatment depends on the occupational therapist, the core value of equality "refers to the desire to promote fairness in interactions with others" (AOTA, 2010, p. S17). The core value of dignity emphasizes "the promotion and preservation of the individuality...of the client, by assisting him or her to engage in occupations that are meaningful to him or her regardless of level of disability" (AOTA, 2010, p. S18). The need to respect the vulnerability of patients and build trust is also expressed in the Code and Ethics Standards in Principle 1, which states,

"Occupational therapy personnel shall demonstrate a concern for the well-being and safety of the recipients of their services." Principle 2 adds, "Occupational therapy personnel shall intentionally refrain from actions that cause harm." Principle 2C also explicitly states that "Occupational therapy personnel shall avoid relationships that exploit the recipient of services…physically, emotionally, psychologically, financially, socially, or in any other manner that conflicts or interferes with professional judgment and objectivity." Principle 3 further demonstrates the concern of occupational therapists for building trust between practitioners and the persons in their care: "Occupational therapy personnel shall respect the right of the individual to self-determination." Under this principle, the importance of collaborating with, gaining informed consent from, and respecting the confidentiality of service recipients is recognized.

As to the second point raised by Pellegrino, occupational therapists do indeed recognize the importance of their training and education. This is emphasized in Principle 5F of the Code and Ethics Standards: "Occupational therapy personnel shall take responsibility for maintaining high standards and continuing competence in practice, education, and research…." The impact of this principle goes beyond just receiving specialized training; occupational therapists seek to maintain competence "by participating in professional development and educational activities." Principle 5G also directs occupational therapists to protect service recipients in the discharge of their knowledge and skill by ensuring that "duties assumed by or assigned to other occupational therapy personnel match credentials, qualifications, experience, and scope of practice." Through these actions, occupational therapists can truly demonstrate that they do not acquire their knowledge for "personal gain, prestige, or power. Rather, the profession holds this knowledge in trust for the good of the sick" (Pellegrino, 1991, p. 114).

Finally, occupational therapists also make a public pledge to promote the well-being of others through the Code and Ethics Standards. The Preamble to the Code and Ethics Standards states, "Members of AOTA are committed to promoting inclusion, diversity, independence, and safety for all recipients in various stages of life, health, and illness and to empower all beneficiaries of occupational therapy" (AOTA, 2010, p. S17). Principle 1 of the Code and Ethics Standards further supports this pledge for the

well-being of the recipients of occupational therapy. Finally, the dedication of occupational therapists to the well-being of those they treat is echoed in the core value of altruism: "the individual's ability to place the needs of others before their own" (AOTA, 2010, p. S17).

This understanding of the duty of health care professionals to treat patients as drawn from the perspective of occupational therapy can provide some guidance for the initial concern of patient abandonment. There is, indeed, a strong claim here to treat all patients to the fullest of one's ability as an occupational therapist. The two limiting factors to this are when a more competent therapist is needed and when the patient's actions make further treatment imprudent. But aside from such cases, the Code and Ethics Standards challenge occupational therapists to act from a higher level of responsibility than the general norms of society. Thus, even though it may be standard practice to refuse to serve customers and clients at one's discretion in business, occupational therapists have a higher standard to follow. Prudential decisions will need to be made about initiating or ceasing treatment when such actions are valid and necessary. However, to avoid the genuine abandonment of patients, occupational therapists must act according to both the letter and the spirit of the Code and Ethics Standards. Kyler (1995) summed up these points well when she wrote,

> As ethical health care practitioners, we are guided by the fundamental belief in the worth of our clients. This belief is based on our social responsibility, as stated in the AOTA Code of Ethics and in the Standards of Practice. An ethical practitioner treats clients and delivers services not simply because of a contractual agreement, but because of a social responsibility to do so. (p. 176)

Conclusion: Abide, Not Abandon

As Purtilo (1993) noted, the actual physical abandonment of patients by health care professionals is no longer as prevalent as it had once been. However, she added that "psychological abandonment often replaces what used to be experienced as the more obvious bodily abandonment of the patient" (p. 156). Psychological abandonment still involves treating a patient, but in such a manner "that the patient becomes a total non-person to the health professional." One of the dangers here is that physical abandonment is rather obvious and can be empirically validated. Psychological abandonment is far more subtle and may even occur without the practitioner's conscious knowledge—for example, as a type of defense mechanism in a difficult case. Nonetheless, even this form of abandonment must be guarded against. But how?

Purtilo (1993) offered a simple, but thought-provoking, suggestion. She explained that the "opposite of abandonment is to stay with or abide with the patient." Learning to abide with those in need, those who are difficult, those whose actions appear immoral to us, and those whom we fear because of their specific health problems will certainly not be easy. However, as Purtilo noted, health care professionals "can overcome their tendency to flee (physically or psychologically) only when the attitude of compassion is combined with an understanding of how much harm is induced by abandonment" (p. 157). Learning to abide with the recipients of occupational therapy may be one of the most important ways to safeguard against patient abandonment.

References

American Medical Association. (1994). American Medical Association's principles of medical ethics. In G. R. Beabout & D. J. Wennemann (Eds.), *Applied professional ethics* (p. 101). New York: University Press of America.

American Occupational Therapy Association. (2010). Occupational therapy code of ethics and ethics standards (2010). *American Journal of Occupational Therapy, 64*(6 Suppl.), S17–S26. http://dx.doi.org/10.5014/ajot.2010.64S17

Arras, J. D. (1991). AIDS and the duty to treat. In T. A. Mappes & J. S. Zembaty (Eds.), *Biomedical ethics* (3rd ed., pp. 115–121). St. Louis, MO: McGraw-Hill.

Dictionary.com. (2011). *Abandon.* Retrieved February 2, 2011, from http://dictionary.reference.com/browse/abandon

Joint Commission on the Accreditation of Healthcare Organizations. (1998, January). *Comprehensive accreditation manual for hospitals* (pp. HR-21–HR-22). Washington, DC: Author.

Jonsen, A. R. (1995). The duty to treat patients with AIDS and HIV infection. In J. D. Arras & B. Steinbock (Eds.), *Ethical issues in modern medicine* (4th ed., pp. 97–106). Mountain View, CA: Mayfield.

Kyler, P. (1995). Ethical commentary—Commentary on Chapter 10, Contracts and Referrals to Private Practice. In D. B. Bailey & S. L. Schwartzberg (Eds.), *Ethical and legal dilemmas in occupational therapy* (pp. 174–176). Philadelphia: F. A. Davis.

Pellegrino, E. D. (1991). Altruism, self-interest, and medical ethics. In T. A. Mappes & J. S. Zembaty (Eds.), *Biomedical ethics* (3rd ed., pp. 113–114). St. Louis, MO: McGraw-Hill.

Purtilo, R. (1993). *Ethical dimensions in the health professions* (2nd ed.) Philadelphia: W. B. Saunders.

Southwick, A. F. (1988). *The law of hospital and health care administration* (2nd ed.). Ann Arbor, MI: Health Administration Press.

USLegal.com. (n.d.). *Patient abandonment law and legal definition.* Retrieved February 2, 2011, from http://definitions.uslegal.com/p/patient-abandonment/

John F. Morris, PhD
Member at Large, Commission on Standards and Ethics (1998–2001)

Chapter 66.

GUIDELINES FOR DOCUMENTATION OF OCCUPATIONAL THERAPY

American Occupational Therapy Association

Documentation of occupational therapy services is necessary whenever professional services are provided to a client. Occupational therapists and occupational therapy assistants[1] determine the appropriate type of documentation structure and then record the services provided within their scope of practice. This document, based on the *Occupational Therapy Practice Framework: Domain and Process* (2nd ed.; American Occupational Therapy Association [AOTA], 2008), describes the components and purpose of professional documentation used in occupational therapy.

AOTA's (2010) *Standards of Practice for Occupational Therapy* states that an occupational therapy practitioner[2] documents the occupational therapy services and "abides by the time frames, format, and standards established by the practice settings, government agencies, external accreditation programs, payers, and AOTA documents" (p. S108). These requirements apply to both electronic and written forms of documentation. Documentation should reflect the nature of services provided and the clinical reasoning of the occupational therapy practitioner, and it should provide enough information to ensure that services are delivered in a safe and effective manner. Documentation should describe the depth and breadth of services provided to meet the complexity of individual client[3] needs. The client's diagnosis or prognosis should not be used as the sole rationale for occupational therapy services.

The purpose of documentation is to

- Communicate information about the client from the occupational therapy perspective;
- Articulate the rationale for provision of occupational therapy services and the relationship of those services to client outcomes, reflecting the occupational therapy practitioner's clinical reasoning and professional judgment; and

---

[1] *Occupational therapists* are responsible for all aspects of occupational therapy service delivery and are accountable for the safety and effectiveness of the occupational therapy service delivery process. *Occupational therapy assistants* deliver occupational therapy services under the supervision of and in partnership with an occupational therapist (AOTA, 2009).

[2] When the term *occupational therapy practitioner* is used in this document, it refers to both occupational therapists and occupational therapy assistants (AOTA, 2006).

[3] In this document, *client* may refer to an individual, organization, or population.

Table 66.1. Common Types of Occupational Therapy Documentation Reports

Process Areas	Type of Report
I. Screening	• Screening Report
II. Evaluation	• Evaluation Report
	• Reevaluation Report
III. Intervention	• Intervention Plan
	• Contact Report Note or Communiqué
	• Progress Report/Note
	• Transition Plan
IV. Outcomes	• Discharge/Discontinuation Report

• Create a chronological record of client status, occupational therapy services provided to the client, client response to occupational therapy intervention, and client outcomes.

Types of Documentation

Table 66.1 outlines common types of documentation reports. Reports may be named differently or combined and reorganized to meet the specific needs of the setting. Occupational therapy documentation should always record the practitioner's activity in the areas of screening, evaluation, intervention, and outcomes (AOTA, 2008) in accordance with payer, facility, and state and federal guidelines.

Content of Reports

I. Screening

A. Documents referral source, reason for occupational therapy screening, and need for occupational therapy evaluation and service.
   1. Phone referrals should be documented in accordance with payer, facility, and state and federal guidelines and include
      a. Names of individuals spoken with,
      b. Purpose of screening,
      c. Date of request,
      d. Number of contact for referral source, and
      e. Description of client's prior level of occupational performance.
B. Consists of an initial brief assessment to determine client's need for an occupational therapy evaluation or for referral to another service if not appropriate for occupational therapy services.

C. Suggested content:
   1. *Client information*—Name/agency; date of birth; gender; health status; and applicable medical/educational/developmental diagnoses, precautions, and contraindications
   2. *Referral information*—Date and source of referral, services requested, reason for referral, funding source, and anticipated length of service
   3. *Brief occupational profile*—Client's reason for seeking occupational therapy services, current areas of occupation that are successful and problematic, contexts and environments that support and hinder occupations, medical/educational/work history, occupational history (e.g., patterns of living, interest, values), client's priorities, and targeted goals
   4. *Assessments used and results*—Types of assessments used and results (e.g., interviews, record reviews, observations)
   5. *Recommendation*—Professional judgments regarding appropriateness of need for complete occupational therapy evaluation.

II. Evaluation

A. Evaluation Report
   1. Documents referral source and data gathered through the evaluation process in accordance with payer, facility, state, or federal guidelines. Includes
      a. Analysis of occupational performance and identification of factors that support and hinder performance and participation, and
      b. Identification of specific areas of occupation and occupational performance to be addressed, interventions, and expected outcomes.

2. Suggested content:
   a. *Client information*—Name; date of birth; gender; health status; medical history; and applicable medical/educational/ developmental diagnoses, precautions, and contraindications
   b. *Referral information*—Date and source of referral, services requested, reason for referral, funding source, and anticipated length of service
   c. *Occupational profile*—Client's reason for seeking occupational therapy services, current areas of occupation that are successful and problematic, contexts and environments that support or hinder occupations, medical/ educational/work history, occupational history (e.g., patterns of living, interest, values), client's priorities, and targeted outcomes
   d. *Assessments used and results*—Types of assessments used and results (e.g., interviews, record reviews, observations, standardized or nonstandardized assessments)
   e. *Analysis of occupational performance*— Description of and judgment about performance skills, performance patterns, contexts and environments, activity demands, outcomes from standardized measures or nonstandardized assessments,[4] and client factors that will be targeted for intervention and outcomes expected
   f. *Summary and analysis*—Interpretation and summary of data as related to occupational profile and referring concern
   g. *Recommendation*—Judgment regarding appropriateness of occupational therapy services or other services.

Note. The intervention plan, including intervention goals addressing anticipated outcomes, objectives, and frequency of therapy, is described in the "Intervention Plan" section that follows.

B. Reevaluation Report
   1. Documents the results of the reevaluation process. Frequency of reevaluation depends on the needs of the setting, the progress of the client, and client changes.
   2. Suggested content:
      a. *Client information*—Name; date of birth; gender; and applicable medical/ educational/developmental diagnoses, precautions, and contraindications
      b. *Occupational profile*—Updates on current areas of occupation that are successful and problematic, contexts and environments that support or hinder occupations, summary of any new medical/educational/ work information, and updates or changes to client's priorities and targeted outcomes
      c. *Reevaluation results*—Focus of reevaluation, specific types of outcome measures from standardized and/or nonstandardized assessments used, and client's performance and subjective responses
      d. *Analysis of occupational performance*— Description of and judgment about performance skills, performance patterns, contexts and environments, activity demands, outcomes from standardized measures or nonstandardized assessments, and client factors that will be targeted for intervention and outcomes expected
      e. *Summary and analysis*—Interpretation and summary of data as related to referring concern and comparison of results with previous evaluation results
      f. *Recommendations*—Changes to occupational therapy services, revision or continuation of interventions, goals and objectives, frequency of occupational therapy services, and recommendation for referral to other professionals or agencies as applicable.

III. Intervention

A. Intervention Plan
   1. Documents the goals, intervention approaches, and types of interventions to be used to achieve the client's identified targeted

---

[4]*Nonstandardized assessment tools* are considered a valid form of information gathering that allows flexibility and individualization when measuring outcomes related to the status of an individual or group through an intrapersonal comparison. Although not uniform in administration or scoring or possessing full and complete psychometric data, nonstandardized assessment tools possess strong internal validity and represent an evidence-based approach to occupational therapy practice (Hinojosa, Kramer, & Crist, 2010). Nonstandardized tools should be selected on the basis of the best available evidence and the clinical reasoning of the practitioner.

outcomes and is based on results of evaluation or reevaluation processes. Includes recommendations or referrals to other professionals and agencies in adherence with each payer source documentation requirements (e.g., pain levels, time spent on each modality).

2. Suggested content:
   a. *Client information*—Name, date of birth, gender, precautions, and contraindications
   b. *Intervention goals*—Measurable and meaningful occupation-based long-term and short-term objective goals directly related to the client's ability and need to engage in desired occupations
   c. *Intervention approaches and types of interventions to be used*—Intervention approaches that include create/promote, establish/ restore, maintain, modify, or prevent; types of interventions that include consultation, education process, advocacy, or the therapeutic use of occupations or activities
   d. *Service delivery mechanisms*—Service provider, service location, and frequency and duration of services
   e. *Plan for discharge*—Discontinuation criteria, discharge setting (e.g., skilled nursing facility, home, community, classroom) and follow-up care
   f. *Outcome measures*—Tools that assess occupational performance, adaptation, role competence, improved health and wellness, improved quality of life, self-advocacy, and occupational justice. Standardized and/or nonstandardized assessments used at evaluation should be readministered periodically to monitor measurable progress and report functional outcomes as required by client's payer source and/or facility requirements.
   g. *Professionals responsible and date of plan*— Names and positions of persons overseeing plan, date plan was developed, and date when plan was modified or reviewed.

B. Service Contacts
   1. Documents contacts between the client and the occupational therapy practitioner. Records the types of interventions used and client's response, which can include telephone contacts, interventions, and meetings with others.

2. Suggested content:
   a. *Client information*—Name; date of birth; gender; and diagnosis, precautions, and contraindications
   b. *Therapy log*—Date, type of contact, names positions of persons involved, summary or significant information communicated during contacts, client attendance and participation in intervention, reason service is missed, types of interventions used, client's response, environmental or task modification, assistive or adaptive devices used or fabricated, statement of any training education or consultation provided, and the client's present level of performance. Documentation of services provided should reflect the complexity of the client and the professional clinical reasoning and expertise of an occupational therapy practitioner required to provide an effective outcome in occupational performance. The client's diagnosis or prognosis should not be the sole rationale for the skilled interventions provided. Measures used to assess outcomes should be repeated in accordance with payer and facility requirements and documented to demonstrate measurable functional progress of the client.
   c. *Intervention/procedure coding* (i.e., CPT^TM),[5] if applicable.

C. Progress Report/Note
   1. Summarizes intervention process and documents client's progress toward achievement of goals. Includes new data collected; modifications of treatment plan; and statement of need for continuation, discontinuation, or referral.
   2. Suggested content:
   a. *Client information*—Name; date of birth; gender; and diagnosis, precautions, and contraindications
   b. *Summary of services provided*—Brief statement of frequency of services and length of time services have been provided; techniques and strategies used; measurable progress or lack thereof using age-appropriate current functional standardized or nonstandardized outcome measures; environmental or task modifications provided; adaptive

---

[5]*CPT* is a trademark of the American Medical Association (AMA). *CPT* five-digit codes, nomenclature, and other data are copyright © 2011 by the AMA. All rights reserved.

equipment or orthotics provided; medical, educational, or other pertinent client updates; client's response to occupational therapy services; and programs or training provided to the client or caregivers

c. *Current client performance*—Client's progress toward the goals and client's performance in areas of occupations

d. *Plan or recommendations*—Recommendations and rationale as well as client's input to changes or continuation of plan.

D. Transition Plan

1. Documents the formal transition plan and is written when client is transitioning from one service setting to another within a service delivery system.

2. Suggested content:

a. *Client information*—Name; date of birth; gender; and diagnosis, precautions, and contraindications

b. *Client's current status*—Client's current performance in occupations

c. *Transition plan*—Name of current service setting and name of setting to which client will transition, reason for transition, time frame in which transition will occur, and outline of activities to be carried out during the transition plan

d. *Recommendations*—Recommendations and rationale for occupational therapy services, modifications or accommodations needed, and assistive technology and environmental modifications needed.

IV. Outcomes

A. Discharge Report—Summary of occupational therapy services and outcomes

1. Summarizes the changes in client's ability to engage in occupations between the initial evaluation and discontinuation of services and makes recommendations as applicable.

2. Suggested content with examples includes

a. *Client information*—Name/agency, date of birth, gender, diagnosis, precautions, and contraindications

b. *Summary of intervention process*—Date of initial and final service; frequency, number of sessions, summary of interventions used; summary of progress toward goals; and occupational therapy

outcomes—initial client status and ending status regarding engagement in occupations, client's assessment of efficacy of occupational therapy services

c. *Recommendations*—Recommendations pertaining to the client's future needs; specific follow-up plans, if applicable; and referrals to other professionals and agencies, if applicable.

Exhibit 66.1. *Fundamentals of Documentation*

- Client's full name and case number (if applicable) on each page of documentation
- Date
- Identification of type of documentation (e.g., evaluation report, progress report/note)
- Occupational therapy practitioner's signature with a minimum of first name or initial, last name, and professional designation
- When applicable, signature of the recorder directly after the documentation entry. If additional information is needed, a signed addendum must be added to the record.
- Cosignature of an occupational therapist or occupational therapy assistant on student documentation, as required by payer policy, governing laws and regulations, or employer
- Compliance with all laws, regulations, and payer and employer requirements
- Acceptable terminology defined within the boundaries of setting
- Abbreviation usage as acceptable within the boundaries of setting
- All errors noted and signed
- Adherence to professional standards of technology, when used to document occupational therapy services with electronic claims or records
- Disposal of records (electronic and traditionally written) within law or agency requirements
- Compliance with confidentiality standards
- Compliance with agency or legal requirements of storage of records
- Documentation should reflect professional clinical reasoning and expertise of an occupational therapy practitioner and the nature of occupational therapy services delivered in a safe and effective manner. The client's diagnosis or prognosis should not be the sole rationale for occupational therapy services.

Each occupational therapy client has a client record maintained as a permanent file. The record is maintained in a professional and legal fashion (i.e., organized, legible, concise, clear, accurate, complete, current, grammatically correct, and objective; see Exhibit 66.1 for more information).

References

American Medical Association. (2011). *Current procedural terminology.* Chicago: Author.

American Occupational Therapy Association. (2006). Policy 1.44. Categories of occupational therapy personnel. In *Policy manual* (2011 ed.). Bethesda, MD: Author.

American Occupational Therapy Association. (2008). Occupational therapy practice framework: Domain and process (2nd ed.). *American Journal of Occupational Therapy, 62,* 625–683. http://dx.doi.org/10.5014/ajot.62.6.625

American Occupational Therapy Association. (2009). Guidelines for supervision, roles, and responsibilities during the delivery of occupational therapy services. *American Journal of Occupational Therapy, 63,* 797–803. http://dx.doi.org/10.5014/ajot.63.6.797

American Occupational Therapy Association. (2010). Standards of practice for occupational therapy. *American Journal of Occupational Therapy, 64*(6, Suppl.), S106–S111. http://dx.doi.org/10.5014/ajot.2010.64S106

Hinojosa, J., Kramer, P., & Crist, P. (2010). *Evaluation: Obtaining and interpreting data* (3rd ed.). Bethesda, MD: AOTA Press.

Authors

Gloria Frolek Clark, MS, OTR/L, FAOTA

Mary Jane Youngstrom, MS, OTR/L, FAOTA

for

The Commission on Practice

Sara Jane Brayman, PhD, OTR/L, FAOTA, *Chairperson Adopted by the Representative Assembly 2003M16*

Edited by the Commission on Practice 2007

Edited by the Commission on Practice 2012

Debbie Amini, EdD, OTR/L, CHT, *Chairperson*

Adopted by the Representative Assembly Coordinating Council (RACC) for the Representative Assembly, 2012

Note. This revision replaces the 2007 document previously published and copyrighted 2008, by the American Occupational Therapy Association in the *American Journal of Occupational Therapy, 62,* 684–690.

Chapter 67.

PROFESSIONAL DRESS AND APPEARANCE

Ashley Fecht, OTD, OTR/L

Don't judge a book by its cover.

Unfortunately, in the health care arena, this old adage does not hold true. As humans, we are driven by what we see. The quality of health care services provided by a health care practitioner may be based partly on a patient's first impression of his or her health care practitioner, including professional appearance. The way people present themselves says a lot about their personal organization and their perceived self-confidence. People who do not take care in their professional appearance may give off the message that they do not respect themselves and do not value their appearance or the job that they are performing. Overall, poor professional appearance affects a health care practitioner's credibility in the eyes of his or her patients.

Professional appearance and dress is an important concept to be communicated and taught to occupational therapy students. Ever-changing trends in fashion often cloud students' understanding of professional dress. An example of this concept is when a female student comes to a presentation at a fieldwork site in a fashionable suit with a skirt that is too short. When confronted about the length of the skirt, the student counters with, "But I look nice."

Though the student's physical appearance is well put together, the length of the student's skirt does not convey a message of professionalism.

If no parameters are given on what is professional, students will defer to what they *think* is professional. This can often differ greatly from the opinions and dress codes of the fieldwork sites where they are assigned for Level I and Level II fieldwork. This is exemplified by a male student wearing a nice pair of jeans, belt, loafers, and a t-shirt to a home health fieldwork experience. The student perceives that he is dressed professionally; however, his fieldwork educator sends him home to change into a polo shirt and khakis because he or she does not deem jeans and a t-shirt professional.

Academic fieldwork coordinators (AFWCs) and fieldwork educators must be prepared to not only teach students how to present themselves professionally but also to enforce dress codes, protocols, and procedures. How students visually present themselves affects the image and reputation of the university or school they attend. Professional appearance also communicates a student's personal organization, self-confidence, and preparation for their learning experience.

Dress codes and other documents regarding professional appearance must be explicit and directive. These documents also must be fluid. The health care environment is always evolving, and professional appearance expectations will inevitably adjust to these changes. Professional dress code documents must include parameters of expected dress and clear procedures of what happens if the dress code is violated. AFWCs and fieldwork educators must be ready to enforce dress code policies and follow up on protocols and procedures for infractions. It is recommended that dress code and professional appearance documents encompass the following areas: grooming, jewelry, perfume and cologne, fingernails, hair, tattoos, clothing, and student or facility identification (Exhibit 67.1).

Teaching students the importance of professional dress and appearance must begin upon their matriculation into an occupational therapy program. Professional dress and appearance should be a part of a student's orientation process and continue to be taught and reinforced throughout academic and fieldwork elements of the occupational therapy program. Methods to teach these concepts should include both overt instruction on the protocols and procedures of professional dress and active learning activities to cement these protocols and procedures into practice. Role playing and activities such as professional dress fashion shows are excellent active learning activities that engage students and teach them the importance of professional dress and appearance.

Exhibit 67.1. *Examples of Language for Professional Dress Code From Touro University, Henderson, Nevada*

Area	Recommended Language
Grooming	Students must arrive clean and well-groomed at the fieldwork site.
Jewelry	Students may not wear any pierced jewelry except for one to two earrings in the lower ear lobes. All other visible piercings must be removed for fieldwork experiences. All jewelry will be minimal and in good taste. Each student must have a watch with a second hand.
Perfume/cologne	No perfume, cologne, or aftershave is allowed.
Fingernails	Nails will be clean and cut short. Artificial nails are not acceptable in hospital environments and may not be acceptable in other health care environments. If allowed by the facility, artificial nails must be short in length with rounded corners.
Hair	Hair should be off the face and shoulders. Longer hair must be contained (e.g., in a pony tail). Facial hair should be well-maintained.
Tattoos	Tattoos must not be visible.
Clothing	Slacks and shirts should be clean with no evidence of tears or frays. Men must wear well-fitting slacks and professional or sports shirts. Women must wear slacks and modest tops that cover midriff, buttocks, and cleavage. The university School of Occupational Therapy polo shirt is provided to each student for use on fieldwork assignments. Shoes must be closed toe; sneakers may be appropriate, depending on the clinical environment. Facilities may allow students to wear scrubs. Scrubs must be in good repair and appropriate to the setting. Some facilities require scrubs of a specific color, which the student will have to obtain.
Identification	All students are expected to wear their student identification. Facilities may issue a specific badge for identification.

Note. From Touro University, Henderson, Nevada student fieldwork handbook. Used with permission.

Ramifications for infractions should include sending the student home from the fieldwork site to correct the dress code or personal appearance violations. A progression of severity of correction should also be included, starting with verbal correction and continuing to written correction. Each instance of a professional dress or professional appearance violation should be documented. If a student demonstrates a continual nonadherence to such policies and procedures, termination of the student from the fieldwork experience should be considered.

In summary, professional dress and appearance is a reflection of students' personal preparation and investment in their education. Students' professional appearance can also affect the reputation and credibility of their occupational therapy program. It is crucial to provide students with the tools to understand professional dress and appearance codes before they embark on Level I and Level II fieldwork experiences. The first step to this process is making sure that an explicit and directive dress code is in place for the occupational therapy program and specifically for the fieldwork aspect of the program. Protocols and procedures regarding professional dress and appearance must be taught and reinforced throughout the educational program. In addition, AFWCs and fieldwork educators must be prepared to enforce dress code and personal appearance infractions, and students must understand the ramifications of these infractions.

Chapter 68.

A FIELDWORK EDUCATOR'S GUIDE TO SOCIAL NETWORKING

Deborah Bolding, MS, OTR/L

Social networking sites can be powerful tools for connecting friends, and may also be used by professionals to develop communities of learning and practice. Some workplaces have guidelines for employees regarding the use of social networking sites, but misunderstandings and misapplications can occur when students transition from the academic setting to the practice arena. This article explores some of the advantages and challenges of using social networking in the workplace, and how fieldwork educators can help mentor "e-professional" behaviors.

The American Occupational Therapy Association has recognized the utility of social networking and created OT Connections (www.OTConnections.org), where occupational therapy practitioners can create and access blogs, forums, and discussion groups related to the profession. Useful applications for social networking in the workplace include collaborating online to develop a group project, or using an online journal club to discuss the clinical applications of a new article.

Practitioners employed by an agency with several sites might use an electronic network to share ideas and resources. Online blogs or discussion groups can supplement evidence-based practice with expertise and judgment about clinical conditions and associated problems. Interns might use

class-protected discussion boards to brainstorm about de-identified clients or problems. However, overlap between personal and professional identities on social networking sites and other forms of electronic communication can elicit questions about their appropriate and ethical use.

Interns who feel confident navigating a variety of social networking sites may want to immediately begin using them at their fieldwork site. Therefore, fieldwork orientation must include information on being an "e-professional" and how public profiles on social networking sites reflect on one's professional presentation and judgment (Thompson et al., 2008). Information about one's political views or sexual orientation, relationship status, use of profanity, or photos depicting inebriation or sexually suggestive behavior might be content shared with close friends. However, this same information is not typically shared *en masse* and unfiltered with one's employer, coworkers, or clients. Interns who want to share this information should use separate personal and professional sites.

The fieldwork educator also needs to consider his or her appropriate and ethical use of social networking sites. For example, the educator could obtain personal information about the intern that influences his or her assessment of the intern's ethics and judgment. Information posted on a website should not be used "unfairly" by fieldwork educators or potential employers (Cain, 2008); however, information posted on unrestricted sites can be considered public information (Lehavot, 2009), making it difficult to respect privacy concerns. Interns may have a reasonable expectation of privacy at networking sites where privacy settings are available and filters enabled. However, consider a scenario where a supervisor or coworker is an alumnus of the intern's school. The fieldwork educator may have ready access to the intern's personal information through this alumni status, even though privacy settings prevent "outsiders" from viewing content.

Other considerations for students in the practice setting are the ethical and legal implications of what they write about clients or situations they observe, and whether the posting violates the privacy rights of clients, codes of conduct, or professional ethics.

To illustrate some of the problems that might occur, consider the following scenarios.

Case Example 1: Lack of Boundaries

Doris is an intern at a large acute care hospital, assigned to the neurology team. After a couple of weeks at the site, she sends "friend" requests to occupational therapists, physical therapists, nurses, and a couple of residents via Facebook. Some of the staff don't recognize her last name, and others don't know how to respond. One lead therapist is asked, "Don't you want to be my friend? Why haven't you answered?"

This scenario illustrates delineation of boundaries in supervisory or team relationships. Potential areas of miscommunication include whether the educator thinks it is appropriate to be "friends" with an intern; which type of social networking site is most appropriate for the setting; individual team members' comfort with social networking; and perhaps even generational issues. "Contacting the preceptor and team to be friends on Facebook may seem like a reasonable request to the intern, who is accustomed to using such networking sites with frequency," suggests one professor, but using these sites is not the norm in most fieldwork settings, and it may even be prohibited.

Mary Barnes, OTR, fieldwork coordinator at Tufts University's Department of Occupational Therapy, notes that she is amenable to using LinkedIn with alumni and fieldwork coordinators. She tells current students that she will decline Facebook friendships for "boundary maintenance" reasons. Another educator writes, "I receive Facebook invites all the time. I simply delete them without worrying that the individual might think I'm not playing nicely in the sandbox."

Social networking provides links to friends of friends. In the scenario above, the intern didn't understand how the implicit social networking rules differ between the college setting and the clinical setting. One solution would be for the internship site to have a policy about the use of social networking sites and discuss it during orientation. E-communication may be misperceived, or inadvertently disrupt working relationships.

Case Example 2: Poor Communication

Josh is in the third week of his internship. He contacts his fieldwork educator via Facebook to ask, "So, how do you really think I'm doing?"

Although Josh asked the question through the messaging feature of Facebook, the question was work related, and not social in nature. The fieldwork educator needs to talk with Josh about his question in person. It could be that he needs reassurance, has questions about his abilities, wants constructive guidance, or is uncomfortable in a supervisory relationship. Although electronic communication is convenient, it loses the majority of context and intent of the message and increases the chance of being misunderstood, due to the lack of rich context (e.g., body language, tone of voice, eye contact) that occurs in face-to-face conversations.

The fieldwork educator can use this situation to meet with Josh face-to-face and model professional communication. Josh can learn that performance information is confidential, and will not be shared through social networking, even at "private" sections of social networking sites. If the fieldwork educator and student are not already meeting regularly, they can establish a time to do so. Josh might be encouraged to reflect on his own skills and needs in written form as a means of increasing his comfort in the supervisory meetings and mutual feedback exchange. The fieldwork educator can reassure him that she will provide both positive and constructive feedback, in a timely way, with specific examples, and that she wants to hear Josh's feedback as well. After they have met face-to-face, they can summarize key points in carefully worded e-mail or electronic documentation, if needed. Hard copy tools such as an interactive journal or shared supervision logs might also be considered.

The fieldwork educator also needs to consider Josh's comfort with verbal communication. Interns need to be able to express their needs and feelings face-to-face for their own professional development, and also to be able to verbally interact with their clients and colleagues.

Case Example 3: Privacy Issues

Luis, a fieldwork educator, visits the Facebook site of his intern, Milena. She has posted the name of the hospital where she is interning in her profile. There's a link to her blog, where she comments, "I'm glad the weekend is here. It's so busy; I didn't have time to see all my patients today. One nurse was really slow getting the pain meds out to the patients, and it made my afternoon crazy. The patients were complaining and I was behind schedule."

Many employers have policies regarding work-related information and expect interns and employees to be aware of and respectful about what they share on networking sites. It may be true that the nurse was late giving the pain medications to her patients, but Milena might not know that one of the nurse's patients needed an emergency ICU transfer. Even if the nurse had no obvious reason for being late, Milena needs to demonstrate appropriate professional behavior, such as discussing the problem with her supervisor and taking a more positive approach. Denigrating a fellow professional in a "public" setting is neither ethical nor an effective team-building behavior.

Milena's description of her fieldwork site may affect her internship and relationship with staff, particularly if she has agreed to an institutional code of conduct that prohibits unauthorized public statements.

Case Example 4: Legalities

David has a 2-week Level I experience in Africa. He writes about his experience on his blog, and includes photographs of the setting and the children.

If David and his fellow students were doing their fieldwork experience at any site in the United States, they would be ethically and legally prevented from displaying photographs of clients on a website without written permission of each person (or in the case of children, their legal guardians). This is because patients' privacy rights are protected by the Health Insurance Portability and Accountability Act (HIPAA; U.S. Department of Health and Human Services, 2009). Is it permissible to post pictures without consent when you are in a country where privacy is not protected by law? Were the subjects of the photographs really "clients" if it was a volunteer experience? These are questions that advisors and students need to discuss before students develop blogs and post pictures about their experiences.

Conclusion

Interns and fieldwork educators need to be proficient in communicating in face-to-face and virtual social and professional networking arenas. Flexibility and a willingness to learn are essential, because the technology and potential uses of that technology will continue to evolve, perhaps even more quickly than policies can be established.

Acknowledgments

The author would like to thank Macy Barnes, OTR, fieldwork coordinator, Tufts University Department of Occupational Therapy; and Laurie B. Kontney, PT, DPT, MS, director of clinical education and clinical associate professor at Marquette University, for their invaluable assistance editing this article; Jaynee Taguchi-Meyer, OTD, academic fieldwork coordinator for occupational therapy, University of Southern California; Darci Hebenstreit, PT, lead therapist at Stanford Hospital; and Kris Tolbert, OTR/L, for their help with case scenarios; and the PT and OT academic fieldwork coordinators who shared information for this article.

References

Cain, J. (2008). Online social networking issues within academia and pharmacy education. *American Journal of Pharmaceutical Education, 72,* 1–2.

Lehavot, K. (2009). "MySpace" or yours? The ethical dilemma of graduate students' personal lives on the Internet. *Ethics and Behavior, 19,* 129–141.

Thompson, L. A, Dawson, K., Ferdig, R., Black, E. W., Boyer, J., Coutts, J., & Black, N. P. (2008). *Journal of General Internal Medicine, 23,* 954–957.

U.S. Department of Health and Human Services. (2009). *Health information privacy.* Retrieved July 26, 2009, from http://www.hhs.gov/ocr/ privacy/hipaa/understanding/index.html

Deborah Bolding, MS, OTR/L, is an education supervisor in clinical services at Stanford Hospital and Clinics in California.

Part 14.

RESOURCES FOR FURTHER LEARNING

OVERVIEW OF PART 14

Donna Costa, DHS, OTR/L, FAOTA

It is hoped that readers of this book will want to continue learning about fieldwork education after reading about the many topics discussed in it. Therefore, Part 14 contains resources that the fieldwork educator may find useful. Chapter 69, "AOTA Fieldwork Educators Certificate Program Workshop" describes the American Occupational Therapy Association Fieldwork Educators Certificate Program, which did not exist when the first edition of this book was published. The content covered in this 2-day course is useful to both the novice fieldwork educator who may not have taught a student yet and the experienced fieldwork educator who has taught many students. At press time, more than 5,000 occupational therapy practitioners have taken this course.

Chapter 70, "Online Fieldwork Educator Training Programs," describes a few of the online training programs that fieldwork educators can access to pursue more knowledge and skills in clinical education. Chapter 71, "Suggested Reading List," contains a list of books that fieldwork educators may find helpful for their professional development.

Chapter 69.

AOTA FIELDWORK EDUCATORS CERTIFICATE PROGRAM WORKSHOP

Donna Costa, DHS, OTR/L, FAOTA

Many occupational therapy practitioners do not feel prepared to take their first fieldwork student. The profession of occupational therapy is approaching its 100th anniversary, and this concern about the lack of preparation to become a fieldwork educator has been echoed for decades. For example, the following story exemplifies the experience of many new fieldwork educators:

> After 1 year of practice, I was informed that I was now ready to serve as a clinical instructor for a student. I was finally comfortable with flexibly managing a full patient caseload and all related activities. Now, without more than a simple proclamation, I was to be assigned to a student for her first clinical experience....Just when I...finally [felt] like I had a handle on performing as a competent practitioner, one more responsibility was being "dumped" on me.
>
> The center coordinator of clinical education had reviewed a copy of the academic program's curriculum, name of academic [fieldwork] coordinator, and the evaluation tool to be used to assess the student's performance for this first clinical experience.

In addition, there was a brief student profile that was written in the student's handwriting, albeit somewhat illegibly, that indicated her address [and] preferred learning style. I was informed that she would be arriving at our clinical facility in 1 week and would need an orientation, "good" patients with whom to practice her skills, and a schedule. The center coordinator asked me if I had any questions. After a brief pause, I quietly replied, "No." Not only did I not know where to begin to ask the first question, but [also] I was absolutely terrified and overwhelmed by the responsibility. I assumed that everyone who was assigned a student after 1 year of clinical practice must be capable to serve as a clinical instructor, and I did not want to respond any differently than my peers.

> Afterwards, I realized that in 1 week I would be responsible for this student's clinical learning experience and I had not a clue as to how to structure an experience or perform a student evaluation....I had only completed a new employee orientation. I knew very little about teaching students in

the clinic other than remembering what it was like to be a student during my clinical experiences. I tried to reflect on what my clinical instructors did during my clinical experiences by posing questions like, How did they provide an orientation to the facility and the specific health care environment? What issues were discussed during the first few days of the experience? What were their expectations for my performance? Did I get a schedule on the first day and what was included on that schedule? What did they do to make me feel more comfortable or uncomfortable? What did I remember most about my clinical supervisors that was positive or negative? Based on my limited discussions with professional peers and my personal reflections, I developed a better, albeit limited, understanding of my perceived roles and responsibilities. All too soon, it was time for me to teach my first student. (Gandy, 1997, pp. 211–213, reprinted with permission)

Since the inception of occupational therapy, the literature has included numerous references about the need for a formalized training program for fieldwork educators. The first mention was in at a conference in 1923, when the Minimum Standards for Courses of Training in Occupational Therapy were established by the American Occupational Therapy Association (AOTA). In 1987, the Representative Assembly of AOTA charged the Commission on Education to explore alternative fieldwork models. In 1989, the Final Report of the Fieldwork Study Committee was issued (Privott, 1998) and formally addressed the need for fieldwork supervision training, stating, "The Committee reiterates and endorses a systematic process for credentialing fieldwork supervisors" (Privott, 1998, p. 416).

Nothing happened with this issue until 1995, when the AOTA Fieldwork for the Future Task Force convened as a result of Resolution E (1992), passed by the Representative Assembly, which requested that "The Intercommission Council (ICC) be charged to conduct a study of Level II fieldwork by reviewing existing data, when indicated, to include, but not limited to…feasibility and implications of accrediting fieldwork instructors" (Privott,

1998, p. 425). This group made a recommendation to "initiate a voluntary credentialing process for clinical fieldwork educators by 1998 consistent with Association policy, review the credentialing process, and phase in mandatory credentialing" (AOTA, 1995, p. 1054). It was not until 2005, however, that the Representative Assembly charged the AOTA president to develop a task force to explore and make recommendations for fieldwork educator resources. Work began on the curriculum for the Fieldwork Educator Certificate Program Workshop (FWECP), which was implemented at the AOTA Annual Conference in 2008. Workshop trainers were identified in pairs (one academic fieldwork coordinator and one fieldwork educator), and train-the-trainer workshops were offered. Since then, more than 5,000 fieldwork educators have participated in the 2-day training.

The curriculum for the FWECP follows the outline of the Self-Assessment Tool for Fieldwork Educator Competency (see Chapter 27) and includes five training modules (introduction, administration, education, supervision, and evaluation) and a summary module. The program contains numerous learning activities to make the learning interactive. Feedback from this program since 2008 has been extremely positive from both novice and experienced fieldwork educators. The FWECP was updated in 2015 to reflect changes in Accreditation Council for Occupation Therapy Education standards and emerging trends in fieldwork education. Academic programs across the country offer the FWECP frequently to ensure that the fieldwork educators they work with are provided with ongoing education. The AOTA website provides registration information and the schedule of courses at http://www.aota.org/Education-Careers/Fieldwork/Workshop.aspx.

Why should you as a fieldwork educator take this course? It can jump start your career as a new fieldwork educator or rejuvenate knowledge and skills of the experienced fieldwork educator. This course provides a comprehensive overview of the theory and practice of fieldwork education, an opportunity to network with other fieldwork educators in your area, and 15 contact hours that you can use for your state's licensing requirements or your National Board for Certification in Occupational Therapy continuing competency requirements.

References

American Occupational Therapy Association. (1924). Minimum standards for courses of training in occupational therapy. *Archives of Occupational Therapy, III*(4), 295–298. Available at http://otsearch.aota.org/files/archives/vol3/VOL3_295-298.pdf

American Occupational Therapy Association. (1995). The 1995 Representative Assembly summary of minutes. *American Journal of Occupational Therapy, 49*(10), 1053–1055. http://dx.doi.org/10.5014.ajot.49.10.1053

Gandy, J. (1997). Preparation for teaching students in clinical settings. In K. Shepherd & G. Jensen (Eds.), *Handbook of teaching for physical therapists* (2nd ed., pp. 39–69). Boston: Butterworth-Heinemann.

Privott, C. (Ed.). (1998). *The fieldwork anthology: A classic research and practice collection.* Bethesda, MD: American Occupational Therapy Association.

Chapter 70.

ONLINE FIELDWORK EDUCATOR TRAINING PROGRAMS

Donna Costa, DHS, OTR/L, FAOTA

Although face-to-face training may seem the ideal vehicle for continuing education opportunities, several online resources have been developed for fieldwork educators and academic fieldwork coordinators (AFWCs).

Preceptor Education Program

The Preceptor Education Program is a free online program aimed at health professionals and students and was developed by the University of Western Ontario. The term *preceptor* is used in Canada instead of *fieldwork educator,* and this program is designed to be used across disciplines. The program contains 8 self-directed modules and can be used by students, AFWCs, and fieldwork educators. Each module takes approximately 30 minutes to complete and includes quick tips, learning activities, and downloadable information. A certificate can be printed at the end of each module to record that it has been completed. Module topics are orientation, developing learning objectives, giving and receiving informal feedback, understanding and fostering clinical reasoning, fostering reflective practice, dealing with conflict, the formal evaluation process, and peer coaching. AFWCs may want to consider using these modules as part of preparing students for fieldwork.

Website: http://www.preceptor.ca/

Preceptor Development Initiative

The Preceptor Development Initiative was developed by the British Columbia Academic Health Council. The term *preceptor* is used in Canada instead of *fieldwork educator.* "E-Tips for Practice Educators" is an online course designed for health professionals who work with students in clinical practice settings. The course includes 8 web-based, interactive education modules to help develop knowledge and skills related to clinical education. The module topics include setting the stage for clinical teaching, learning in the practice education setting, teaching skills, fostering clinical reasoning, giving feedback, the evaluation process, supporting the struggling student, and strategies for resolving conflict.

Website: http://www.practiceeducation.ca/

Queensland Occupational Therapy Fieldwork Collaborative

This collaborative's website contains a "Clinical Educator's Resource Kit" that is aimed specifically at occupational therapy fieldwork educators. Five sections include preplacement considerations, setting up and maintenance, approaches to clinical education, feedback and evaluation, and students experiencing difficulty.

Chapter 71.

SUGGESTED READING LIST

Donna Costa, DHS, OTR/L, FAOTA

Readers of this book may find themselves challenged by some of the material and wanting to learn more on several topics. There is a relatively small collection of books related to fieldwork education; the best reads are included in this chapter.

Clinical Supervision in Occupational Therapy: A Guide for Fieldwork and Practice (Costa, 2007)

This book addresses the process and practice of clinical supervision, linking it to the occupational therapy knowledge base, providing a theoretical and philosophical framework, and forging a connection between the theory and practice of clinical education and supervision. For occupational therapy and occupational therapy assistant students, this book encourages an active learning experience. For new practitioners, it identifies a body of knowledge not learned in school. For fieldwork educators, it assists with self-assessment and encourages creating a professional development plan to further refine supervision skills. For managers

of practice settings, it provides a theoretical base for the administrative, supportive, and educational functions of clinical supervision. The book includes an 18-minute DVD produced by occupational therapy fieldwork students with 5 clinical scenarios that show situations between students and supervisors, followed by suggested discussion questions.

Collaborative Clinical Education: The Foundation of Effective Health Care (Westberg & Jason, 1992)

This book is an older but classic text aimed at people who are now, and who intend to become, clinical teachers in the health professions. Its primary focus is the teaching of medical students and residents, but the principles discussed apply equally to teaching students in other health professions. The main focus is on the process of teaching—the strategies and tactics involved in helping others learn—and the authors discuss the generic steps, strategies, and principles of effective teaching that apply in any clinical setting.

Fundamentals of Clinical Supervision, 5th Edition (Bernard & Goodyear, 2013)

This is a classic and comprehensive textbook on the subject of clinical supervision. It emphasizes central themes from a variety of mental health professions and covers supervision models, supervision modalities, administrative issues, and professional concerns. This 5th edition covers the latest research and more discussion about second-generation models of supervision, includes a new section on triadic supervision, and examines new technology.

Handbook of Teaching and Learning for Physical Therapists (Jensen, 2012)

Although this book is written for physical therapy, it has great applicability for teaching occupational therapy. It is divided into 2 sections: teaching in academic environments and teaching in clinical environments. Each chapter includes case studies that highlight chapter discussion.

Innovations in Allied Health Education (McAllister, Peterson, & Higgs, 2010)

This book presents a wide-ranging, international overview of innovations in fieldwork education in 3 allied health disciplines: speech therapy, physical therapy, and occupational therapy. It presents theoretical foundations and outcomes of a range of approaches used in fieldwork education. The book covers new models, locations and modes of delivery, and teaching and learning strategies for fieldwork education. It also discusses emerging possibilities for future fieldwork education.

Occupational Therapy Fieldwork Survival Guide: A Student Planner (Napier, 2010)

This book is aimed at the occupational therapy student who is transitioning from the classroom to Level II fieldwork. It is a combination handbook and self-organizer containing a review of a variety of topics such as time management, teamwork, and

occupational therapy practice issues as they relate to fieldwork success.

Role Emerging Occupational Therapy: Maximising Occupation Focused Practice (Thew, Edwards, Baptiste, & Molineux, 2011)

This text explores emerging innovative directions for occupational therapy, with a focus on the theory and application of role-emerging fieldwork placements. It discusses how occupation-focused practice can be applied to a wide variety of settings and circumstances to improve the health and well-being of a diverse range of people.

The Fieldwork Anthology: A Classic Research and Practice Collection (Privott, 1998)

This book is out of print, but interested readers may be able to find a used copy. It is a great historical read and presents a chronology of U.S. fieldwork education through a collection of selected papers.

The Occupational Therapy Handbook: Practice Education (Polglase & Treseder, 2012)

This British textbook was written specifically for occupational therapy students and newly qualified occupational therapists and educators. Many developments in fieldwork and practice education have refocused on the value the profession places on occupation, particularly in role-emerging placements and expanding areas of practice, and are discussed in this text. This book is also available in an e-format (Kindle).

Transforming Practice Through Clinical Education, Professional Supervision and Mentoring (Rose & Best, 2005)

This book is an incredible resource, combining the 3 interrelated topics of clinical education, professional supervision, and mentoring into 1 book. It is multidisciplinary in its focus and goes beyond student supervision, also discussing supervision of professionals in the workplace and the emerging importance of mentoring for ongoing professional development.

References

Bernard, J., & Goodyear, R. (2013). *Fundamentals of clinical supervision* (5th ed.). Upper Saddle River, NJ: Pearson.

Costa, D. (2007). *Clinical supervision in occupational therapy: A guide for fieldwork and practice.* Bethesda, MD: AOTA Press.

Jensen, G. (Ed.). (2012). *Handbook of teaching and learning for physical therapists* (3rd ed.). Philadelphia: Saunders.

McAllister, L., Peterson, M., & Higgs, J. (2010). *Innovations in allied health education.* Boston: Sense.

Napier, B. (2010). *Occupational therapy fieldwork survival guide: A student planner.* Bethesda, MD: AOTA Press.

Polglase, T., & Treseder, R. (2012). *The occupational therapy handbook: Practice education.* Keswick, UK: M&K.

Privott, C. (Ed.). (1998). *The fieldwork anthology: A classic research and practice collection.* Bethesda, MD: American Occupational Therapy Association.

Rose, M., & Best, D. (2005). *Transforming practice through clinical education, professional supervision and mentoring.* New York: Churchill Livingstone.

Thew, M., Edwards, M., Baptiste, S., & Molineux, M. (Eds.). (2011). *Role emerging occupational therapy: Maximising occupation focused practice.* Hoboken, NJ: Wiley-Blackwell.

Westberg, J., & Jason, H. (1992). *Collaborative clinical education: The foundation of effective health care.* New York: Springer.

SUBJECT INDEX

Note: Page numbers in *italic* refer to exhibits, figures, learning activities, and tables.

CITATION INDEX

Note: Page numbers in *italic* refer to tables.